Kem B[...]

1402 SW 59th #2225

OKC, OK 73119

CLEFT PALATE SPEECH

Second Edition

BETTY JANE McWILLIAMS, Ph.D.

Professor of Communication Disorders
Director, Cleft Palate–Craniofacial Center
University of Pittsburgh
Pittsburgh, Pennsylvania

HUGHLETT L. MORRIS, Ph.D.

Professor of Speech Pathology
Department of Otolaryngology—
Head and Neck Surgery
Department of Speech Pathology and Audiology
The University of Iowa
Iowa City, Iowa

RALPH L. SHELTON, Ph.D.

Professor, Department of Speech and Hearing Sciences
University of Arizona
Tucson, Arizona

1990

B.C. DECKER INC. • Philadelphia • Toronto

Publisher

B.C. Decker Inc
One James Street, South
Hamilton, Ontario L8P 4R5

B.C. Decker Inc
320 Walnut Street
Suite 400
Philadelphia, Pennsylvania 19106

Sales and Distribution

United States and Puerto Rico
Mosby-Year Book Inc.
11830 Westline Industrial Drive
Saint Louis, Missouri 63146

Canada
Mosby-Year Book Limited
5240 Finch Avenue E., Unit 1
Scarborough, Ontario M1S 5A2

Australia
McGraw-Hill Book Company Australia Pty. Ltd.
4 Barcoo Street
Roseville East 2069
New South Wales, Australia

Brazil
Editora McGraw-Hill do Brasil, Ltda.
rua Tabapua, 1.105, Itaim-Bibi
Sao Paulo, S.P. Brasil

Colombia
**Interamericana/McGraw-Hill
de Colombia, S.A.**
Carrera 17, No. 33-71
(Apartado Postal, A.A., 6131)
Bogota, D.E., Colombia

Europe, United Kingdom, Middle East and Africa
Wolfe Publishing Limited
Brook House
2–16 Torrington Place
London WC1E 7LT England

Hong Kong and China
McGraw-Hill Book Company
Suite 618, Ocean Centre
5 Canton Road
Tsimshatsui, Kowloon
Hong Kong

India
Tata McGraw-Hill Publishing Company, Ltd.
12/4 Asaf Ali Road, 3rd Floor
New Delhi 110002, India

Indonesia
Mr. Wong Fin Fah
P.O. Box 122/JAT
Jakarta, 1300 Indonesia

Japan
Igaku-Shoin Ltd.
Tokyo International P.O. Box 5063
1-28-36 Hongo, Bunkyo-ku,
Tokyo 113, Japan

Korea
Mr. Don-Gap Choi
C.P.O. Box 10583
Seoul, Korea

Malaysia
Mr. Lim Tao Slong
No. 8 Jalan SS 7/6B
Kelana Jaya
47301 Petaling Jaya
Selangor, Malaysia

Mexico
**Interamericana/McGraw-Hill de Mexico,
S.A. de C.V.**
Cedro 512, Colonia Atlampa
(Apartado Postal 26370)
06450 Mexico, D.F., Mexico

New Zealand
McGraw-Hill Book Co. New Zealand Ltd.
5 Joval Place, Wiri
Manukau City, New Zealand

Portugal
Editora McGraw-Hill de Portugal, Ltda.
Rua Rosa Damasceno 11A–B
1900 Lisboa, Portugal

Singapore and Southeast Asia
McGraw-Hill Book Co.
21 Neythal Road
Jurong, Singapore 2262

South Africa
Libriger Book Distributors
Warehouse Number 8
''Die Ou Looiery''
Tannery Road
Hamilton, Bloemfontein 9300

Spain
McGraw-Hill/Interamericana de Espana, S.A.
Manuel Ferrero, 13
28020 Madrid, Spain

Taiwan
Mr. George Lim
P.O. Box 87–601
Taipei, Taiwan

Thailand
Mr. Vitit Lim
632/5 Phaholyothin Road
Sapan Kwai
Bangkok 10400
Thailand

Venezuela
Editorial Interamericana de Venezuela, C.A.
2da. calle Bello Monte
Local G-2
Caracas, Venezuela

NOTICE

The authors and publisher have made every effort to ensure that the patient care recommended herein, including choice of drugs and drug dosages, is in accord with the accepted standards and practice at the time of publication. However, since research and regulation constantly change clinical standards, the reader is urged to check the product information sheet included in the package of each drug, which includes recommended doses, warnings, and contraindications. This is particularly important with new or infrequently used drugs.

Cleft Palate Speech, Second Edition

ISBN 1–55664–238–5

Library of Congress catalog card number: 89–51244

10 9 8 7 6 5 4

To our mentors and friends:

JACK MATTHEWS, Ph.D.
University of Pittsburgh

D.C. SPRIESTERSBACH, Ph.D.
The University of Iowa

JAMES F. BOSMA, M.D.
The Johns Hopkins University

And to our patients and our students
from whom we continue to learn.

PREFACE TO THE FIRST EDITION

This book was begun at least five years ago. Hugh Morris asked Ralph Shelton and Betty Jane McWilliams to join him in revising *Cleft Palate and Communication* by Spriestersbach and Sherman (1968). We all had thoughts about what we would like to see in a textbook about cleft palate written for speech pathologists and other professional people concerned in the management of disordered speech. Many meetings, telephone calls, and letters led us to the decision to write our own book and to broaden the base to include other malformations of the craniofacial complex. In the process, we had to resolve conflicting goals and develop a plan acceptable to us all. Finally, we adopted an outline which we knew would be modified as we progressed and divided the initial tasks among us. Hugh Morris was to write the chapters in the first three sections, Betty Jane McWilliams the section on development and the chapters on language and voice, and Ralph Shelton the section and clinical chapters on velopharyngeal valving and articulation.

We circulated rough drafts many times; much rewriting was done by all of us; and portions of text were expanded, cut, or moved from one chapter to another. Massive editing was done and illustrations and art work were executed and assembled. Betty Jane prepared and coordinated the material and worked with the publisher during the publication process. We wondered a time or two if our long and cherished friendship could survive the impossible task of three authors in three widely separated parts of the country writing one book presenting an integrated view. Our friendship has survived, and the book has been published. We do not all agree with every statement made in the book, and we have tried to point out some of our differences. We all do agree, however, that working in this area of speech pathology is a privilege, and we are excited about sharing it with you in the expectation that you will generate new knowledge and find better ways than we have set forth here. The state of the art in 1984 *requires* that you join us in the effort to bring better communication skills to patients with clefts and other craniofacial abnormalities.

We have enjoyed remarkable support during the writing of this book from our institutions, our friends, and our families, who have listened to our lamentations, encouraged us when we needed it, and refrained from asking if we were *still* writing. We are grateful to them all.

From the onset of this project, Brian Decker has worked with us, encouraged and prodded us, and served as coordinator and mediator. We appreciate his remarkable assistance and are especially pleased with his choice of editor, Mary K. Maudsley. With her background in linguistics and her sensitivity for the English language, she has been a fine colleague.

Special thanks are extended to staff members at the Cleft Palate Center, University of Pittsburgh. They read manuscript, made valuable suggestions, helped find illustrations, reviewed drawings, and offered wise counsel. Helen Baum, Ellen Cohn, Ph.D., Michelle Ferketic, M.S., William S. Garret, M.D., Kenneth Garver, M.D., Dennis Hurwitz, M.D., Linda Jardini, M.S., Jack Matthews, Ph.D., Ross Musgrave, M.D., Robert Mundell, Ph.D., Jack Paradise, M.D., Sylvan Stool, M.D., and Linda Vallino, M.S. all made major contributions.

From the University of Iowa, doctoral candidate Mary Hardin and staff member Janet Beckwith spent long hours reading and working with the manuscript. We appreciate their assistance.

We are especially indebted to Jeanne K. Smith, M.A. and D.R. Van Demark, Ph.D., who took extra clinical duty so that Hugh could devote time to the project.

The Speech and Hearing Sciences Department at the University of Arizona participated in many ways, particularly in the reading of manuscript and in providing support for the project. Our appreciation goes to Daniel R. Boone, Ph.D., Richard F. Curlee, Ph.D., Thomas J. Hixon, Ph.D., William R. Hodgson, Ph.D., Rebecca McCauley, Ph.D., and Paul H. Skinner, Ph.D.. From the Faculty of Rehabilitation Medicine, University of Alberta, Anne H.B. Putnam, Ph.D. and Frank B. Wilson, Ph.D. made major contributions, particularly during Ralph Shelton's sabbatical spent with them in Edmonton.

We thank Mary Anne Witzel, Ph.D., Hospital for Sick Children, Toronto, for the help she provided in getting permission to adapt several illustrations and R. Bruce Ross, D.D.S., Editor, *The Cleft Palate Journal*, for his great generosity in allowing us to use illustrations published in the *Journal* over the past 20 years.

John Coulter, medical illustrator, earned our gratitude for the execution of art work and for the efficiency and speed with which he accomplished it. We are especially appreciative to him for making available original drawings from other sources for reproduction in this book.

Finally, we acknowledge the invaluable support of the National Institute of Dental Research (N.I.D.R.), the arm of the National Institutes of Health with responsibility for funding research in craniofacial abnormalities. Much of the research reviewed in this book, including our own, would not have been possible had N.I.D.R. not made the decision more than 20 years ago to emphasize the importance of cleft lip and palate and related disorders. We pay special tribute to Richard Christiansen, D.D.S., M.S.D., Ph.D. whose wise leadership at N.I.D.R. we valued and continue to appreciate now that he has moved on to become Dean of the School of Dentistry at the University of Michigan.

Betty Jane McWilliams, Ph.D.
Hugh Morris, Ph.D.
Ralph Shelton, Ph.D.
February, 1984

ADDENDUM

The Second Edition was not as difficult to execute as the first, but we could not have done it as well or as quickly without the cooperation of Helen Baum, University of Pittsburgh; Janet Beckwith, The University of Iowa; and Agnes McIvor and Carol McMaster of B.C. Decker Inc. We thank them for their invaluable assistance and also extend our gratitude to Brian Decker for his continued professional and personal interest and support.

B.J.McW.
H.L.M.
R.L.S.
October, 1989

CONTENTS

THE NATURE OF THE PROBLEM

1 | CLEFT LIP, CLEFT PALATE AND RELATED DISORDERS

Cleft lip and palate and related disorders assume many forms. They are malformations that occur in utero and are present at birth. Deformities similar to these congenital defects can come about later in life as a result of severe injuries to the oral structures or from ablative surgery, usually for the treatment of malignant tumors. Some problems associated with these acquired deformities resemble those that result from congenital abnormalities. However, treatment will differ. For example, communication problems that arise from severe injury or surgery are quite different from those that arise from congenital defects since communication skills were previously normal. Since this is not true for patients born with congenital malformations, both treatment and outcome may differ in the two groups.

The term "cleft" accurately describes the major deformities under consideration. The upper lip may be open on one or both sides, and the palate or roof of the mouth may be divided so that the oral and nasal cavities are coupled. Infrequently more extensive clefts may affect the face, the nose, the eyes, and related structures. These openings represent a developmental failure or disruption in the midface and oral cavity, and they have profound implications in the lives of those who are so affected.

TYPES OF CLEFTS

Cleft Lip

A cleft of the lip involves only soft tissue and extends through the red part of the lip, or vermilion border, into the upper portion of the upper lip toward the nostril. If the cleft is incomplete, it may be only a minor notch or may extend almost to the nostril. If it is complete, it will include all of the lip and continue into the floor of the nostril.

A cleft lip may be *unilateral*, only one side is affected (Fig. 1.1), or *bilateral*, both sides are affected (Fig. 1.2). If the cleft is unilateral, it most commonly occurs on the left. Cleft lip is usually but not always accompanied by a cleft of the alveolus or dental arch. Usually the cleft extends completely through the arch but it may also be minimal and consist only of a slight notch. Cleft lip can occur with or without cleft palate.

A bilateral complete cleft of the lip and alveolus, usually accompanied by cleft palate, is an extensive defect in which the central portion of the upper lip and alveolus are attached to the tip of the nose as in the infant profile shown in Figure 1.2.

Since the architecture of the nose is closely related to the upper lip and the midface, a complete cleft of the lip, whether it be unilateral or bilateral, has adverse effects on the nose. Indeed, so closely are the lip and nose related that many surgeons refer to the cleft lip and nose deformities as if they were a single entity. The effect is a partial collapse or flattening of the nose and a flaring of the alar base on the side of the cleft. The resulting misshapen nostril can be a significant visual clue to the existence of the deformity even after lip repair. However, some patients with minimal defects and excellent results from lip surgery may have little if any nose deformity.

The patient with cleft lip may also have a short columella, which is the strip of tissue between the base and the tip of the nose. Such a defect is almost universal in complete bilateral cleft lips and is often so severe that primary

1

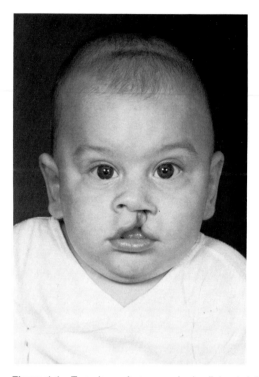
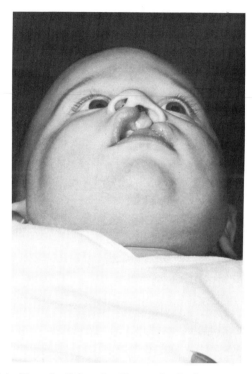

Figure 1.1 Two views of an unrepaired unilateral cleft lip and palate. (From the University of Iowa collection.)

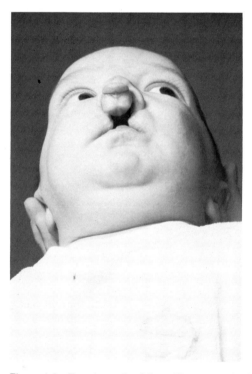
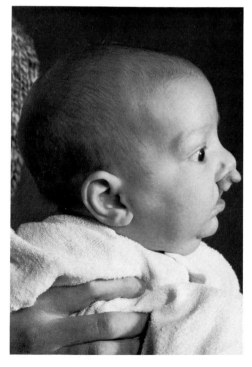

Figure 1.2 Two views of an infant with an unrepaired bilateral cleft lip and palate. Note the premaxilla attached to the tip of the nose. (From the University of Iowa collection.)

surgery for the repair of the lip does not correct the nostril deformity, and subsequent surgery is necessary for cosmetic improvement.

Cleft Palate

In the normal individual, the palate serves as the partition between the nasal and the oral cavities. The anterior two-thirds of the palate make up the hard palate, commonly referred to as the roof of the mouth. The bone underlying the mucosa is composed of the maxillary and the palatine bones of the skull. The alveolar ridge, a part of the prepalate, partially encircles the hard palate and consists primarily of supporting structures for the teeth. The soft palate or velum consists of the posterior one-third of the palate. This structure has no bony underlay and is composed of muscle and mucosa. The hard palate is intact and stationary. When separation of the oral and nasal cavities is required, as in swallowing, yawning, and most speech tasks, the soft palate moves superiorly and posteriorly in concert with the posterior and lateral pharyngeal walls, to occlude the velopharyngeal portal. This portal couples the oral and nasal cavities when the palate is at rest as in nasal breathing.

A complete cleft of the lip and palate extends from the external lip posteriorly through the alveolar arch and the hard and soft palates. The soft palate and the uvula are split (Fig. 1.3). The nasal septum is usually attached to the larger of the two palatal segments in unilateral clefts but is not attached to either segment in bilateral clefts.

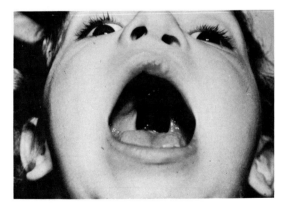

Figure 1.3 Intraoral view of an unrepaired cleft palate. (From the University of Iowa collection.)

In both cases, the inferior aspect of the septum frequently can be seen during examination of the oral structures.

Isolated cleft palate, without cleft lip, also varies in severity. It may include all of the hard palate posterior to the incisive foramen and the soft palate; it may involve only a small portion of the posterior part of the soft palate; or it may be between these two extremes (Fig. 1.4). The simplest defect is the bifid uvula which many people refer to as a "double uvula". In reality, it is two halves that never fused. In and of itself, it is not usually symptomatic. In isolated cleft palate the nasal septum is not attached to either segment, but is at the midline and can be seen during physical examination if the cleft is wide enough and includes the hard palate.

Facial Clefts

Facial clefts take a variety of forms as can be seen in Figure 1.5 from Millard (1976), who described several different types. These deformities are very rare, but speech pathologists should know about them.

Submucous Cleft Palate

In submucous cleft palate, the palate appears to be structurally intact, but there usually are both bony and muscular deficits (Calnan, 1954; Weatherley-White et al., 1972; Velasco et al., 1988). The defect is associated with a triad of symptoms including a bony notch in the hard palate, a bluish line at the midline of the soft palate, and a bifid uvula. The bony notch can be seen or felt where normally the posterior nasal spine is found along the posterior border of the hard palate. The notch, or bony cleft, is not always observable during routine examination but can often be detected by manual palpation. Sometimes, however, this notch is deep and wide. Figure 1.6 shows such a cleft. The submucous cleft of the hard palate is not functionally significant, but the muscular deficit found in the soft palate often is. This muscular cleft, covered only by oral mucosa, is seen as a bluish line through the length of the soft palate. The levator muscles in these cases are often found to be inserted into the hard palate instead of interdigitating to form the normal levator sling. This condition foreshortens

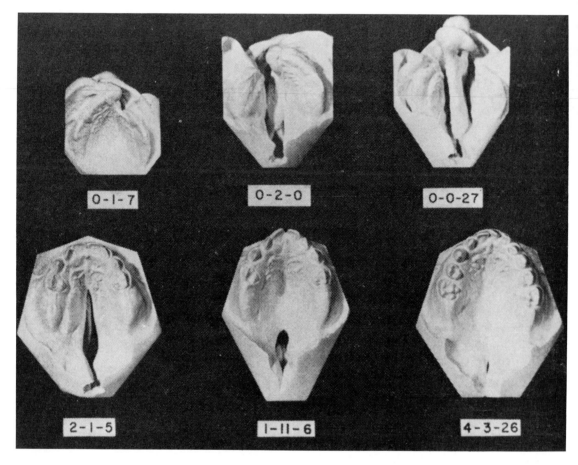

Figure 1.4 Casts of various types of unoperated clefts of the lip and/or palate. Casts 0-20 and 0-0-27 clearly show the status of the nasal septum in unilateral and bilateral defects. Casts 2-1-5, 1-11-6, and 4-3-26 show varying degrees of isolated cleft palate. (From Meskin LH, Pruzansky S, Gullen WH. An epidemiologic investigation of factors related to the extent of facial clefts. I. Sex of patient. Cleft Palate J 1968;5:25.)

the functional soft palate and creates a further complexity, which may contribute to velopharyngeal incompetence requiring surgery. Unlike overt clefts, submucous cleft palates (to be described later), often go undiagnosed unless speech problems reflect the need for diagnostic study.

SIGNIFICANT VARIATIONS IN THE SEVERITY OF THE CLEFT

The traditional basis for describing the severity of a cleft has been cleft type. One attribute of cleft type is length. The assumption is that a complete cleft of the lip, alveolus, and hard and soft palates is more severe than an incomplete

cleft and that a bilateral complete cleft is more severe than a unilateral complete cleft. An incomplete cleft lip is usually less difficult to repair than is a complete cleft lip; and surgical results for a cleft involving only the soft palate tend to be somewhat better than for a unilateral complete cleft of the lip and palate.

Another important variable in determining the severity of deformity is the width of the cleft. Since surgery for the majority of clefts of the lip and palate uses soft tissue from areas adjacent to the cleft, a wide cleft is more difficult to manage than is a narrow cleft because the amount of soft tissue available may be deficient. Consequently, a relatively short cleft of either the lip or palate may be severe because the cleft is very wide. An

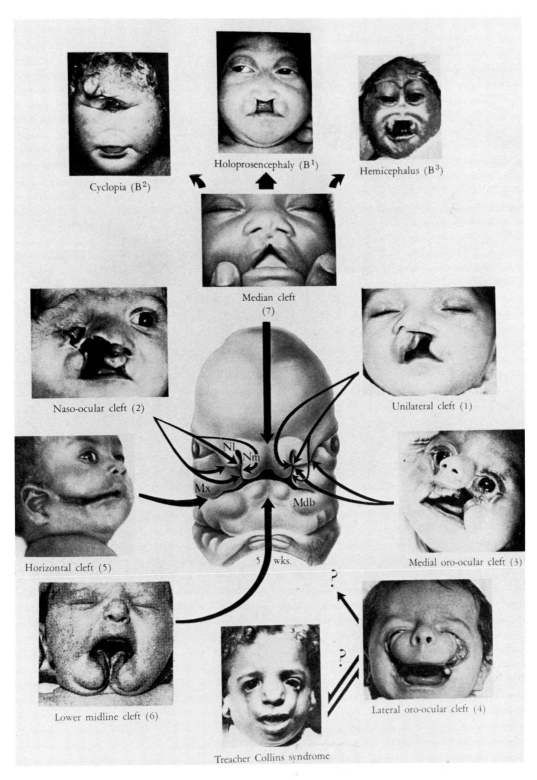

Figure 1.5 Rare facial clefts and their origins. (From Millard DR. Cleft craft. Vol 1. Boston: Little, Brown, 1976.)

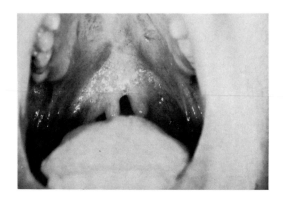

Figure 1.6 A submucous cleft palate with deep bony notch in the hard palate, thin, attenuated raphe in the midline of the soft palate, and a bifurcation of the uvula extending slightly into the soft palate. (From McWilliams BJ. Communication problems associated with cleft palate. In: Van Hattum RJ, ed. Communication disorders, an introduction. New York: Macmillan, 1980.)

example of such a cleft is the incomplete palatal cleft that may be described as horseshoe-shaped.

Other Cleft-Related Deformities

In addition to the problems just described, a variety of other related defects may occur. A minor variation of this type is a congenital hairline "scar" on the lip. While the upper lip has the appearance of a surgically repaired cleft lip, there has never been a cleft, and treatment is not usually indicated. Another such defect is congenitally missing lateral incisors (Meskin et al., 1965). The assumption is that the incisor is missing because of a disturbance in the part of the alveolus where a cleft would have appeared had one occurred. Some writers have considered this to be a frequent occurrence in families with histories of clefts. However, Woolf et al., (1965) and Chosack and Eidelman (1978) did not support this assumption. Missing or deformed lateral incisors are not uncommon, and they cannot be directly associated with clefts.

Other conditions have been explored to determine if they are microforms of cleft palate. These include various dental anomalies, skeletal variations, and facial asymmetries. These microforms would presumably be linked to an increased risk of producing offspring with clefts. However, Fraser (1971) considered most of the studies to be flawed in their designs and, thus, of little practical importance. A major difficulty in conducting studies of this type is arriving at a satisfactory definition of microform.

Clefts of the lip and palate are highly variable, ranging from a relatively easy to manage deficit, with few long-range implications, to an extensive defect with serious adverse effects. The heterogeneity of the defect demands that treatment and research be based on accurate classification of the defects.

Congenital Palatopharyngeal Incompetence (CPI)

Descriptions of congenital palatopharyngeal incompetence (CPI) have been presented by Calnan (1956 and 1971a,b), Randall et al. (1960), Blackfield et al. (1962) Fara and Weatherley-White (1977), and Croft et al. (1978). Some authors also use the term occult cleft palate to refer to the same disorder.

As the term suggests this condition is present from birth and results in velopharyngeal incompetence for speech, although no overt or submucous cleft is present. Like submucous cleft palate, the defect is usually diagnosed after speech develops (Morris et al., 1982) and hypernasality is heard.

On visual inspection, the hard and soft palates may appear to be adequate in bulk, length, and motility. Yet, speech characteristics are consistent with those associated with velopharyngeal incompetence. Closer examination of the physical valving mechanism by multiview videofluoroscopy or endoscopy, both described in Chapter 11, reveals that the velopharyngeal valve does not close during speech. Although data about the extent of velopharyngeal incompetence in these patients are scant, both clinical experience and clinical reports indicate valving deficits that range from borderline to severe incompetence.

A number of anatomical and physiological conditions which contribute to the disorder have been identified. They include congenitally short palate, reduced palatal bulk, a deep or enlarged pharynx, malinsertion of the levator muscles, and combinations of these. Some writers have included submucous cleft palate and bifid uvula in this classification, but we consider these to be true variations of cleft palate. Others have included neuromotor deficits of the palate and pharynx because they obviously can result in velopharyngeal incompetence in the absence of cleft palate. We prefer to treat these problems as a separate entity, fully recognizing that these motor problems are indeed responsible for severe and difficult-to-manage velopharyngeal incompetence associated with cleft-like speech.

Children with CPI can be divided into two groups on the basis of the age at which the speech symptoms are first expressed. One group experiences difficulty from the onset of speech, and the other suffers speech deterioration as a consequence of adenoidectomy (Gibb, 1958; Lubit, 1967; Calnan, 1971b; Mason, 1973; Jackson et al., 1980; Morris et al., 1982; and Cotton and Nuwayhid, 1983). In the second group, the adenoid pad apparently plays a significant role in compensating for the velopharyngeal incompetence which, therefore, goes undiagnosed. It is important to understand that the adenoidectomy does not cause the velopharyngeal incompetence. The incompetence is simply unmasked by the removal of the adenoid tissue, a procedure that can be tolerated by people who do not have CPI (Calnan, 1956; Subtelny and Koepp-Baker, 1956; and Gibb, 1958).

This discussion raises the issue of whether CPI patients or others develop velopharyngeal dysfunction as a result of normal adenoidal involution (shrinkage). No data of this sort, to our knowledge, have been reported for CPI patients, but are available for other subject groups. Siegel-Sadewitz and Shprintzen, (1986) observed 20 normal children, five children with cleft palate, and five children with submucous clefts for 10 years and found no instance of developing insufficiency. Morris et al. (in press) reported that 7 of 39 cleft palate subjects showed evidence of deteriorating velopharyngeal function with progressive decrease in midsagittal adenoidal bulk.

Kaplan (1975) described four different origins of velopharyngeal incompetence in patients who do not have clefts:

1. Anatomic disproportion with normal palatal function. These patients have short soft or hard palates or deep nasopharynxes (Fig. 1.7).
2. Muscle dysfunction with normal proportions (Fig. 1.7:2,4).
3. Intermediate. These patients have both anatomic disproportions and muscle dysfunction (Fig. 1.7:3).

4. Indeterminate. These patients do not fit clearly into any of the other three categories.

Clues to the origin of CPI or occult cleft palate, as this condition has been called under some circumstances, were also provided by Kaplan (1975). He believed that such children frequently have aberrant facial characteristics that are related to mesodermal deficiencies, a major factor in the embryology of cleft palate. Kaplan studied 41 patients with submucous cleft palates, 23 with occult submucous cleft palates, and 167 with other problems, most of whom he thought had occult clefts or other microforms which were missed because of a lack of appreciation of this condition. The unusual facial features which he found included:

1. maxillary hypoplasia—dish face (75%)
2. lip deformity at the vermilion border (75%)
3. drooping of the oral commissure (25%)
4. dynamic facial muscle abnormality (25%)
5. external ear abnormality (10%)
6. alveolar arch abnormalities (5%)

Figure 1.8 shows three of these deformities.

Kaplan performed surgery on 26 patients with classic submucous clefts. All of these patients had insertion of the levator muscles into the hard palate rather than into the midline soft palate raphe. In most cases, 75 to 90 percent of the muscle was inserted into the palatine bone. Occult submucous cleft palate can be suspected but not finally diagnosed until the levators are dissected at the time of surgery. (Fig. 1.9).

Kaplan's work supported that of Chaco and Yules (1969) who demonstrated electromyographically an absence of motor units in the midline of the palates of patients with velopharyngeal incompetence of unknown origin.

Fara and Weatherley-White (1977) discussed the "syndrome of developmental shortening of the palate". They stated that only a small number of these patients have submucous cleft palates, which they included in the syndrome. This shortening may well be the result of muscle malinsertion. Fara and Weatherley-White also reported that patients with this "syndrome" have unique facial features: a wide root of the nose, narrow palpebral fissures, narrow external auditory canals and nasal airways, and hyposemia. The upper lip is often vertically shortened and the

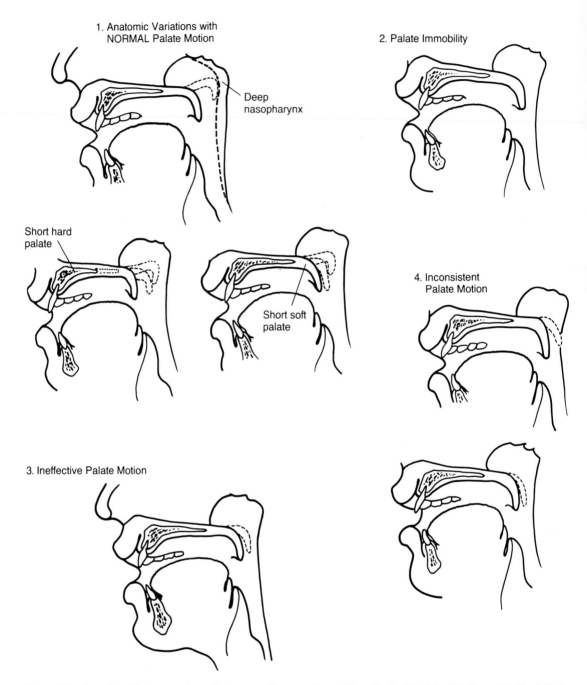

Figure 1.7 Grouping of factors causing velopharyngeal incompetence. (From Kaplan EN, Jobe RP, Chase RA. Flexibility in surgical planning for velopharyngeal incompetence. Cleft Palate J 1969; 6:166–174.)

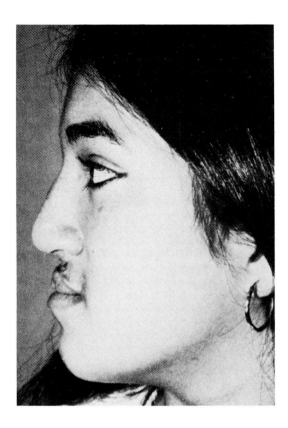

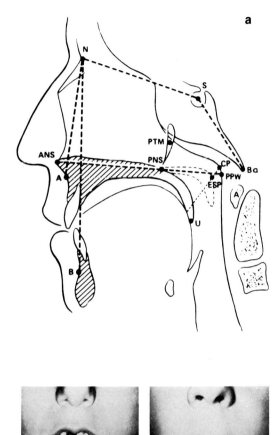

philtrum poorly defined. The lobules are short **b**
and diagonally directed.

Croft et al. (1978) also presented data on the
occult submucous cleft palate. Their 20 patients **c**
all had hypernasal speech, normal palatal morphology on oral examination, and small central
gaps in the velopharyngeal sphincter on multiview
videofluoroscopy. These patients were evaluated
endoscopically, and the movements of the velopharyngeal sphincter were recorded during connected speech. These patients had orifice areas
during connected speech of 1.0 mm^2 to 12.0 mm^2.
The most striking physical finding was a midline
v-shaped defect and the absence of the musculus
uvular bulge on the nasal surface of the velum.
This latter finding was present in all 20 subjects.
Twenty normal control subjects all demonstrated
uvular bulge.

This study supplied another bit of evidence
pointing to muscle deficiencies in these patients
and to the probability that Cotton and Nuwayhid
(1983) were accurate in considering these "occult
clefts" to represent a continuum of submucous

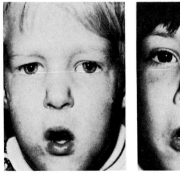

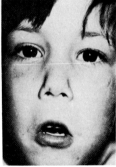

Figure 1.8 (a) The "dish face" maxillary hypoplasia.
Cephalometric measures of SNA and hard palate length
are normal. (b) Lip contour deformity ("gull wing") along the
vermilion border. (c) Drooping of the oral commissure in a
convex lip orifice instead of horizontal. The frown-like
appearance is probably due to facial muscle dysfunction.
(From Kaplan EN. The occult submucous cleft palate. Cleft
Palate J 1975;12:356.)

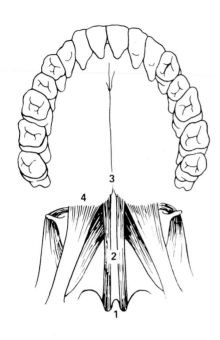

Figure 1.9 Representation by Kaplan (1975) of four classic signs of submucous cleft palate: 1. bifid uvula; 2. furrow along the midline of the soft palate; 3. bony notch in hard palate; 4. insertion of levator and other palate muscles onto hard palate instead of the midline.

cleft palate. A case might be made for establishing a cleft continuum which would include overt clefts and all of the variations that have been presented here.

CLASSIFICATION

There is considerable variability among clinicians and researchers in their methods for classifying cleft lip and palate (Berlin, 1971). Sometimes the most simple classification of cleft type (cleft lip only, cleft lip and palate, cleft palate only) is satisfactory to the purpose. Frequently, however, a more descriptive system is required.

A system in common use is that described by Veau (1931), that provides distinction among four types: cleft of the soft palate only (Group 1); cleft of the soft and hard palate extending to the incisive foramen (Group 2); complete unilateral

cleft of the lip, alveolus, and hard and soft palates (Group 3); and complete bilateral clefts of the lip, alveolus, and hard and soft palates (Group 4). A disadvantage of the Veau system is that it does not provide for isolated clefts of the lip or alveolus or for partial clefts.

Kernahan and Stark (1958) recommended a classification based on embryological development that includes two major categories (Fig. 1.10). Clefts of the primary palate include those that involve structures *anterior to the incisive foramen*. Clefts of the secondary palate occur in structures *posterior to the incisive foramen* and may affect both the hard and soft palates or only some part of the soft palate. These clefts are also described as complete or incomplete or total or

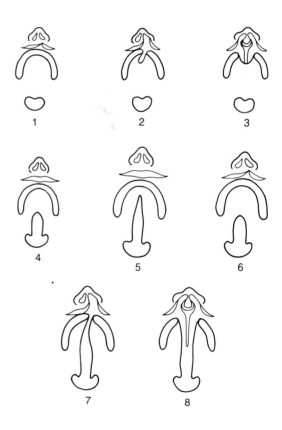

Figure 1.10 Classification of cleft lip and palate by Kernahan and Stark. Clefts of the primary palate: (1) subtotal (2) unilateral (3) bilateral. Clefts of the secondary palate: (4) subtotal (5) total. Clefts of the primary and secondary palates: (6) unilateral, subtotal (7) unilateral total (8) bilateral. (From Kernahan DA, Stark RB. A new classification for cleft lip and cleft palate. Plast Reconstr Surg 1958; 22:435.)

subtotal. Clefts involving both the lip and palate are classified as clefts of both the primary and secondary palates. Provision is made for unilateral, median, and bilateral clefts that are complete (total) or incomplete (subtotal).

Olin (1960) provided for diversity in a system that included clefts of the lip (Group 1) with eight subdivisions; clefts of the palate only (Group 2) with four subdivisions; and clefts of the lip and palate (Group 3) with eight subdivisions (Fig. 1.11).

The American Cleft Palate-Craniofacial Association has sponsored two classification projects. The first (Harkins et al., 1962) yielded a much more elaborate system than any that had preceded it. It made direct provision for such problems as congenital scarring, short palates with no overt clefts, submucous cleft palates, prepalate protrusion or rotation, vomer attachment, and facial clefts. It also emphasized the width of clefts, one of the factors in severity.

A still more complicated system was proposed by Whitaker et al. (1981). It was designed for classifying disorders of the cranium and face, but includes clefts also. Craniofacial defects are discussed in greater detail in Chapter 2.

Recently, Kriens (in press) provided a useful review of literature about several classification systems and proposed one that facilitates documentation for both clinical and research purposes.

No single system has been universally accepted, and none is universally used. The reason for this is that these defects vary widely, and clinicians often resort to descriptive terms and drawings to provide the specificity required in individual cases.

INCIDENCE

A safe, conservative estimate of incidence appears to be approximately one in every 750 live

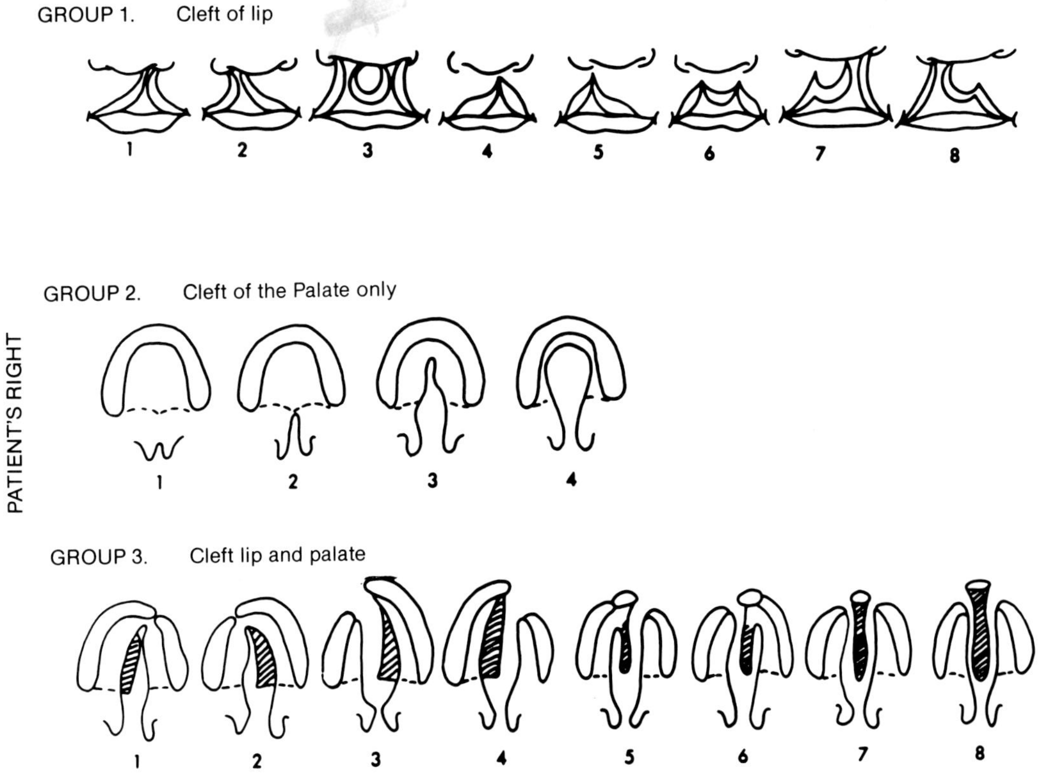

Figure 1.11 A classification of cleft lip and palate. The nasal septum is represented by the stippled area. (From Olin WH. Cleft lip and palate rehabilitation. Springfield, IL: CC Thomas, 1960.)

births, although there are some indications that the rate may be even higher than that figure. Rintala (1982) reports an incidence rate of 1/462 in Finland and Jensen et al. (1988), 1/529, in Denmark. Hook (1988) reviews two data sets from Hungary (Czeizel, 1984) and the United States (Myrianthopoulos and Chung, 1974) and reports overall rates of 1/645 and 1/625, respectively.

The estimate of one in 750 does not include certain minimal expressions of the defect such as bifid uvula, which has an incidence rate of one in 80 Caucasians (Gorlin et al., 1976) or submucous cleft palate and congenital palatal incompetence, which are rarely diagnosed at birth. Weatherley-White et al. (1972) examined 10,836 school-aged children and found evidence of submucous cleft in one in 1200.

Source of Data

One method of collecting data about the incidence of clefts and other congenital malformations is the inspection of birth certificates. Birth certificates are reliable only if the physical examinations performed at birth were accurate and if the recording of them was without error. Cleft lip by itself and cleft lip associated with cleft palate are likely to be seen during the initial physical examination because the cleft lip is obvious. Isolated cleft palate, however, is probably under-reported because it is less obvious and requires more careful assessment. As detection of an abnormality becomes more difficult, errors in reporting increase. Another source of error in the use of birth certificates is failure to indicate whether the data included both live- and still-births. This is a crucial distinction since the incidence of clefts among live births is likely to be lower than it is for stillbirths, which may result from multiple congenital malformations (Vanderas, 1987; Hook, 1988).

The most reliable data combine information from birth certificates and hospital records. This is the approach used by Fogh-Andersen (1942), Tretsven (1963), and Bardanouve (1969). Even then, however, under-reporting remains a significant problem. Meskin and Pruzansky (1967) found that the birth certificates did not report the clefts in 29.4% of their cases and that more than 50% of isolated palatal clefts were not shown. Ivy (1957) was one of the first to recognize this

problem, and he recommended the use of a 20% correction factor to provide for under-reporting.

Racial Difference

There is considerable variation in the frequency of clefts from one racial group to another. The best data available concerns the frequency of cleft lip, with or without cleft palate. Excellent data about these differences came from a project supported by the World Health Organization (WHO) and reported by Stevenson et al. (1966). These and other data were critically reviewed and summarized by Leck (1977), Ross and Johnston (1972), and Oka (1979). A recent review of available findings was provided by Vanderas (1987). On the basis of data reported in some 65 papers, he concludes that North American Indians show the highest incidence rates (as high as 3.74/1000), followed by the Japanese (0.82 to 3.36), the Chinese (1.45 to 4.04/1000), the Whites (1.00 to 2.69/1000), and the Blacks (0.18 to 1.67/1000). He attributes these differences to environmental and genetic factors, or a combination of both. Similar trends are reported by Chavez et al. (1989). Oka (1979) concluded that, overall, there is a distinct racial gradient in the incidence of cleft lip with or without cleft palate and a minor difference in the incidence of isolated cleft palate.

Change in Occurrence Rates

There are some indications, still to be confirmed, that the rate of occurrence may now be higher than it once was in certain populations (Fogh-Andersen, 1961; Jensen et al., 1988). One explanation may be that with better medical treatment more pregnancies come to term and more high-risk infants, among them, those with clefts, survive, thrive, and live to adulthood. Second, more sophisticated treatment probably results in adults with clefts who look, speak, and interact more normally, thus making it more likely than was once the case that they will produce children. Both of these factors could increase the size of the genetic pool that carries the cleft trait. As a result, proportionately more children with clefts are born. On the other hand, it may be that the apparent increase in occurrence is merely the result of improved diagnosis, a more efficient system for reporting birth defects in general, and more people seeking correction of defects of this type. This seems especially probable in the highly industrialized parts of the world. There are some findings that suggest a reverse trend. Data collected in Pennsylvania reflect a gradual decline, for the years 1973 through 1981 (Cohn et al., 1984), to 1 in 975 births. Similar findings have been reported by Briggs (1976). Further investigation is needed to indicate whether the incidence may be increasing in some areas and decreasing in others.

Sex Difference

It is well established that cleft lip with or without cleft palate occurs about twice as often in males as in females and that the males tend to have more severe deformities than the females. However, the reverse is true for isolated cleft palate. More girls than boys are affected with this type of cleft (Warkany, 1971). Oka (1979) analyzed data from 26 studies published between 1951 and 1976 in various parts of the world, including 10,885 subjects with cleft lip with or without cleft palate. Of these, 62% were male, and 38% were female. The sex ratio was reversed, however, for isolated cleft palate. There were 4004 cases with this deformity. Of these, 57.3% were female, while only 42.7% were male. Similar results have been recently reported by Jensen et al. (1988). The reasons for the higher prevalence among females is not well understood, but it may be related to male-female differences in the timing of development of the lip and palate. Burdi and Silvey (1969) found female embryos to be delayed by about 1 week in comparison to males. While this may be true, differing genetic factors may also contribute. Gorlin et al. (1976) pointed out that, when the collective cases of submucous cleft palate described by Calnan (1954) and Gylling and Soivio (1965) are analyzed, over 50% appear to have occurred in males. This is surprising since overt isolated cleft palate is more common in females. In order to resolve the questions raised by these figures, carefully designed and executed studies are required.

Differences in Cleft Type

There is considerable evidence of differences in incidence rates according to cleft type. Hanson and Murray (in press) indicate that cleft palate

occurs in 1/1000 term newborns and cleft palate alone in 1/2000. They note the importance of racial and ethnic groups in estimating frequency of occurrence, as do Hook (1988) and Chavez et al. (1989).

It follows that there are also differences among the various cleft types. In his classic study of incidence, Fogh-Andersen (1942) suggested that, of the total group of patients with clefts, 25% have cleft lip only; 50% have cleft lip and palate; and 25% have cleft palate only. Although there are differences in percentages from one report to another, most are consistent with that distribution. Greene et al. (1964) analyzed the birth records of 4451 infants with clefts. Cleft lip constituted 27.2% of the cases, cleft lip and palate 44.3%, and cleft palate 28.5%. Similarly, Jensen et al. (1988) report distribution among 678 Danish children as follows: cleft lip only, 33.5%; cleft lip and palate, 39.1%; and cleft palate only, 27.4%. On the other hand, there is recent evidence that more children with isolated cleft palates are now being seen in clinics. McWilliams (personal communication) reported that of her patients with palatal clefts about 49% were isolated cleft palate, and about 51% were clefts of the lip and palate. This varies from year to year, but hovers around a one-to-one ratio. This may be peculiar to this one particular center, which treats complex cases and tends to attract children with multiple handicaps.

Other Congenital Malformations

Three general conclusions can be drawn from the available findings: (1) individuals with clefts have additional congenital malformations more frequently than the general population; (2) cleft palate alone is associated more often with other anomalies than cleft lip, with or without cleft palate; and (3) there is considerable variability in the findings, depending on the population studied (for example, stillbirths or live births) and the way in which that data are collected.

In an early study, Greene et al. (1964) examined all live birth certificates recorded for four states from 1956 through 1960. They found that 15% of 4451 infants with clefts had at least one congenital anomaly (by their definition) in addition to the cleft, while only 0.8% of the records of 17,859 controls showed that at least one anomaly was present. The occurrence of additional malformations by cleft type was as follows: isolated cleft lip, 7%; cleft lip and palate, 14%; and isolated cleft palate, 24%. Spriestersbach et al. (1962) examined 111 patients with clefts for other malformations rather than depending on clinical records as the source of information. They reported associated defects in 16% of individuals with cleft lip with or without cleft palate and in 51% of the cases with cleft palate only.

Pannbacker (1968) reviewed clinical records for 100 patients with cleft palate or congenital palatal incompetence (CPI). Nearly one in three were reported to have an associated anomaly, with higher incidence in cleft palate only (29.6%) than cleft lip only (28.5%) or cleft lip and palate (26.3%). Six of the nine CPI patients had an associated malformation.

Gorlin et al. (1976) reported that although children with complete clefts of the lip and palate are not exempt from other malformations, isolated palatal clefts are much more frequently accompanied by other congenital anomalies. They indicate also that children with bilateral complete clefts of the lip and palate are at higher risk for associated malformations than are those with unilateral complete clefts. McWilliams and Matthews (1979) found that 14% of the children with unilateral cleft lip and palate had additional birth defects, in contrast to 34% of those with isolated cleft palate. These latter findings are based on a Caucasian population. Honda (1978) reviewed 356 Japanese patients with clefts and found associated congenital anomalies in only 21 or 5.9%.

Shprintzen et al. (1985) reviewed clinical records for 1000 patients examined from 1976 through 1982 and reported an incidence rate of associated anomalies of 63.4%. They found more anomalies in the patients with cleft palate only than in those with cleft lip, with or without cleft palate. Jensen et al. (1988) showed a relatively low occurrence of associated anomalies: 4.5% in 602 patients, not including Pierre Robin syndrome. The distribution of associated anomalies between the two major cleft types was nearly equal (14 in cleft lip with or without cleft palate, and 12 in cleft palate only). They comment that their figure may underestimate the true frequency, since stillbirths and early deaths are excluded from their sample.

Jones (1988) evaluated 428 consecutive patients. She reported that 54.7% of the 139 isolated cleft palate patients had a "multiple malformation syndrome", as did 14.3% of the 259 patients with cleft lip with or without cleft palate. Of the CPO

group, 14 were found to have Stickler syndrome, which had not been previously recognized in 12.

Many types of associated malformations have been reported. Warkany (1971) noted mental retardation, congenital heart disease, clubfoot, absence of the radius and thumb, renal anomalies, microphthalmia, microcephaly, and dwarfism. Greene et al. (1964) reported syndactyly, congenital heart disease, malformed ears, spina bifida, polydactyly, clubfoot, and micrognathia concurrent with cleft defects. In the study by Honda (1978), the anomaly most frequently associated with clefts was Pierre Robin syndrome with strabismus.

McWilliams and Matthews (1979) related types of congenital abnormalities to cleft type. They found that 18% of the subjects with isolated palatal clefts had some type of syndrome, whereas none of the subjects with complete clefts of the lip and palate had an identifiable syndrome. Among the children who had other associated defects, 70% of those with isolated palatal clefts had skeletal deformities, which were never found in the children with complete clefts of the lip and palate. Defects of the urinogenital system occurred in 36% of the cases with isolated palatal clefts associated with other defects and not at all in complete clefts. Gastrointestinal defects, on the other hand, accounted for 31% of the deformities occurring in children with complete clefts and for only 17% of those associated with isolated palatal clefts. The authors suggested that these data, based on 226 subjects, should be interpreted with caution and that more extensive investigations in this area are necessary. Geis et al. (1981) screened 282 patients by physical examination and chest x-ray films, followed by ECG and cardiology examination if indicated. The overall prevalence rate of congenital heart disease was 6.7%, with variability in rates among cleft types. The 26 Danish subjects with associated anomalies reported by Jensen et al. (1988) showed a variety of anomalies; also, four of the 13 subjects with cleft lip with or without cleft palate showed a syndrome, as did seven of the 12 subjects with cleft palate only.

We have referred several times in this discussion to syndromes. A syndrome, as used here, is a cluster of malformations that occur together with the result that people suffering from the same syndrome look more like each other than they do like the other members of their own families. Fraser (1970), Warkany (1971), Gorlin et al. (1971,

1976), Cohen (1978), Pashayan (1983), and Jones (1988) all have provided information about syndromes in general and about those including orofacial clefting. Cohen (1978) reported that there are 154 syndromes which include clefting as one of several features. Goodman and Gorlin (1983) have published an illustrated guide of 200 malformations of children, including syndromes, with and without clefts. Jung (1989) provides information about genetic syndromes in communication disorders, including cleft lip and palate. The speech pathologist must understand that, in patients with several malformations, management of those that are life-threatening takes precedence over the others. For instance, palatoplasty would be delayed until risks imposed by a congenital heart defect were minimized. In addition, the nature and extent of the other malformations influence both treatment planning and prognosis. The presence of a syndrome may also be of major importance in considering genetic factors in etiology of a cleft. Additional syndromes involving the craniofacial complex are discussed in Chapter 2.

EMBRYOLOGY

Since cleft lip and palate must be understood in the context of human embryology, some attention is needed to the overall process of embryonic and fetal development (Fig. 1.12). Cleft lip and palate is the result of developmental variations that occur primarily during the embryonic period, which ends at about 8 weeks of gestation, and the very early fetal period, which follows immediately. Normal embryonic development of the face and the embryogenesis of cleft lip with or without cleft palate and of isolated cleft palate are relatively well understood (Patten, 1961; Ross and Johnston, 1972; Nishimura et al., 1977; Rogers, 1977; Krogman, 1979; Stool and Mundell, 1983; Johnston and Sulik, 1984; Sperber, 1981).

Changes in Visual Characteristics From Three To Nine Weeks

At 3 to 4 weeks of embryonic life, the structures are still so undifferentiated that there is

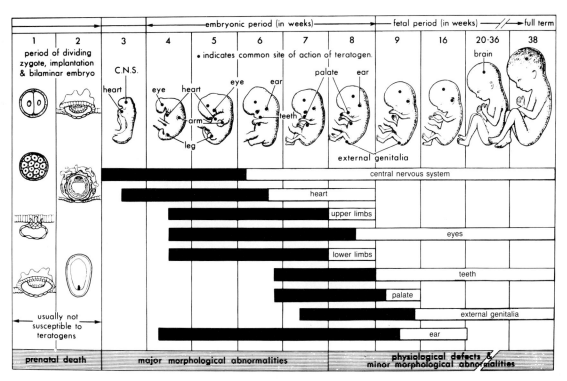

Figure 1.12 Schematic illustration of the sensitive or critical periods in human development. (From Moore KL. Before we are born: basic embryology and birth defects. 2nd ed. Philadelphia: WB Saunders, 1983.)

not an identifiable face. Only those elements that will eventually form the face can be seen. Figure 1.13A shows the anterior neuropore and the primitive brain covered by a membrane. The eyes have not yet developed but can be seen as bulges on each side of the head. A stomadeum will later become the oral and nasal cavities.

At 5 to 6 weeks great changes have occurred, and the face begins to become apparent. Figure 1.13B shows the first or mandibular branchial

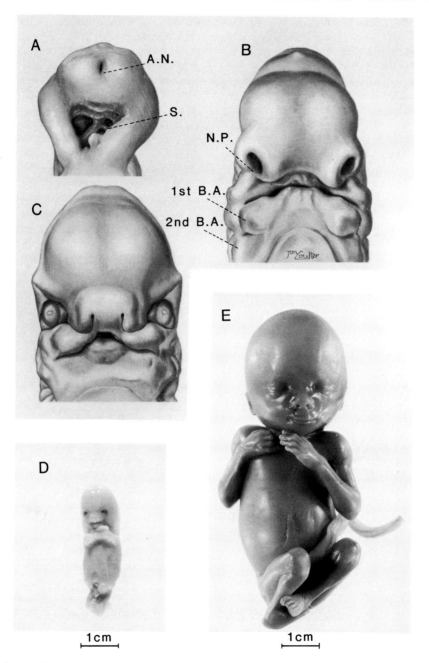

Figure 1.13 Prenatal facial development. (A) An embryo of three to four weeks. AN, anterior neuropore; S, stomadeum. (B) An embryo of five to six weeks. NP, nasal pit; lst BA, first branchial arch; 2nd BA, second branchial arch. (C) An embryo of 7 to 8 weeks. (D) A fetus of 8 to 9 weeks. (E) A fetus of 3 to 4 months. (From Stool S, Mundell R. Phylogenetic aspects and embryology. In: Bluestone CD, Stool SE, eds. Pediatric otolaryngology. Vol 1. Philadelphia: WB Saunders, 1983:6.)

arch and the second or hyoid branchial arch from which the structures comprising the mid and lower face will arise. The base of the tongue will be formed in the region of the third branchial arch, which is not seen in this drawing, while the anterior two-thirds of the tongue forms in the region of the first branchial arch. At this stage, the nasal pits, which will help form the nose, can be seen on either side of the face. Students often mistake these high, widely separated structures for primitive eyes.

Figure 1.13C shows the embryo at 7 to 8 weeks when the nose, eyes, and mouth are fully recognizable but are not as well defined as they are at 8 to 9 weeks (Fig. 1.13D). Note that this latter photograph shows a nose with a broad bridge and eyes that are wide-set as in hypertelorism. This appearance is normal at this stage of development, but with additional growth the eyes will continue to move away from each other as the rest of the head also grows to create the configuration we recognize as normal. Disruption in this process results in hypertelorism, a frequent characteristic of craniofacial abnormalities.

Stool and Mundell (1983) pointed out that the rapid growth that occurs during the embryonic period is marked by differential development. There is enlargement or rearrangement of previous forms as well as the appearance of new configurations. They noted that this concept is difficult for students to grasp because illustrations of embryonic stages are usually shown in drawings of equal size (Fig. 1.14). Figures 1.13D and 1.13E make the size comparison they referred to.

There are a number of theories of how the structures with which we are concerned develop embryologically. We shall discuss one that is widely accepted today.

Neural Crest Theory Of Development

Critical to the development of the face is the formation of neural crest cells around the anterior neuropore (Johnston, 1975; Johnston and Sulik, 1984). These cells are composed of ectoderm, which is the outermost layer of the three primary germ layers of the embryo. (The middle layer is the mesoderm, and the inner layer the entoderm.) These cells, which migrate at different rates, give rise to a variety of connective and nervous tissues of the skull, the branchial arches, and, ultimately, the face. Cells which form the frontonasal process arise from the forebrain fold and move quickly

into the area that will become the nose and adjacent structures. Cells which form the right and left maxillary processes and the mandible have further to travel and so take longer to reach the branchial arches (Krogman, 1973). The mesenchymal tissue, which is formed by the migrating cells, provides for most of the bone and soft tissue that make up the face. Patten (1961) suggested that "when a mesenchymal cell has arrived where it is destined to settle down, it declares its nature by differentiating into the specialized cell type dictated by its inherent developmental potency". Figure 1.15 illustrates this process. If this migration of neural crest cells fails to take place and there is an absence or inadequacy of mesoderm, clefts and other facial abnormalities may result (Stark, 1961, 1977).

Development Of The Primary Palate

Through the mechanism just described, the frontonasal process is differentiated to form the medial nasal process between the nasal pits and, lateral to them, the lateral nasal processes. Krogman (1979) considered the resulting tissue beneath each nostril to be representative of the first separation between the oral and nasal cavities. This early structure will become the primary palate. It contains the prolabium, the premaxilla, and the four maxillary incisor teeth. This separation occurs during the sixth week, a critical period in the development of the lip and, thus, in events that could be responsible for cleft lip and some cleft palates.

In summarizing the literature on this topic, Krogman (1979) concluded that clefts of the lip are caused by the premature cessation of epithelial fusion so that the epithelial wall is too short as it comes into the nasal cavity. Thus, the frontal nasal process and one or both of the lateral maxillary processes fail to unite to complete the upper lip. Krogman's summation of the literature was consistent with the report of Töndury (1961), who related lip clefts to failure of epithelial fusion of the swellings circumscribing the nasal pocket, causing a complete cleft lip, and to arrested epithelial fusion resulting in an epithelial wall that is too short as it comes into the oral cavity, causing a "simple" or incomplete cleft lip. In discussing the epithelial wall Töndury said that, in the development of the nasal cavity, there is a zipper-like seam between the two nasal swellings. This seam, ultimately, dissolves and is replaced by

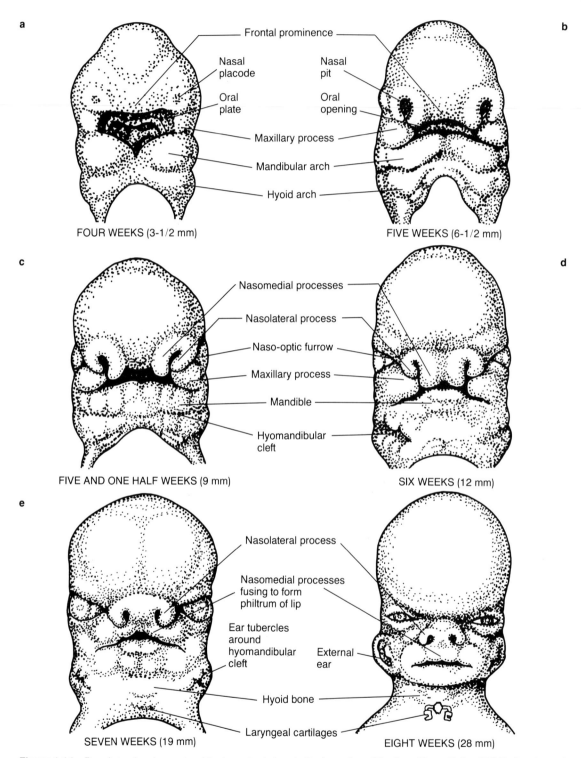

Figure 1.14 Drawings showing some of the important steps in the formation of the face. (From Patten BM. Embryology of the palate and the maxillofacial region. In: Grabb WC, Rosenstein SW, Bzoch KR, eds. Cleft lip and palate: surgical, dental, and speech aspects. Boston: Little, Brown, 1971:23.)

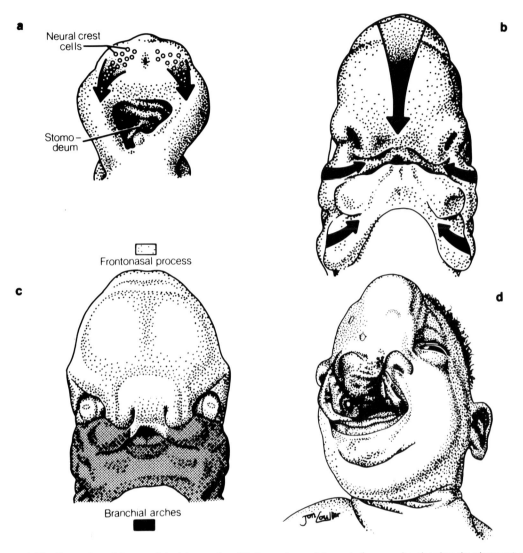

Figure 1.15 Formation of the craniofacial complex. (A) An embryo of three to four weeks showing development and beginning migration of neural crest cells. (B) Migration of neural crest cells to the forebrain and the branchial arches. (C) Contributions to the face of the frontonasal process and branchial arches. (D) Deformity caused by failure of neural crest cell migration. (From Stool SE, Mundell R. Phylogenetic aspects and embryology. In: Bluestone CD, Stool SE, eds. Pediatric otolaryngology. Vol 1. Philadelphia: WB Saunders, 1983:8.)

mesenchyme. Töndury also described cleft lips with "bridges," often referred to as Simonart's bands. These occur if the epithelial wall is defectively laid down and is maintained beyond the normal time. These bands may also be the remnants of a cleft lip cyst.

Stark (1961) suggested that the cleft lip deformity includes all structures anterior to the incisive foramen because he considered these anatomical parts to be embryologically different from those posterior to it. He believed that lip clefts are invariably the result of mesodermal deficiencies, a theory also expressed by Veau (1931).

Development Of The Secondary Palate

Complete separation of the oral and nasal cavities is accomplished when the primary and secondary palates fuse to create continuous structures. Early in development, the rapidly growing tongue occupies the oral space and pushes into the nasal cavity. As shown in Figure 1.16, the palatal shelves, springing from the maxillary processes bilaterally, are in a vertical position on either side of the tongue. During the seventh and eighth weeks, the tongue drops, and the palatal shelves elevate from a vertical to a horizontal position in a plane above the tongue and below the nasal septum (Avery, 1973). This elevation begins at the back of the palate and moves forward to the front (Stark, 1961). The shelves continue their growth, now moving toward each other to the midline. Krogman (1979) likened this process to "two horizontal sliding doors . . . closing at the center." As the shelves meet, fusion begins, proceeding from *front* to *back*, opposite from the direction of the palatal elevation (Fig. 1.17).

The "medial triangle" of the prepalate, lying as it does between the elevated shelves, fuses with them to complete the contour of the maxillary arch. At the same time, the nasal septum grows downward and fuses with the palate, completing the separation of the two nostrils (Patten, 1961, 1971). Patten placed the completion of the fusion of the hard palate at 8 weeks based upon the work of Fulton (1957). Others place it at about 9 weeks. Most of the development of both the hard and soft palates has been completed by the end of the tenth week although final closure of the uvula occurs later, certainly by the twelfth week. Figure 1.18 illustrates the process. However, in some fetuses, openings between the palatal shelves posteriorly have been observed as late as the tenth week. Thus, the completion of the entire process may be as late as 12 weeks. Stark (1961) stated that any impedance in development from the seventh to the twelfth week of gestation may interrupt the elevation and fusion of the palatal shelves and produce the "persistence of the original cleft in the roof of the mouth." This is indicative of variation from one fetus to another. Differences in the time of shelf elevation were shown by Kraus et al. (1966). Obviously, the later any disruption of the developmental process occurs, the more minor the defect will be.

The development of the soft palate has received less attention than has that of the hard palate. Stark (1961) stated that the two structures develop simultaneously. Researchers differ in their views of how the closure of the soft palate occurs. Some say little or nothing about it; others

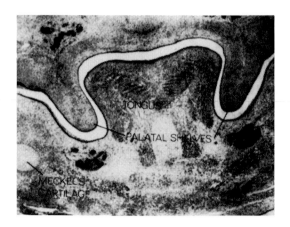

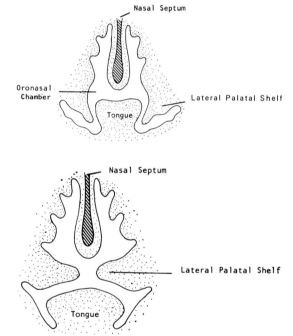

Figure 1.16 Photomicrograph and schematic representations of tongue and palatal shelf positions in embryo. (From Sperber GH. Craniofacial embryology. 3rd ed. Dental Practictioner Handbook, No. 15. Bristol: Wright, 1981.)

imply that the fusion responsible for completion of the hard palate continues through the velum or soft palate; still others describe velar closure as a process of "merging" (Burdi, 1968). Fusion and merging are illustrated in Figure 1.19.

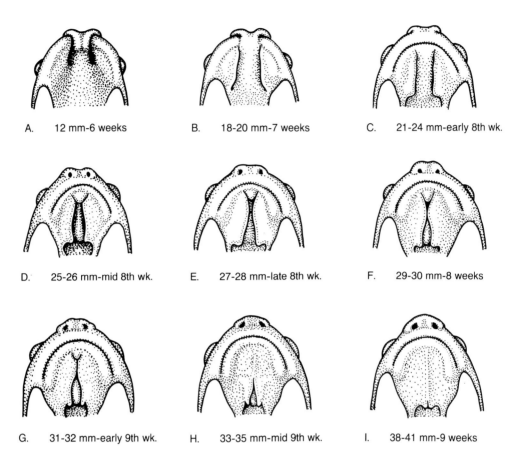

A.   12 mm-6 weeks   B.   18-20 mm-7 weeks   C.   21-24 mm-early 8th wk.

D.   25-26 mm-mid 8th wk.   E.   27-28 mm-late 8th wk.   F.   29-30 mm-8 weeks

G.   31-32 mm-early 9th wk.   H.   33-35 mm-mid 9th wk.   I.   38-41 mm-9 weeks

Figure 1.17 Graphic summary of palatal fusion. The measurements and estimated ages should be regarded as averages as there is considerable variability among specimens. (A) 12mm—6 weeks; (B) 18-20mm—7 weeks; (C) 21-24mm—early 8th week; (D) 25-26 mm—mid 8th week; (E) 27-28 mm—late 8th week; (F) 29-30 mm—8 weeks; (G) 31-32 mm—early 9th week; (H) 33-35 mm—mid 9th week; (I)38-41 mm—9 weeks. (From Patten BM. Embryology of the palate and the maxillofacial region. In: Grabb WC, Rosenstein SW, Bzoch KR. Cleft lip and palate: surgical, dental, and speech aspects. Little, Brown, 1971:31.)

Facial Clefts

Figures 1.5 and 1.15D are thought to be the result of massive failure of neural crest cell migration. The embryological mechanisms responsible for these severe malformations are much the same as they are for clefts in general, but they are more profound and involve the failure of several different structures to unite. For example, the oblique cleft, naso-ocular type, shown in Figure 1.5(2) results from failure of the medial nasal process, the lateral nasal processes, and the maxillary prominences to unite with each other. The horizontal cleft shown in Figure 1.5(5) is the result of failure of the maxillary and mandibular prominences to merge. Figure 1.5(4) however, cannot be explained on the basis of this model (Millard, 1976).

Factors That Interfere With Development

Defects in neural crest formation and migration can result in mesenchyme deficiencies, which in turn can lead to clefts of the primary palate. Ross and Johnston (1972) and Johnston and Sulik (1984) discussed the factors that result in clefts of

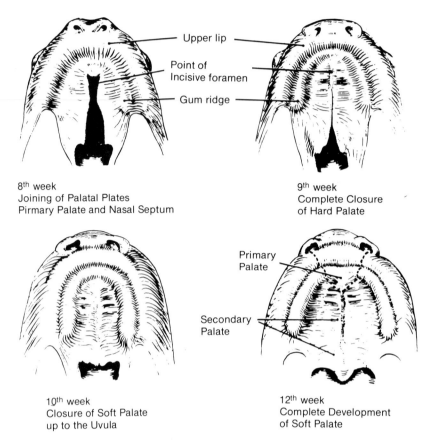

Upper lip

Point of
Incisive foramen

Gum ridge

8th week
Joining of Palatal Plates
Pirmary Palate and Nasal Septum

9th week
Complete Closure
of Hard Palate

Primary
Palate

Secondary
Palate

10th week
Closure of Soft Palate
up to the Uvula

12th week
Complete Development
of Soft Palate

Figure 1.18 Palatal joining, which takes place as a wedge-shaped closure from front to back. (A) 8th week. Joining of palatal plates, primary palate and nasal septum. (B) 9th week. Complete closure of hard palate. (C) 10th week. Closure of soft palate up to the uvula. (D) 12th week. Complete development of soft palate. (From Bzoch KR, Williams WN. Introduction, rationale, principles, and related basic embryology and anatomy. In: Bzoch KR. Communicative disorders related to cleft lip and palate. Boston: Little, Brown, 1979:11.)

the secondary palate relative to size and elevation of the palatine shelves, lowering of the tongue, width of the primitive oronasal cavity, and malfunction of the fusion process.

Fraser (1971) referred to the elevation of the palatal shelves as a "threshold character." This means that there are variations in the timing of shelf elevation, and some of the delays may be so serious that, by the time the shelves are horizontal, they are too far apart for fusion ever to occur, and a cleft is the result. The threshold is the point beyond which fusion will not be possible. Delay in shelf elevation may not create clefts if the embryo is programmed for early elevation, but it can be disastrous for the embryo programmed for shelf elevation at or beyond the threshold zone. Figure

1.20 is a hypothetical diagram of this phenomenon.

Krogman (1979) presented a causal model related to structure and function (Fig. 1.21). The structure category has to do with the interrelated *forms* of the "cranial-facial-palatal complex," while the function category has to do with the *manner* in which the parts behave as they interact with each other.

ETIOLOGY

Understanding the etiology of cleft lip and palate is complicated and difficult, particularly in specific cases. Certainly, there are serious techno-

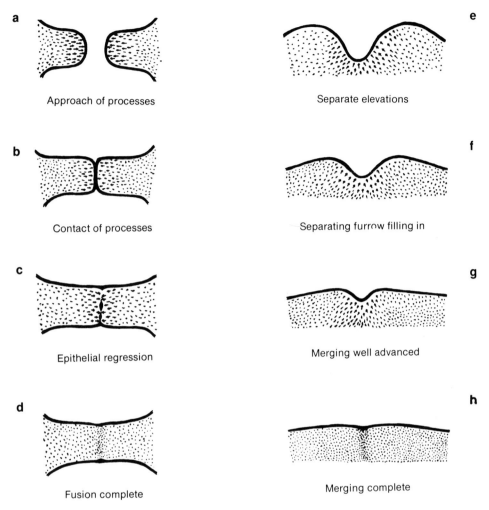

a Approach of processes

b Contact of processes

c Epithelial regression

d Fusion complete

e Separate elevations

f Separating furrow filling in

g Merging well advanced

h Merging complete

Figure 1.19 Diagrams contrasting the process of fusion as it occurs, for example, in the palatal shelves, with the process of merging as it occurs in the formation of the mandibular arch or in the frontal region of the embryonic head. The short arrows suggest the directions in which mesenchymal cell movements are most marked. (A) Approach of processes; (B) Contact of processes; (C) Epithelial regression; (D) Fusion complete; (E) Separate elevations; (F) Separating furrow filling in; (G) Merging well advanced; (H) Merging complete. (From Patten BM. Normal development of the facial region. In: Pruzansky S, ed. Congenital anomalies of the face and associated structures. Springfield, IL: CC Thomas, 1961:35.)

logical limitations to the methods available for studying this issue. There are great variations in the "normal" developmental processes and serious ethical considerations in the study of human reproduction.

Our purpose is to provide speech pathologists with a background that will enable them to be helpful to patients and families, recognizing that expert counseling about etiology should always be made available and that many family histories demand direct referral for such counseling even when the families themselves do not make the request.

Most clinicians are in agreement that genetic background plays a significant role in these malformations. Most also agree that various environmental factors influence cleft formation, despite a lack of evidence that clearly relates animal and human pathogenesis (Niebyl et al., 1985).

There seems also to be consensus that cleft lip with or without cleft palate is etiologically and

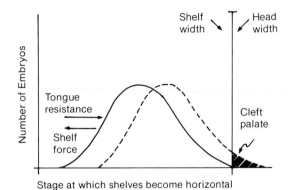

Figure 1.20 Hypothetical diagram illustrating some of the factors involved in palate closure. If the developmental stage at which the palatal shelves become horizontal is delayed sufficiently, the shelves will be too far apart to meet, and a cleft palate will result. (From Fraser FC. Etiology of cleft palate. In: Grabb WC, Rosenstein SW, Bzoch KR. Cleft lip and palate: surgical, dental, and speech aspects. Boston: Little, Brown, 1971.)

Inadequacy of
Palatal Processes:
Time and Size Factors
(too late or too
small)

Tongue Position:
Spatial, Timing ⟶ STRUCTURAL ⟵ Cranial Factors:
Shape, Growth

CLEFT
PALATE
and
CLEFT
LIP

Secondary Rupture: ⟶ FUNCTIONAL ⟵ Failure of
"Epithelial Pearls" Epithelial De-
(connecting bands of generation:
tissue in the line of Inclusion Cysts.
the cleft) Mesoderm Growth
Failure

Inadequacy of
"Shelf Force":
Innate Medialward
Movement Inhibited

Figure 1.21 A schematic representation of possible factors in the development of clefts. (From Krogman WM. Craniofacial growth: prenatal and postnatal. In: Cooper HK, Harding RL, Krogman WM, Mazaheri M. Millard RT, eds. Cleft palate and cleft lip: a team approach to clinical management and rehabilitation of the patient. Philadelphia: WB Saunders, 1979: 32.)

genetically different from isolated cleft palate. Most of the reliable developmental data available are about cleft lip, with or without cleft palate. Less is known about isolated cleft palate save that individuals with that condition have a higher

incidence of additional congenital malformations than has the group with clefts of the lip with or without cleft palate.

Genetic Factors

As indicated above, there is general agreement that genetic factors are of primary importance in the etiology of clefts. However, Fraser (1971) wrote that the evidence has been obscured by failure to distinguish among cleft types in such investigations and by falsely assuming that a positive family history is indicative of genetic variations, whereas a negative history is not. A cleft may be genetic in nature, even if there is no evidence that the defect has ever been expressed before in the family lines of the patient.

We have a relatively good, if far from complete, understanding of the developmental disruptions that result in clefts. We are less secure in our ability to determine *why* the disruptions occur and what can be done to prevent them. However, a considerable amount of information, much of it derived from animal studies, is available and leads to formulation of hypotheses about the causes of clefts and related disorders. These hypotheses can be tested in a variety of ways, but it remains difficult, however, to apply knowledge of this type to the individual family.

As indicated by Fraser (1970), genetic studies in human subjects are difficult for a variety of reasons, not the least of which is the nature and mobility of people. It may be impossible to construct an accurate family history that includes several generations. In spite of these obvious obstacles to understanding the genetics of clefting, especially in individual cases, it is important that we refrain from assuring parents that their child's cleft is "not hereditary." It is very probable that genetic factors played a significant role.

Fraser (1971) divided the genetic factors underlying clefts into two major categories: mutant genes and chromosomal aberrations. Mutant genes are responsible for some clefts that are associated with certain rare syndromes. Taken together, these syndromes account for a small percentage of all clefts. However, every major treatment center regularly sees patients with these complex problems. These syndromes may be autosomal dominant or autosomal recessive. If they are dominant, only one parent must carry the trait in order for it to be expressed in offspring in one out of two births. Examples of syndromes with an autosominal dominant mode of inheritance are ectodermal dysplasia, Waardenburg syndrome, craniofacial dysostosis, lip-pit syndrome. Some of these will be considered in detail in Chapter 2.

In a syndrome that is recessive, both parents must carry the trait or it will not be expressed in their offspring. This illustrates one of the complexities of genetic patterns in humans. A parent may carry a recessive trait and never know it unless that same trait is also present in the other parent. Both could be at increased risk for producing cleft offspring with syndromes, and both could have negative family histories. For detailed discussion of the approximately 154 syndromes that may be associated with clefting, see Rubin (1967), Gorlin et al. (1971), Gorlin et al. (1976), Cohen (1978), and Jones (1988), among others. An additional valuable source for students is the slide-audio-tape collection demonstrating the physical aspects of a number of syndromes prepared by Gellis and Feingold (1976).

Chromosomal aberrations are occasionally involved in clefts that are associated with other even more major congenital malformations. Each somatic cell contains 23 pairs of chromosomes, making a total of 46. Abnormalities in these chromosomes produce a variety of different anomalies. The best known of the autosomal defects is trisomy 21 or Down syndrome, which includes oral-facial variations but rarely cleft palate (0.5%). Down syndrome is often associated with an extra #21 chromosome (trisomy meaning three instead of the usual two). Some patients with Down syndrome have a translocation, meaning that a fragment of one chromosome is shifted to another. Others are mosaics, meaning that 10 to 50% of the cells have 46 chromosomes, and the rest have 47. This variation is transmittable from parent to child when one parent is a carrier. Maternal age is a factor in Down syndrome, ranging from one in 2000 births at age 25 to one in 40 at age 45. When one such child has been born, the risk is two to three times greater in subsequent pregnancies (Rubin, 1967).

Trisomy 13 usually involves a nondisjunction in chromosome 13. Nondisjunction is the failure of two homologous chromosomes or chromatids to pass to separate cells, with the result that one "daughter" cell has two chromosomes or chromatids and the other has none. Cleft lip with or without cleft palate occurs in 60 to 70% of the cases of trisomy 13, and micrognathia in over 80 percent (Gorlin et al., 1976). This is a rare condition occurring only once in 6000 births, and no risk data are available. Chromosomal disorders are usually marked by multiple, major congenital abnormalities. Some are so rare that risk figures cannot be projected.

Environmental Teratogens

Environmental teratogens are agents that act upon the developing child to create malformations. Fraser (1971) discussed these under the general heading of genetics because he believed that these teratogens interact with susceptible genotypes. This is a reasonable assumption when it is remembered that only a fraction of women who are exposed to various medications or other teratogens do, in fact, produce malformed offspring.

A variety of teratogens have been identified as causing clefting and other malformations in laboratory animals (Wilson and Fraser, 1977). Infections, diseases, irradiation, environmental chemicals, maternal metabolic and endocrine imbalances, drugs, and nutritional deficiencies and excesses have all been implicated. However, not much is known about the effects of these teratogens in the human. Fraser (1971) listed only two, the rubella virus and thalidomide. Both of these are known to cause severe malformations, but they account for only a small proportion of clefts. Warkany (1971) also concluded that few cases of clefting are clearly attributable to exogenous causes. However, there is increasing suspicion that certain drugs and environmental pollutants may be important hazards during pregnancy, and considerable research about these issues is now underway. An example is a report by Safra and Oakley (1976) concerning the possible teratogenic effects of valium taken by women very early in pregnancy. Dilantin is another of the drugs thought to be responsible for clefts in the offspring of susceptible women.

In light of this information, many physicians, as a general philosophy, advise pregnant women to avoid drugs, environmental chemicals, x-ray, alcohol, or other possible toxic agents as far as possible. Excessive use of even aspirin and caffeine are possible sources of danger. Diet and nutrition during pregnancy are likely to be important factors, but definitive information about them is not yet available. Certainly, the pregnant woman should avoid exposure to rubella and other childhood diseases and should consult her physician immediately if she suspects that such exposure has occurred.

Multifactorial Inheritance

Fraser (l963, 1970, 1971, 1977) believed that the great majority of clefts are caused by multifactorial inheritance; Carter (1970) has also reviewed this topic. This etiological theory is the most widely accepted explanation that has been proposed to date, although it is not universally accepted. Bixler (1981) interpreted the available data to mean that cleft lip with or without cleft palate and cleft palate are both etiologically heterogeneous and that, therefore, it is improbable that any single etiological model will ever be fully satisfactory.

The theory of multifactorial inheritance suggests that there are many genes that contribute to clefting. Individually they are of minor importance, but their joint interaction with negative environmental factors may mean that a given embryo will reach the threshold of abnormality described earlier.

Counseling About Etiology

All members of cleft palate teams and all speech pathologists, whether they are members of teams or not, should have basic information about the knowns and unknowns about the etiology of clefts, and should be prepared to provide simple information to patients and their families, keeping in mind that genetic counseling should be provided by specially trained counselors. (See Broder and Trier, 1985, for an informative report about the effectiveness of such counseling.)

Speech pathologists should appreciate the risk factors that may be involved for people with family histories of clefting. Fraser (1971) presented two tables that are helpful in this regard (Tables 1.1 and 1.2). While there is always a much higher chance that normal rather than cleft offspring will be produced in families with histories of clefting, parents and patients are entitled to know what the

TABLE 1.1 Frequency of Cleft Lip With or Without Cleft Palate (CLP) in Relatives of Persons with CLP, and of Cleft Palate (CP) in Relatives of Persons with CP

Frequency	Proband Has CLP		Proband Has CP	
	%	Total	%	Total
Siblings	4.1	2972	2.9	1078
Children	3.4	325	6.8	146
Uncles & aunts	0.6	9437	0.4	3294
Nephews & nieces	1.0	1058	0.0	248
First cousins	0.4	13,656	0.2	6563

From Fraser FC. Etiology of cleft lip and palate. In: Grabb WC, Rosenstein SW, Bzoch KR, eds. Cleft lip and palate; surgical, dental, and speech aspects. Boston: Little, Brown, 1971:61.

risks are, understanding that the unknown aspects of etiology prevent precise predictions in individual cases.

Speech pathologists must never overstep the bounds of their very limited training and experience in genetics. They can serve a vital need by helping families find a genetic counselor. These counselors can usually be found in teaching hospitals that treat children or specialize in obstetrics. State Departments of Health can also provide information about the availability of genetic counseling.

Clinics must not only make genetic counseling available but, for the protection of the clinic, should keep dated and signed clinical notes to show: that the matter has been approached, the nature of the information provided, recommendations made, and the response of the parents.

Our position is that the parents and the patient ought to have every opportunity to explore the etiology of the cleft and to be as well informed as possible about the likelihood of future clefts or other malformations in the family. Some parents and some patients seem to be content with general information and will decide against seeking more specific direction if there appears to be no special reason for doing so. Others are motivated to learn as much as possible about the etiology. All, however, should understand that such help is available. The decision about whether or not to have children must be made by the parents or patient as they consider

TABLE 1.2   Risks for Cleft Lip, With or Without Cleft Palate (CL±CP), and Cleft Palate (CP).

Situation	Proband Has CL±CP	Proband Has CP
Frequency of defect in the general population	0.1%	0.04%
My spouse and I are unaffected.		
We have an affected child		
What is the probability that our next baby will have the same condition if:		
We have no affected relatives?	4%	2%
There is an affected relative?	4%	7%
Our affected child also has another malformation?	2%	2%
My spouse and I are related?	4%	—
What is the probability that our next baby will have some other sort of malformation?	Same as general population	
We have two affected children.		
What is the probability that our next baby will have the same condition?	9%	1%
I am affected (or my spouse is).		
We have no affected children.		
What is the probability that our next baby will be affected?	4%	6%
We have an affected child.		
What is the probability that our next baby will be affected?	17%	1⁵%

From Fraser FC. Etiology of cleft lip and palate. In: Grabb WC. Rosenstein SW, Bzoch KR, eds. Cleft lip and palate: surgical, dental, and speech aspects. Boston: Little, Brown, 1971:63.

risk, their own feelings, and other issues peculiar to them.

Summary

The congenital malformation of cleft lip and palate is not caused by a single factor or a simple system of maldevelopment. Genetic factors are basic and must always be considered, particularly in questions of family planning. Embryological environmental factors are probably important, but their identity in the human is not yet clear. A multifactorial model, including the impact of both genetic and environmental factors, appears to be appropriate. Whatever the causes, they must have impact early in pregnancy, since the palatal structures are completed by 9 to 12 weeks of fetal life. Parents of the affected child or adults with clefts may find the lack of clarity about etiology confusing and unsatisfactory, but more definitive information is usually not available unless specific syndromes encompassing several malformations are present. The speech pathologist who works with patients with clefts must be prepared to participate with other members of the specialty team in general counseling about etiology, but all need to be alert to the need for professional genetic counseling and for making all patients aware that such referral sources are available.

REFERENCES

Avery JK. Prenatal facial growth. In: Moyers RE, ed. Handbook of orthodontics. 3rd ed. Chicago: Year Book, 1973:27.

Bardanouve VT. Cleft palate in Montana: a 10-year report. Cleft Palate J 1969;6:213.

Berlin AJ. Classification of cleft lip and palate. In: Grabb WC, Rosenstein SW, Bzoch KR, eds. Cleft lip and palate: surgical, dental, and speech aspects. Boston: Little, Brown, 1971:66.

Bixler D. Genetics and clefting. Cleft Palate J 1981;18:10.

Blackfield HM, Miller ER, Owsley JQ, Lawson LI. Cine-fluorographic evaluation of patients with velopharyngeal dysfunction in the absence of overt cleft palate. Plast Reconstr Surg 1962;30:441.

Briggs RM. Vitamin supplementation as a possible factor in the incidence of cleft lip/palate deformities in humans. Clin Plast Surg 1976;3:647.

Broder H, Trier WC. Effectiveness of genetic counseling for families with craniofacial anomalies. Cleft Palate J 1985;22:157.

Burdi AR. Distribution of midpalatine cysts: a reevaluation of human palatal closure mechanisms. J Oral Surg 1968;26:41.

Burdi AR, Silvey RG. Sexual differences in closure of the human palatal shelves. Cleft Palate J 1969;6:1.

Calnan JS. Submucous cleft palate. Br J Plast Surg 1954;6:264.

Calnan JS. Diagnosis, prognosis, and treatment of "palato-pharyngeal incompetence" with special reference to radiographic investigations. Br J Plast Surg 1956;8:265.

Calnan JS. Congenital large pharynx: a new syndrome with a report on 41 personal cases. Br J Plast Surg 1971a;24:263.

Calnan JS. Permanent nasal escape in speech after adenoidectomy. Br J Plast Surg 1971b;24:197.

Carter CO. Multifactorial inheritance revisited. In: Fraser FC, McKusick VA, eds. Congenital malformations. Amsterdam: Excerpta Medica, 1970:227.

Chaco J, Yules RB. Velopharyngeal incompetence post tonsillo-adenoidectomy. Acta Otolaryngol 1969; 68:276.

Chavez GF, Cordero JF, Bećerra JE. Leading major congenital malformations among minority groups in the United States, 1981–1986. J Am Med Assoc 1989;261:205.

Chosak A, Eidelman E. Cleft uvula: prevalence and genetics. Cleft Palate J 1978;15:63.

Cohen MM Jr. Syndromes with cleft lip and cleft palate. Cleft Palate J 1978;15:306.

Cohn ER, McWilliams BJ, Knapp DM, Garrett WS. The team approach to cleft care in the Commonwealth of Pennsylvania. J Pennsylvania Speech-Language-Hearing, Vol XVI, Sept 1983. J Pennsylvania Dental Association, May 1984.

Cotton R, Nuwayhid NS. Velopharyngeal insufficiency. In: Bluestone CD, Stool SE, eds. Pediatric otolaryngology. Vol. 2. Philadelphia: WB Saunders, 1983:1521.

Croft CB, Shprintzen RJ, Daniller A, Lewin ML. The occult submucous cleft palate and the musculus uvulae. Cleft Palate J 1978;15:150.

Czeizel A. Re "Incidence and prevalence as measures of the frequency of birth defects." Am J Epidemiol 1984; 119:141.

Fara M, Weatherley-White RCA. Cleft palate: submucous cleft palate. In: Converse JM, ed. Reconstructive plastic surgery: principles and procedures in correction, reconstruction and transplantation. Vol 4. 2nd ed. Philadelphia: WB Saunders, 1977;2104.

Fogh-Andersen P, ed. Inheritance of harelip and cleft palate: contribution to the elucidation of the etiology of the congenital clefts of the face. Copenhagen: Nyt Nordisk Forlag Arnold Busck, 1942.

Fogh-Andersen P. Incidence of cleft lip and palate: constant or increasing? Acta Chir Scand 1961;122:106.

Fraser FC. Hereditary disorders of the nose and mouth. In: Human genetics: Proc 2nd Internal Cong Human Genet. Vol 3. Instituto G Mendel, Rome, 1963:1852.

Fraser FC. The genetics of cleft lip and cleft palate. Am J Hum Genet 1970;22:336.

Fraser FC. Etiology of cleft lip and palate. In: Grabb WC, Rosenstein SW, Bzoch KR, eds. Cleft lip and palate: surgical, dental, and speech aspects. Boston: Little, Brown, 1971:54.

Fraser FC. Interactions and multiple causes. In: Wilson JC, Fraser FC, eds. Handbook of teratology: general principles and etiology. Vol 1. New York: Plenum Press, 1977:445.

Fulton JT. Closure of the human palate in embryo. Am J Obstet Gynecol 1957;74:179.

Geis N, Seto B, Bartoshesky L, Lewis MB, Pashayan HM. The prevalence of congenital heart disease among the population of a metropolitan cleft lip and palate clinic. Cleft Palate J 1981;18:19.

Gellis SS, Feingold M. Syndromes in pediatrics. (a slide and audio tape.) New York: Medcome, 1976.

Gibb AG. Hypernasality (rhinolalia aperta) following tonsil and adenoid removal. J Laryngol Otol 1958;72:433.

Goodman RM, Gorlin RJ, eds. The malformed infant and child: an illustrated guide. New York: Oxford University Press, 1983.

Gorlin RJ, Cervenka J, Pruzansky S. Facial clefting and its syndromes. In: Bergsma D, ed. 3rd Conference on the Clinical Delineation of Birth Defects: Part XI Orofacial Structure. Birth Defects: Original Article Series 1971;1:3.

Gorlin RJ, Pindborg JJ, Cohen MM. Syndromes of the head and neck. New York: McGraw-Hill, 1976.

Greene JC, Vermillion JR, Hay S, Gibbens SF, Kerschbaum S. Epidemiologic study of cleft lip and cleft palate in four states. J Am Dent Assoc 1964;68:387.

Gylling U, Soivio AI. Submucous cleft palates: surgical treatment and results. Acta Chir Scand 1965;129:282.

Hanson JW, Murray JC. Genetic aspects of cleft lip and palate. In: Bardach J, Morris HL, eds. Multidisciplinary management of cleft lip and palate. Philadelphia: WB Saunders, in press.

Harkins CS, Berlin A, Harding RL, Longacre JJ, Snodgrasse RM. A classification of cleft lip and palate. Plast Reconstr Surg 1962;29:31.

Honda M. A clinical study on cleft lip and/or palate, 1978; statistical observations. J Jap Cleft Palate Assoc 1978;3:50.

Hook EB. "Incidence" and "prevalence" as measures of the frequency of congenital malformations and genetic outcomes: application to oral clefts. Cleft Palate J 1988;25:97.

Ivy RH. Congenital anomalies as recorded on birth certificates in the Division of Vital Statistics of the Pennsylvania Department of Health, for the period 1951-1955, inclusive. Plast Reconstr Surg 1957;20:400.

Jackson IT, McGlynn MJ, Huskie CF. Velopharyngeal incompetence in the absence of cleft palate: results of treatment in 20 cases. Plast Reconstr Surg 1980;66:211.

Jensen BL, Kreiborg S, Dahl E, Fogh-Andersen P. Cleft lip and palate in Denmark, 1976-1981: epidemiology, variability, and early somatic development. Cleft Palate J 1988;25:258.

Johnston MC. The neural crest in abnormalities of the face and brain. In: Bergsma D, ed. Morphogenesis and malformation of face and brain. Birth Defects: Original Article Series II. 1975;7:1.

Johnston MC, Sulik KK. Embryology of the head and neck. In: Serafin D, Georgiade NG, eds. Pediatric plastic surgery. St. Louis: CV Mosby, 1984:184.

Jones KL. Smith's recognizable patterns of human malformation. 4th ed. Philadelphia: WB Saunders, 1988.

Jones MC. Etiology of facial clefts: prospective evaluation of 428 patients. Cleft Palate J 1988;25:16.

Jung JH. Genetic syndromes in communication disorders. Boston: Little, Brown, 1989.

Kaplan EN. The occult submucous cleft palate. Cleft Palate J 1975;12:356.

Kernahan DA, Stark RB. A new classification for cleft lip and cleft palate. Plast Reconstr Surg 1958;22:435.

Kraus BS, Kitamura H, Latham RA, eds. An atlas of developmental anatomy of the face. New York: Harper and Row, 1966.

Kriens O. Documentation of cleft lip, alveolus, and palate. In: Bardach J, Morris H, eds. Multidisciplinary management of cleft lip and palate. Philadelphia: WB Saunders, in press.

Krogman WM. Craniofacial growth and development: an appraisal. J Am Dent Assoc 1973;87:1037.

Krogman WM. Craniofacial growth: prenatal and postnatal. In: Cooper HK, Harding RL, Krogman WM, Mazaheri M, Millard RT, eds. Cleft palate and cleft lip: a team approach to clinical management and rehabilitation of the patient. Philadelphia: WB Saunders, 1979:23.

Leck I. Correlations of malformation frequency with environmental and genetic attributes in man. In: Wilson JG, Fraser FC, eds. Handbook of teratology: comparative, maternal, and epidemiologic aspects. Vol 3. New York: Plenum Press, 1977:243.

Lubit EC. Before an adenoidectomy. Stop! look!, and listen! N Y State J Med 1967;67:681.

Mason RM. Preventing speech disorders following adenoidectomy by preoperative examination. Clin Pediatr 1973;12:405.

McWilliams BJ. Personal communication.

McWilliams BJ, Matthews HP. A comparison of intelligence and social maturity in children with unilateral complete clefts and those with isolated cleft palates. Cleft Palate J 1979;16:363.

Meskin LH, Gorlin RJ, Isaacson RJ. Abnormal morphology of the soft palate. II. The genetics of cleft uvula. Cleft Palate J 1965;2:40.

Meskin LH, Pruzansky S. Validity of the birth certificate in the epidemiological assessment of facial clefts. J Dent Res 1967;46:1456.

Millard DR. Cleft craft: the evaluation of its surgery. The unilateral deformity. Boston: Little, Brown, Vol 1, 1976.

Morris HL, Miller-Wroblewski SK, Brown CK, Van Demark DR. Velarpharyngeal status in cleft patients with expected adenoidal involution. Ann Otol Rhinol Laryngol, in press.

Morris HL, Krueger LJ, Bumsted RM. Indications of congenital palatal incompetence before diagnosis. Ann Otol Rhinol Laryngol 1982;91:115.

Myrianthopoulos NC, Chung CS. Congenital malformations in singletons: epidemiologic survey. In: Bergsma D, ed. Congenital malformations in singletons: epidemiologic survey. Birth Defects Original Article Series 1974;10:1.

Niebyl JR, Blake DA, Rocco LE, Baumgardner R, Mellits ED. Lack of maternal, metabolic, endocrine, and environmental influences in the etiology of cleft lip with or without cleft palate. Cleft Palate J 1985;22:20.

Nishimura H, Sembe R, Tanimura T, Tanaka O. Prenatal development of the human with special reference to craniofacial structures: an atlas. DHEW Publication No. (NIH) 77-946. Bethesda: Public Health Service, 1977.

Oka SW. Epidemiology and genetics of clefting: with implications for etiology. In: Cooper HK, Harding RL, Krogman WM, Mazaheri M, Millard RT, eds. Cleft palate and cleft lip: a team approach to clinical management and rehabilitation of the patient. Philadelphia: WB Saunders, 1979;108.

Olin WH. Cleft lip and palate rehabilitation. Springfield: CC Thomas, 1960.

Pannbacker M. Congenital malformations and cleft lip and palate. Cleft Palate J 1968;5:334.

Pashayan HM. What else to look for in a child born with a cleft of the lip and/or palate. Cleft Palate J 1983;20:54.

Patten BM. The normal development of the facial region. In: Pruzansky S, ed. Congenital anomalies of the face and associated structures. Springfield: CC Thomas, 1961:41.

Patten BM. Embryology of the palate and the maxillofacial region. In: Grabb WC, Rosenstein SW, Bzoch KR, eds. Cleft lip and palate: surgical, dental, and speech aspects. Boston: Little, Brown, 1971:21.

Randall P, Bakes FP, Kennedy C. Cleft palate-type speech in the absence of cleft palate. Plast Reconstr Surg 1960;25:484.

Rintala A, Stegars T. Increasing incidence of clefts in Finland: reliability of hospital records and central register of congenital malformations. Scand J Plastic Reconstr Surg 1982;16:35.

Rogers BO. Embryology of the face and introduction to craniofacial anomalies. In: Converse JM, ed. Reconstructive plastic surgery: principles and procedures in correction, reconstruction and transplantation. Vol 4. 2nd ed. Philadelphia: WB Saunders, 1977:2296.

Ross RB, Johnston MC, eds. Cleft lip and palate. Baltimore: Williams & Wilkins, 1972.

Rubin A, ed. Handbook of congenital malformations. Philadelphia: WB Saunders, 1967.

Safra MJ, Oakley GP. Valium: an oral cleft teratogen? Cleft Palate J 1976;13:198.

Shprintzen RJ, Siegel-Sadewitz VL, Amato J, Goldberg RB. Anomalies associated with cleft lip, cleft palate, or both. Am J Med Genet 1985;20:585.

Siegel-Sadewitz VL, Sphrintzen RJ. Changes in velopharyngeal valving with age. Intern J Pediatr Otorhinolaryngol 1986;11:171.

Spriestersbach DC, Spriestersbach BR, Moll KL. Incidence of clefts of the lip and palate in families with children with clefts and families with children without clefts. Plast Reconstr Surg 1962;29:392.

Stark RB. Embryology, pathogenesis and classification of cleft lip and cleft palate. In: Pruzansky S, ed. Congenital anomalies of the face and associated structures. Springfield: CC Thomas, 1961:66.

Stark RB. Embryology of cleft palate: In: Converse JM, ed. Plastic and reconstructive surgery: principles and procedures in connection, reconstruction, and transplantation. Vol 4. 2nd ed. Philadelphia: WB Saunders, 1977:1941.

Stevenson AC, Johnston HA, Stewart MI, Golding DR. Congenital malformations: a report of a study of series of consecutive births in 24 centres. Bull WHO 1966;34(Suppl 9):9.

Stool SE, Mundell RD. Phylogenetic aspects and embryology. In: Bluestone CD, Stool SE, eds. Pediatric otolaryngology. Vol 1. Philadelphia: WB Saunders, 1983:3.

Subtelny JD, Koepp-Baker H. The significance of adenoid tissue in velopharyngeal function. Plast Reconstr Surg 1956;17:235.

Töndury G. On the mechanism of cleft formation. In: Pruzansky S, ed. Congenital anomalies of the face and associated structures. Springfield: CC Thomas, 1961:85.

Tretsven VE. Incidence of cleft lip, and palate in Montana Indians. J Speech Hear Dis 1963;28:52.

Vanderas AP. Incidence of cleft lip, cleft palate, and cleft lip and palate among races: a review. Cleft Palate J 1987; 24:216.

Veau V. Division palatine. Paris: Masson, 1931.

Velasco MG, Yzunza A, Hernandez X, Manquez C. Diagnosis and treatment of submucous cleft palate: a review of 108 cases. Cleft Palate J 1988;25:171.

Warkany J. Congenital malformations; notes and comments. Chicago: Year Book, 1971.

Weatherley-White RCA, Sakura CY Jr, Brenner LD, Stewart JM, Ott JE. Submucous cleft palate: its incidence, natural history and indications for treatment. Plast Reconstr Surg 1972;49:297.

Whitaker LA, Pashayan HA, Reichman J. A proposed new classification of craniofacial anomalies. Cleft Palate J 1981;18:161.

Wilson JC, Fraser FC, eds. Handbook of teratology. General principles and etiology. Vol 1. New York: Plenum Press, 1977.

Woolf CM, Woolf RM, Broadbent TR. Lateral incisor anomalies: microforms of cleft lip and palate? Plast Reconstr Surg 1965;35:543.

2 | PATTERNS OF MALFORMATION ASSOCIATED WITH CLEFTING

Some children may have clefts that are associated with other malformations that can be classified as syndromes or placed in other categories that can have major implications for diagnosis, treatment, genetic counseling, outcome, and life expectancy. This chapter emphasizes a few of the conditions that are associated with clefts and that affect other craniofacial structures as well. The reader is reminded, however, that there are literally hundreds of syndromes that are associated with communication disorders of various types. Since diagnosing and treating patients with these conditions offer expanding opportunities to speech-language pathologists (Peterson, 1973; Elfenbein et al., 1981; Sparks and Millard, 1981; Peterson-Falzone, 1982; Siegel-Sadewitz and Shprintzen, 1982; McWilliams, 1983; Witzel, 1983; Sparks, 1984; Schaefer and Sullivan, 1986; Jung, 1988; Peterson-Falzone, 1988); this material serves as an introduction for interested students.

TERMINOLOGY

A *syndrome* can be defined as a group of symptoms regularly occurring together and appearing to be causally related. Jones (1988) refers to these as "multiple localized defects." When those symptoms involve the craniofacial complex, the features commonly shared by affected individuals result in their close resemblance to each other even though there is no family relationship. In the three editions of their book, Smith (1976, 1982)

and Jones (1988) note the predictability of characteristics found in syndromes in the title *Recognizable Patterns of Human Malformation*. Sometimes an unusual group of symptoms, never previously reported, is found in one individual and is designated as a "provisionally unique" syndrome, pending reports of other similar cases.

Association is a term applied when two or more abnormalities occur together more often than would be expected by chance, but without yet having been designated as a syndrome. *Sequence* refers to conditions involving characteristics that occur together, one of which is basic to the others. Jones (1988) describes this as "a single localized anomaly plus its subsequently derived structural consequences."

Craniofacial has reference to malformations that affect the head at or above the upper eyelid (cranio-) and those affecting structures at or below the lower eyelid (facial) (Tessier, 1976; Whitaker et al., 1981). Thus strictly defined, craniofacial malformations affect both the cranium and the face. However, because of overlapping treatment needs, patients with disorders involving only the cranium or only the face and oral cavities are now often described as having craniofacial malformations.

OCCURRENCE

While there are many different syndromes involving the craniofacial complex, they occur relatively infrequently, although occurrence rates

31

differ from one syndrome to another. The frequency of clefting in relevant syndromes may range from very rare to frequent or usual.

Cohen (1978) listed 154 syndromes associated with clefting. Smith (1982) pointed to 17 conditions frequently associated with cleft lip with or without cleft palate and to 18 others with occasional occurrence. In the 1988 edition (Jones, 1988), those numbers were increased to 19 and 28 respectively. Cleft palate or bifid uvula was reported to occur frequently in 13 conditions and occasionally in 25 (Smith, 1982). In the most recent edition (Jones, 1988), those figures have risen to 22 and 47 respectively.

Gorlin et al. (1976) provide an extensive discussion of clefting and of some of the associated abnormalities, including syndromes, in their classic book, currently undergoing revision. Reference to Chapter 10 will remind readers that associated malformations are common in children with clefts, especially in isolated palatal clefts and in those with velopharyngeal incompetence in the absence of overt clefts. Thus, it is mandatory that all children with these problems be carefully assessed. Many will be found to have syndromes.

ETIOLOGY

There are several ways of thinking about the etiology of these complex birth defects. Jones (1988) describes the types of malformations found in morphogenesis in terms of poor tissue formation, which may result in multiple localized defects, classified as malformation syndromes or associations. Such malformations are thought to spring from a single cause, which may be a chromosomal abnormality, a mutant gene disorder, or an environmental teratogen (Jones, 1988). In contrast, other defects, such as cleft lip and cleft palate without other congenital anomalies are thought to have a polygenic-multifactorial etiological basis, which means that they are brought about by the interaction of several genes with environmental factors as described in Chapter 1.

The malformation may be a single localized defect, or the single localized defect may be responsible for other structural consequences, in which case there would be a malformation sequence.

A deformation or a deformation sequence is related to some mechanical force that alters the morphogenesis of an otherwise normal embryo or fetus, whereas a disruption or disruption sequence occurs when a normal embryo or fetus is subjected to some destructive event such as vascular problems or infections.

It is clear that malformations have different root causes from either deformations or disruptions. Since malformation syndromes may be caused by chromosomal or genetic factors, they can often be found in other family members and may be associated with an increased recurrence risk for the parents and for the affected individual. Thus, genetic counseling in these cases is based upon the syndrome rather than upon the cleft.

Chromosomal Abnormalities

It is estimated that 0.5% of all live births have some type of chromosomal variation (Jung, 1988). Cohen (1978) lists 29 chromosomal syndromes that have clefting as one of their features. Normal human cells contain 23 pairs of chromosomes, a normal *karotype*, one of each pair coming from the mother and one from the father. In some cases, there may be extra chromosomes, as in Down syndrome, or trisomy 21. Individuals with Down syndrome have 47 chromosomes, the extra chromosome being number 21. Thus, the designation *trisomy* to indicate three instead of two number 21 chromosomes.

Other possible variations include changes in the structure of chromosomes from such things as breakage. *Translocations* or the movement of chromosomal material from one place to another may occur as may *deletions* or *duplications* of chromosomal parts.

The recurrence risk varies widely for chromosomal abnormalities. For many, the risk is less that 1% if both parents have normal chromosomes. If a phenotypically normal parent is a carrier for a balanced translocation, the risk that offspring will have an unbalanced rearrangement varies, but is usually 5 to 10%. In some instances, however, the risk may be significantly higher. Obviously, genetic counseling is required when chromosomal abnormalities are present.

Gene Abnormalities

Each chromosome in each pair will have gene determinants similarly located to those of its mate or allele. The exceptions to this are the X and Y chromosomes which determine sex. Any chromosome other than the sex chromosomes are called autosomes, and they carry autosomal-linked genes. If a defective gene is contributed by one parent but not by the other, it may or may not be expressed in the offspring. If it is autosomal dominant, the contribution from one parent will reproduce the defect, so there is a 50% risk of having an affected child. When there is clearly no previous family history of the defect, the first child may have been a sporadic event, and the risk for future children may be significantly reduced even though the affected child will have a 50% chance of reproducing the syndrome. Cohen (1978) identifies 35 cleft-associated syndromes that are autosomal dominant.

If the defective gene is autosomal recessive, it will not be expressed unless both parents carry the altered gene, in which case there is a 25% chance of expression with each pregnancy. The altered gene may, however, be passed on to make carriers of 50% of their offspring, who are not at increased risk for bearing children with the defect unless their partners also carry the defective gene. Cohen (1978) includes 39 autosomal-recessive syndromes that have clefting as a possible feature.

It is important to know that it is not always possible to determine recurrence risks for syndromes with or without clefts. A number remain obscure as to their genesis.

This brief coverage is intended only to prepare students to read about the specific syndromes that are discussed in the pages that follow, not in any way to substitute for courses in genetics or for reading in depth on this topic.

ASSOCIATED PROBLEMS

Communication Problems

Communication problems resulting from a variety of causes and combinations of causes occur in most, but not all, patients with craniofacial abnormalities. Reviews of these problems have been provided by Siegel-Sadewitz and Shprintzen, 1982; McWilliams, 1983; Witzel, 1983; Sparks, 1984; Schaefer and Sullivan, 1986; Jung, 1988; Peterson-Falzone, 1988. A general overview is presented below prior to discussion of several representative syndromes.

Speech patterns have not been exhaustively investigated in large numbers of patients with various diagnoses; but information that is available is reasonably consistent. It has been known for a long time that major deformities of the orofacial structures are often associated with articulation disorders that are functionally related to the structural deficits (Bloomer, 1971, 1973). All of the reports referred to in the previous paragraph and our own clinical observations indicate considerable variation in speech production among these patients, depending upon the severity of their structural anomalies as well as upon psychosocial, neurological, and sensory integrity.

Generally, these individuals show orally distorted consonants related to malocclusions and to other associated abnormalities. Articulation may be further compromised by phonological deficits, learning disabilities, mental retardation, hearing impairments, or some combination of these. Hypernasality or various forms of audible nasal escape resulting from velopharyngeal incompetence with or without palatal clefts may also be present, or hyponasality may result from reduced pharyngeal depth or increased nasal resistance from other causes.

Language disorders in children with craniofacial syndromes have not been systematically studied. However, it is clear that such problems occur with greater frequency than in a normal population. They are alluded to in various publications about specific syndromes (Elfenbein et al., 1981; McWilliams, 1983; Sparks, 1984; Jones, 1988; Jung, 1988), and an increasing number of articles describing language behavior in specified syndromes are appearing. Mental retardation, learning disabilities, and hearing loss may complicate our understanding of language disorders in this population.

Hearing impairments are found frequently in both children and adults (Selder, 1973). Stool and Houlihan (1977) stated that any child with marked facial deformity is assumed to have a hearing loss until it is determined otherwise. While these losses are often conductive in nature, sensorineural losses secondary to deformities of the inner ear must also be ruled out. Bergstrom (1978) placed the incidence of hearing loss in this group of patients, including those with clefts, at 88%.

Crysdale (1981) pointed out that congenital conductive hearing loss is an intrinsic component of many craniofacial syndromes. Some of these losses are related to microtia, whereas others represent what he calls "invisible" deformities that result in a delay in identification. Some of these hidden anomalies are ossicular deformities, stapedial fixation, or tympanic membranes that are small and oblique with abnormal landmarks.

Identifying hearing losses is highly relevant in treatment planning because they may significantly influence development if they are sufficiently severe and because many can be successfully treated.

Mental Development

Mental development is often a major issue both in the diagnosis and the outcome of major craniofacial abnormalities. Nearly half of the syndromes listed by Siegel-Sadewitz and Shprintzen (1982) are reported to be *frequently* or *probably* associated with cognitive disorders. Some syndromes are associated with malformations of the brain resulting in mental retardation in 100% of affected children. Within any one of a number of other syndromes, the range may extend from normal intelligence through very severe mental retardation. Thus, some syndromes are invariably associated with some degree of mental retardation and others are not. DeMeyer et al. (1964) believed that the face predicts the brain. For example, hypotelorism (close-set eyes) is often associated with mental retardation, whereas hypertelorism is less likely to be related to mental retardation unless it is extreme and is an isolated facial abnormality. Since those rules of thumb do not invariably apply, speech pathologists and other specialists must be careful to avoid making assumptions about intelligence in the absence of careful psychological and neuropsychological testing. When developmental problems, including mental retardation and learning disabilities, are present, however, they cannot be ignored in treatment planning.

Psychosocial Factors

Psychosocial factors have also been examined. Patients with craniofacial anomalies usually have remarkable appearances that set them apart from their peers and to which society responds negatively since high value is placed on physical appearance. Clifford (1979) and Stricker et al. (1979) described the impact of these disfiguring conditions on the patient and the family. They indicated the importance of assessing the psychosocial aspects of these anomalies in estimating the

potential effects of cosmetic surgery. These anomalies are serious to the patient and the family, and they affect socialization, education, family life, vocational choice, and, certainly, communication skills.

Pertschuk and Whitaker (1987) note that research over more than 20 years demonstrates that appearance is a potent and pervasive social variable and that attractiveness brings with it a number of social advantages, whereas unattractiveness fosters social disadvantages. Research reported in Chapter 8 is equally applicable here. Pertschuk and Whitaker reported psychosocial data on two groups of children between the ages of 6 and 13, one treated for craniofacial problems before the age of 4 and the other in the process of being treated. The children treated early were similar to normal children on data derived from questionnaires completed by the children, their parents, and their classroom teachers. Presurgical testing of the untreated group demonstrated poorer self concepts, greater anxiety, more introversion, more behavioral problems at home and at school, and significantly more negative social encounters than were found in the treated group. Even after surgery, these psychosocial problems persisted. These data suggest a definite advantage for children who come to craniofacial surgery early rather than late.

Pertschuk and Whitaker also evaluated more than 60 patients between the ages of 14 and 50 prior to surgical correction of congenital craniofacial malformations. Semistructured patient interviews and unspecified measurements of self concept, extroversion, anxiety, depression, social adjustment, and psychiatric symptomatology were used. Almost half of the patients had an abnormal score on one or more tests. Over 30% had abnormal scores on two or more tests. Half of these subjects had entirely normal test profiles. The authors' impression was that lesser deformities tended to be associated with more nearly normal test scores. In spite of these latter findings, nearly all of the patients reported having to contend with social penalties including teasing, which peaked around junior high school; social isolation in high school; and staring and remarks from strangers. A majority reported self consciousness in social situations, especially when meeting new people. Emotional disturbance was rarely incapacitating, and professional help was almost never sought. Pertschuk and Whitaker question if such help might have been beneficial.

Overall, there is considerable pain attached to having significant craniofacial abnormalities, even though the actual adjustments that are ultimately made will differ widely from person to person. This is an area that must be considered in planning and executing treatment.

TREATMENT

The best initial approach to treatment is to modify the facial and oral structures to correct facial disfigurement to the extent possible and permit improved function, including speech production. Craniofacial surgery (Tessier, 1967, 1970, 1971, 1974; Whitaker and Randall, 1974; Jackson et al., 1982; Jackson, 1983; Marsh, 1986; Tulsane and Tessier, 1986; Whitaker and Hurwitz, in press) offers at least a partial solution to some of the more profound anomalies. Since syndromes affect many aspects of life, treatment is best carried out in an interdisciplinary setting similar to that described in Chapter 3. The craniofacial team, however, will ideally include more different specialists than are normally required for the management of clefts. In almost all cases of marked deformity requiring surgical correction, a team of surgeons will be needed. The exact make-up of the team will depend upon the problem, but it is usual to include a plastic surgeon, a neurosurgeon, an ophthalmological surgeon, an oral surgeon, and an orthodontist. These specialists examine, diagnose, plan, and treat in a cooperative manner, using information provided by the otolaryngologist who sometimes joins the surgical team; the speech pathologist, audiologist, psychologist, psychiatrist, geneticist, and others may be included as case requirements dictate.

Surgery to correct these deformities is extensive, time-consuming, and expensive. Twenty years ago almost none of these procedures were done, and people with major defects of this type were doomed to live with their deformities. Today, craniofacial surgery is available to most patients who want it. The work is usually done in large centers with a wide array of specialists, related services, and facilities. A brief overview of surgical procedures is provided in Chapter 4.

Following surgery, the team will have long-term involvement in assessing results and providing any continuing care that may be necessary, including attention to communication and psychosocial problems.

SYNDROMES ASSOCIATED WITH CLEFTING

Students are urged to review Cohen's work (1978) for information about some of the syndromes associated with clefting. The tables incorporated in the article provide an easy reference and will help to direct additional reading. Appropriate references appear at the end of his article.

In addition to this information, we discuss in detail some of the major syndromes that speech-language pathologists are likely to encounter in their practices.

Pierre Robin or Robin Sequence and Stickler Syndrome

Pierre Robin sequence is so called because it is thought that the small mandible is the major deformity that interferes with the descent of the tongue into the oral cavity to permit the elevation of the palatal shelves necessary for the completion of the palate (Latham, 1966; Gorlin et al., 1976). Thus, the cleft palate is a secondary rather than an initiating deformity.

The primary features of Robin sequence are mandibular hypoplasia (micrognathia or small lower jaw) accompanied by glossoptosis (retrusion of the tongue into the pharyngeal airway) and, usually, a mid-line posterior cleft of the palate. Other abnormalities that may occur include congenital heart problems, digital anomalies, eye and ear defects, and developmental deficits.

Robin sequence presents a major problem of diagnosis since it is sometimes a part of the symptom complex of a number of other syndromes (Pashayan and Lewis, 1984). An example is Stickler syndrome (Fig. 2.1). Elster (1983) compared the family histories of seven children with Stickler syndrome and 26 with Robin sequence, 71% of whom had family histories similar to the Stickler families, so may well have been misdiagnosed.

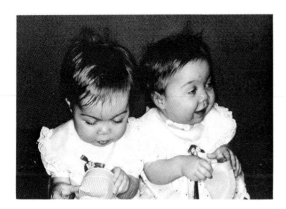

Figure 2.1 Twins with Stickler syndrome. Both babies have had tracheotomies for airway malformations in addition to those related to Pierre Robin.

Stickler syndrome is autosomal dominant with highly variable expression (Stickler, 1965; Herrmann et al., 1975; Jones, 1988). This syndrome involves skeletal abnormalities, arthritis, severe myopia (usually before age 10), retinal detachment, cataracts, or both in addition to the anomalies associated with Robin sequence. Most clinics now routinely explore the possibility of Stickler syndrome in children with Robin sequence.

Embryology and Etiology

As noted above, the initiating factor in Robin sequence that is not related to another syndrome is assumed to be the small mandible. Gorlin et al. (1976) attributed it to arrested embryonic development. Smith (1982) and Jones (1988) suggest that the small mandible may arise from mechanical constraint, which causes the chin to be compressed thus limiting its growth prior to palatal closure. The small mandible forces the tongue into a posterior position so that closure of the posterior palate is impaired. The associated cleft is usually U-shaped. Cleft lip does not occur in this sequence (Gorlin et al., 1976). Postnatally, the mandible continues to develop so that many but not all children with Pierre Robin do not appear to have unusually small mandibles by the age of about 5 years, even though measurements usually continue to be below average.

Little is known about hereditary factors in Robin sequence by itself. When Robin is associat-

ed with another syndrome, the recurrence rates will depend upon the syndrome.

Major Hazards

Airway obstruction is a major hazard to babies with Robin sequence during the first few months of life. Paradise (1983) stated that, because the tongue lies in an abnormally posterior position, it is unusually susceptible to the negative pressures of both deglutition and inspiration. The tongue tends to be aspirated and to be held in the hypopharynx in a ball-valve manner so that the upper airway is obstructed. The traditional view of this retracted tongue was that it fell back into the pharynx because of the small oral space. This thinking is now being replaced by the negative-pressure theory (Goldberg and Eckblom, 1962; Fletcher et al., 1969; Mallory and Paradise, 1979).

In severe cases, these babies may die of asphyxia. More often, they suffer from a milder but chronic obstruction, which may lead to cor pulmonale (Jersaty et al., 1969; Cogswell and Easton, 1974; Greenwood et al., 1977; Mallory and Paradise, 1979; Paradise, 1983) or to congestive heart failure (Shah et al., 1970; Mallory and Paradise, 1979). Airway obstruction either resolves spontaneously or improves notably by 4 to 6 months of age, probably as the result of progressive improvement in tongue control, with maturation (Mallory and Paradise, 1979; Paradise, 1983).

Until the resolution of the problem, infants experiencing respiratory difficulty may be kept in a prone position so that gravity will influence the tongue to fall forward, away from the airway. If this approach is unsuccessful, a tracheotomy may be required. Occasionally, the tongue is sutured to the lower lip in order to keep it forward out of the airway (Randall, 1977). This procedure is used less frequently today than it once was. Although other more complex procedures have been suggested, they are not usually required.

Feeding problems, as described in Chapter 8, apply to the child with Robin sequence. However, they are made more complex by the glossoptosis. In some cases, feeding can be accomplished in the prone position. In others, a nasogastric tube may be introduced temporarily.

Developmental problems occur frequently in children with Robin sequence. They are at increased risk for minimal brain dysfunction and often have learning disabilities.

Hearing losses are common since there are associated palatal clefts (see Chapter 6).

Communication deficits are usually related to the cleft or to the minimal brain dysfunction that is sometimes present. This is especially true for the child with Robin sequence in association with some other syndrome (Pashayan and Lewis, 1984). Delayed onset of language is common, and significant language disorders are often found.

Apert Syndrome (Acrocephalosyndactyly)

The primary and invariable features of Apert syndrome are craniosynostosis (premature closure of the sutures of the skull, especially the coronal suture) and syndactyly of the hands and feet (webbing between fingers and toes, often

from the base of the digits to the tips with fusion of bones and nails). Thumbs are often broad and turned away from the midline. The forehead is high, steep, and broad, and the occiput is flattened. The eyes are widely spaced (hypertelorism) with an antimongoloid slant and exophthalmos (protrusion of the eye balls). A saddle or a beak-like nose is sometimes present. Midfacial deficiency and a narrow pharyngeal airway are typical, along with facial asymmetry and crowded teeth (Fig. 2.2). Of special interest is the configuration of the palate. It may be very high and narrow, and

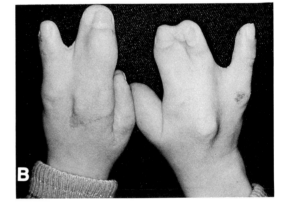

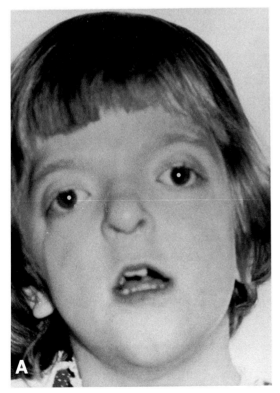

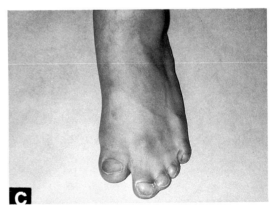

Figure 2.2 (A) Facial features of a child with Apert syndrome; associated deformities of the hand (B); and of the foot (C).

the maxillary arch may appear to be overdeveloped or swollen. The true palate is so narrow that it looks like an unusual cleft, but an actual cleft of the hard palate is not usually present. Clefts of the soft palate, however, occur in about 30% of the cases. The hard palate tends to be short and the soft palate long and thick (Peterson and Pruzansky, 1974; Peterson-Falzone et al., 1981).

Prevalence

Gorlin et al. (1976) indicated that Apert syndrome occurs once in every 169,000 live births; but, because of the high infant-mortality rate, only one in 2,000,000 people in the general population has the condition.

Etiology

It has been suggested that the causal factors leading to Apert syndrome occur prior to the fifth or sixth week of intrauterine life as the result of a hereditary defect in the tissues which separate the various bone anlagen from one another. Anlagen is the earliest discernable indication of an organ or part. Gorlin et al. (1976) indicated that this theory (Park and Powers, 1920) offers a plausible explanation for the combination of problems in these patients.

Most cases (Gorlin, 1976; Jones, 1988) appear to be sporadic, with older paternal age being a factor (Cohen, 1975; Jones, 1988). Since the syndrome is autosomal dominant, affected individuals have a 50% likelihood of producing children with the same condition.

Major Hazards

Psychosocial problems, as in all craniofacial syndromes, are of major concern. See the discussion on this topic earlier in this chapter. Suffice it to say here that surgical management of these problems early in life as opposed to later in life appears to minimize psychosocial problems, although, given society's response to facial disfigurement, it is not likely to eliminate them.

Functional limitations imposed by the hand deformities are common, although modern surgical techniques can improve function remarkably. The authors know of one young man who is successfully employed as an auto mechanic and of a young woman who is developing fine needlework skills.Esthetically, however, the hands remain remarkable.

Conductive hearing losses are found frequently (Elfenbein et al., 1981; Jones, 1988; Peterson-Falzone, 1988). These losses are related to several different causes, including deformities of the stapes and oval window, fixation or crowding of the nasopharynx (Peterson-Falzone, 1988), and palatal clefts.

Mental retardation, once thought to be typical of Apert syndrome, is now less frequently found since early surgery to relieve increased intracranial pressure is more commonly available. In our experience, however, problems of mental development are complex, and children with Apert syndrome must be carefully evaluated. Educational planning is essential since there are often evidences of borderline capabilities complicated by learning disabilities. Many older patients who have not had the benefit of modern treatment techniques, including educational opportunities, appear to be more significantly retarded than they may in reality have needed to be.

Communication problems are usual. Early in life, there is likely to be overall language development commensurate with mental abilities, with delayed onset of expressive language. As verbal output increases, certain predictable problems, described below, become apparent.

The narrow pharyngeal airway and increased nasal resistance result in hyponasality for most individuals with Apert syndrome. The effects of cleft palate, if present, are often masked by this concomitant condition. In addition to the speech problems, children with Apert syndrome should be watched for signs of sleep apnea and for educational problems related to chronic fatigue.

The midfacial hypoplasia and Class III dental malocclusion lead to habitual tongue protrusion into the lower dental arch, chronic mouth breathing, and distortion of sibilants. Clinical experience has not demonstrated any exception to this. Peterson (1973) referred to these problems as obligatory in view of the maxillary-mandibular arch relationships, and Elfenbein et al. (1981) also found them to be present.

Other articulation errors, some related to structure, may occur in some cases. Peterson (1973) described one patient who produced /t/ and /d/ by positioning the tongue blade against the lower border of the upper incisors; /f/ was a lingualabial fricative and /v/ a bilabial fricative. These articulatory behaviors are undoubtedly compensations for structural anomalies, but they are not as common as are the sibilant distortions.

Vowels may also be somewhat distorted because of the crowding of the oral and pharyngeal cavities (Peterson-Falzone, 1988).

Apert obviously creates communication problems that are rarely treatable by behavioral therapies. Midface advancement can provide both improved appearance and a deeper pharyngeal airway, often resulting in the elimination of hyponasality—although in some cases it may also place the patient at risk for velopharyngeal incompetence with hypernasality, which will then require treatment. Creating improved relationships between the mandible and maxilla may serve to improve sibilant articulation spontaneously or provide an environment conducive to improvement with speech therapy. Psychotherapy or some form of counseling should be considered mandatory, particularly prior to surgical correction for older patients, who may have unrealistic expectations of what the surgery will accomplish in their lives.

Crouzon Syndrome (Craniofacial Dysostosis)

Crouzon syndrome is much like Apert syndrome but is less severe, and there is no involvement of the hands and feet. Midfacial hypoplasia is characteristic. The upper lip is short, the lower lip tends to droop, and the nose is sometimes beak-like. The orbits of the eyes are shallow, and this is the most consistent clinical finding (Jones, 1988). Exophthalmos, as in Apert syndrome, is secondary to the orbital defect. Hypertelorism is very common. About 80% of these cases have optic nerve defects, and other eye anomalies may also be present. The shape of the head depends upon which sutures have closed prematurely. The palate is usually narrow and high and may be cleft. There is a Class III occlusion with open bite and a reduced pharyngeal airway.

Etiology

Crouzon syndrome results from premature closure of some cranial sutures. Its expression depends upon which sutures close early, when the process begins, and how fast it progresses. It is transmitted in an autosomal dominant manner. We have recently seen an infant whose mother is affected and who represents the sixth generation of his maternal line to have authenticated Crouzon syndrome (Fig. 2.3). Jones (1988) notes that

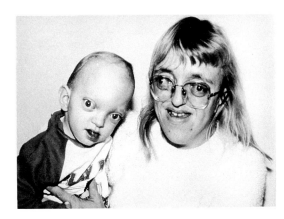

Figure 2.3 A mother and son with Crouzon's disease. This boy represents the sixth documented generation in the maternal line to have Crouzon syndrome.

about one-fourth of all cases have negative family histories, and Gorlin et al. (1976) suggested the need to study large numbers of these fresh mutations to learn whether or not older fathers are at increased risk of producing children with Crouzon syndrome. Obviously, genetic counseling is a necessity.

Major Hazards

Psychosocial problems in two adults with Crouzon syndrome were described by Cohn et al. (1985). Each had two children with the same syndrome in addition to several other family members with it as well. In depth interviews revealed that these two adults shared many life experiences. Both described their childhoods as marked by teasing and social isolation; both felt that vocational and heterosexual options had been limited; both saw themselves as different from others; both were alternately angry at society for demanding physical attractiveness and eager to demonstrate to society that they had value; both minimized the negative impact of their deformities; both described their efforts to live meaningful lives in spite of their deformities; both were aware of a gradual process, beginning in childhood, of learning to accept their differences instead of running away or feeling angry; both were proud that they had overcome their handicaps; both had consciously tried to develop values beyond physical appearance; both wanted to protect their affected children from suffering the same pain they had experienced; both expressed strong, positive feelings about having surgical correction for their children.

The authors concluded: that these adults frequently tried to present an overly positive picture of themselves to clinicians; that they had concerns that were different from parents without such malformations; that they also had needs akin to those of parents in general; that they had complex attitudes about physical attractiveness; that they needed help in separating their own feelings about their malformations from the feelings of their children. This work indicates that Crouzon syndrome is associated with psychosocial problems that may not be paralyzing in nature but that appear to have a marked impact on attitudes toward life. Again, counseling should be provided whenever possible if only to verify that life is as satisfying as possible under the circumstances, which do seem to make a difference.

Conductive hearing loss of a nonprogressive nature is present in about half of the cases and is probably related to anomalies of the middle ear. Jung (1988) provides a brief overview of this topic. When there is an associated cleft palate, the occurrence of conductive hearing loss rises accordingly.

Mental retardation is sometimes present and may be secondary to an increase in intracranial pressure. Identical twins known to us demonstrate this. One has a seizure disorder with mental retardation and motor deficits; the other is bright normal.

Communication problems vary more widely in Crouzon syndrome than they do in Apert syndrome. Some individuals with Crouzon syndrome have essentially normal speech; others have mild speech problems that appear to be unrelated to their oral structures; and still others have relatively severe deviations similar to those found in Apert syndrome. Peterson (1973) described two children with mildly impaired speech and one who had a severe disorder. The severely affected child had to carry his head in an extended position in order to maintain an adequate nasopharyngeal airway for breathing. (This condition results in audible breathing that is distracting in a communicative exchange and may increase the frequency of respiratory infections and of sleep disturbances including sleep apnea.) This child also had oral distortions of fricatives and affricatives, especially sibilants and inconsistent distortions of /r/ and /l/. Most of these errors were thought to be related to abnormal tongue place-

ment mandated, as in Apert syndrome, by the faulty maxillomandibular relationships. Later, Elfenbein et al. (1981) also reported sibilant distortions in one patient with Crouzon syndrome.

McWilliams (1983) wrote of structurally-related sibilant distortions in four cases, a brother and sister (with an affected mother) and twin boys (with an affected father). These 4 children all had denasalization of /m/, /n/, and /ŋ/ and consistent mouth breathing necessitated by the shallowness of the pharynx.

Treacher Collins Syndrome (Mandibulofacial Dysostosis, Franceschetti-Zwahlen-Klein Syndrome)

Treacher Collins is marked by malar hypoplasia with or without a cleft in the zygomatic bone, mandibular hypoplasia, macro- or microstomia, malformation of the auricles, defects of the external auditory canal, cleft palate, antimongoloid slant of the palpebral fissures, colobomo of the lower eyelid, projection of scalp hair onto the cheek, and occasional skin tags between the ear and the mouth (Fig. 2.4).

Etiology

Treacher Collins syndrome varies widely in its expressivity to the extent that it has sometimes been misdiagnosed (Jones, 1988). However, it is autosomal dominant with close to 100% penetrance, which refers to the frequency with which the genotype is expressed. About 60% of the cases represent fresh mutations (Rubin, 1967; Jones, 1988). This high percentage of cases without known family histories of Treacher Collins syndrome could be the result of missed diagnoses. The malformations of Treacher Collins syndrome occur early in development, probably around 7 weeks (Rogers, 1977). Jones (1988) reports an excess of affected offspring from affected females and of normal offspring from affected males.

Major Hazards

Many infants with Treacher Collins syndrome die before or at birth. Those who survive are at risk for problems in several different areas. Johnston et al. (1981) described an 8-year-old boy with Treacher Collins syndrome complicated by

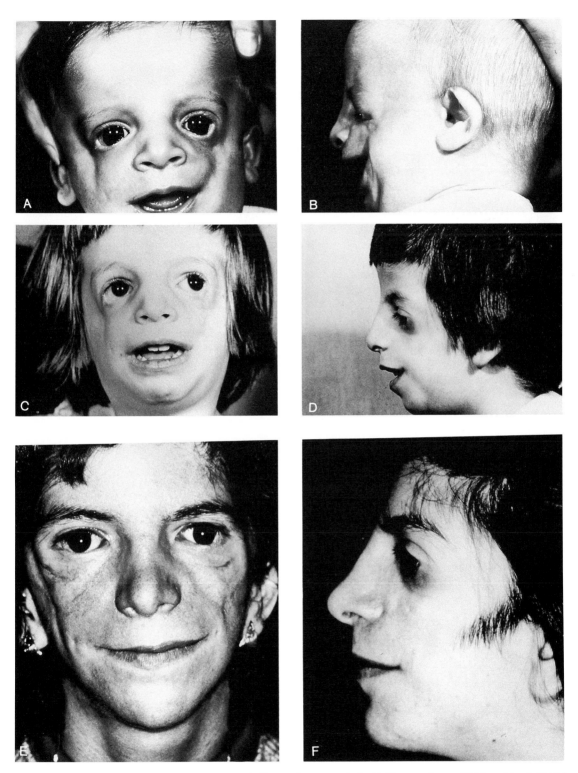

Figure 2.4 Full-face and profile views of Treacher Collins syndrome, as a baby (A,B), at age 5 years (C,D), and in adulthood after 10 operations (E,F).

obstructive sleep apnea, which was eliminated by surgical advancement of the mandible. Other problems include those discussed below.

Psychosocial problems are probably similar to those in other craniofacial malformations, but many patients with this syndrome do quite well and are able to put their intelligence to work positively for them. They encounter the added burden of coping with the hearing losses described in the next paragraph.

Conductive hearing losses are typical of patients with Treacher Collins syndrome. It is customary now to fit these babies with hearing aids at birth in order to minimize the effects of early auditory deprivation. When there is a microtic ear, that defect is quite obvious, especially in boys, and can be an added psychological hazard since it seems to prompt added questions and comments. However, these patients, if their losses cannot be reversed by surgery, as is sometimes possible, generally do very well with hearing aids.

Mental retardation is rare in patients with Treacher Collins syndrome, but untreated hearing losses may sometimes lead to erroneous identification of mental retardation as a major problem. It is essential that careful diagnostic assessment be carried out as protection against disastrous errors of this type.

Communication problems arise primarily from conductive hearing loss or from velopharyngeal incompetence associated with palatal clefts. Malocclusions are notable in some but not all patients and, if present, may also be influential in the etiology of communication deficits.

Hemifacial Microsomia (Facio-Auriculo-Vertebral Spectrum)

It has been suggested that hemifacial microsomia and Goldenhar syndrome may be gradations in severity of a similar error in morphogenesis (Gorlin et al., 1976; Jones, 1988). While bilateral facial assymetries of the type described below do occur, 80% are unilateral (Gorlin et al., 1976; Converse et al., 1977; Jones, 1988). Dupertius and Musgrave (1959) reported a unilateral to bilateral ratio of 6 to 1. The condition occurs once in every 3,000 to 5,000 births, and the male-to-female ratio is 3:2 (Gorlin, 1976; Jones, 1988). Outstanding characteristics of the syndrome include hypoplasia of the malar, maxillary, and

mandibular regions, especially of the ramus and condyle of the mandible and the temporomandibular joint; lateral cleft-like extension of the corner of the mouth; hypoplasia of facial musculature; microtia; preauricular tags, pits, or both; middle-ear anomalies; malfunction of the tongue and soft palate; clefts of the lip or palate; heart or renal malformations, among others (Jones, 1988; Converse et al., 1977). Gorlin et al. (1976) placed the occurrence of heart anomalies as high as 45 to 55% (Fig. 2.5).

Etiology

Hemifacial microsomia springs primarily from the first and second branchial arches (Converse, 1977; Jones, 1988). However, Gorlin et al. (1976) make the point that "terms such as first arch syndrome, first and second branchial arch syndrome, and hemifacial microsomia impart the erroneous impression that involvement is limited to facial structures when in fact, cardiac, renal, and skeletal anomalies..." may also occur. Gorlin et al. (1976) suggest that the etiology is unresolved and probably complicated. Jones (1988) agrees. There is marked variability in the many sporadic cases that occur, but there are also familial occurrences, which, according to Gorlin et al., suggest etiologic heterogeneity.

Major Hazards

These deformities are so variable and may be so mild that there is often no unusual hazard except in the psychosocial areas. In other cases, the defects may be incompatible with life or constitute severe disfigurement with marked functional variations.

Conductive hearing losses are especially prevalent on the affected side, and they may range from very mild to the upper limits of conductive involvement, especially if microtia is present. There may also be anomalies of the middle ear in 30 to 50% of the cases (Gorlin, 1976). Thus, hearing losses should be routinely suspected.

Mental retardation is uncommon in hemifacial microsomia. Jones (1988) indicates that about 13% have IQs below 85.

Communication problems, like the deformity itself, range from no perceptible problem to severe, usually depending upon the extent of the orofacial anomaly. In severe asymmetries, articulation may be significantly compromised, and

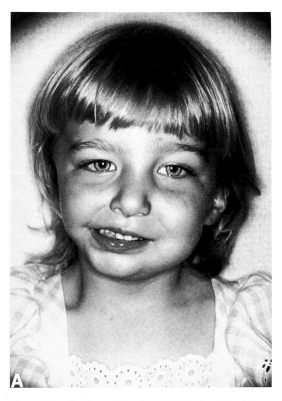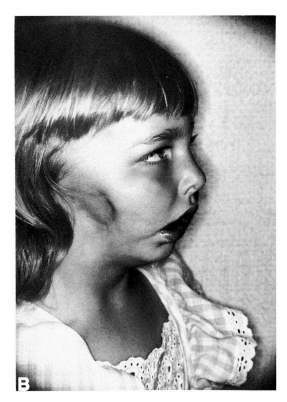

Figure 2.5 Full-face (A) and profile (B) of a child with hemifacial microsomia.

there may be alterations in oral resonance resulting from changes in the position and extent of the oral opening. Nasal resonance may be increased by asymmetrical movement in the soft palate with velopharyngeal incompetence occurring, per-haps, on only one side of the velopharyngeal valve. This condition is apparently rare even when the movement of the valving structures is asymmetrical. This topic is well reviewed by Peterson-Falzone (1988).

Shprintzen Syndrome (Velo-Cardio-Facial Syndrome)

This syndrome, described by Shprintzen et al. (1978, 1981) is of special interest to speech-language pathologists because of the universality of language deficits and learning disabilities combined with palatal clefts or congenital velopharyngeal incompetence. Other features include small stature, usually below the tenth percentile; prominent nose, often with a broad, square nasal root and a narrow alar base; narrow palpebral fissures; malar deficiency; vertical maxillary excess with a long face; a retruded chin, sometimes with a class II malocclusion; microcephaly in 40 to 50%; slender hands and digits; and cardiac anomalies in about 84% of the cases. Jones (1988) also describes hypotonia in infancy (Fig. 2.6).

Shprintzen syndrome is variable in its expression, and geneticists do not always agree about its diagnosis, which is true also of a number of other syndromes with wide variability and physical features that are less precise than in such syndromes as those previously described. For this reason, speech pathologists must avoid jumping to unwarranted conclusions about any child in whom Shprintzen syndrome has been diagnosed or is suspected.

Etiology

This is an autosomal-dominant syndrome with most of the reported cases occurring sporadically.

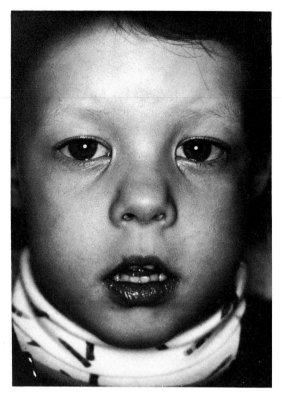

Figure 2.6 A child with Velo-Cardio-Facial syndrome. Her features include velopharyngeal incompetence, pulmonary atresia, ventriculoseptal defect, seizure disorder, emerging learning disabilities with average intelligence, bilateral epicanthal folds, wide nasal root, micrognathia, long face, and long fingers.

Psychosocial problems have not been described in detail, but Jones (1988) suggests that children with the syndrome may have social skills that surpass their mental abilities. Several patients known to us have shown notably poor social judgment and have encountered marked problems in their peer relationships. They often appear to be somewhat unresponsive and to lack variety in facial expression. More information is needed about the origins of these characteristics.

Conductive hearing losses are consistent with the occurrence of palatal clefts. Shprintzen et al. (1981) found hypoplasia of the cartilage of the eustachian tube and marked reduction in the size of the nasopharyngeal lumen of the eustachian tube. These authors reported one subject who had a sensorineural hearing loss.

Mental retardation was present in 16 of 39 patients described by Shprintzen (1981). One fell

into the trainable classification, and all the others were educable. Ten of the 16 were microcephalic. All of the subjects demonstrated some form of perceptual impairment. Golding-Kushner et al. (1985) described these children as appearing somewhat more capable in the preschool years than their later academic performances suggest. Their cognitive behavior remains concrete, and they have notable difficulty with mathematical concepts. Jones (1988) describes these patients as demonstrating somewhat perseverative behavior and refers also to concrete patterns of thinking secondary to mental retardation. This concreteness may in some cases be more marked than mental abilities would seem to warrant.

Communication problems are characteristic, with delayed onset of expressive language and evidences of language impairment thereafter. The speech pattern is marked by the influences of the cleft or the congenital velopharyngeal valving deficits, which may be complicated by motor impairment as well. These children are often diagnosed after considerable therapy has been undertaken to correct language delays and hypernasality. It is surprising that some speech-language pathologists are still caught in the trap of treating without diagnosing, often to the detriment of the child. It is clear that these children have multiple impairments that are better managed if they are assessed in their totality rather than in bits and pieces.

SUMMARY

The speech-language pathologist is required to treat communication disorders that require information about a variety of craniofacial syndromes, only a few of which have been reviewed in this chapter. These complex malformations affect the entire craniofacial complex or parts thereof. They range in severity from slight to marked and very often are transmitted to subsequent generations in a predictable manner.

These anomalies, depending upon their severity, have various effects on feeding, breathing, early development, intelligence, social competence, educational capabilities, hearing, and communication skills. They are best treated by an interdisciplinary team of specialists, including the speech-language pathologist and audiologist. Some form of surgical intervention is usually required, and behavioral therapies alone cannot be expected to succeed.

Students are urged to explore syndromes in greater depth, either in formal courses or by reading and observing independently. A careful clinician will always consider the possibility of a syndrome when evaluating any child with a communication problem, especially if velopharyngeal incompetence or unusual physical characteristics are apparent.

REFERENCES

Bergstrom L. Congenital and acquired deafness in clefting and craniofacial syndromes. Cleft Palate J 1978;15:254.

Bloomer HH. Speech defects associated with dental malocclusions and related abnormalities. In: Travis LE, ed. Handbook of speech pathology and audiology. Englewood Cliff, NJ: Prentice-Hall, 1971:715.

Bloomer HH, Hawk AM. Speech considerations: speech disorders associated with ablative surgery of the face, mouth, and pharynx — ablative approaches to learning. In: Wertz RT, ed. Orofacial anomalies and research implications. ASHA Reports No. 8, 1973:42.

Clifford E. Psychologic aspects of craniofacial anomalies. In: Converse JM, McCarthy JG, Wood-Smith D, eds. Symposium on diagnosis and treatment of craniofacial anomalies. St. Louis: CV Mosby, 1979:12.

Cogswell JJ, Easton DM. Cor pulmonale in the Pierre Robin syndrome. Arch Dis Child 1974;49:905.

Cohn ER, Hesky EM, Bradley WF, McWilliams BJ, Hurwitz DJ, Wallace SB. Life response to Crouzon's disease. Cleft Palate J 1985;22:123.

Cohen MM Jr. An etiologic and nosologic overview of craniosynostosis syndromes. In: Bergsma D, ed. Malformation syndromes. Amsterdam: Excerpta Medica, 1975.

Cohen MM. Syndromes with cleft lip and cleft palate. Cleft Palate J 1978;15:306.

Converse JM, McCarthy JG, Wood-Smith D, Coccaro PJ. Craniofacial microsomia. In: Converse JM, ed. Reconstructive plastic surgery. Vol 4. Philadelphia: WB Saunders, 1977:2359.

Crysdale WS. Otorhinolaryngologic problems in patients with craniofacial anomalies. Otolaryngol Clin North Am 1981;14:145.

DeMeyer W, Zeman W, Palmer CG. The face predicts the brain. Diagnostic significance of median face anomalies for holoprosencephaly (arrhinencephaly). Pediatrics 1964;34:256.

Dupertius SM, Musgrave RH. Experiences with the reconstruction of the congenitally deformed ear. Plast Reconstr Surg 1959;23:361.

Elfenbein JL, Waziri M, Morris HL. Verbal communication skills of six children with craniofacial anomalies. Cleft Palate J 1981;18:59.

Elster B. The risk of Stickler syndrome in infants born with Pierre Robin anomalad. Essay for Master's degree. School of Public Health, University of Pittsburgh, 1983.

Fletcher MM, Blum SL, Blanchard CL. Pierre Robin syndrome pathophysiology of obstructive episodes. Laryngoscope 1969;79:547.

Goldberg MH, Eckblom RH. The treatment of the Pierre Robin syndrome. Pediatrics 1962;30:450.

Golding-Kushner K, Weller G, Shprintzen R. Velo-cardio-facial syndrome: language and psychosocial profile. J Craniofac Genet Dev Biol 1985;5:59.

Gorlin RJ, Pindborg JJ, Cohen MM. Syndromes of the head and neck. 2nd ed. New York: McGraw-Hill, 1976.

Greenwood RD, Waldman JD, Rosenthal A, et al. Cardiovascular abnormalities associated with Pierre Robin anomaly. Pediatr Dig 1977;19:31.

Herrmann J, France JD, Spranger JW, Opitz JM, Wiffler C. The Stickler syndrome (hereditary arthro-ophthalmopathy). Birth Defects, Original Article Series, 1975;11:76.

Jackson IT. The wide world of craniofacial surgery. J Oral Maxillofac Surg 1983;41:103.

Jackson IT, Munro IR, Salyer KE, Whitaker LA, eds. Atlas of craniofacial surgery. St. Louis: CV Mosby, 1982.

Jeresaty RM. Huszar RJ, Basw S. Pierre Robin syndrome. Am J Dis Child 1969;117:710.

Johnston C, Taussig LM, Koopmann C, Smith P, Bjelland J. Obstructive sleep apnea in Treacher Collins syndrome. Cleft Palate J 1981;18:39.

Jones KL. Smith's recognizable patterns of human malformation. 4th ed. Philadelphia: WB Saunders, 1988.

Jung JH. Genetic syndromes in communication disorders. Boston: Little, Brown, 1988.

Latham RA. The pathogenesis of cleft palate associated with the Pierre Robin syndrome. Br J Plast Surg 1966; 19:205.

Marsh JL, ed. Long-term results of craniofacial surgery. Cleft Palate J 1986;23:Suppl I.

McWilliams BJ. Speech problems associated with craniofacial anomalies. In: Costello JM, ed. Recent advances: speech disorders. San Diego: College Hill Press, 1983.

Mallory SB, Paradise JL. Glossoptosis revisited: on the development and resolution of airway obstruction in the Pierre Robin syndrome. New observations from a case with cor pulmonale. Pediatrics 1979;64:946.

Paradise JL. Primary care of infants and children with cleft palate. In: Bluestone CD, Stool SE, eds. Pediatric otolaryngology. Philadelphia: WB Saunders, 1983:924.

Park EA, Powers GF. Acrocephaly and scaphocephaly with symmetrically distributed malformations of the extremities. Am J Dis Child 1920;20:235.

Pasyayan HM, Lewis MB. Clinical experience with the Robin sequence. Cleft Palate J 1984;21:270.

Pertschuk MJ, Whitaker LA. Psychosocial considerations in craniofacial deformity. Clin Plast Surg 1987;14:163.

Peterson SJ. Speech pathology in craniofacial malformations other than cleft lip and palate. In: Wertz RT, ed. Orofacial anomalies: clinical and research implications. ASHA Reports No. 8, 1973:111.

Peterson S, Pruzansky S. Palatal anomalies in the syndromes of Apert and Crouzon. Cleft Palate J 1974;11:394.

Peterson-Falzone SJ. Resonance disorders in structural defects. In: Lass NJ, McReynolds LV, Northern JL, Yoder DE, eds. Speech, language and hearing. Vol II. Philadelphia: WB Saunders, 1982.

Peterson-Falzone SJ. Speech disorders related to craniofacial structural defects: Part 2. In: Lass NJ, McReynolds LV, Northern JL, Yoder DE, eds. Handbook of speech pathology and audiology. Toronto: BC Decker, 1988.

Peterson-Falzone SJ, Pruzansky S, Parris PJ, Laffer JL. Nasopharyngeal dysmorphology in the syndromes of Apert and Crouzon. Cleft Palate J 1981;18:237.

Randall P. The Robin anomalad: micrognathia and glossoptosis with airway obstruction. In: Converse JM, ed. Reconstructive plastic surgery. Vol 4. Philadelphia: WB Saunders, 1977:2235.

Rogers BO. Embryology of the face and introduction to craniofacial anomalies. In: Converse JM, ed. Reconstructive plastic surgery. Vol 4. Philadelphia: WB Saunders, 1977:2296.

Rubin A, ed. Handbook of congenital malformations. Philadelphia: WB Saunders, 1967.

Schaefer L, Sullivan MD. The speech-language pathologist's role on the craniofacial team. Ear Nose Throat J 1986;65:346.

Selder A. Hearing disorders in children with otocraniofacial syndromes. In: Wertz RT, ed. Orofacial anomalies: clinical and research implications. ASHA Reports No. 8, 1973:95.

Shah CV, Pruzansky S, Harris WS. Cardiac malformations with facial clefts. Am J Dis Child 1970;119:238.

Shprintzen RJ, Goldberg RB, Lewin ML, Sidoti EJ, Berkman MD, Argamaso RV, Young D. A new syndrome involving cleft palate, cardiac anomalies, typical facies, and learning disabilities: velo-cardio-facial syndrome. Cleft Palate J 1978;15:56.

Shprintzen RJ, Goldberg RB, Young D, Wolford L. The velo-cardio-facial syndrome: a clinical and genetic analysis. Pediatrics 1981;67:167.

Siegel-Sadewitz V, Shprintzen RJ. The relationship of communication disorders to syndrome identification. J Speech Hear Dis 1982;47:338.

Smith DW. Recognizable patterns of human malformation. 2nd ed. Philadelphia: WB Saunders, 1976.

Smith DW. Recognizable patterns of human malformation. 3rd ed. Philadelphia: WB Saunders, 1982.

Sparks SN. Birth defects and speech-language disorders. Boston: Little, Brown, 1984.

Sparks SN, Millard S. Speech and language characteristics of genetic syndromes. J Comm Dis 1981;14:411.

Stickler GB, Belau PG, et al. Hereditary progressive arthro-ophthalmopathy. Mayo Clin Proc 1965;40:433.

Stool SE, Houlihan R. Otolaryngologic management of craniofacial anomalies. Otolaryngol Clin North Am 1977;20:41.

Stricker G, Clifford E, Cohen LK, Giddon DB, Meskin LH, Evans CA. Psychosocial aspects of craniofacial disfigurement. Am J Orthod 1979;76:410.

Tessier P. Osteotomies totals de la face: syndrome de Crouzon, syndrome d'Apert, oxycephalie, scaphocephalie, turricephalie. Ann Chir Plast 1967;12:273.

Tessier P. The treatment of facial dysmorphology particularly of craniofacial dysostosis (CFD) Crouzon and Apert disease, total osteotomy and sagittal displacement. Chirurgie 1970;96:667.

Tessier P. The definitive plastic surgical treatment of the severe facial deformities of craniofacial dysostosis: Crouzon's and Apert's disease. Plast Reconstr Surg 1971;48:419.

Tessier P. Experiences in the treatment of orbital hypertelorism. Plast Reconstr Surg 1974;53:1.

Tessier P. Anatomical classification of facial, cranio-facial, and latero-facial clefts. J Maxillofac Surg; 1976;4:69.

Tulasne JF, Tessier PL. Results of the Tessier integral procedure for correction of Treacher Collins syndrome. In: Marsh JL, ed. Long-term results of craniofacial surgery. Cleft Palate J 1986;23(suppl 1):40.

Whitaker LA, Hurwitz DJ. Principles and methods of management. In: Bluestone CD, Stool S, eds. Pediatric otolaryngology. 2nd ed. Philadelphia: WB Saunders, in press.

Whitaker LA, Pashayan H, Reichman J. A proposed new classification of craniofacial anomalies. Cleft Palate J 1981;18:161.

Whitaker LA, Randall P. The developing field of craniofacial surgery. Pediatrics 1974;54:571.

Witzel MA. Speech problems in craniofacial anomalies. Comm Dis 1983;4:45.

3 | DELIVERY OF CARE

INTERDISCIPLINARY TREATMENT

Patients who have various types of clefts, congenital palatopharyngeal insufficiency, or orthognathic-craniofacial anomalies have many different and complex problems that are interrelated and must be treated as such. These intricate interrelationships demand cooperation among the professional people responsible for the care of these patients. Specialists who combine their talents in one setting to provide this care are usually referred to as a cleft palate, craniofacial, orofacial, or dentofacial team, among many possible designations. Descriptions of cleft palate teams, their objectives, and functions have been provided by Koepp-Baker (1955, 1963, 1979), Bleiberg and Leubling (1971), Falk (1971), Morris et al. (1978), Krogman (1979), Morris (1980), and Holve (1985). Whitehouse (1965) discussed management teams in more general terms. All of these authors pointed to the better integrated care received by patients and the benefits derived by professional people from team work.

Integrated Management

Krogman (1979) credited HK Cooper, founder of the Lancaster Cleft Palate Clinic, with having advanced the concept of team care for cleft lip and palate and related disorders in the early 1930s. Cooper (1953) noted that in the past care had often been dispersed and uncoordinated:

For many years the cleft palate patient has been treated by various specialists, by the surgeon, by the dentist, by the speech therapist, each working separately, trying with the skill of his profession to solve the problem from that standpoint alone. Some have been successful, many have not.

Cooper went on to describe the early beginnings of interdisciplinary treatment programs. He emphasized that specialists should work side by side in a truly cooperative manner:

True integration starts with a meeting of the minds of the individuals who first examine the patient together and then agree on a program for treatment. The error to be avoided has been stated simply: 'Men do not plan to fail, they fail to plan'.

Cooper illustrated his team by showing all specialties as the spokes in a wheel with the child as the hub, the center of all activities.

Team Members

We think there is general agreement that contemporary standards for treatment of cleft lip and palate and related disorders require contributions from a number of specialists. That is because of the widespread effects of this kind of birth defect. These specialists include the surgeon, speech pathologist, orthodontist, otolaryngologist, prosthodontist, general dentists, psychologist, and pediatrician. Some state cleft palate programs require only that recognized teams have board-certified (or the equivalent) specialists in plastic surgery, dentistry, and speech pathology, and these specialists are often thought of as the core members of the team. The exact composition of a specific team depends upon its mission and purpose. In addition to those identified above, we consider the social worker, audiologist, and clinical geneticist to be crucial. A cooperating radiologist should be available for special cases; a nurse is used extensively by some teams (Scheuerle et al., 1984). Access to psychological and mental health services is also necessary (Broder and Richman, 1987). The patient and the parents complete the make-up of the team. Many teams include experienced mothers and fathers as extensions of their professional staffs.

If the team is involved in the care of patients with craniofacial anomalies, a neurologist, neurosurgeon, ophthalmic surgeon, and pediatric anesthesiologist will also be required.

Advantages of Team Care

Clinical care by a management team has major benefits in the more efficient integration of the various types of treatment. That is especially the case when there is necessary interaction among aspects of treatment (e.g., the surgeon may act on the speech pathologist's findings, social history reported by the social worker may result in deferment of elective physical management).

Another relevant aspect of the issue is that the patient's needs change over time. In Table 3.1, Krogman used data from the Lancaster protocol to illustrate various aspects of treatment from the prenatal period to adulthood. These changing needs can best be dealt with in the structure of a management team.

Other practical advantages to team care include: (1) the family can often see a number of specialists at one appointment; (2) follow-up can be managed in a controlled system; (3) the family associates all aspects of care with one program; and (4) only one contact has to be made if emergencies arise.

There are advantages also for the specialists involved. They enjoy mutual intellectual stimulation, learn new approaches to problem solving, do research together, publish together, and broaden their professional horizons. The professional interaction growing out of interdisciplinary care led to the formation in 1943 of the American Cleft Palate-Craniofacial Association. (We note with pride that, according to Wells, 1979, four speech pathologists — Herbert Koepp-Baker, Eugenet T. McDonald, Gladys Fish, and Margare Raabe — were among the founders of that organization).

A possible disadvantage to team care is that the family must relate to many specialists rather than to one individual. Some teams avoid that hazard by having one person establish an especially close relationship with a particular child and family. This person may change with the changing needs of the patient over time.

Team Leadership

The question of team leadership is one that often presents a major hurdle as teams are organized. This can usually be resolved in a pragmatic manner in accordance with local circumstances. Leadership may be decided on the basis of administrative policy within an institution, the time commitments of staff members, the size of the program, or the interests of the participants.

Team Function

Most teams come together in one setting for the purpose of examining patients. The team members may work either separately or together. By discussion and cooperative decision-making, they define problems and devise sequenced treatment strategies. These teams or clinics provide both initial evaluations and follow-up care for as long and as often as required. Modifications of the treatment plan may be indicated when growth and development cause some change in the patient or the protocol. Patient care extends from birth to early adulthood. For some individuals, particularly those wearing various types of dental prosthetic appliances, it may be a lifetime proposition. Some teams assemble in a formal way only once a month. Others have several team clinics every week, with additional services provided as needed.

Changing Needs Over Time

Krogman (1979) has indicated how patient's needs change over time (Table 3.1). For example, the feeding problems that are present at birth are soon resolved, but the need for ear and dental care may persist for a lifetime. The ages and services presented by Krogman are taken from the Lancaster protocol. While their plan is generally applicable, other clinics address different aspects with more or less emphasis. For example, in some programs, the audiologist may introduce impedance testing at 6 months rather than at 2-1/2 years; developmental testing may more frequently be carried out; educational counseling may be included; and radiology may be more visible. Much depends upon the talents and interests of the team members. Such differences serve to strengthen rather than to weaken the care of patients.

Interpreting Findings to the Family

When a number of specialists have examined a patient at one time or at different times on the same day and have coordinated their findings and

TABLE 3.1 The Function of the Cleft Palate Team with the Changing Needs of Patients From Birth Through Adulthood

Age In Years	Overall Summary
Prenatal	History of gestation of maternal health; close supervision first trimester. If FH+, counseling of parents, especially by geneticist and social worker. This is time of great developmental speed. Cleft may or may not be part of syndrome involving many structures developing at time cleft occurs. Embryonic period (3 lunar months) = differentiation; fetal period (7 lunar months) = growth.
Birth	Pediatrician discusses cleft condition with parents, with cooperation of geneticist and social worker. Surgeon discusses cleft type and advises of operative procedures. Dental specialist appraises arch relationships, especially in bilateral cleft palates; checks for associated orodental anomalies. Growth researcher obtains data on prenatal history, including maternal health; confers with geneticist regarding family pedigree; evaluates degree adjacent structures (on time-linked basis) are involved in the dysplastic effects of the cleft.
B–1:0	Pediatrician advises on feeding (problem) and dietary regimen; watches child's health and early development. Surgeon closes lip ("rule of 10") at c. 0:3. Dental specialist secures models, x-ray head films, and height and weight at 0:3, 0:6, and 1:0. Genetic pedigree secured, evaluated. Social worker counsels on family situation. Pediatrician, surgeon, dental specialist, geneticist, and social worker coordinate family counseling. Growth researcher evaluates craniofacial status at birth; follows growth progress first year. ENT specialist continues ear observations. Audiologist begins hearing tests via "noise" response at 0:6; gets family hearing history. Earliest speech = "babbling." Speech pathologist and surgeon discuss possible VP insufficiency and incompetence. Child progresses through several early stages of speech and language development in preparation for use of the first true words, which appear about first birthday.
1:0–2:0	Pediatrician continues role in health and nutrition. Surgeon evaluates effect of lip repair. Hard palate closed 1:2, soft palate 1:6, in conference with dental specialist. Speech pathologist evaluates VP structure and function; confers with dental specialist on possible prosthesis. Dentist and growth researcher work together on craniofacial arch relationship, etc., and follow growth pattern. Geneticist and social worker counsel as before. ENT watches ear condition. Audiologic hearing tests. Speech specialist, surgeon, and dentist work together in VP evaluation, and with growth researcher evaluate x-ray films of oropharyngeal development. Child's vocabulary goes from c. 10 to c. 270 words by 2:0.
2:0–6:0	Pediatrician's role is the same. Surgeon has follow-up role; works with speech pathologist on effect of surgery on VP function. Dental specialist notes oral segmental relations, with reference to crossbite and malocclusion (with orthodontist); casts and x-rays taken annually. Genetic role slight. Social worker notes preschool child's development of attitudes toward self and peer relations; continues role as counselor. Growth researcher follows craniofacial growth for progress in postoperative "catch-up" trend; growth pattern analyzed. ENT specialist continues services. Audiologist begins audiometric and impedance tests at 2:6; hearing evaluated in terms of cleft type. Speech data are recorded for articulation, voice quality, etc. Speech specialists, surgeon, dentist, and growth researcher work closely together. Period of rapid speech and language growth.
6:0–12:0	Pediatrician's role as in 2:0–6:0. Surgical follow-up for possible need of secondary repair of lip, palate, or nose. Residency program* begins: dentistry, speech, social work closely interrelated. Dental specialist and orthodontist teamed closely with growth researcher. Role of geneticist not significantly changed. Growth focuses on more rapid craniofacial growth of "pre-pubertal" acceleration. ENT specialist continues. Audiologist and speech specialist work together; progress in speech and hearing noted. Speech therapy as required. Cineradiography taken for oropharyngeal form and function. Speech matures to adult levels at 7–8 years. Grammar is refined and vocabulary expanded.
12:0–18:0	Surgical follow-up on lip and nose; focus on orthodontic care. Geneticist may give premarital counseling. Social worker begins intensive study of attitude development in adolescence and in child to parent relationship. Growth researcher works with dentistry, speech, orthodontics. ENT and audiology continue as in 6:0–12:0. Speech therapy and counseling as indicated.
18:0+ Adult	Health in hands of general practitioner. Surgical role moot. Dental care probably by general dentist. Geneticist and social worker counsel mostly in premarital and marital terms, mainly regarding risk and parent to child relationships. Hearing and speech as needed. Speech is mature; vocabulary continues to expand.

*No longer a part of the Lancaster program. (From Krogman WM. The cleft palate team in action. In: Cooper HK, Harding RL, Krogman WM, Mazaheri M, Millard RT, eds. Cleft palate and cleft lip: a team approach to clinical management and rehabilitation of the patient. Philadelphia: WB Saunders, 1979:147.)

recommendations, it is easy for the family to be uncertain of who is recommending what and how it is to be carried out. For this reason, the interpretation of findings and recommendations and family counseling have a high priority. There are several approaches to this problem. One requires each specialist to interpret anything relating to his or her specialty. While this method is commonly used and works well for many teams, especially for those that are tightly integrated, it may be confusing to families, and that must be taken into account in deciding on a procedure. Some patients or families may need a single person who will help them to receive, integrate, analyze, and act upon the various types of information given.

This counselor has an important obligation. He or she must understand the team's recommendations, must be able to put them into the perspective of the patient's and family's situation, and must communicate them in a manner that the patient and parents can act upon. The recommendations must also be made with an understanding of the resources available to that particular patient and family. Finally, the exit conference must be conducted in a way that makes clear to family members that they are important parts of the team and have options available to them. Some clinics regularly use one person to fill this counseling role. Some make regular use of written recommendations, which are given to the family at the conclusion of the conference so that they can review the recommendations under less trying circumstances.

Another approach to this problem is to select the counselor or counselors according to the major focus of the recommendations being made. For example, in one of our clinics, the plastic surgeon and speech pathologist, together, routinely discuss with parents velopharyngeal incompetence, its implications for speech, and the treatment being recommended.

Cultural Differences

In an interesting discussion of the craniofacial team and the Navajo patient, Smoot et al. (1988) remind us of the vital importance of cultural influences in the delivery of health care, including that for cleft lip and palate. A similar message was delivered by Strauss and Meyerson (1989) who chaired a panel on treatment of birth defects across cultures in the United States. We need more reports of this kind about various cultural groups in order to develop constructive and efficient delivery systems.

The Role of Community Personnel

As indicated elsewhere in several discussions, the special management team for cleft palate or any other disease or disorder depends heavily on resources in the local community. For example, the family doctor and dentist and the school speech pathologist provide important care for general needs and often, aspects of the cleft lip and palate. As a consequence, the lines of communication between these practitioners and members of the team must be strong. Unquestionably, community personnel have a vital role in assisting a family with a new baby with a cleft or other craniofacial disorder to obtain appropriate treatment. That is especially the case when the family, or even some of the professional personnel, has had little or no personal experience with the disorder. To meet all these needs, continuing education programs about the disorders for members of the health, education, and welfare professions are especially important (Morris 1983; Mitchell et al., 1984; Scheuerle et al., 1984; Middleton et al., 1986).

THE SPEECH PATHOLOGIST ON THE CLEFT PALATE TEAM

The speech pathologist has an important and, at times, difficult role on the cleft palate team. A major purpose of surgery for clefts and other problems is to provide a mechanism consistent with normal speech. As a consequence, many of the issues discussed by the team, such as timing of palatal surgery, the necessity for secondary surgery, and the need for alteration in dental relationships, are related to information provided by the speech pathologist.

In the deliberations of the team, the speech pathologist must always be the advocate of the patient in the matter of speech proficiency. She or he must assert and vigorously defend the patient's right to the very best oral communication skills possible. Compromise of that objective is acceptable only on the basis of persuasive arguments such as other treatment requirements, anatomical or physiological limitations, parental or patient preference, family circumstances, or other conditions that appear to take precedence. For example, for certain patients, palatoplasty may be delayed for reasons of maxillofacial growth even though the delay may interfere with the development of communication skills. An orthodontic appliance may interfere seriously with certain aspects of speech production but be badly needed for functional and cosmetic reasons. An adenoidectomy may result in velopharyngeal incompetence with consequent nasalization of speech, but may be indicated for medical and audiologic reasons. The speech pathologist must function in close harmony with other team members on these issues so that incongruous or contradictory messages are not communicated to patients and families.

Frequently, in working with a team, and in interdisciplinary efforts in general, the question arises about standards to be used for defining "normal" speech. Sometimes the speech pathologist may feel defensive when fellow team members offer opinions about whether an individual patient's speech is "normal" or "acceptable." We must resist the notion that special training is required for making decisions about the normality of speech. After all, the objective of our profession is to assist patients to acquire verbal communication skills that will not distinguish them from their peers. Who better to help us determine these standards than the physician, the dentist, the nurse, the teacher, and certainly the family? We have special training to determine the type of disorder, its etiological foundations, and the preferred treatment, but we must never forget that the final speech outcome must pass muster with the average listener.

On the other hand, the speech pathologist must be straightforward with other team members about speech as he or she hears it. It is not acceptable for the speech pathologist to retreat from a position or fail to communicate concerns simply out of fear that others may disagree. Each member of the team must be the expert in his or her own field, and that applies to the speech pathologist as well as to all the others. As speech pathologists, we must be in a peer relationship with other team members, have the courage to express our convictions, and know when and how to compromise.

THE SPEECH PATHOLOGIST IN OTHER SETTINGS

The speech pathologist working apart from the other members of a team may have special problems in relating to the team. In many instances, the cleft palate team depends on practitioners in the patient's home community for important aspects of ongoing treatment. For example, the local pediatrician provides general health care; the local otolaryngologist may monitor and treat ear disease; the local orthodontist may do the orthodontic work; and the speech pathologist, perhaps in a school setting, local hospital or clinic, or private practice, may provide speech and language therapy. All of these people are important members of the expanded cooperating management team, but are removed geographically from their colleagues. This separation makes communication among the team members more difficult. Written reports then become necessary, and this demands that the right to privacy of the patient and family be protected by being certain to have properly signed releases.

Close cooperation between the speech pathologist in the local community and the speech pathologist on the team is a major requisite for effective and efficient management of the patient's communication disorders. The team's findings must be conveyed to the speech pathologist so that appropriate therapy can be carried out. In turn, information about the patient's response to speech therapy is needed to confirm or question the results of other diagnostic testing. Hence, reports about therapy must be made available to the speech pathologist on the team when crucial decisions are being made about such matters as diagnosis and management of velopharyngeal incompetence. The burden for maintaining communications is on both persons and must be attended to carefully.

The speech pathologist in the field must think as a member of the team and thus refrain from making specific recommendations for treatment that may be inconsistent with the overall plan. For example, an occasional speech pathologist will become concerned with a facial scar, discuss it with the child, and inform the parents that they should return to the team to have it revised. The team is then faced with a sizable counseling problem if the child is quite young and there are sound reasons for delaying further surgery. However, it is not only legitimate but highly appropriate to raise questions of this sort directly with the team and to provide them with the reasons for the special concern and interest.

Another pitfall to avoid is making a specific diagnosis in the absence of the information necessary to do so. It is far better to tell a parent that there are questions about velopharyngeal function and that a referral to a team is necessary than it is to say that the child definitely has a submucous cleft palate.

It is important also to remember that the team has responsibility for the child's treatment and must expect that speech pathologists in the field will cooperate with them by raising questions about matters that are unclear or that are not agreed upon. Some teams, for example, do not want a child to have speech therapy for a number of months following pharyngeal-flap surgery. While the speech pathologist must understand the team's thinking, he or she also must reserve the right to disagree and to discuss the issues with the team. It is ill-advised, however, in the best interests of the child, to undertake therapy unilaterally.

The other side of this coin is that the cooperating speech pathologist has important rights. One is the expectation that the team will welcome him or her into the extended team as a peer and will honor professional autonomy and integrity. McWilliams (1982) has addressed some of these problems.

TREATMENT RESOURCES

Speech pathologists working in public schools, independent clinics, or private practices must be well informed about resources for referrals in their vicinity. State and local treatment programs are best identified through a specialist who works with these disorders. Almost every teaching hospital in the United States has a cleft palate team, and the coordinator of the team will be useful in describing available services. In addition, speech pathologists should know about services offered through their local State Department of Health, and contacts should be made there so that those resources will always be available.

Families should be aware that teams are not available in most small communities and that traveling to a clinic is almost always necessary. This is not unique to craniofacial problems, but is sometimes the excuse for not seeking assistance when it is required. Getting such parents to accept these referrals can be difficult, but the speech pathologist frequently serves as an important facilitator.

The speech pathologist should try to visit the special centers where patients with clefts and other problems are treated, to observe and get acquainted. Visits should be planned ahead, but most clinics welcome such expressions of interest and concern.

THE COST OF TREATMENT

As for other serious diseases and disorders, treatment for cleft lip and palate and other abnormalities of the face and head is expensive. This is true because of the number of highly trained specialists who provide treatment over a period of years and because hospitalization is required at least once. We know of one child with very severe facial clefts who has had 53 operations in 13 years. This is unusual, but it serves to emphasize the extent of the problem and the great costs that can accrue.

Morris and Tharp (1978) estimated how much surgery, dentistry, and speech pathology would cost for three hypothetical patients with a range of treatment requirements. Using their 1977 data, with a 10% yearly increase during the past decade, present day estimated costs range from $35,000 for a patient with a relatively minor defect, to $85,000 for a patient with a more extensive problem. Even these figures did not include indirect costs such as travel expenses, loss of earnings, and child care for siblings, all of which can be substantial when the family lives a fair distance from the treatment center. Another cost that the family may or may not be expected to share is the expense of operating an interdisciplinary clinic. McWilliams (personal communication) compiled figures for budgetary purposes at the University of Pittsburgh and found that the cost per patient in that clinic for the fiscal year 1983-84 was $500 for team visits and special services. Since children visit clinics until they are 18 to 20 years old, the costs for that aspect of care should reach $10,000 per patient, exclusive of dental and surgical treatment.

How do families manage to pay these costs? If they have no assistance from health insurance or government health care programs, it can be very difficult. Private health insurance is a major source of help, and most underwriters now provide such support if the individual policy was in effect when the child with the cleft was born. Even so, many of these policies apply only when the patient is hospitalized. Outpatient diagnosis and procedures for otitis media, audiologic evaluations, speech and language studies, pediatric examinations, and psychological evaluations are frequently not covered.

Dental treatment is not covered by most insurance policies, and even when dental coverage is available, it is usually limited. Thus, dental expense can be a significant problem for families, since most children with cleft lip and palate require extensive orthodontic work over a period of years if optimal occlusion and facial growth are to be obtained. This care is expensive as is prosthetic management when that is required.

Speech and language intervention, including therapy, is frequently available as part of the public schools' programs for preschool and school-age children who have special needs. When that is the case, these services are provided at no direct cost to the family. However, sometimes these programs may not be satisfactory to the needs of an individual child or family, and assistance is sought from a speech pathologist in a community hospital or private practice, on a fee-for-service basis. In many cases, these services are not included in health insurance plans.

Financial aid can be obtained from various state and federal agencies. Morris and Tharp (1978) obtained information about such programs available in 44 states and through federal programs. The sources included Crippled Children's Services or similar programs under other names, Medicaid, Vocational Rehabilitation, special state and county programs, Champus (a program for military dependents), federal grants, Indian Health Service, and local teaching hospitals and clinics.

Some years ago teaching hospitals and clinics and state Crippled Children's Services, which receive federal aid through grants for Maternal and Child Health Services, provided substantial financial support for these patients. Most teaching hospitals, particularly those connected with public universities, had plans by which patients who met reasonable economic criteria could obtain diagnosis and treatment at costs that were substantially reduced or free. However, during the past decade, many of these assistance programs have been changed and the extent of support reduced. Some of these budgetary losses have been compensated for by other federal and state programs such as Medicaid, but not to a satisfactory extent. Many states have, however,

maintained their State Cleft Palate Programs even in the face of shrinking funds. They now receive aid through block grants from Maternal and Child Health and can themselves decide how to spend the money. Many parents are working to see that funds are allocated for cleft care.

Morris and Tharp also listed a number of private sources of assistance. These included the teaching hospitals and clinics referred to earlier, Easter Seal agencies, March of Dimes, civic and service clubs, and donated professional services. These resources may become more important as others decrease, but are probably not significant at this time.

Identifying avenues for obtaining financial assistance for the patient with cleft lip and palate is important and deserves serious consideration in health-care planning (Morris and Morris, 1980).

Several states have passed laws requiring that complete care for cleft lip and palate be provided under the terms of any health insurance policies written in those states. Such legislation is now pending in a few other states, and it offers hope for the future.

INTERESTED ORGANIZATIONS

The primary national organizations that are especially interested in craniofacial abnormalities, including clefts, are the American Cleft Palate-Craniofacial Association (ACPA)[1] referred to earlier and the Cleft Palate Foundation (CPF).[1] These two closely related groups are dedicated to the study and treatment of cleft lip and palate and related disorders, with membership from all of the professions that are referred to in this book. ACPA holds an annual meeting, usually in the spring, at which a variety of scientific papers are presented. This association publishes a *Newsletter* as well as the *Cleft Palate Journal*. Students are welcomed at annual meetings and as *Journal* subscribers. CPF is primarily an educational organization which emphasizes public and parent concerns, publishes educational materials, and provides information for public consumption via the newspapers, television, and radio.

At least two states have organizations of craniofacial teams to provide coordination of services with that state: Illinois (Will and Aduss, 1987) and Pennsylvania.

The March of Dimes Birth Defects Foundation[2] also has an interest in these disorders. They provide support for research and educational activities and publish public educational material.

SUMMARY

We believe that diagnosis and treatment of craniofacial disorders including cleft lip and palate are provided more effectively and efficiently by an interdisciplinary team that includes a variety of specialists, has a strong organizational structure, and meets face-to-face on a regular basis. All members, including the speech pathologist, must work to achieve the best communication possible among themselves and with the patient and family. Good communication and respect among team members are vital to the creation and maintenance of a superior clinical program.

Cleft lip and palate and related disorders are expensive to treat, and the costs are increasing at the same alarming rate, as they are for health care in general. Faced with a cumulative cost of something in excess of $50,000, families may be badly in need of assistance. Limited funds are available in many states, but they are unevenly distributed. Although further development of private and public insurance plans is expected to be helpful, in the meantime, many families find themselves under severe financial stress.

---

[1]Both ACPA and CPF can be addressed at 1218 Grandview Avenue, Pittsburgh, Pennsylvania 15211.

[2]1275 Mamaroneck Avenue, White Plains, New York 10605.

REFERENCES

Bleiberg AH, Leubling HE. Parents' guide to cleft palate habilitation: the team approach. New York: Exposition Press, 1971.

Broder H, Richman L. An examination of mental health services offered by cleft/craniofacial teams. Cleft Palate J 1987; 24:158.

Cooper HK. Integration of services in the treatment of cleft lip and cleft palate. J Am Dent Assoc 1953; 47:27.

Falk ML, ed. A cleft palate team addresses the speech clinician. Springfield: CC Thomas, 1971.

Holve LM. An ideal cleft palate-craniofacial team for comprehensive longitudinal patient care (editorial). Cleft Palate J 1985; 22:235.

Koepp-Baker H. The multidisciplinary approach to the treatment of the child with cleft palate. J Internat Coll Surg 1955; 24:3.

Koepp-Baker H. Cleft palate. Multidisciplinary management. In: Morris HL, ed. Cleft lip and palate: criteria for physical management. Iowa City: University of Iowa Press, 1963:21.

Koepp-Baker H. The craniofacial team. In: Bzoch KR, ed. Communicative disorders related to cleft lip and palate. Boston: Little, Brown, 1979:52.

Krogman WM. The cleft palate team in action. In: Cooper HK, Harding RL, Krogman WM, Mazaheri M, Millard RT, eds. Cleft palate and cleft lip: a team approach to clinical management and rehabilitation of the patient. Philadelphia: WB Saunders, 1979:145.

McWilliams BJ. Personal communication.

McWilliams BJ. State of the art—an opinion—the trouble with speech pathology. Cleft Palate J 1982; 19:281.

Middleton GF, Lass NJ, Starr P, Pannbacker M. Survey of public awareness and knowledge of cleft palate. Cleft Palate J 1986; 23:58.

Mitchell CK, Lott R, Pannbacker M. Perceptions about cleft palate held by school personnel: suggestions for in-service training development. Cleft Palate J 1984; 21:308.

Morris HL. The structure and function of interdisciplinary health teams. In: Salinas CF, Jorgenson RJ, eds. Dentistry in the interdisciplinary treatment of genetic diseases. Birth Defects: Original Article Series, Vol 16. No. 5. New York: Alan R Liss, 1980:105.

Morris HL. The needs of children with cleft lip and palate: a comprehensive view. Division of Developmental Disabilities, University Hospital School, The University of Iowa, Iowa City, IA 1983.

Morris HL, Jakobi P, Harrington D. Objectives and criteria for the management of cleft lip and palate and the delivery of management services. Cleft Palate J 1978; 15:1.

Morris HL, Morris JM. A beam of light through the fog. Cleft Palate J 1980; 17:334.

Morris HL, Tharp R. Some economic aspects of cleft lip and palate treatment in the United States in 1974. Cleft Palate J 1978; 15:167.

Scheuerle J, Olsen S, Guilford AM, Redding B, Habal MB. A survey of nursing care for parents and infants with cleft lip and palate. Cleft Palate J 1984; 21:110.

Strauss RP, Meyerson MD. Panel discussion: treatment and maltreatment of birth defects across cultures in the United States. Annual Convention of the American Cleft Palate-Craniofacial Association, San Francisco 1989.

Smoot EC III, Kucan JO, Cope JS, Aase JM. The craniofacial team and the Navajo patient. Cleft Palate J 1988; 25:395.

Wells CG. The American Cleft Palate Association: its first 36 years. Cleft Palate J 1979; 16:86.

Whitehouse FA. Teamwork as a dynamic system. Cleft Palate J 1965; 2:16.

Will LA, Aduss MK. Illinois Association of Craniofacial Teams: a new state organization. Cleft Palate J 1987; 24:339.

4 | SURGICAL MANAGEMENT

It is our purpose to acquaint the reader with the surgical management of cleft lip and palate and related anomalies. This will be done from the perspective of the speech pathologist, who should understand some of the underlying principles of surgery, some of the complications and special problems that may be associated with it, the limitations of surgical solutions, and the responsibilities that the speech pathologist and the surgeon share. Technical descriptions of cleft surgery prepared by surgeons are provided in various texts, including recent ones by Millard (1976, 1977, 1980), Serafin and Georgiade (1984), and Bardach and Salyer (1987).

LIP SURGERY

The repair of the cleft lip, or cheilorrhaphy, is usually the first stage of surgical reconstruction when the baby has both cleft lip and cleft palate. It is an event that parents anticipate with mixed emotions. They are eager to have their child's face made whole, but they may fear the procedure and worry about having the baby cared for by someone else. Nevertheless, the surgery is a major event in their lives, and they rarely allow their concerns to stand in the way of having the cleft repaired. Some parents are comforted by the presence during the surgery of another parent who has gone through the same experience; others want to be alone. Participants on cleft palate teams try to be supportive but also to honor the feelings of the family. The speech pathologist should be alert to these feelings and needs and assist the family in any way possible. However, technical questions about surgery and hospitalization should be directed to the surgical and nursing staff.

The Goals of Lip Surgery

Musgrave and Garrett (1977) indicated that the overall goal is the normal appearance of the lip and nostril in infancy and throughout childhood, adolescence, and adulthood. They listed seven goals of surgery for the repair of cleft lip: (1) accurate skin, muscle, and mucous-membrane union; (2) symmetrical nostril floors; (3) symmetrical vermilion border; (4) slight eversion of the lip; (5) a minimal scar, which, through contraction, will not interfere with the accomplishment of the other four goals; (6) preservation of the Cupid's bow and the vermilion-cutaneous ridge; and (7) symmetry of the nostrils as well as of the nostril floors.

Age of Surgery

In theory, lip repair can be carried out at almost any age. However, for a variety of reasons, it is usually performed when the baby is about 3 months old (Osborn and Kelleher, 1983). The age will vary somewhat from surgeon to surgeon and from baby to baby. Many surgeons do not like to undertake the surgery before the baby conforms to the "rule of tens" (Wilhelmsen and Musgrave, 1966), that is, the child weighs at least 10 pounds, has a hemoglobin of at least 10 grams and a white count no higher than 10,000, and is at least 10 weeks of age. In addition, the baby should be in good general health when the procedure is done. There are several reasons for delaying surgery beyond the newborn period. Peet (1969) wrote that a better technical result is achieved if the repair occurs after the neonatal period. Musgrave and Garrett (1977) reported that many surgeons prefer to delay the surgery until the parents have lived with their baby long enough to understand and accept the cleft and what will be involved in managing it. This time to adjust may help the parents to develop a realistic attitude about the results and benefits of surgery and to be accepting of the inevitable scar. The speech pathologist should be aware also that the repair of the cleft lip may be delayed beyond 3 months if the baby has other problems that are of higher priority than the correction of the lip deformity. These prevailing attitudes to the contrary, however, some surgeons are repairing cleft lip in the first few days of life. Data about outcome when this is done are yet to be developed.

Surgical Procedures

Rogers (1967) provided an interesting review of the historical evolution of plastic and reconstructive surgery, including techniques for repair of cleft lip. The development of methods for anesthesia and infection control in the latter part of the 19th century were of course major advances. Thereafter, surgeons could design operations that were more complicated and took longer to carry out. Since they knew more about controlling infection, the results were improved over those that had been achieved in earlier times.

Figure 4.1 shows a baby with a unilateral complete cleft lip before and after surgical repair. There are relatively few basic surgical procedures for use in lip repair, but there are several variations on each one. The major approaches are four: the straight-line closure, the triangular flap, the quadrilateral flap, and the rotation-advancement. Quadrilateral flaps are rarely used today.

The Rose-Thompson repair (Fig. 4.2) is an example of a straight-line procedure reserved for minimal clefts. This technique is usually unsatisfactory for more extensive clefts because it sacrifices too much tissue, creates a short lip, and destroys the Cupid's bow (Ross and Johnston, 1972; Musgrave and Garrett, 1977; Harding, 1979).

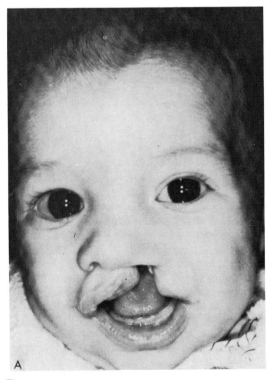
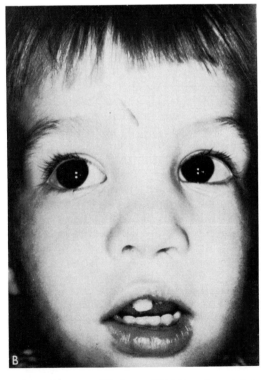

Figure 4.1 An infant with a unilateral cleft lip before and after surgery. (From Musgrave RH, Garrett WS. The unilateral cleft lip. In: Converse JM, ed. Reconstructive plastic surgery. Vol 4. Philadelphia: WB Saunders, 1977:2030.)

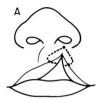 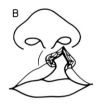 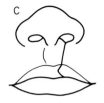

Figure 4.2 The Rose-Thompson lip repair is a straight-line procedure not often used for extensive clefts.

Figure 4.3 shows the triangular-flap procedure introduced by Tennison (1952), and modified by Randall (1959). This operation, or one of its many variations, is still commonly used and is incorporated into the Skoog (1958) technique. The use of triangular flaps in lip repair probably originated in the mid-1800s but was not widely adopted until the early 1950s. Many surgeons prefer the triangular flap because it wastes little or no tissue and produces a full lip with a natural Cupid's bow. However, the lip may become elongated on the cleft side, and this deformity is difficult to correct.

The rotation-advancement (Millard, 1971, 1976, 1984) (Fig. 4.4) is now commonly used for the repair of unilateral clefts (Musgrave and Garrett, 1977). Millard first performed the operation during the Korean War on a 10-year-old boy with an unrepaired unilateral cleft lip and introduced the operation in 1955 at the First Interna-

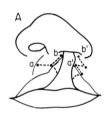 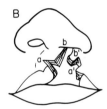 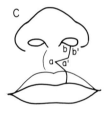

Figure 4.3 An illustration of a triangular-flap surgical procedure for lip repair.

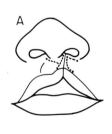 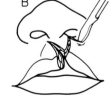 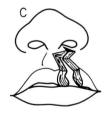

 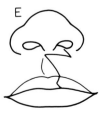

Figure 4.4 The Millard rotation-advancement technique of lip repair.

tional Congress on Plastic Surgery. The rotation-advancement technique is described as highly flexible in that it permits the surgeon to make modifications during the execution of the surgery. The resulting scars are ideally situated to minimize visibility; disproportionate growth is not often a problem; the lip is symmetrical; and revisions are simpler than with other approaches. Millard's various modifications of the technique make it appropriate for incomplete, complete, and wide clefts alike (Harding, 1979).

The procedures just described are used for the repair of unilateral cleft lips and have been adapted for bilateral clefts as well. However, bilateral clefts present unusual complications, some of them quite severe. (Millard, 1977; Georgiade et al., 1984; Bardach and Salyer, 1987). The premaxilla and the prolabium are likely to be attached to the tip of the nose; the columella may be almost nonexistent; and the maxillary arch may be collapsed behind the premaxilla (Figure 4.7).

In order to minimize such problems, some-

times, prior to lip surgery, an attempt is made to create a better alignment of the separated structures. Several methods have been reported. One is an intraoral dental prosthetic appliance, such as that described by Hotz (1969) and Hotz and Gnoinski (1979). Another is a device for the application of external pressure to the premaxilla (Fig. 4.5). Still another is a lip adhesion, which is the surgical closure of both sides of the nostril floor and of the upper part of the lip (Fig. 4.6), described by Randall (1965) and recently by Millard (1984).

The bilateral cleft lip is sometimes repaired in two stages, first one side then the other, but both sides can also be repaired in the same operation. Figure 4.7 shows a child with a bilateral cleft lip before and after surgery.

The surgeon chooses the surgical procedure on the basis of his or her preference, the type of cleft, the extent of the cleft including its width, and whether or not there appears to be adequate tissue for use in the repair. The operation is carried out under general anesthesia, usually using the

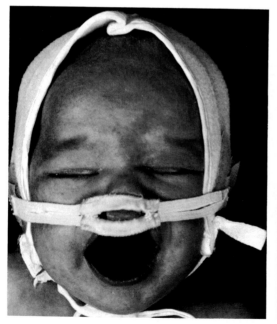 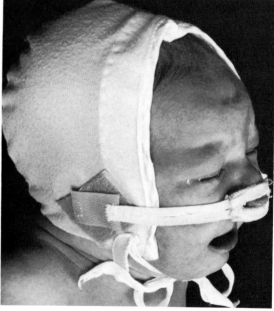

Figure 4.5 Head cap to which 1/4-inch elastic is attached using Velcro or hooks and eyes to allow adjustment of tension. The band is retained in place more easily when split so that one piece goes over the prolabium and one piece below it. A piece of smooth material protects the lip from the rough elastic. Traction is used continuously, except when feeding. When started at birth, effective repositioning may be anticipated within 1 to 3 months, at which time the lip can be repaired. (From Cronin TD. The bilateral cleft lip with bilateral cleft of the primary palate. In: Converse JM, ed. Reconstructive plastic surgery: principles and procedures in construction, reconstruction and transplantation. 2nd ed. Vol 4. Philadelphia: WB Saunders, 1977:2052.)

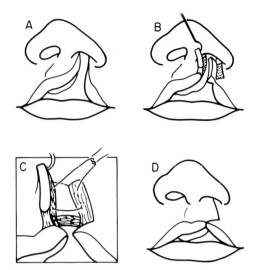

Figure 4.6 A complete cleft of the lip is modified to create an incomplete cleft by the Randall-Graham lip adhesion operation. (Adapted from: Musgrave RH, Garrett WS. In: Converse JM, ed. Plastic and reconstructive surgery: principles and procedures in correction, reconstruction and transplantation. Philadelphia: WB Saunders, 1977:2033.)

oral endotracheal tube. See Bloch (1984) for a useful discussion of anesthesia for the pediatric patient.

Postoperative Care

Most surgeons advocate use of antibiotic ointment on the sutures as a precaution against infection. In addition several methods are used to shield the wound and to reduce tension along the suture line. Millard (1976, 1984) uses an appliance to prevent application of adhesive tape to the sutures. Bardach and Salyer (1987) use paper tape for suture support, particularly for the unilateral cleft lip.

It is also common practice for the baby to be placed in arm restraints of some sort after the operation in order to control arm and hand movements, which could damage the repair (Millard, 1976, Musgrave and Garrett, 1977).

Bardach and Salyer (1987) recommend massage of the scar following lip repair to keep the "scar soft and the lip pliable" (p. 19), as do Georgiade et al. (1984).

Careful feeding practices must be used for as long as 3 weeks postoperatively. Either a bulb syringe or a medicine dropper is commonly utilized. Cereal and other soft foods can be mixed with the formula if indicated. Each surgeon has preferences in this regard, so feeding will vary somewhat from one setting to another.

Surgical Complications

There are a number of possible complications associated with cleft lip surgery. Wilhelmsen and Musgrave (1966) listed pneumonia, partial or complete surgical breakdown, postoperative hemorrhage, diarrhea, otitis media, and mild upper respiratory infections. They reported complications in 13.4% of their series of 585 cleft lip operations from 1950 to 1964 inclusive. Infection is of major concern because it may be responsible for dehiscence of tissues and the development of fistulas. For this reason, precautions are taken to avoid repairing the lip if there is any evidence of infection prior to surgery.

Bromley et al. (1983) assessed morbidity of cleft lip repairs performed on 135 patients during a 15-year period. There were no deaths in the series and no instances of postoperative hemorrhage or sepsis. Minor wound separation was the complication most often observed. They reported that major morbidity, such as complete wound dehiscence, aspiration pneumonia, and severe respiration depression, was slightly more common in patients who had lip repair during the first week of life than in those who had repair later.

Secondary Lip and Nose Surgery

Many if not most patients require secondary surgery to improve the appearance of the lip scar, alter certain aspects of the lip if necessary, bring the two sides of the lip and nose into symmetry with each other, elevate the nostril, or remove undesirable flair. Such work is usually delayed until the child is older in order to permit optimal growth to take place. The age when surgery of this type is undertaken depends upon many factors that the surgeon and cleft palate team take into account (Converse et al. 1977a).

PALATAL SURGERY

Cleft palate and its management vary from patient to patient just as cleft lip does. There are a variety of surgical techniques that are appropriate

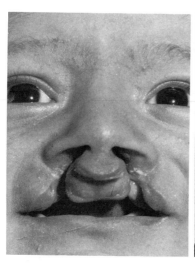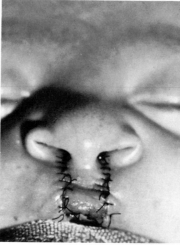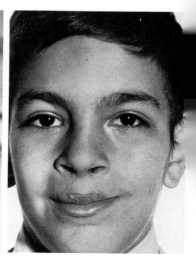

Figure 4.7 Complete bilateral cleft lip with protrusion of the premaxilla, before and after repair. (From Cronin TD. The bilateral cleft lip with bilateral cleft of the primary palate. In: Converse JM, ed. Reconstructive and plastic surgery. 2nd ed. Vol 4. Philadelphia: WB Saunders, 1977:2066.)

for the initial closure of the palate, often referred to as "primary surgery." We shall discuss some of these approaches and their underlying principles in sufficient detail to provide the background necessary for a basic appreciation of palatal closure and for further independent exploration of the literature.

The Goals of Palatal Surgery

The major reason for performing surgery to close a cleft palate is to create a velopharyngeal valving mechanism that is capable of separating the oral from the nasal cavities during speech. Added benefits to the patient when this mechanism is functioning properly include easier intake of food, reduction in the number of upper-respiratory infections, and improvement to the status of the middle ear. In addition, parents probably experience a psychological lift when the cleft is corrected. These are all important advantages, but they never replace speech adequacy as the primary goal of surgery. Without closure of the cleft in the palate by some means, the patient faces a lifetime of impaired ability to communicate. For this reason, the speech pathologist is concerned with the nature of surgery for the repair of cleft palate and with the outcome as reflected by the patient's speech.

Age of Surgery

There seems to be general agreement among most surgeons that primary cleft palate surgery can be performed effectively before the child is 2 years of age (Osborn and Kelleher, 1983), and many perform the surgery even earlier, between 9 and 12 months. Having said that, however, it is important for speech pathologists to be aware of the controversial nature of issues surrounding the age of palatal repair. Surgeons avoid an operation at any age if the health or the survival of the patient is at risk. As with cleft lip, surgery for cleft palate is likely to be delayed if there is any evidence of infection that might compromise postoperative recovery or if there are other malformations that may be life-threatening or must take priority over the cleft palate. While palatal surgery is desirable, it is in the final analysis, an elective procedure that can, and sometimes should, be delayed.

Another issue pertains to the circumstances under which the best technical result can be obtained. For example, some surgeons prefer to delay the operation on the premise that the cleft may narrow with age. Others may want to wait for increased dimensions in an unusually small oral cavity. Decisions about these and other similar problems must be made by the surgeon, who has the ultimate surgical responsibility for the patient. However, other team members, including the speech pathologist, may have relevant observations, which the surgeon will want to take into account when the age of surgery is decided. Compromise is possible, and it does occur.

Parental preference may be another factor in the timing of palatal surgery. Some parents may refuse surgery or may want to delay it because of fear, religious beliefs, or other family problems. Others may insist that the surgery be done earlier than is desirable. Parents with these attitudes are candidates for careful counseling by the surgeon and the speech pathologist.

In addition to these influences on surgical age, there are two other major sources of controversy. They have to do with how surgery affects the growth and development of the maxillofacial complex and the conditions under which normal speech can be anticipated. Ideally, it is desirable to repair the palate sufficiently early to permit the child to develop normal speech while, at the same time, avoiding adverse effects on growth and development of the maxillary arch and the midface.

Historically, the suspicion that early cleft palate surgery is harmful to subsequent facial growth and development stems from work such as that by Graber (1949, 1950, 1954). The hypothesis has since been examined by a number of investigators, among them Dahl (1970), Ross and Johnston (1972), Krogman et al. (1975), Krogman (1979), and Ross (1987).

Prior to the 1987 report by Ross, which we consider of landmark status, the consensus was that early surgery was indeed harmful to growth and development. The main questions to be answered were ones like how harmful? when might the extent of damage be lessened? and what are the important variables to consider in further consideration of the relationship between age of surgery and facial growth?

The ambitious and comprehensive study by Ross provides considerable information about these questions, including the one about timing. His report is arguably the most relevant publication about the topic ever made and merits careful study by the serious scholar. Briefly his strategy was to invite clinicians from 13 treatment centers to provide cephalometric records from their various patient groups for his analysis. Identification about the patient and treatment received was also provided; only patients with complete unilateral cleft lip and palate were included in the sample, for whom 1600 cephalometric radiographs were available. Data from 16 treatment groups were available; in addition, a serial control group of noncleft children for the Burlington Growth Study, University of Toronto, was used for comparison purposes. Differences in treatment among the various centers permitted evaluation of several treatment strategies, among them variations in timing of cleft palate surgery.

Specifically he evaluated dimensions of maxillofacial development for five groups: early palatal surgery (at or before 11 months); medium (between 12 and 20 months); late (between 21 and 33 months); delayed (early soft palate followed by hard palate repair between 4 and 9 years); and unoperated. Subject groups ranged in number from 35 to 211.

Ross summarizes his findings in this way:

The overall conclusion must be that there is not a great deal of difference in facial growth related to the age of hard and soft palate repair, but the data seemed to favor early repair in the first year of life as having a slight advantage over the medium and delayed hard palate repair groups, and the late repair group results were not as good.

He writes further:

The arguments circulated on the age at which to operate seem to focus on whether to operate early for speech purposes at the expense of facial growth, or to delay hard palate surgery for optimum growth at the expense of speech. This study demonstrates rather clearly and conclusively that facial growth is **not** *the issue, and if anything, early repair provides better facial growth than does the delayed hard palate repair. (p. 62).*

The Ross data are not the last word about the relationship between timing of cleft palate surgery and subsequent facial growth and development. There still are issues to be addressed. One is whether his findings hold also for females and for other cleft types. Another is whether children at risk for growth deficiency can be identified early and treated in a way so as to minimize the risk. A third is whether some children may show "lags" and "catch-ups" in growth patterns, related to surgical timing, that are not reflected in Ross's data and their clinical significance.

A larger issue, not specifically related to timing of surgery, is the relationship between a statistical difference and a perceptual difference. We are not yet clear about the degree to which a cephalometric measurement, significantly different from the normal, would be reflected in perceptible difference. Such information is badly needed to give perspective to the research findings.

On the other hand, the investigation reported by Ross is extremely impressive, and the data are persuasive that the dangers of harming facial growth by early cleft palate surgery are not as great as formerly thought.

The available data about age at palatoplasty and subsequent speech proficiency come from ten studies: Veau (1933), Jolleys (1954), McWilliams (1960), Peet (1961), Lindsay et al. (1962), Holdsworth (1963), Morris (1978), Dorf and Curtin (1982), Randall et al. (1983), and Hardin et al. (in prep). Nine of the ten studies indicate that better speech proficiency is more often demonstrated when palate surgery is performed early than late. Certainly there are differences in methodology among the studies, especially with regard to the criterion measure of speech proficiency, but the consistency of finding is impressive and persuasive.

There are some remaining questions to be answered. One is about the strength of the relationship. Another is whether the relationship is linear throughout infancy and childhood, or whether there is an optimal age for palate surgery, an age at which the provision of normal velopharyngeal function is crucial for the development of normal speech and language skills (Kemp-Fincham et al., in press). Further investigation is needed.

Further investigation is needed also to provide additional information about the nature of the relationship between the two variables. That is, why might earlier palatal surgery be more often associated with normal speech than later surgery?

Perhaps there are three separate hypotheses to be tested. The first is that the physiologic potential of the muscles comprising the velopharyngeal valving mechanism is irretrievably lost by delay in moving them into normal relationships with each other. A test of this first hypothesis is to determine whether early palatoplasty results in physiological velopharyngeal competence more frequently than does later palatoplasty.

The second hypothesis is that, when palatoplasty, and hence any possibility of normal velopharyngeal functioning, is delayed until after the child has begun to talk, the resulting speech patterns are apt to be defective because of the abnormal velopharyngeal anatomy and physiology. A test of this hypothesis is to determine whether early palatoplasty results in normal patterns of speech more frequently than does later palatoplasty.

The third hypothesis states that delay in palatoplasty ensures that the child will have defective articulation patterns and that the defective articulation will impair intelligibility sufficiently to curtail normal language development. This hypothesis presumes that language learning is facilitated by the ability of parents and others to understand the child's early attempts at verbal communication. This hypothesis can be tested by determining whether overall language skill is depressed when speech intelligibility is poor during the developmental years.

The distinctions among the three hypotheses are important since they focus on different aspects of oral communication: the ability to control oral and nasal features of speech (velopharyngeal function); speech production skills (speech articulation); and speech-language learning in general.

Data from several of these 10 studies cited address the two latter hypotheses that focus on behavior, specifically the notion of whether abnormal speech production patterns are learned when palate surgery is delayed. However, most of the available data seem to address both physiologic and behavioral status. It is reasonable to do so, since the desired end product is normally oral and normally articulated speech.

There would be special relevance to data that examine speech variables and growth variables simultaneously as a function of age at palate surgery. We know of only one such report, that by Jolleys (1954). He found better speech results in his patients who had surgery before 2 years of age and no differences in maxillofacial development. More data of this type are badly needed.

We take the position that the speech pathologist must be aggressive in informing other members of the management team that early surgery is more likely to give better speech results than is late surgery. However, we also want to avoid maxillofacial deformities because a clinically significant malocclusion is frequently a hazard to speech production. Furthermore, cosmetic appearance is important to the patient, and certainly growth deficits are difficult and expensive to treat. We must all join in our efforts to discover ways of meeting the several goals of palatoplasty to everyone's satisfaction. The ideal age for palatal closure remains controversial, and the age selected will depend upon the philosophy of the surgeon and the treatment team responsible for the child's care. Although that age is likely to be between 12 and 18 months, there are many exceptions. The speech pathologist who understands the reasons for these differences in clinical practice will be better able to work with the team and to be supportive to parents.

This seems an appropriate time to indicate that consideration is being given to methods of in utero (prenatal) surgery that might be applicable to cleft lip and palate (Sullivan, 1989; Harrison, 1989). These methods are still experimental but have proven satisfactory in the prenatal surgical repair of other structural deformities. Of particular interest is the finding that in utero surgical wound healing is characterized by less scar tissue formation than surgery performed after birth. For obvious reasons this is a complex matter since it involves prenatal detection of the cleft and the social and ethical issues that follow (Strauss and Davis, 1989). However, these technological advances are very real and will have great future impact on the diagnosis and treatment of many birth defects, including cleft lip and palate.

Surgical Procedures

Our purpose here is to provide general information about several surgical procedures commonly used in North America for primary cleft palate surgery. More specific and technical information can be found in a number of articles, chapters, and texts written by surgeons, including Grabb et al. (1971), Converse (1977), Millard (1980), Serafin and Georgiade (1984), Bardach and Salyer (1987), and Bardach and Morris (in press).

The main focus is on three procedures, the V-Y retroposition, the von Langenbeck, and delayed hard palate closure, sometimes referred to as primary veloplasty; additionally we consider more briefly several other procedures that have been described by various authors.

V-Y Retroposition

Sometimes called the Oxford technique, the Wardill-Kilner, or the Veau-Wardill-Kilner procedure, there are a number of variations of this basic surgical design. Calnan (1971) traced the V-Y

procedure now in general use to Veau and considered the modifications introduced by Kilner and Wardill to be significant.

The procedure (Fig. 4.8) involves the surgical preparation of two *unipedicle* or single-base flaps of palatal mucoperiosteum, the soft tissue on both sides of the palatal cleft. The flaps are then elevated from the bony palate and retropositioned so that the cleft defect is covered with soft tissue and the length of the soft palate increased. For patients with clefts that extend through the alveolar ridge, a somewhat more elaborate approach is used (Calnan, 1971). This technique appears to yield a higher success rate as measured by speech results than any other technique that has been studied, although there is considerable variability in the data.

A limitation of this and other procedures is that the actual gain in palatal length is not as great postoperatively as it is during surgery because of contraction of scar tissue. Another disadvantage is that the relatively large surfaces of denuded bone in the anterior palate may result in maxillary growth deficits, particularly in the anterior- posterior direction. Some surgeons have discarded the procedure in favor of simpler, more conservative methods (Harding, 1979).

The two-flap palatoplasty (Bardach and Salyer, 1987) was designed to counteract some of these limitations. It also involves two single base flaps, with special emphasis on closure of the anterior cleft, in order to prevent fistula formation.

The island flap is used in combination with the V-Y procedure (Millard, 1963, 1980; Millard et al. 1970). It uses a flap of palatal mucoperiosteum and provides for dissection of the levator muscles from the hard palate: both maneuvers are designed to increase and maintain palatal length.

von Langenbeck

Lindsay (1971) provided an historical review of the procedure, indicating that it probably originated in the middle 1800s. This makes it the oldest known surgical technique for the repair of palatal clefts. A lateral incision is made on both sides of the palate along the alveolar ridge (Fig. 4.9). The margins of the cleft are pared, and two mucoperiosteal palatal flaps are elevated. These flaps are *bipedicle*, that is, they have two attachments, one anterior and the other posterior. The two soft-tissue margins of the cleft palate are then

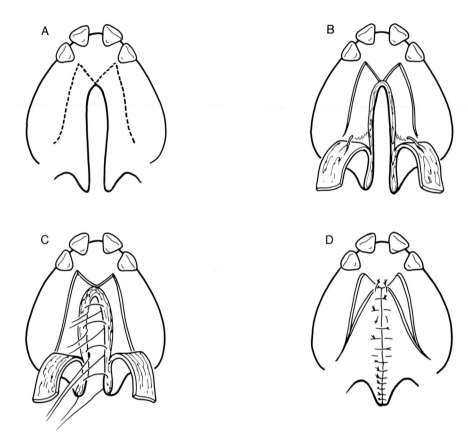

Figure 4.8 The V-Y retroposition procedure for the repair of palatal clefts. Note the two unipedicle flaps. (Adapted from Stark RB. Cleft palate. In: Converse JM, ed. Reconstructive plastic surgery: principles and procedures in correction, reconstruction and transplantation. 2nd ed. Vol 4. Philadelphia: WB Saunders, 1977:2096.)

approximated and sutured. This maneuver is simplified by the relaxation of tissues created by the incisions, which also serve to reduce tension on the united palate. Bone denudation occurs at the lateral margins of the palate, on both sides, extending the length of the hard palate. Modifications of the von Langenbeck are used also for palatal clefts that extend through the alveolar ridge.

A theoretical limitation of this procedure is that not much palatal lengthening can be expected because of the bipedicle nature of the flaps. In addition, the lateral areas of bone denudation may result in collapse of the maxillary arch.

Delayed Hard Palate Closure (Fig. 4.10)

As the name indicates, the soft palate cleft is repaired first, sometimes at the time of the cleft lip surgery, and the hard palate surgery is delayed.

Apparently described first by Schweckendiek (1966, 1978), the method has been reported also by Fara and Brousilova (1969), Perko (1984), Campo-Paysaa and Ajacques (1983) Jackson et al. (1983), Meijer and Cohen (in press), and a number of authors in the impressive volume about treatment results, edited by Gnoinski (1986). The rationale for the procedure is to unify the soft palate musculature at an early age to promote normal velopharyngeal function, and to delay hard palate surgery to avoid or minimize damage to subsequent maxillofacial development (Witzel et al. 1984). Although there is variability among surgeons in age of veloplasty, most perform the procedure during the first year of life, some at 3 months of age, in combination with lip surgery. The majority of surgeons report hard palate surgery during the preschool years, but Schweckendiek typically delays that stage even longer, until age 13 (Bardach et al. 1984a). Sometimes a

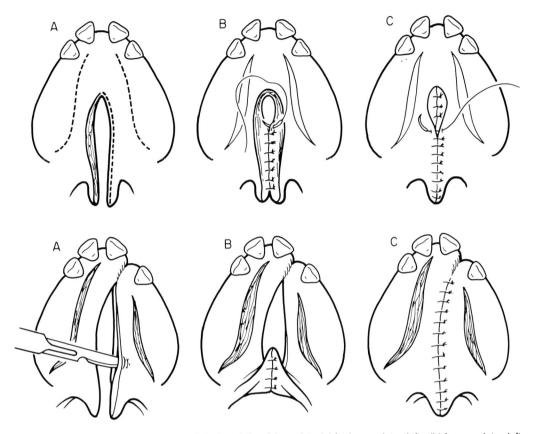

Figure 4.9 The von Langenbeck method of closing clefts of the palate (a) for incomplete clefts; (b) for complete clefts.

dental prosthetic appliance is constructed to cover the anterior cleft palate until hard palate surgery.

There is considerable controversy about whether, in the presence of the anterior cleft, the restoration of the velum is sufficient to promote eventual normal velopharyngeal function and speech production patterns. As we shall see in later discussion there are some data about that question.

Primary Pharyngeal Flap

This procedure has been used by a few surgeons as a means of ensuring improved speech. It will be discussed under the heading of secondary surgery since that is the usual purpose of the pharyngeal flap.

Structuring the Levator Sling

Although not technically a procedure for the closure of a palatal cleft, many surgeons incorpo-

rate it with either the V-Y or the von Langenbeck. Muscle separation has been recognized for many years as one feature of clefts involving the soft palate. Uniting these muscles has long been viewed as a necessary part of palatal repair. However, only recently have efforts been made to create the levator sling as it is found in the normal palate (Chapter 31 in Millard 1980). In patients with clefts, the levator and the palatopharyngeus muscles are attached to the posterior margin of the hard palate instead of mingling together in the palatal aponeurosis. Removing those muscles from the hard palate and bringing them together in the soft palate appears to create added length in the palate. Braithwaite (1964) described this procedure and indicated that it would maintain palatal length. Kriens (1969, 1970) referred to an end-to-end muscle union in midline as an intravelar veloplasty, a technique that is used increasingly today (Trier and Dreyer, 1984; Marsh et al, 1989). Fara et al. (1970a and b) also focused

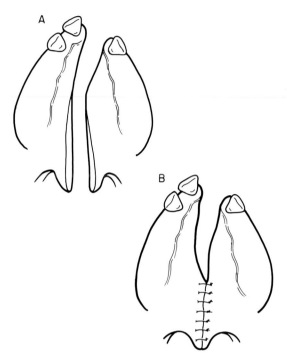

Figure 4.10 Delayed hard palate closure in which the soft palate is closed first and repair of the hard palate is delayed to a later age.

attention on the levator sling. Garrett (personal communication) considered the procedure to be more relevant to successful palatal repair than the choice of technique for palatoplasty.

Other Procedures

The island flap, described by Millard (1963, 1970) has been referred to earlier. Another procedure is the Z- plasty, described by Furlow (1978, 1986) and used by Randall et al. (1986).

Alveolar Bone Grafting

Many patients whose clefts extend through the alveolus (the gum ridge) have repair in adolescence by bone graft. By such treatment, the patient may acquire better dental occlusion of significance in the production of fricatives and affricates, especially the sibilants. Rationales and procedures for this kind of surgery are described by Bergland et al. (1986) and Vig et al. (in press).

Postoperative Care

The postoperative care of babies who have undergone palatal surgery can be difficult because the surgery is undertaken when the children are too young for explanation and too old for easy control. Many surgeons want to avoid allowing the child to suck from a bottle and suggest dropper or cup feeding. Liquids are recommended for at least 48 hours after surgery; then pureed foods can be introduced. Arm restraints are used for a short time as they are with lip surgery, and the baby is usually placed in a mist tent for a day or two to provide a moist environment. Sedation is sometimes required immediately after surgery, particularly for very active babies.

Explaining these procedures to parents before the surgery will help them feel more comfortable with the care their baby is receiving. Otherwise, they may be anxious because they are afraid that extreme or unusual measures are being taken. Speech pathologists can often effectively alert parents about what to expect. However, counseling of this type should be undertaken only when it is acceptable to the surgeon. In addition, there must be understanding of the procedures to be used in a particular case. Those presented here are meant to show the kinds of things to be considered. They provide general rather than specific guidelines.

There are many possible complications associated with surgical repair of the palate (see Wray et al., 1979 and Moore et al., 1988 for recent reports). They are much like those that occur with lip repair and are not usually of major consequence, although every precaution is taken to avoid even minor negative events in the postoperative period. We shall discuss mortality and oronasal fistulas, two topics about which there are considerable data.

Mortality Rate

Fortunately, todays parents can be assured about the safety of the operation, although they can be given no guarantees as to its results. Prior to the 1940s and the advent of endotracheal anesthesia, survival was of some concern, primarily because the anesthesia was not sufficiently sophisticated to permit the surgeon to do as careful and meticulous surgery as is possible today. Musgrave (1969) reviewed early reports about cleft palate surgery and found mortality rates ranging from 2 to 7%. Other summaries have been consistent with these percentages. For example, Calnan (1971) reported that no deaths occurred in a series of 245 palatal procedures. Wray et al. (1979) reported no deaths in 47 patients, as did Moore et al. (1988) in 196 patients. Today, death as the result of palatal closure is very rare.

Oronasal Fistula

Another surgical complication of major concern is an oronasal (sometimes called palatal) fistula (Fig. 4.11). Musgrave (1969) reviewed the early literature about postsurgical fistula formation and found rates of "surgical failure" of between 2% and 80%. He quoted Davis (1931) as having estimated that 70 to 80% of operations for cleft palate were failures because of surgical breakdown. Since that time things have improved remarkably. Oneal (1971) reviewed more recent findings and found the incidence of failure to be between zero and 21%. Schultz (1986) reported that 22% of 199 patients had postoperative fistulas, of which half were symptomatic.

Clefts involving the soft palate seem less likely to develop a fistula following surgical repair than do more extensive deformities. Peer et al. (1954) found no fistulas associated with soft palate repair as compared to a 14.8% occurrence rate for other types of clefts. Lindsay (1971) reported no fistulas in his series of clefts of the palate only as compared to 15% for unilateral and 20% for bilateral clefts.

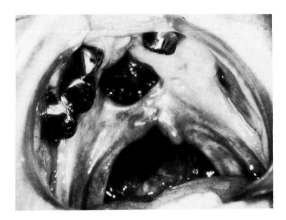

Figure 4.11 A large anterior oronasal fistula combined with a short palate.

the palate only as compared to 15% for unilateral and 20% for bilateral clefts.

The type of surgical repair may influence the occurrence of a fistula. Van Demark (1974a and b) found that 47% of a group of Danish children who had had V-Y procedures at a mean age of 24.6 months had a fistula, whereas only 10% of an Iowa group who had had von Langenbeck operations at an average of 37.2 months developed a fistula. Morris (1978) found a fistula in 3% of 101 patients who had had the Demjen modification of the V-Y technique in which the neurovascular bundle is severed in order to obtain palatal length.

Abyholm et al (1979) reviewed 1108 patients who had had von Langenbeck procedures between 1954 and 1969 and found a fistula in 18%. The lowest occurrence rate, 3.5%, was associated with incomplete palatal clefts. Cosman and Falk (1980) reported that surgical closure of the hard palate in patients who had undergone repair of the soft palate at an early age, as in the Schweckendiek technique, resulted in a fistula rate of 65%, which the authors described as "embarrassingly high."

Oneal (1971) suggested that the combined effects of certain palatoplasty techniques and the severity of the defect may be important in the etiology of a palatal fistula. Since both of these factors have been implicated, this conclusion appears to have merit. Preoperative upper respiratory infection has also been identified as a significant factor in the etiology of fistulas (Musgrave and Bremner, 1960; Oneal, 1971). Musgrave and Bremner (1960) found an overall rate of "healing difficulty" in 7.7% of 780 cases. However, these healing difficulties were associated with an oronasal fistula in only 5% of the cases. Large fistulas occurred in only 1.5% of the 780 cases.

Moore (1988) reports postsurgical fistulas in 11 (6%) of 196 patients, more frequently in those who had received Wardill-Kilner palatoplasty, and less frequently in those who received perioperative antibiotics. Morris et al. (1989) report no fistulas in 45 patients who had two-flap palatoplasty, nor did they find any fistulas in a later study of 58 patients who had unilateral cleft lip and palate with two-flap palatoplasty (Bardach et al., in press).

These reports suggest that a fistula may occur in any surgical series and that the prevalence, even today, varies widely from surgeon to surgeon, from cleft type to cleft type, and perhaps from procedure to procedure.

Symptoms associated with an oronasal fistula have been extensively discussed in the literature. Many writers and most clinicians and speech pathologists indicate that, in some cases, liquids escape from the oral cavity through the fistula into the nose during swallowing. Lehman et al. (1978) observed that food may become impacted in a fistula and cause malodor. Even a small fistula, they reported, may cause loss of suction and may interfere with the retention of dentures. In addition, the nasal mucosa adjacent to the fistula may hypertrophy with resulting increase in nasal discharge. Lindsay (1971) observed nasal secretions flowing down into the mouth through fistulas. He recognized that young children are more likely to present symptoms of these types than are older children or adults, many of whom have learned to compensate and thus avoid some of the disturbances. These symptoms can be distressing and a source of embarrassment. Speech pathologists may encounter children who do not want to eat in the presence of other children because they are embarrassed by a trickle of chocolate milk or some food seeping out of their noses. The speech pathologist can be effective in helping children handle such situations and in educating their peers to understand, so that social pressures are reduced.

A palatal fistula may also result in the nasalization of speech. There is some question about how large the fistula must be to affect speech perceptually. Shelton and Blank (1984) noted a loss of intraoral air pressure for large fistulas but not systematically for those of small or moderate size. Henningsson and Isberg (1987) report that a fistula 4.5 mm^2 in area influences speech and resonance. In a later paper (in press) they report that their clinical experience indicates that a fistula of "only a few mm^2" can have such an effect also. It is clear that each patient must be individually assessed to determine the extent of the influence of an existing palatal fistula. Treatment for an oronasal fistula is indicated if distressing symptoms are present, and is covered briefly in the section on secondary surgery.

Caution must be exercised in diagnosing deficiency of the velopharyngeal valving mechanism, for possible pharyngeal flap surgery, in the presence of an oronasal fistula. That is because, in many cases, it is difficult to separate the effect of the fistula from the effect of a deficient mechanism. As a general statement, it seems better to repair the fistula first, then evaluate the velopharyngeal mechanism for possible surgery.

Assessment of Surgical Results

The results of palatal repair are commonly assessed first by the status of speech and then by the adequacy of maxillofacial development. The rationale for using these two measures was described earlier when the timing of surgery was considered. Because the major purpose of palatal closure has been speech outcome, that is the focus here. The major goal of surgery to close the hard palate is to separate the oral from the nasal cavities so that the structures are not under undue tension and so that fistulas do not develop. The objective is to accomplish the major goal without sacrificing facial growth. The major goal of surgery to close the soft palate is to ensure that palatal length, bulk, muscle arrangement, and movement are sufficient to work cooperatively with the pharyngeal walls to achieve closure of the velopharyngeal port during speech. A patient able to do that has velopharyngeal competence. When the patient is not able to achieve closure, velopharyngeal incompetence, inadequacy, or dysfunction is present.

McWilliams (in press) has provided a comprehensive review of investigations designed to determine the speech results associated with different surgical procedures. Although the criteria for judging success were often vague, the results were surprisingly consistent. At least 15 investigations evaluated speech outcome in relationship to the V-Y procedure. Success rates ranged from lows of 21 and 42% (Blocksma et al., 1975; Lindsay, 1971) to a high of 95% (Braithwaite, 1964). The mean success rate for the 15 studies was 67%, with two falling between 60 and 70% (Greene, 1960; Calnan, 1971; Dreyer and Trier, 1984; Marsh et al., 1989); four between 70 and 80% (Battle, 1967; Evans and Renfrew, 1974; Krause et al., 1975, 1976; Morris 1978); and five between 80 and 95% (McWilliams, 1960; Braithwaite, 1964; Trauner and Trauner, 1967; McEvitt, 1971; Musgrave et al., 1975). Nine of the 15 studies, a solid majority, report success rates of over 70%.

Eight reports have presented data on the von Langenbeck procedure. Success rates ranged from 47% (Bardach et al., 1984b) to 73% (Musgrave et al., 1975), with a mean of 58%. Three studies reported success rates, usually not well specified, between 47 and 60% (McEvitt, 1971; Blocksma et al., 1975; and Krause et al., 1975, 1976; Bardach et al. 1984b). The most frequent success rate is between 50 and 60%. Dreyer and Trier (1984) report a much higher success rate (91%) when they combined the von Langenbeck and levator reconstruction.

There is variation also in obtained speech results associated with early closure of the soft palate and delayed closure of the hard palate. Schweckendiek (1978) found that 57% of his patients had "normal" speech as judged by intelligibility. Cosman and Falk (1980), using clinical judgments, concluded that only 34% of their patients had "acceptable" speech. Bardach et al. (1984a) used a battery of tests to determine velopharyngeal competence and classified only 6 (16%) of 43 patients operated by Schweckendiek as having velopharyngeal competence and 16 (37%) as having marginal competence. Noordhoff et al. (1987) reported data for Mandarin-speaking children from Taiwan who had soft palate closure before 18 months and hard palate surgery at 6 years, as compared to normal preschool children. The children with clefts had significantly poorer speech production skills than the comparison group. Meijer and Cohen (in press) report good results for 65% of their 116 patients, evaluated by the Iowa method (Morris 1978; Bardach et al. 1984a, 1984b). Van Demark et al. (1989) used the Iowa method also to evaluate 37 patients treated by the Zurich approach (Hotz et al., 1986). He reported that 94.5% of the patients were judged clinically to show normal or marginally normal velopharyngeal function for speech. Further, nearly every subject showed good speech production skills. By any standard, these are remarkable findings and indicate that the primary veloplasty strategy can be used successfully with careful treatment and close follow-up.

In conclusion, the available data indicate that any one of several surgical procedures for primary palatoplasty, when performed by experienced surgeons, can be expected to yield normal or nearly normal velopharyngeal physiology for speech about 75% of the time. On balance, the V-Y retroposition, or some modification of it, appears to be used most often. Certainly it should be apparent that research of this kind is difficult to conduct because so many variables seem impor-

tant and because experimental control of some of these variables is frequently problematic at best. Thus, we must depend on imperfect data gathered whenever there is the opportunity, searching for trends if not definitive results. Important variables to consider in the design of the investigation are: cleft type, age of surgery, the type of surgery, and other forms of intervention being utilized. Sample size should be large enough to ensure both valid and reliable data. When possible, prospective studies such as that reported by Marsh et al. (1989) should be conducted.

Of particular concern is the need to include a wide range of patients representing a random sample of the population available for study. Clinical researchers are often troubled by the tendency of patients with notable problems to remain in the caseload, whereas those whose treatment has been successful fail to return for subsequent examinations because they are not interested in further treatment. To study only the former group of patients is to eliminate those with satisfactory results.

Subjects who are selected to participate in studies of outcome should be old enough to cooperate in the testing required and should have speech that is free from developmental disorders unrelated to the success or failure of surgery. Beyond that, careful, systematic methods of evaluation of speech and of velopharyngeal function are required if the data are to be meaningful. There are a number of approaches to consider in this evaluation, and these are discussed in detail in Chapters 16 through 19.

SECONDARY PALATAL SURGERY FOR VELOPHARYNGEAL INCOMPETENCE

We have seen that about one in four patients who have primary surgery for the correction of palatal clefts fails to achieve velopharyngeal competence. Since there are no methods of speech therapy that result in the achievement of velopharyngeal closure, additional physical management— surgical or dental—will be required in most cases if normal or near-normal speech is to be realized by these patients. Dental prostheses, sometimes used to correct incompetence, are described in Chapter 5. However, the majority of cases of velopharyngeal incompetence are managed surgically rather than prosthetically. In the centers with which we are associated, it is rare for a prosthesis to be selected over surgery if conditions warrant surgical intervention. Several commonly used secondary surgical procedures that have been designed to improve velopharyngeal competence are presented here so that speech pathologists will be aware of them and of what they can accomplish. A useful description of several of these procedures, from the surgeon's perspective together with excellent illustrations is provided in Chapter 8 of Bardach and Salyer (1987).

Pharyngeal Flap

The pharyngeal flap procedure is widely used and appears to be successful. It was probably first described about 1875 but was not in common use until the 1950s. Since that time, the pharyngeal flap has received wide attention and has been the topic of many investigations.

A pharyngeal flap is created by elevating a unipedicle soft-tissue flap from the posterior pharyngeal wall. As shown in Figure 4.12, the flap can be inferiorly or superiorly based, the latter orientation being the one preferred by most surgeons. One end of the flap remains attached to the pharyngeal wall, while the other is sutured to or sandwiched between the two layers of the palate to bridge and partially occlude the velopharyngeal space. On each side of the flap, there is a lateral opening, which permits nasal breathing,

nasal drainage, and nasalization of speech when that is appropriate. The goal is for these two lateral ports to close during speech that requires velopharyngeal closure. This is accomplished by mesial movement of the lateral pharyngeal walls (Morris and Spriestersbach, 1967; Skolnick and McCall, 1972; Shprintzen et al., 1979) in concert with any movement that may be present in the soft palate. Zwitman (1982a, b) studied the pharyngeal flap mechanism by oral endoscopy. On the basis of his observations, he distinguished between lateral wall and posterolateral wall movements. He compared the latter to the phenomenon of Passavant's ridge. In 18 patients with normal oral resonance he noted various combinations of velar (palatoflap), lateral wall, and posterolateral pharyngeal wall movements.

There is controversy as to whether the palatoflap structure moves as one component in the velopharyngeal valving mechanism in patients who have had pharyngeal flaps. Shprintzen et al. (1979) reported that the 120 patients they examined by multiview videofluoroscopy and nasopharyngoscopy showed no such movement. On the other hand, Tuttle (1969) found that the lack of palatoflap movement was associated with defective speech more often than when movement occurred. More information is required on this issue.

A crucial problem in constructing a soft-tissue flap is that the flap must be wide enough and at the proper level to permit closure of the two

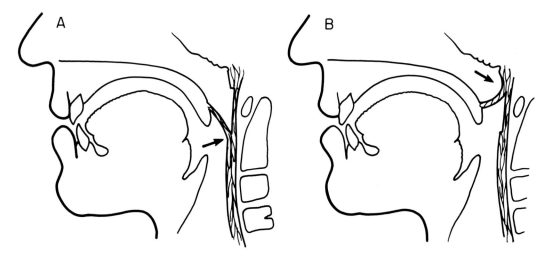

Figure 4.12 (a) An inferiorly-based pharyngeal flap. (b) A superiorly-based pharyngeal flap.

lateral ports during speech by action of the pharyngeal walls. At the same time, the flap must not be so wide that the lateral ports are occluded or too small for effective nasal respiration. If this is the case, the patient will be a persistent mouth breather, will probably have hyponasality and denasalized nasal consonants, and may suffer from sleep disturbances ranging in severity from severe snoring to sleep apnea.

Orr et al., (1987) report that airway obstruction immediately after pharyngeal flap surgery is resolved in most patients within 3 months. More data of this sort are urgently needed.

The conventional method for obtaining proper flap width appears to be visual inspection at the time of surgery. Most surgeons probably make the flap as wide as the surgical field permits, assuming that with normal shrinkage after surgery it will not be too wide.

Another means of attempting to control the size of the lateral ports is the placement of a catheter in the port during the surgery (Hogan, 1973; Hogan et al., 1977), shown in Figure 4.13. The presumption in this approach is that the dynamic nature of the palatoflap structure and of the lateral pharyngeal walls will close the portals appropriately during speech. The catheter represents the desired port size; the surgeon works around it, fashioning the flap so that the two openings between the flap and the pharyngeal wall will be neither larger nor smaller than the catheter. Special precautions are taken to avoid postoperative shrinkage. They used two catheters, each 10 mm^2 in size, based on data by Warren and Devereau (1966) and Isshiki et al. (1968). Recent data reported by McWilliams et al., (1981) indicated that a velopharyngeal opening of 20 mm^2 results in seriously defective speech. In addition it seems likely that the technique is not as precise as the authors claimed because the size of the lateral ports and the position of the flap change following surgery as a result of the healing process.

Some attention has been given to varying the construction of pharyngeal flaps based on judgments about the clinical needs of the patient. Shprintzen et al. (1979) reported the results of a study designed to evaluate the effectiveness of three procedures for the construction of pharyngeal flaps. Sixty patients were assigned in random order to one of five surgeons. The surgeon then selected the procedure to be used. Another 60 patients had surgery later than the first 60 and were assigned to one of the three procedures on

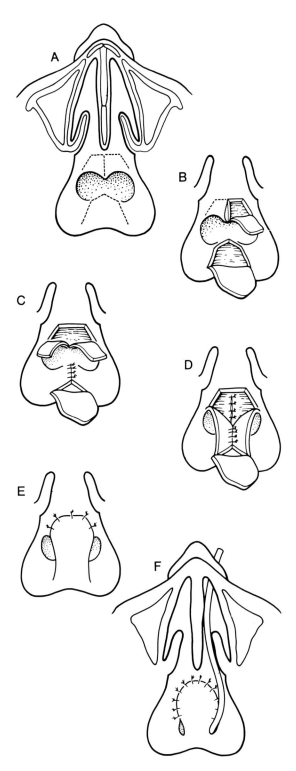

Figure 4.13 Control of lateral ports in surgery for pharyngeal flaps as suggested by Hogan et al. (1977).

the basis of preoperative findings about the mechanism as seen on multiview videofluoroscopy and through nasopharyngoscopy. Results obtained when a surgical procedure was assigned on the basis of the preoperative examination were superior to those achieved when the procedures were selected by the randomly assigned surgeons. The authors also reported that all 120 subjects achieved closure of the lateral ports solely on the basis of "medial movement of the lateral pharyngeal walls." They did not comment about the need for the lateral-wall movement to coincide with the flap as it elevates along with a dynamic palate. Zwitman (1982b) also made suggestions about specific methods of constructing pharyngeal flaps in order to make the best use of varying degrees and kinds of preoperative movement in the velopharyngeal structures.

It should be pointed out that surgical opinion differs in how high or how low in the pharynx the pharyngeal flap is elevated. This is true for either a superiorly based or an inferiorly based flap. The position of the flap may be important in relation to the maximum excursion of the lateral pharyngeal walls. If no movement is present, a high, broad, superiorly based flap generally is more effective in improving the separation between the oral and nasal cavities than is a narrow flap lower in the pharynx. These are variables that have not been carefully studied in relation to speech and that are worthy of continuing investigation.

Age at Surgery

When the flap is a secondary procedure, the age at surgery is likely to be between 6 and 12 years (McWilliams, in press), as soon as possible after the diagnosis of velopharyngeal incompetence is made. The major factor is that the patient must be old enough to cooperate well during diagnosis, must have sufficient verbal expressive ability to provide an adequate speech sample, and must demonstrate stable patterns of velopharyngeal activity. A six-year-old child is usually old enough for valid decisions to be made about the need for a flap. It can be done earlier than that in children who can be successfully evaluated at younger ages. Much depends upon the individual child.

Surgery for older patients is technically possible, but some surgeons feel that the results are less positive the older the patient is when the flap is constructed. There are few reliable data about age as it relates to the success of a pharyngeal flap.

Riski (1979) found better development of articulation skills in children who had the surgery before rather than after the age of 6 years. Tuttle (1969) reported that improvement in speech occurred at all ages, but that it was more pronounced before 8 years of age.

Complications

Nylen and Wahlin (1966) and Graham et al. (1973) have reported complications associated with pharyngeal flaps. Nylen and Wahlin found airway complications in connection with bleeding in 14 of 103 patients (14%). In 11 of the 14, bleeding was satisfactorily checked; tracheotomy was necessary in four; and there was one death. Graham et al. described complications in 46 of 222 patients. Seven of the 46 had hemorrhages; seven required tracheotomy; and partial or complete separation of the flap occurred in 18. Persistent and significant nasal obstruction was found in 12 patients, and there was one death. These complications seem excessive in light of today's clinical experience. Thurston et al. (1980) found significant nasal obstruction in eight of 85 patients, all of whom benefited from revisions of the pharyngeal flaps.

Assessment of Surgical Results

Facial Growth and Development

Three studies have been reported about patterns of facial growth following pharyngeal flap surgery: Subtelny and Pineda Nieto (1978), Keller et al. (1988), and Semb and Shaw (in press). The rationale of the investigations was that, according to Semb and Shaw, the procedure "may adversely affect subsequent development . . . by inducing functional adaptations in facial form secondary to increased airway resistance . . . (and) by anteroposterior maxillary growth restraint (p.2)." Taken together, the three data sets seem to address the question well and yield essentially negative results. On the basis of present information, the concern about facial growth following the construction of a pharyngeal flap appears to be unwarranted.

Speech Results

As indicated by McWilliams (in press), research conducted in this country and abroad over the past 20 years has shown that patients are not harmed by the operation and that, almost without exception, their speech is significantly improved. Clinical judgments of speech have been used most commonly in these studies; some have employed physiologic techniques to assess velopharyngeal closure. Terminology to describe speech following a pharyngeal flap has ranged from such adjectives as "normal," "satisfactory," "improved," or "average." Such descriptions are frequently difficult to interpret. However, most of the studies reviewed employed one or more speech pathologists to make the judgments that led to the global clinical conclusions about speech status. "Normal" speech occurred in varying percentages of patients, ranging from 33% (Bernstein, 1967) to 100% when the pharyngeal flap was combined with palatal lengthening (Shprintzen, et al. 1979). Eight additional investigations reported from 34 to 92% success after a pharyngeal flap, with a mean of 72% (Smith et al., 1963; Skoog, 1965; Owsley et al., 1966, 1970; Bucholz et al., 1967; Bernstein, 1975; Smith et al., 1985; Trier, 1985; and Van Demark and Hardin, 1985). Engstrom et al (1970) used listener judgments and intelligibility tests to assess postoperative improvement, which was noted in 79% of 68 cases. How many of these were normal speakers or had adequate velopharyngeal valving is not clear.

Shprintzen et al. (1979) compared results achieved with the pushback procedure (palatal lengthening) combined with the pharyngeal flap, the sandwich pharyngeal flap, and the split-return with the flap. Normal speech was found in all nine of the subjects who had the pushback, in 72% of those who had sandwich flaps (another 24% were hyponasal while only 3% were hypernasal); and in 77% of patients who had the split-return. In the latter group, 18% were hyponasal, and 4% had hypernasality. In this series, the pushback procedure combined with the pharyngeal flap eliminated hypernasality without creating hyponasality, an obvious advantage.

Surgical Failures

These are associated with two clinical outcomes. One is the case in which the flap is too narrow or is improperly positioned so that the lateral pharyngeal walls cannot close the lateral portals, with the result that velopharyngeal incompetence persists. The other outcome is when

the flap is too wide, and the nasal airway is partially or completely obstructed.

When the flap is too narrow, the most attractive approach is to consider widening the flap or reducing the size of the lateral ports by some other means. Such surgery may be somewhat complex and technically difficult. Three reports about procedures designed for this purpose have been provided by Cosman and Falk (1975), Owsley et al. (1976), and Gray (in press). Another alternative is to use some injectible material for the purpose of narrowing the port; procedures of this sort are still in the experimental stages. When the flap is improperly positioned, usually too low in the pharynx, revision is sometimes carried out, but data about outcome are lacking.

When the flap is too wide, speech is hyponasal, and the patient may be an habitual mouth breather, with snoring occurring during sleep. In the more severe case, there may be indications of sleep apnea that warrant further investigations by special sleep studies or other physical examinations. Fortunately these extreme cases do not occur frequently. However, the speech pathologist must be alert for them.

When there are significant indications of obstruction of the nasal airway, surgical revision may be indicated. Some surgeons dilate the lateral ports, or they may reduce the width of the flap (Gray, in press). Sometimes, if the flap is new, revision may be delayed in the hope that the flap will narrow, that growth will increase the size of the airway, or that more lateral movement of the lateral pharyngeal walls will be demonstrated over time. Dentists concerned with mouth breathing may urge flap revision somewhat sooner. However, revision should only rarely be considered for at least a year after surgery. In doing flap revisions, care must be taken to avoid increasing the lateral ports more than is desirable to avoid recurrence of velopharyngeal incompetence.

Primary Versus Secondary Pharyngeal Flap Surgery

The pharyngeal flap was originally designed as a primary procedure but was seldom used. Only later did it become popular as a secondary technique. However, several surgeons have incorporated the pharyngeal flap into their primary palatal repairs (Conway 1951; Stark and DeHaan, 1960; Cox and Silverstein, 1961; Bucholz et al.,

1967; Stuteville et al., 1970; Stark and Frileck, 1971; and Dalston and Stuteville, 1975).

Primary pharyngeal flap surgery is controversial (Bingham et al., 1972). Those who favor its use as a primary procedure argue that there is no reason to take the risk that the primary palatoplasty will not yield velopharyngeal competence. As we have seen, that appears to be the case for about one in every four patients, and they usually require pharyngeal flaps later in life. Advocates of primary pharyngeal flaps believe that, for those patients, the delay in providing competence results in several years of unnecessarily impaired speech. They argue that delay may result in compensatory speech patterns that will require extensive and expensive speech therapy even after normal velopharyngeal function is achieved. This, of course, is precisely the same issue that was discussed in connection with the age of primary palatal repair.

On the other hand, specialists who oppose primary pharyngeal flap surgery contend that although the procedure seems to be successful and has few adverse side effects, it does result in abnormal speech and respiratory physiology and should not be used unless it is required, that is, after the first procedure has failed to produce velopharyngeal valving integrity. They comment that, when the technique is incorporated into the primary procedure, it is employed in patients for whom the need cannot be demonstrated. That means that at least three out of every four patients who have the procedure would not have required the flap since primary palatoplasty alone would have been sufficient. An overriding argument against the procedure is that the results are not generally better than the best outcomes reported for more traditional techniques. In addition, the possibility of habitual mouth breathing, possible long-term growth abnormalities, and undesirable respiratory deficits cannot be ignored even though there is scant evidence pointing to these side effects. On the other hand, airway obstruction resulting from lateral ports that are too small can be rather easily corrected. Consequently, at this time, the decision about whether to employ the primary pharyngeal flap depends on the preference of the surgeon. If we could predict prior to surgery those children at high risk for postoperative velopharyngeal incompetence, it might be possible to incorporate pharyngeal flaps with primary closure in those patients.

Primary pharyngeal flaps have been assessed in relationship to speech results in four studies. One (Stark et al., 1969) combined the primary pharyngeal flap with the von Langenbeck "before the onset of speech" in 32 children, all of whom were reported to have developed speech that was "average or above." Another (Bingham et al., 1972) compared 10 children who had had the V-Y procedure with 10 who had had primary pharyngeal flaps and found "less hypernasality in the primary flap group." Curtin et al (1973) compared two groups of 10 patients who had had pharyngeal flaps at a mean age of 15 years. One group had the operation as a primary procedure and the other as a secondary technique to correct residual hypernasality. No differences in outcome were found in the two groups. Dalston and Stuteville (1975) found either no hypernasality or minimal hypernasality in 94% of their 50 cases.

The primary pharyngeal flap is not a commonly used procedure except in older patients as in the study by Curtin et al. (1973). Yet, the limited data available point to the success of the technique.

Pharyngoplasty

In addition to the pharyngeal flap, several other procedures have been designed for the treatment of velopharyngeal incompetence.

One type of procedure is the lateral pharyngoplasty. This procedure is somewhat the reverse of the pharyngeal flap, designed to narrow the velopharynx, leaving a smaller central orifice. Reports have been made by Orticochea (1968, in press) and Jackson and Silverton (1977), Roberts and Brown (1983) and Jackson (in press). Orticochea (1983) indicates that his procedure is moderately successful, with best results achieved in patients who are younger and who have less severe clefts. Roberts and Brown (1983) report improvement in eight of their 10 patients and conclude that the procedure is useful for selected patients. Jackson (in press) reports a success rate of about 90%. He indicates also that the procedure is not suitable for all patients who show velopharyngeal dysfunction and that patients should be carefully selected for best results.

In another type of procedure, nontoxic substance is positioned in or injected into the posterior pharyngeal wall to provide a permanent pseudoadenoidal pad, which has the effect of narrowing the pharynx and improving the likelihood that velopharyngeal closure will occur.

Materials such as paraffin have been tried with poor results. Hagerty and Hill (1960, 1961) did the pioneer work in this country on pharyngeal augmentation following studies of pharyngeal physiology. Blocksma (1963, 1964) introduced implantations using synthetic materials such as silicone and Lewy et al. (1965), Smith and McCabe (1977), Kuehn and Van Demark (1978), and Furlow et al. (1982) used Teflon. There have been more recent reports about the use of dacron wool/silicone gel bag (Brauer et al., in press), cartilage (Trigos et al., 1988), and proplast (Wolford et al., 1989).

These techniques appear to work relatively well (normal speech ranging from 18 to 83% with "improvement" occurring in all but about 25%) if patients are selected carefully. However, several factors must be considered in the selection process. First, the palate must be mobile and well coordinated. The reason for this is that advancing the posterior pharyngeal wall cannot compensate for a palate that moves poorly or that is uncoordinated. Secondly, the velopharyngeal gap must not be large because there is a quantitative limit to the amount of material that can be injected into the pharyngeal walls. Augmentation methods cannot be expected to be successful if the velopharyngeal space in lateral view is larger than 3 or 4 millimeters. Indeed even that gap may be too great. Bluestone et al. (1968a,b) found that the procedure was most successful when subjects had videofluoroscopic evidence of a light touch closure in lateral projection, with a very close approximation when the neck was extended.

The most important message to be gained from this discussion of procedures designed to correct velopharyngeal incompetence that remains after primary surgery or that occurs for other reasons is that it is no longer necessary from a technical point of view for patients to suffer from the continuing effects of nasalized speech. Surgical techniques exist for the correction of such problems, and they are successful.

CLOSURE OF ORONASAL FISTULA

As indicated earlier, surgical failure of palatoplasty can result in an oronasal fistula. Sometimes the fistula is readily apparent; other times it is discovered only by close examination. In some patients the appearance of an oronasal fistula seems related to maxillary expansion by ortho-

dontics. It is possible that expansion could break down a surgical repair, but more probably an existing fissure only becomes more evident as a result of the orthodontic treatment (Ross and Johnston, 1972).

When the fistula is clinically significant for either speech or nasal regurgitation, it should be closed. In most cases surgical repair is the treatment of choice (Musgrave and Bremner 1960; Holdsworth 1963; Oneal 1971; Jackson et al., 1976; Lehman et al., 1978; Bardach and Salyer, 1987; Schultz, 1989). Although many can be operated successfully, surgery for others is sometimes difficult because of size and location, poor blood supply, or scar tissue from earlier surgery.

Management by prosthesis is indicated for some patients, especially if a dental prosthesis is recommended for esthetic, occlusal, or speech purposes, or if surgery is considered difficult. Residual alveolar clefts may also be treated by prosthesis, although many such defects are closed by alveolar bone grafts. Typically, alveolar defects do not result in nasalization of speech.

On a related matter, the speech pathologist needs to consider the impact of the unrepaired hard palate on speech following delayed closure of the hard palate. Obviously this is a residual cleft, not a postsurgical fistula, but the opening may need to be covered, usually by prosthesis, to prevent acquisition of abnormal speech production patterns.

Evaluation and treatment of an oronasal fistula must be conducted on an individual basis since there is such variety among patients. The deciding factors are impact of the fistula on speech, whether surgery is indicated, and dental status. With careful attention, a fistula can be successfully treated.

CRANIOFACIAL AND MAXILLOFACIAL SURGERY

Earlier discussion in Chapter 2 indicates the complexity of craniofacial disorders and hence the need for careful treatment, including surgery. Contemporary craniofacial surgery is based on the work of Tessier and his colleagues (Tessier et al., 1967; Tessier 1967, 1971) although credit is due Sir Harold Gillies for the first craniofacial surgical procedure (Gillies and Harrison, 1950). Tessier's first craniofacial operation was done in 1965. Since that time, several craniofacial centers have been developed in the United States and abroad. Craniofacial surgery is complex, time-consuming, and demanding, and it must be performed under special conditions with properly trained personnel working in ideal facilities. This means that such surgery will not be carried out except in highly specialized centers.

To qualify as "craniofacial," at least one orbit must be involved in the surgery. If that is not the case and the correction involves structures at or below the lower eyelid, it is referred to as maxillo-facial surgery. Both maxillofacial and craniofacial surgery are custom-designed to correct variations in the mandible, the maxilla and midface, the molar region, the orbits, and the cranium, either individually or in combination. The surgery involves work on the bones of the face and head. Osteotomies and bone grafts are carried out in order to reduce or increase the size of various structures, change the relationships among structures, reposition various parts of the face, remold the bones of the skull, and create symmetry out of asymmetry. The procedures may be intracranial, in some cases, as well as extracranial (Converse et al., 1977 a,b,c; McCarthy et al., 1984; Marsh, 1986).

Craniofacial Team

Craniofacial surgery requires participation by several types of surgeons, including an ophthalmologist when the orbit of the eye is involved, and a neurosurgeon, when there is intracranial surgery. The orthodontist is also an important member of the team, particularly in describing structural aspects of the disorder, in estimating the effects of treatment on subsequent growth and in evaluating the results of treatment. Of specific importance in planning surgery are recent developments in computer-assisted imaging techniques that yield information in three dimensions (Marsh and Vannier 1983, 1986).

Surgical Procedures

General information about craniofacial surgical procedures is provided by Christiansen and Evans (1975), Converse et al. (1974, 1977b,c, 1979), Jackson et al. (1982), and Marsh and Vannier (1985).

Three Le Fort techniques form a basis for both maxillofacial and craniofacial surgery. The nature of the procedure selected depends upon the extent of the maxillary deformity, the portion of the maxilla that is affected, the type of malocclusion, and the degree to which other facial structures are involved. Osteotomies involving the maxilla are based on the fracture classification described by Le Fort in 1901. A Le Fort I is a low maxillary osteotomy, and a Le Fort II is described as a pyramidal naso-orbito-maxillary osteotomy, and a Le Fort III is a high maxillary osteotomy. In this latter procedure, the midface is detached from the cranium through the base of the nose, orbits, and pterygoid space.

The Le Fort I procedure is frequently used to advance the maxilla in patients with midfacial deficiencies associated with cleft palate. As seen in Figure 4.14, the maxilla may be advanced, retracted, rotated, or tilted. Converse et al. (1977) said that this procedure and variations of it are among the most frequently performed operations for the correction of maxillary deformities. Figure 4.15 shows the Le Fort I procedure. Note that, in addition to advancing the maxilla, bone grafts have been used. Wiring, and intermaxillary fixation are employed to stabilize the correction until healing takes place. Onlay bone grafts can be incorporated to improve facial contour.

There is general concern about the possibility of developing velopharyngeal incompetence as a result of maxillary advancement for the patients with and without cleft palate. Generally surgeons inform the patient and parents of the possibility of deterioration in speech, but do not do a pharyngeal flap unless the need is apparent after the intermaxillary appliances have been removed and healing is complete.

Witzel (1981) reported the use of a diagnostic battery of tests designed to predict postsurgical velopharyngeal incompetence. She reported that deterioration in nasal resonance, nasal air emission, and velopharyngeal closure occurred in 16% of 70 patients who had the Le Fort I. Of those who developed velopharyngeal valving problems, 81% had clefts. She concluded that the postoperative speech outcome could be predicted from the presurgical speech and valving evaluations. Figure 4.16A shows the preoperative status of a patient with borderline valving. Figure 4.16B shows the improved maxillary-mandibular relationships and the resulting velopharyngeal incompetence.

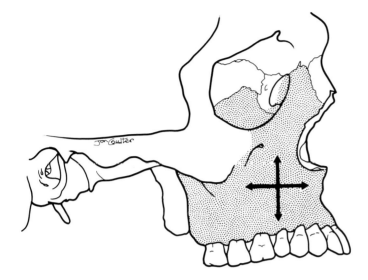

Figure 4.14 Directions in which the maxilla may be advanced, retracted, rotated, or tilted during a Le Fort I procedure. (From Witzel MA. Orthognathic defects and surgical correction: the effects on speech and velopharyngeal function. Doctoral dissertation. University of Pittsburgh, 1981. Adapted by permission of Mary Casey, Department of Visual Education, Hospital for Sick Children, Toronto)

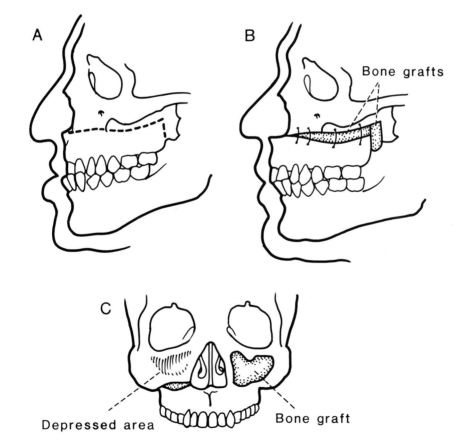

Figure 4.15 Details of the Le Fort I surgical procedure. (From Converse JM, et al. Deformities of the jaws. In: Converse JM, ed. Reconstructive plastic surgery: principles and procedures in correction, reconstruction and transplantation. Vol 3. Philadelphia: WB Saunders, 1977:1288.)

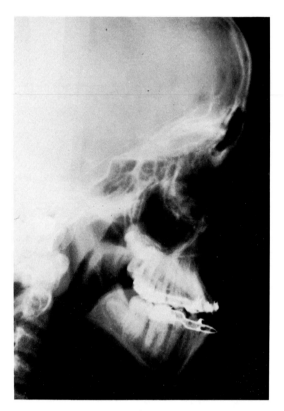 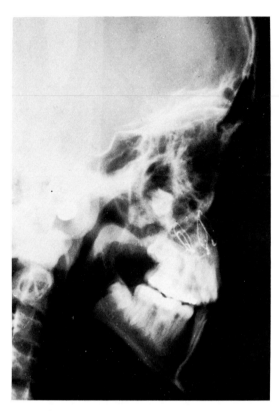

Figure 4.16 A. Preoperative lateral radiograph showing prognathia, negative maxillary incisor overjet and negative overbite and borderline velopharyngeal closure. B. Same patient one year after Le Fort I maxillary advancement. Note improved maxillary-mandibular relationships and resulting velopharyngeal incompetence. (From Witzel MA. Orthognathic defects and surgical correction: the effects on speech and velopharyngeal function. Doctoral dissertation. University of Pittsburgh, 1981. Adapted by permission of Mary Casey, Department of Visual Education, Hospital for Sick Children, Toronto)

Converse et al. (1977c) reported a personal communication from Schwartz (1976) in which he provided pre- and postsurgical information for nine patients who had midface advancements that included the maxilla. None developed hypernasality, and velopharyngeal orifice areas as measured by aerodynamic techniques never exceeded 5 mm^2.

The Le Fort II is more extensive than the Le Fort I and includes the upper portion of the nose and the medial orbital wall. Figure 4.17 shows the procedure. As can be seen, the deformity of the nose has been corrected along with the maxilla.

The Le Fort III formed the foundation for Tessier's original design for craniofacial surgery. This is extensive surgery and involves stripping the soft tissue from the underlying facial bones from the forehead to the maxilla. In this procedure, the eyes are attached only at the apex of the orbit and

the nasolacrimal apparatus, leaving the orbits free to be moved to a new position. If the surgery is to involve alteration of the bones of the skull or deep orbit, it will be considered to be intracranial, and the brain will be exposed and protected during the procedure. Figure 4.18 outlines a Le Fort III procedure. Figure 4.19 shows a patient with Goldenhar syndrome and hypertelorism prior to surgery and 3 years later.

Figure 4.20 shows a patient with Crouzon disease prior to and following craniofacial surgery. Both a Le Fort I and a Le Fort III were carried out. In addition to an improvement in appearance, this boy had a decrease in strabismus, an increase in the size of the nasal airway, a decrease in hyponasality, and an improvement in occlusion.

Craniofacial surgery involving the Le Fort III procedure is even more highly specialized than

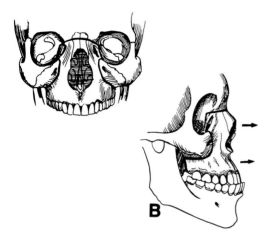

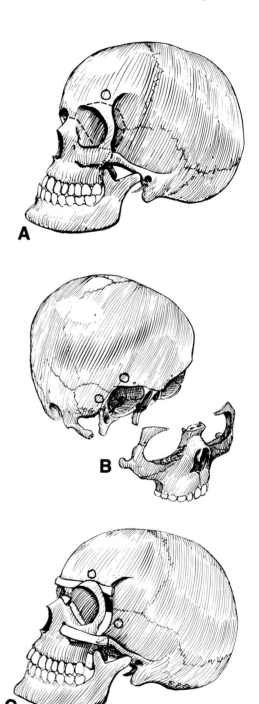

Figure 4.17   The Le Fort II osteotomy. A. Outline of the Le Fort II osteotomy. The osteotomy crosses the upper portion of the nasal bones, extends along the medial orbital wall above and behind the lacrimal groove, medial to the intraorbital foramen downward and laterally, below the zygomatic process of the maxilla to the pterygomaxillary junction. B. Lateral view of the osteotomy. (From Converse JM, et al. Deformities of the jaws. In: Converse JM, ed. Reconstructive plastic surgery: principles and procedures in correction, reconstruction and transplantation. 2nd ed. Vol 4. Philadelphia: WB Saunders, 1977:2480.)

the other two procedures. Facial procedures incorporating the Le Fort I or mandibular advancements, setbacks, or repositioning are done much more frequently and in more clinical settings by both plastic and oral surgeons. Since all of these structural alterations influence the speech mechanism, the speech pathologist is an important participant both prior to and following surgery.

Results of Surgery

Students who have not had personal experience with extensive surgery of this nature may expect that the results will change a person with marked craniofacial problems into one who is normal in appearance. While that is not the case, the improvement is usually notable, and function is sometimes remarkably altered for the better. These are worthy goals and can make a significant difference in the quality of life of the patient. The various illustrations in this chapter will help readers come to terms with what can be expected from these procedures.

Figure 4.18   The Le Fort III surgical procedure. A. Osteotomy lines including sites of burr holes for midface advancement: B. Osteotomy achieved: C. Bone grafts in place and midface advanced. (From Whitaker LA. Principles and methods of management. In: Bluestone CD, Stool SE, eds. Pediatric otolaryngology. Philadelphia: WB Saunders, 1983.)

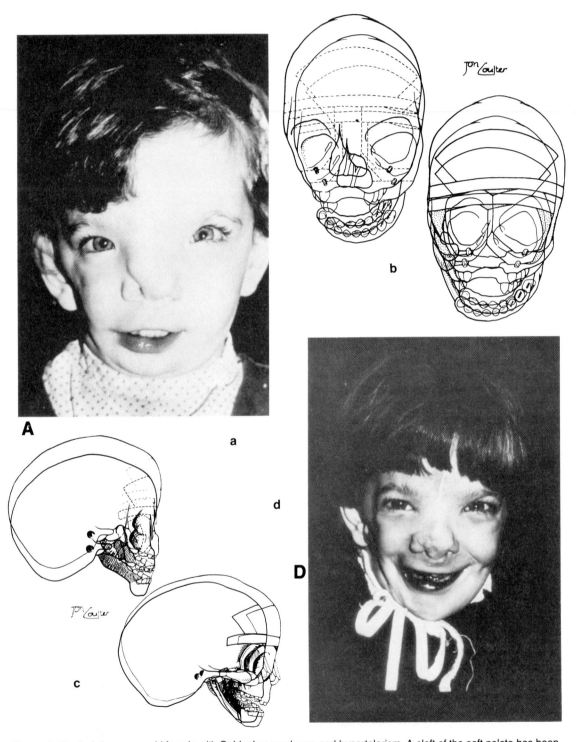

Figure 4.19   A. A three-year-old female with Goldenhar syndrome and hypertelorism. A cleft of the soft palate has been repaired. (The patient has a cleft through the right ala. There is a cleft in the zygomatic arch, absence of the ascending ramus of the mandible, and a hypoplastic right parotid gland. The right labial commissure is laterally displaced: B. Frontal view before and after correction of hemifacial microsomia and hypertelorism. The orbits were moved closer together and bone grafts were used to reconstruct the zygomatic arch, the ascending ramus of the mandible and the nasal bridge: C. Lateral view of the correction: D. The postoperative result 3 years after the corrective surgery. (Reproduced by permission of Dennis Hurwitz, M.D.)

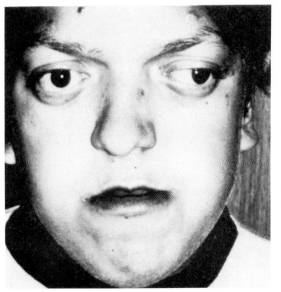
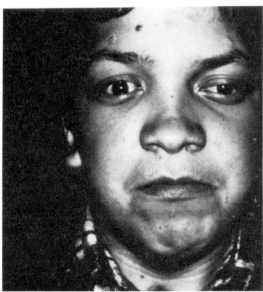

A

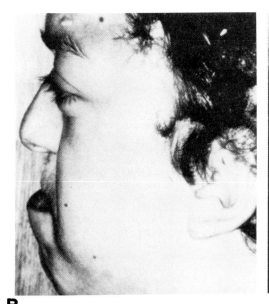
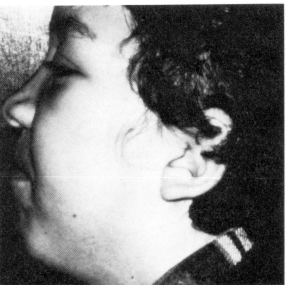

B

Figure 4.20 A. Full face views of 13-year-old male with Crouzon disease prior to surgery and one year after craniofacial surgery: B. Profile views prior to surgery and one year following craniofacial reconstruction: C. Preoperative view of dental malocclusion. There is an Angle Class III dental relationship due to maxillary hypoplasia: D. The dental occlusion 1 year after midfacial and orbital advancement: E. Diagram of skeletal reconstruction and bone grafting. There was a craniofacial dysfunction along the posterior maxilla and pterygomaxillary fissure. Transverse osteotomy (Le Fort I) of the maxillary allowed for anterior facial lengthening. (Parts C, D, and E on page 82) (Reproduced by permission of Dennis Hurwitz, M.D.)

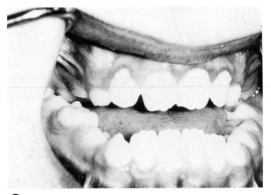

C

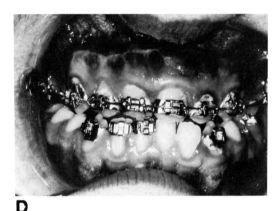

D

As indicated earlier, patients who qualify for craniofacial and maxillofacial surgery vary in communication abilities, ranging from normal to severe impairment. Those with impairment demonstrate a variety of problems in speech, language, and hearing. For this reason the speech pathologist who works with a craniofacial team needs considerable training and experience.

REFERENCES

Abyholm FE, Borchgrevink HHC, Eskeland G. Palatal fistulae following cleft palate surgery. Scand J Plast Reconstr Surg 1979; 13:295.

Bardach J, Morris HL, eds. Multidisciplinary management of cleft lip and palate. Philadelphia: WB Saunders, in press.

Bardach J, Morris HL, Olin WH. Late results of primary veloplasty: the Marburg project. Plast Reconstr Surg 1984a; 73:207.

Bardach J, Morris HL, Olin W, McDermott-Murray J, Mooney J, Bardach E. Late results of multidisciplinary management of unilateral cleft lip and palate. Ann Plast Surg 1984b; 12:235.

Bardach J, Salyer K. Surgical techniques in cleft lip and palate. Chicago: Year Book, 1987.

Bardach J, Morris HL, Gundlach K, et al. The Iowa-Hamburg project: late results of multidisciplinary management at the Iowa Cleft Palate Center. In: Bardach J, Morris HL, eds. Multidisciplinary management of cleft palate. Philadelphia: WB Saunders, in press.

Battle RJV. Speech results of palatal repair when performed before two years of age. Trans 4th Internat Cong Plast Reconstr Surg 1967; 425.

Bergland O, Semb G, Abyholm FE. Elimination of residual alveolar cleft by secondary bone grafting and subsequent orthodontic treatment. Cleft Palate J 1986; 23:175.

Bernstein L. Treatment of velopharyngeal incompetence. Arch Otolaryngol 1967; 85:67.

Bernstein L. A modified pharyngeal flap operation. Trans Am Acad Ophthalmol Otolaryngol 1975; 80:14.

Bingham HG, Suthunyarat P, Richards S, Graham M. Should the pharyngeal flap be used primarily with palatoplasty? Cleft Palate J 1972; 9:319.

Bloch EC. Anesthesia for the pediatric patient undergoing plastic surgery. In: Serafin D, Georgiade NG, eds. Pediatric plastic surgery. Vol 1. St. Louis: CV Mosby, 1984:50.

Blocksma R. Correction of velopharyngeal insufficiency by

silastic pharyngeal implant. Plast Reconstr Surg 1963; 31:268.

Blocksma R. Silicone implants for velopharyngeal incompetence: a progress report. Cleft Palate J 1964; 1:72.

Blocksma R, Leuz CA, Mellerstig KE. A conservative program for managing cleft palates without the use of mucoperiosteal flaps. Plast Reconstr Surg 1975; 55:160.

Bluestone CD, Musgrave RH, McWilliams BJ, Crozier PA. Teflon injection pharyngoplasty. Cleft Palate J 1968a; 5:19.

Bluestone CD, Musgrave RH, McWilliams BJ. Teflon injection pharyngoplasty—status 1968. Laryngoscope 1968b; 78:558.

Braithwaite E. Cleft palate repair. In: Gibson T, ed. Modern trends in plastic surgery. London: Butterworths, 1964:30.

Brauer RO, Fox DR, Humphreys MD. Augmentation of the posterior pharyngeal wall. In: Bardach J, Morris HL, eds. Multidisciplinary management of cleft lip and palate. Philadelphia: WB Saunders, in press.

Bromley GS, Rothaus KO, Goulian D. Cleft lip: morbidity and mortality in early repair. Ann Plast Surg 1983; 10:214.

Bucholz RB, Chase RA, Jobe RP, Smith H. The use of the combined palatal pushback and pharyngeal flap operation: a progress report. Plast Reconstr Surg 1967; 39:554.

Calnan JS. V-Y pushback palatorrhaphy. In: Grabb WC, Rosenstein SW, Bzoch KR, eds. Cleft lip and palate: surgical, dental, and speech aspects. Boston: Little, Brown, 1971:422.

Campo-Paysaa A, Ajacques JC. Early veloplasty in the treatment of cleft lip and palate. (French). Chir Pediatr 1983; 24:305.

Christiansen RL, Evans CA. Habilitation of severe craniofacial anomalies—the challenge of new surgical procedures: An NIDR workshop. Cleft Palate J 1975; 12:167.

Converse JM. Reconstructive plastic surgery: principles and procedures in correction, reconstruction and transplantation. Philadelphia: WB Saunders, 1977.

Converse JM, Hogan VM, Barton FE. Secondary deformities of cleft lip, cleft lip and nose, and cleft palate. In: Converse JM, ed. Reconstructive plastic surgery: principles and procedures in correction, reconstruction and transplantation. 2nd ed. Vol 4. Philadelphia: WB Saunders, 1977a:2165.

Converse JM, Kawamoto HK, Wood-Smith D, Coccaro PJ, McCarthy JC. Deformities of the jaws. In: Converse JM, ed. Reconstructive plastic surgery: principles and procedures in correction, reconstruction and transplantation. Vol 3. Philadelphia: WB Saunders, 1977b:1288.

Converse JM, McCarthy JG, Wood-Smith D, Coccaro PJ. Principles of craniofacial surgery. In: Converse JM, ed. Reconstructive plastic surgery: principles and procedures in correction, reconstruction and transplantation. Vol 4. Philadelphia: WB Saunders, 1977c:2427.

Converse JM, McCarthy JG, Wood-Smith D, eds. Symposium on diagnosis and treatment of craniofacial anomalies. Vol 20. St. Louis: CV Mosby, 1979.

Converse JM, Wood-Smith D, McCarthy JG, Coccaro PJ. Craniofacial surgery. Clin Plast Surg 1974; 1:499.

Conway H. Combined use of the push-back and pharyngeal flap procedures in the management of complicated cases of cleft palate. Plast Reconstr Surg 1951; 7:214.

Cosman B, Falk AS. Pharyngeal flap augmentation. Plast Reconstr Surg 1975; 55:149.

Cosman B, Falk AS. Delayed hard palate repair and speech deficiencies; a cautionary report. Cleft Palate J 1980; 17:27.

Cox JB, Silverstein B. Experiences with posterior pharyngeal flap for correction of velopharyngeal insufficiency. Plast Reconstr Surg 1961; 27:40.

Cronin TD. The bilateral cleft lip with bilateral cleft of the primary palate. In: Converse JM, ed. Reconstructive plastic surgery. 2nd ed. Vol 4, Philadelphia: WB Saunders, 1977.

Curtin JW, Subtelny JD, Nobuo O, Subtelny JD. Pharyngeal flap as a primary and secondary procedure. Cleft Palate J 1973; 10:1.

Dahl E. Craniofacial morphology in congenital clefts of the lip and palate. Acta Odont Scand 1970; 28(Suppl 57):1.

Dalston RM, Stuteville OH. A clinical investigation of the efficacy of primary nasopalatal pharyngoplasty. Cleft Palate J 1975; 12:177.

Davis AD. Role of orthodontia following cleft lip and palate surgery. Pacific Dent Gaz 1931; 39:571.

Dorf DS, Curtin JW. Early cleft palate repair and speech outcome. Plast Reconstr Surg 1982; 70:74.

Dreyer TM, Trier WC. A comparison of palatoplasty techniques. Cleft Palate J 1984; 21:251.

Engstrom K, Fritzell B, Johanson B. A study of speech improvement following palatopharyngeal flap surgery. Cleft Palate J 1970; 7:419.

Evans D, Renfrew C. The timing of primary cleft palate repair. Scand J Plast Reconstr Surg 1974; 8:153.

Fara M, Brousilova M. Experiences with early closure of velum and later closure of hard palate. Plast Reconstr Surg 1969; 44: 134.

Fara M, Dvorak J. Abnormal anatomy of the muscles of palatopharyngeal closure in cleft palate: anatomical and surgical considerations based on the autopsies of 18 unoperated cleft palates. Plast Reconstr Surg 1970a; 46:488.

Fara M, Sedlackova E, Klaskova O, Hrivnakova J, Chmelova A, Supacek L. Primary pharyngo fixation in cleft palate repair; a survey of 46 years experience with an evaluation of 2073 cases. Plast Reconstr Surg 1970b; 45:449.

Furlow LT Jr. Cleft palate repair: preliminary report on lengthening and muscle transposition by z-plasty. Presented at the Annual meeting of the Southeastern Society of Plastic and Reconstructive Surgeons. Boca Raton, FL May 16, 1978.

Furlow LT Jr. Cleft palate repair by double opposing z-plasty. Plast Reconstr Surg 1986; 78:724.

Furlow LT, Williams WN, Eisenback CR, Bzoch KR. A long term study on treating velopharyngeal insufficiency by Teflon injection. Cleft Palate J 1982; 19:47.

Georgiade GS, Georgiade NG, Latham RA. The bilateral cleft lip. In: Serafin D, Georgiade NG, eds. Pediatric plastic surgery. Vol I. St. Louis: CV Mosby, 1984:281.

Gilles H, Harrison SH. Operative correction by osteotomy of recessed malar maxillary compound in a case of oxycephaly. Br J Plast Surg 1950; 3:123.

Gnoinski W, ed. Early treatment of cleft lip and palate. Toronto: Hans Huber, 1986.

Grabb WC, Rosenstein SW, Bzoch KR, eds. Cleft lip and palate: surgical, dental, and speech aspects. Boston: Little, Brown, 1971.

Graber TM. Craniofacial morphology in cleft palate and cleft lip deformities. Surg Gynecol Obstet 1949; 88:359.

Graber TM. Changing philosophies in cleft palate management. J Pediatr 1950; 37:400.

Graber TM. The congenital cleft palate deformity. J Am Dental Assoc 1954; 48:375.

Graham WP III, Hamilton R, Randall P, Winchester R, Stool S. Complications following posterior pharyngeal flap surgery. Cleft Palate J 1973; 10:175.

Gray S. Airway obstruction and apnea in cleft palate patients. In: Bardach J, Morris HL, eds. Multidisciplinary management of cleft lip and palate. Philadelphia: WB Saunders, in press.

Greene MCL. Speech analysis of 263 cleft palate cases. J Speech Hear Dis 1960; 25:43.

Hagerty RF, Hill MJ. Pharyngeal wall and palatal movement in postoperative cleft palates and normal palates. J Speech Hear Res 1960; 3:59.

Hagerty RF, Hill MJ. Cartilage pharyngoplasty in cleft palate patients. Surg Gynecol Obstet 1961; 112:350.

Hardin MA, Van Demark DR, Morris HL. Longitudinal speech results of cleft palate patients. In preparation

Harding RL. Surgery. In: Cooper HK, Harding RL, Krogman WM, Mazaheri M, Millard RT, eds. Cleft palate and cleft lip: a team approach to clinical management and rehabilitation of the patient. Philadelphia: WB Saunders, 1979; 163.

Harrison M. An overview of wound healing and future perspectives in fetal surgery: Experiences and future directions of the UCSF team (program abstract). Annual meeting of the American Cleft Palate-Craniofacial Association. San Francisco, 1989.

Henningsson G, Isberg A. Influence of palatal fistulae on speech and resonance. Folia Phoniatrica 1987; 39:183.

Henningsson G, Isberg A. Palatal fistulas and speech production. In: Bardach J, Morris HL, eds. Multidisciplinary management of cleft lip and palate. Philadelphia: WB Saunders, In press.

Hogan VM. A clarification of the surgical goals in cleft palate speech and the introduction of the lateral port control (L.P.C.) pharyngeal flap. Cleft Palate J 1973; 10:331.

Hogan VM, Schwartz MF, Valauri AJ. Velopharyngeal incompetence. In: Converse JM, ed. Reconstructive plastic surgery: principles and procedures in correction, reconstruction and transplantation. 2nd ed. Vol 4. Philadelphia: WB Saunders, 1977:2268.

Holdsworth WG. Cleft lip and palate. 3rd ed. New York: Grune and Stratton, 1963.

Hotz MM. Pre and early postoperative growth-guidance in cleft lip and palate cases by maxillary orthopedics (an alternative procedure to primary bone grafting. Cleft Palate J 1969; 6:368.

Hotz MM, Gnoinski WM. Effects of early maxillary orthopedics in coordination with delayed surgery for cleft lip and palate. J Maxillofac Surg 1979; 3:201.

Hotz M, Gnoinski W, Perko M, Nussbaumer H, Hof E, Haubensak R. The Zurich approach, 1964 to 1984. In: Gnoinski W, ed. Early treatment of cleft lip and palate. Toronto: Hans Huber, 1986:42.

Isshiki N, Honjow I, Morimoto M. Effects of velopharyngeal incompetence upon speech. Cleft Palate J 1968; 5:297.

Jackson IT. Pharyngoplasty: Jackson technique. In: Bardach J, Morris H, eds. Multidisciplinary management of cleft lip and palate. Philadelphia: WB Saunders, in press.

Jackson MS, Jackson IT, Christie FB. Improvement in speech following closure of anterior palatal fistulas with bone grafts. Br J Plast Surg 1976; 29:295.

Jackson I, McLennan G, Scheker L. Primary veloplasty or primary palatoplasty: Some preliminary findings. Plast Reconstr Surg 1983; 72:153.

Jackson IT, Munro IR, Salyer KE, Whitaker LA. Atlas of craniomaxillofacial surgery. St. Louis: CV Mosby, 1982.

Jackson IT, Silverton JS. The sphincter pharyngoplasty as a secondary procedure in cleft palates. Plast Reconstr Surg 1977; 59:518.

Jolleys A. A review of the results of operations on cleft palates with reference to maxillary growth and speech function. Br J Plast Surg 1954; 7:229.

Keller BG, Long RE, Gold ED, Roth MD. Maxillary dental arch dimensions following pharyngeal-flap surgery. Cleft Palate J 1988; 25:248.

Kemp-Fincham SI, Kuehn DP, Trost-Cardamone JE. Speech development and the timing of primary palatoplasty. In:Bardach J, Morris HL, eds. Multidisciplinary management of cleft lip and palate. Philadelphia: WB Saunders, in press.

Krause CJ, Tharp RF, Morris HL. A comparative study of results of the von Langenbeck and V-Y pushback palatoplasties. Cleft Palate J 1976; 13:11.

Krause CJ, Van Demark DR, Tharp R. Palatoplasty: a comparative study. Trans Am Acad Ophthal Otolaryngol 1975; 80:551.

Kriens OB. An anatomical approach to veloplasty. Plast Reconstr Surg 1969; 43:29.

Kriens OB. Fundamental anatomic findings for an intravelar veloplasty. Cleft Palate J 1970; 7:27.

Krogman WM. Craniofacial growth: prenatal and postnatal. In: Cooper HK, Harding RL, Krogman WM, Mazaheri M, Millard RT, eds. Cleft palate and cleft lip: a team approach to clinical management and rehabilitation of the patient. Philadelphia: WB Saunders, 1979:23.

Krogman WM, Mazaheri M, Harding RL, Ishiguro K, et al. A longitudinal study of the craniofacial growth pattern in children with clefts as compared to normal, birth to six years. Cleft Palate J 1975; 12:59.

Kuehn DP, Van Demark DR. Assessment of velopharyngeal competency following Teflon pharyngoplasty. Cleft Palate J 1978; 15:145.

Lehman JA Jr, Curtin P, Haas DG. Closure of anterior palatal fistulae. Cleft Palate J 1978; 15:33.

Lewy R, Cole R, Wepman J. Teflon injection in the correction of velopharyngeal insufficiency. Ann Otol Rhinol Laryngol 1965; 74:874.

Lindsay WK. von Langenbeck palatorrhaphy. In: Grabb WC, Rosenstein SW, Bzoch KR, eds. Cleft lip and palate: surgical, dental, and speech aspects. Boston: Little, Brown, 1971; 393.

Lindsay WK, LeMesurier AB, Farmer AW. A study of the speech results of a large series of cleft palate patients. Plast Reconstr Surg 1962; 29:273.

Marsh JL, ed. Long-term results of craniofacial surgery. Cleft Palate J 1986; 23(Suppl 1).

Marsh JL, Vannier MW. The "third" dimension in craniofacial surgery. Plast Reconstr Surg 1983; 71:759.

Marsh JL, Vannier MW. Comprehensive care for craniofacial anomalies. St. Louis: CV Mosby, 1985.

Marsh JL, Vannier MW. Cranial base changes following surgical treatment of craniosynostosis. Cleft Palate J 1986; 23(Suppl 1):9.

Marsh JL, Grames LM, Holtman B. Intravelar veloplasty: a prospective study. Cleft Palate J 1989; 26:46.

McCarthy JG, Epstein F, Sadove M, Grayson B, Zide B. Early surgery for craniofacial synostosis: an 8-year experience. Plast Reconstr Surg 1984; 73:521.

McEvitt WG. The incidence of persistent rhinolalia following cleft palate repair. Plast Reconstr Surg 1971; 47:258.

McWilliams BJ. Cleft palate management in England. Speech Pathol Ther 1960; 3:3.

McWilliams BJ, Glaser ER, Philips BJ, et al. A comparative study of four methods of evaluating velopharyngeal adequacy. Plast Reconstr Surg 1981; 68:1.

McWilliams BJ. The long-term speech results of primary and secondary surgical correction of palatal clefts. In: Bardach J, Morris HL, eds. Multidisciplinary management of cleft lip and palate. Philadelphia: WB Saunders, in press.

Meijer R, Cohen S. Two-stage palatoplasty and evaluation of speech results. In: Bardach J, Morris HL, eds. Multidisciplinary management of cleft lip and palate. Philadelphia: WB Saunders, in press.

Millard DR. The island flap in cleft palate surgery. Surg Gynecol Obstet 1963; 116:297.

Millard DR, Batstone JHF, Heycock MH, Bensen JF. Ten years with the palatal island flap. Plast Reconstr Surg 1970; 46:540.

Millard DR. Rotation-advancement in the repair of bilateral cleft lip. In: Grabb WC, Rosenstein SW, Bzoch KR, eds. Cleft lip and palate: surgical, dental, and speech aspects. Boston: Little, Brown, 1971; 305.

Millard DR, ed. Cleft craft: the evolution of its surgery. The unilateral deformity. Vol I. Boston: Little, Brown, 1976.

Millard DR, ed. Cleft Craft: the evolution of its surgery. Bilateral and rare deformities. Vol 2. Boston: Little, Brown, 1977.

Millard DR, ed. Cleft craft: the evolution of its surgery. Alveolar and palatal deformities. Vol 3. Boston: Little, Brown, 1980.

Millard DR. The unilateral cleft lip. In: Serafin D, Georgiade NG, eds. Pediatric plastic surgery. Vol I. St. Louis: CV Mosby, 1984:268.

Moore MD, Lawrence WT, Ptak JJ, Trier WC. Complications of primary palatoplasty: a twenty-one year review. Cleft Palate J 1988; 25:156.

Morris HL. Velopharyngeal competence and the Demjen W/V-Y technique. In: Morris HL, ed. The Bratislava project: some results of cleft palate surgery. Iowa City: University of Iowa Press, 1978; 49.

Morris HL, Bardach J, Van Demark DR, Jones DL, Sharkey SG. Results of two-flap palatoplasty with regard to speech production. Eur J Plast Surg 1989; 12:19.

Morris HL, Spriestersbach DC. The pharyngeal flap as a speech mechanism. Plast Reconstr Surg 1967; 39:66.

Musgrave RH. Presidential address: 1969. Cleft Palate J 1969; 6:361.

Musgrave RH, Bremner JC. Complications of cleft palate surgery. Plast Reconstr Surg 1960; 26:180.

Musgrave RH, Garrett WS. The unilateral cleft lip. In: Converse JM, ed. Reconstructive plastic surgery: principles and procedures in correction, reconstruction and transplantation. Vol 4. 2nd ed. Philadelphia: WB Saunders, 1977:2016.

Musgrave RH, McWilliams BJ, Matthews HP. A review of the results of two different surgical procedures for the repair of clefts of the soft palate only. Cleft Palate J 1975; 12:281.

Noordoff MS, Kuo J, Wang F, Huang H, Witzel MA. Development of articulation before delayed hard-palate closure in children with cleft palate: a cross-sectional study. Plast Reconstr Surg 1987; 80:518.

Nylen B, Wahlin A. Post-operative complications in pharyngeal flap surgery. Cleft Palate J 1966; 3:347.

Oneal RM. Oronasal fistulas. In: Grabb WC, Rosenstein SW, Bzoch KR, eds. Cleft lip and palate: surgical, dental, and speech aspects. Boston: Little, Brown, 1971:490.

Orr WC, Levine NS, Buchanan RT. Effect of cleft palate repair and pharyngeal flap surgery on upper airway obstruction during sleep. Plast Reconstr Surg 1987; 80:226.

Orticochea M. Construction of a dynamic muscle sphincter in cleft palate. Plast Reconstr Surg 1968; 41:323.

Orticochea M. A review of 236 cleft palate patients treated with dynamic muscle sphincter. Plastic Reconstr Surg 1983; 71:180.

Orticochea M. The dynamic muscle sphincter of the pharynx. In: Bardach J, Morris H, eds. Multidisciplinary management of cleft lip and palate. Philadelphia: WB Saunders, in press.

Osborn JM, Kelleher JC. A survey of cleft lip and palate surgery taught in plastic surgery training programs. Cleft Palate J 1983; 20:166.

Owsley JQ, Lawson LI, Chierici GJ. The re-do pharyngeal flap. Plast Reconstr Surg 1976; 57:180.

Owsley JQ, Lawson LI, Miller ER, Blackfield HM. Experience with the high attached pharyngeal flap. Plast Reconstr Surg 1966; 38:232.

Owsley JQ, Lawson LI, Miller ER, Harvold EP, Chierici G, Blackfield HM. Speech results from the high attached pharyngeal flap operation. Cleft Palate J 1970; 7:306.

Peer LA, Hagerty RF, Hoffmeister FD, Collito MB, Manly RS. An evaluation of the Warren Davis osteo-plastic technique in cleft palate repair. Plast Reconstr Surg 1954; 14:1.

Peet E. The Oxford technique of cleft palate repair. Plast Reconstr Surg 1961; 28:282.

Peet E. Cleft lip and palate. In: Rob C, Smith R, eds. Operative surgery. Philadelphia: JB Lippincott, 1969:75.

Perko M. Closure of the hard palate in unilateral cleft palate cases following previous closure of the soft palate according to the Widmaier-Perko technique. Chir Testa e Coll 1984; 1:9.

Randall P. A triangular flap operation for the primary repair of unilateral clefts of the lip. Plast Reconstr Surg 1959; 23:331.

Randall P. A lip adhesion operation in cleft lip surgery. Plast Reconstr Surg 1965; 35:371.

Randall P, LaRossa D, Fakhree SM, Cohen MA. Cleft palate closure at 3 to 7 months of age: a preliminary report. Plast Reconstr Surg 1983; 71:624.

Randall P, LaRossa D, Solomon M, Cohen M. Experience with the Furlow double-reversing Z-plasty for cleft repair. Plast Reconstr Surg 1986; 77:569.

Riski JE. Articulation skills and oral-nasal resonance in children with pharyngeal flaps. Cleft Palate J 1979; 16:421.

Roberts TMF, Brown SJ. Evaluation of a modified sphincter pharyngoplasty in the treatment of speech problems due to palatal insufficiency. Ann Plast Surg 1983; 10:209.

Rogers BO. The historical evolution of plastic and reconstructive surgery. In: Wood-Smith D, Parowski PC, eds. Nursing care of the plastic surgery patient. St. Louis: CV Mosby.

Ross RB. Treatment variables affecting facial growth in complete unilateral cleft lip and palate. Cleft Palate J 1987; 24:5.

Ross RB, Johnston MC. Cleft lip and palate. Baltimore: Williams & Wilkins, 1972.

Schultz RC. Management and timing of cleft palate fistula repair. Plast Reconstr Surg 1986; 78:739.

Schultz RC. Cleft palate fistula repair: Improved results by the addition of bone. Arch Otolaryngol Head Neck Surg 1989; 115:65.

Schwartz MF. Personal communication to Converse JM, Kawamoto HK. Wood-Smith D, Coccaro PJ, McCarthy JG, 1976.

Schweckendiek W. Primary veloplasty. In: Schuchardt K, ed. Treatment of patients with clefts of lip, alveolus and palate. Stuttgart: Thieme, 1966:85.

Schweckendiek W. Primary veloplasty: long-term results without maxillary deformity. A twenty-five year report. Cleft Palate J 1978; 15:268.

Semb G, Shaw W. The influence of pharyngeal flap on facial growth. In: Bardach J, Morris H, eds. Multidisciplinary management of cleft lip and palate. Philadelphia: WB Saunders, in press.

Serafin D, Georgiade NG, eds. Pediatric plastic surgery. Vol 1. St. Louis: CV Mosby, 1984.

Shelton RL, Blank JL. Oronasal fistulas, intraoral air pressure, and nasal air flow during speech. Cleft Palate J 1984; 21:91.

Shprintzen RJ, Lewin JL, Croft CB, et al. A comprehensive study of pharyngeal flap surgery: Tailor made flaps. Cleft Palate J 1979; 16:46.

Skolnick ML, McCall GN. Velopharyngeal competence and incompetence following pharyngeal flap surgery: a video-fluoroscopic study in multiple projections. Cleft Palate J 1972; 9:1.

Skoog T. A design for the repair of unilateral cleft lips. Am J Surg 1958; 95:223.

Skoog T. The pharyngeal flap operation in cleft palate. Br J Plast Surg 1965; 18:265.

Smith JK, Huffman WC, Lierle DM, Moll KL. Results of pharyngeal flap surgery in patients with velopharyngeal incompetence. Plast Reconstr Surg 1963; 32:493.

Smith JK, McCabe BF. Teflon injection in the nasopharynx to improve velopharyngeal closure. Ann Otol Rhinol Laryngol 1977; 86:559.

Smith BE, Skef Z, Cohen M, Dorf DS. Aerodynamic assessment of the result of pharyngeal flap surgery: a preliminary investigation. Plast Reconstr Surg 1985; 76:402.

Stark RB, DeHaan CR. The addition of a pharyngeal flap to primary palatoplasty. Plast Reconstr Surg 1960; 26:378.

Stark RB, DeHaan CR, Frileck SP, Burgess PD. Primary pharyngeal flap. Cleft Palate J 1969; 6:381.

Stark RB, Frileck S. Primary pharyngeal flap and palatorrhaphy. In: Grabb WC, Rosenstein SW, Bzoch KR, eds. Cleft lip and palate: surgical, dental, and speech aspects. Boston: Little, Brown, 1971:404.

Strauss RP, Davis JU. Prenatal detection and fetal surgery of clefts and craniofacial abnormalities in humans: social and ethical issues (program abstract). Annual meeting of the American Cleft Palate-Craniofacial Association. San Francisco, 1989.

Stuteville OH, Pirruoceelo FW, Janada CA, Sullivan MR, Pandya N. Pharyngeal flap. 309 cases: anatomical, physiological and operative considerations. 49th Annual Meeting of the Society of Plastic and Reconstructive Surgery. Colorado Springs. 1970.

Subtelny JC, Pineda Nieto R. A longitudinal study of maxillary growth following pharyngeal flap surgery. Cleft Palate J 1978; 15:118.

Sullivan WG. In-utero cleft lip repair in the mouse without an incision (program abstract). Annual meeting of the American Cleft Palate-Craniofacial Association. San Francisco, 1989.

Tennison CW. The repair of the unilateral cleft lip by the stencil method. Plast Reconstr Surg 1952; 9:115.

Tessier P. Osteotomies totales de la lace. Syndrome de Crouzon Syndrome d' Apert. Orycephales, scaphocephales. turricephales. Ann Chir Plast 1967; 12:273.

Tessier P. The definitive plastic surgical treatment of the severe facial deformities of craniofacial dysostosis, Crouzon's and Apert's Disease. Plast Reconstr Surg 1971; 48:419.

Tessier P, Guiot G, Rougerie J, Delbet JP, Pastoriza J. Osteotomies cranio-naso-orbito-faciales. Hypertelorisme. Ann Chir Plast 1967; 12:103.

Thurston JB, Larson DL, Shanks JC, Bennett JE, Parson RW. Nasal obstruction as a complication of pharyngeal flap surgery. Cleft Palate J 1980; 17:148.

Trauner R, Trauner M. Results of cleft palate operations. Plast Reconstr Surg 1967; 39:168.

Trier WC. The pharyngeal flap operation. Clin Plast Surg 1985; 12:697.

Trier WC, Dreyer TM. Primary von Langenbeck with levator reconstruction: rationale and technique. Cleft Palate J 1984; 21:254.

Trigos I, Ysunza A, Gonzalez A, Vazquez M. Surgical treatment of borderline velopharyngeal insufficiency using homologous cartilage implantation with videonasopharyngoscopic monitoring. Cleft Palate J 1988; 25:167.

Tuttle GA. A teleradiographic investigation of the correlates of normal voice quality in patients having pharyngeal flaps. Doctoral dissertation, University of Pittsburgh, 1969.

Van Demark DR. Assessment of articulation and velopharyngeal competence for children with cleft palate. Tale og Stemme 1974a; 34:107.

Van Demark DR. A comparison of articulation abilities and velopharyngeal competency between Danish and Iowa children with cleft palate. Cleft Palate J 1974b; 11:463.

Van Demark DR, Gnoinski W, Hotz MM, Perko M, Naussbaumer H. Speech results of the Zurich approach in the treatment of unilateral cleft lip and palate. Plast Reconstr Surg 1989; 83:605.

Van Demark DR, Hardin MA. Longitudinal evaluation of articulation and velopharyngeal competence of patients with pharyngeal flaps. Cleft Palate J 1985; 22:163.

Veau V. 1933. In: Morley M, ed. Cleft palate and speech. 5th ed. Baltimore: Williams & Wilkins, 1962:81.

Vig KL, Fonseca RJ, Turvey TA. Bone grafting of the cleft maxilla. In: Bardach J, Morris HL, eds. Multidisciplinary management of cleft palate. Philadelphia: WB Saunders, in press.

Warren DW, Devereau JL. An analog study of cleft palate speech. Cleft Palate J 1966; 3:103.

Wilhelmsen HR, Musgrave RH. Complications of cleft lip surgery. Cleft Palate J 1966; 3:223.

Witzel MA. Orthognathic defects and surgical correction: The effects on speech and velopharyngeal function. Doctoral dissertation, University of Pittsburgh, 1981.

Witzel MA, Salyer KE, Ross RB. Delayed hard palate closure: the philosophy revisited. Cleft Palate J 1984; 21:263.

Wolford LM, Oelschlaeger M, Deal R. Proplast as a pharyngeal wall implant to correct velopharyngeal insufficiency. Cleft Palate J 1989; 26:119.

Wray RC, Dann J, Holtmann BA. Comparison of three technics of palatorrhaphy: in-hospital morbidity. Cleft Palate J 1979; 16:42.

Zwitman DH. Velopharyngeal physiology after pharyngeal flap surgery as assessed by oral endoscopy. Cleft Palate J 1982a; 19:36.

Zwitman DH. Oral endoscopic comparison of velopharyngeal closure before and after pharyngeal flap surgery. Cleft Palate J 1982b; 19:40.

5 | DENTAL PROBLEMS

The patient with cleft lip and palate is likely to have significant dental problems that require the attention of various specialists in dentistry. Treatment is likely to be both long and costly. Individual teeth in the area of the cleft may be missing or malpositioned. The upper or maxillary arch may not fit well with the lower or mandibular arch, a misfit usually referred to as malocclusion. There may be problems in arch width and length. There is some controversy about the specific causes of these deformities, but it is generally agreed that they are, in part, the direct result of clefting and that they may be exacerbated by the surgery required for the correction of the cleft lip and palate.

DENTAL DEVELOPMENT

An excellent description of dental developmental patterns and mechanisms for the general population is provided by Burdi and Moyers (1988). The speech pathologist with special interest in oral structure malformation needs to be familiar with that kind of material.

Loevy and Aduss (1988) provide a review of the literature about dental development in patients with clefts as well as some findings about tooth maturation in the group. Both their data and the data reports they review (Bohn, 1963; Jordon et al., 1966; Ranta, 1971, 1972; Prahl-Andersen, 1976) indicate delayed development for certain gender and cleft type subgroups. For example, their data indicate no differences from the normal for girls for any cleft type, but a delay in boys for all cleft types combined, and an even more striking delay for boys with unilateral cleft lip and palate. They offer no explanation for the findings but indicate that further study with larger sample sizes is indicated.

EARLY DENTAL CARE

The child with a cleft or other orofacial anomaly has a special need for early dental monitoring to ensure appropriate treatment as it is required. The relationships in early childhood among the primary teeth and between the two dental arches are important bases for later development, as are healthy and strong teeth, which are required for the orthodontics needed by most cleft patients. Good dental hygiene and dental restorations, important for all children, are mandatory for children with clefts. Dental care is especially necessary in the mixed-dentition stage. Every young child with a cleft should be seen regularly by a pediatric dentist.

MALOCCLUSION AND ORTHODONTIC TREATMENT

Many children and adults in the general population as well as in the cleft population have malocclusions. In general, the same methods for diagnosis and treatment are used for both groups, but there are certain differences in the nature of the disorders and, often, in the design and timing of treatment. General principles of orthodontics, such as described by Moyers (1988), provide the foundation necessary for understanding the problems encountered in people with clefts. Bloomer (1971) and Starr (1979) have written essays on dental deformities specifically for the speech pathologist.

A General Review

The term *malocclusion* refers to an improper relationship between the two dental arches. Figure 5.1 provides orientation for tooth placement in

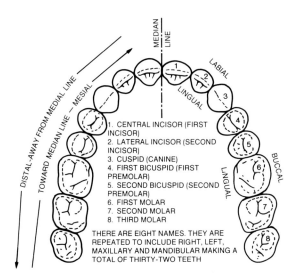

1. CENTRAL INCISOR (FIRST INCISOR)
2. LATERAL INCISOR (SECOND INCISOR)
3. CUSPID (CANINE)
4. FIRST BICUSPID (FIRST PREMOLAR)
5. SECOND BICUSPID (SECOND PREMOLAR)
6. FIRST MOLAR
7. SECOND MOLAR
8. THIRD MOLAR

THERE ARE EIGHT NAMES. THEY ARE REPEATED TO INCLUDE RIGHT, LEFT, MAXILLARY AND MANDIBULAR MAKING A TOTAL OF THIRTY-TWO TEETH

Figure 5.1 Permanent teeth in an adult dental arch, showing arrangement and terms of orientation. (From Bloomer HH. Speech defects associated with dental malocclusions and related abnormalities. In: Travis LE, ed. Handbook of speech pathology and audiology. Englewood Cliffs, NJ: Prentice-Hall, 1971.)

the adult maxillary arch and introduces the terminology used to discuss dental relationships. Many orthodontists use a classification system originally described by Edward H. Angle (1907). As shown in Figures 5.2 and 5.3, the maxillary arch is normally slightly larger than the mandibular arch and so to some extent fits over it. In Angle's system, the primary reference point for defining normal occlusion is the relationship between the maxillary and mandibular first molars in which the mesiobuccal cusp of the first maxillary permanent molar occludes with the buccal groove of the mandibular first permanent molar. There are several types of malocclusion that the speech pathologist should recognize. Figure 5.4 shows the Angle classification. In Class I (neutroclusion), the arch relationship is normal, but there is misalignment of individual teeth. In Class II (distoclusion), the mandibular arch is positioned posteriorly to the maxillary arch. As a consequence, the maxillary arch protrudes. Patients with bilateral clefts of the lip and protruding premaxillae frequently show this kind of arch relationship, at least anteriorly. In Class III (mesioclusion), the converse is true. The mandibular

arch is positioned anteriorly to the maxillary arch. In these patients, the mandibular arch protrudes. Patients with clefts who have severe midfacial deficiency frequently show this type of arch relationship.

When incisal contact does not occur, a condition known as *openbite* is seen. An *overbite* may be either mandibular or maxillary and refers to the overlapping of the teeth vertically (Fig. 5.5). The horizontal space between the teeth in the two arches is called *overjet* when the maxillary incisors are *labial* to the mandibular incisors. If the maxillary incisors are *lingual* to the mandibular incisors, the condition is known as *underjet*.

The dental arches may also be in *crossbite* relationship, in which case the arches, which may or may not be of normal size, are misaligned. For example, a common type of crossbite is that in which the maxillary arch fits inside the mandibular arch. Crossbite of only the anterior or posterior relationship is sometimes observed. Crossbite is frequently seen in patients with cleft lip and palate (Fig. 5.6).

Determining the causes of dental malocclusion in the general population may be difficult. Discussions by Graber (1966) and Foster (1975) indicated three major etiological groupings: congenital, genetic, and acquired. There is often considerable interaction among the three.

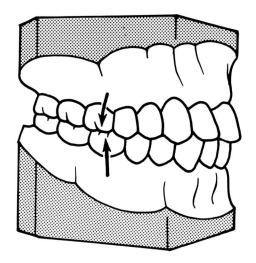

Figure 5.2 Normal occlusion. Arrows indicate normal occlusal relationship. (From Bloomer HH. In: Travis LE, ed. Handbook of speech pathology and audiology. Englewood Cliffs, NJ: Prentice-Hall, 1971.)

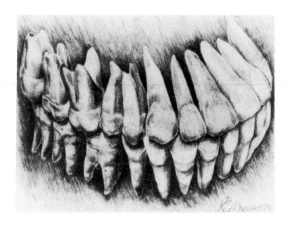

Figure 5.3 Ideal alignment and occlusion of all 32 permanent teeth. (From Hall DJ, Warren DW. Orthodontic problems in children. In: Bluestone CD, Stool SE, eds. Pediatric otolaryngology. Vol II. Philadelphia: WB Saunders, 1983:959.)

Individuals with congenital orofacial or craniofacial anomalies such as cleft lip and palate frequently have malocclusions. The malocclusion may be the result of a lack of continuity of the maxillary arch, as when there is a cleft, or it may be the result of a congenital deformity affecting subsequent growth, as is seen in some of the craniofacial anomalies described in Chapter 2.

There is substantial evidence that genetic factors are important in occlusion, although the precise mechanisms are not well understood. Heredity plays a major role in determining the morphology of skeleton and muscle, both of which are crucial in formulating occlusal relationships. Of particular concern is tooth size in relation to jaw size. The situation in which teeth are too large for the space provided by the jaw is likely to be genetic in nature and is a frequent underlying factor in malocclusion. Other such genetic dental factors are congenitally missing teeth or supernumerary (extra) teeth.

Acquired malocclusion is caused by extrinsic factors that are usually difficult if not impossible to identify. One example might be the possible effects of cleft lip and palate surgery. Other examples are physical injury or disease to the jaws that results in malocclusion and injury or disease suffered at an early age that disturbs subsequent

development. Nutrition factors may affect dental eruption and, hence, occlusion. Premature loss of the primary teeth is often cited as contributory to malocclusion. There are also suggestions, some of them strong, that patterns of oral function, including aberrant tongue habits, may cause malocclusion. Although we sometimes see evidence of such patterns in children with cleft lip and palate, these are not central to our present discussion.

Diagnosis and Treatment

We will not discuss in detail the process of diagnosis and treatment for malocclusion. For information about this topic as it relates to cleft palate, see Ross and Johnston (1972), Mazaheri (1979), and Section IX, "Orthodontic Treatment of Cleft Lip and Palate," in Bardach and Morris (in press).

In general terms, diagnosis and treatment are best conducted by the orthodontist, although the general dentist, the pediatric dentist, and the oral and maxillofacial surgeon also contribute.

The above discussion indicates the complexity of malocclusion. Certain children, particularly those with clefts, require periodic observation as well as treatment at a young age. Others are probably best treated during their adolescent years. Treatment may also be effective during the adult years, although ideally the goal is to correct problems before adulthood. Patients with clefts may need orthodontic treatment in childhood, adolescence, and young adulthood.

Orthodontic techniques vary in complexity according to the nature and extent of the disorder (Graber and Swain, 1985; Moyers, 1988). Conventional procedures are directed toward the goal of applying small amounts of pressure on the tooth to be moved and using the other appropriately positioned teeth as the anchor for the pressure (Figs. 5.7 and 5.8). An anchor outside the mouth may sometimes be necessary, in which case a head strap on the forehead, the top of the head, or the back of the neck is used.

Another orthodontic procedure is designed for arch expansion (Fig. 5.9). The assumption here is that under certain conditions the palatal segments can be moved to a position that facilitates normal occlusion. This procedure is used with moderate frequency for young children with clefts, particularly in cases where the maxillary

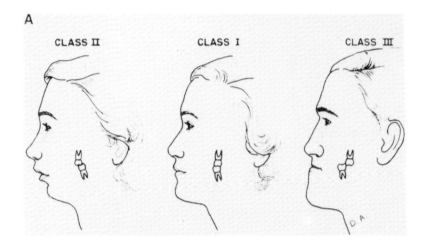

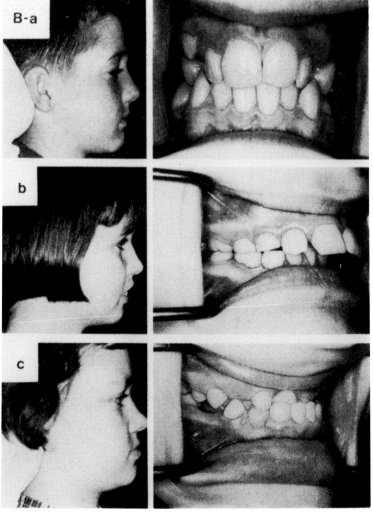

Figure 5.4 A. Angle classification. Facial profile and molar relationship; note how the two change together. It would be difficult, for example, to have a Class III molar relationship in a Class II profile. B. the relationship of the soft-tissue profile to the occlusion. a. a balanced profile with a Class I malocclusion. b. a retrognathic profile and the Class II malocclusion. Note how the lips reflect the overjet of the incisors. c. a Class III malocclusion. Here, the lip posture clearly indicates the presence of a Class III malocclusion. (From Moyers RE. Handbook of orthodontics. 4th ed. Chicago: Year Book, 1988:185.)

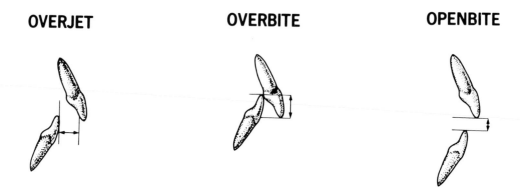

OVERJET   **OVERBITE**   **OPENBITE**

Figure 5.5   Schematic illustration of the terms overjet, overbite, and open bite. Overjet is the horizontal projection of the upper incisors in front of the lower incisors. Overbite is the extent to which the upper anterior teeth overlap the lower in a vertical direction. Open bite is the vertical distance between the upper and lower incisors when they do not overlap. (From Hall DJ, Warren DW. Orthodontic problems in children. In: Bluestone CD, Stool SE, eds. Pediatric otolaryngology. Vol II. Philadelphia: WB Saunders, 1983:966.)

arch has collapsed or narrowed. Orthodontic appliances for arch expansion of this type are positioned inside the dental arch, often fitting across the hard palate.

These orthodontic techniques are based on the premise that small, steady amounts of pressure over time will result in tooth movement or, in some cases, arch expansion. It follows that such techniques must be carefully monitored to avoid undesired results. For that reason, the orthodontist often needs to examine the patient at frequent intervals.

It should also be obvious that there are distinct limitations to these techniques. Banding and related procedures are effective in moving individual teeth but are not useful in changing skeletal relationships. As a consequence, they are of limited use when there is marked skeletal malocclusion between the maxillary and mandibular arches.

Surgical orthodontics for some occlusal disorders have been given increased attention during the past decade. These techniques employ surgical manipulation to advance, retrude, or realign the maxilla or mandible, sometimes with appropriate bone grafts to provide supplemental bony tissue. These techniques are generally used by plastic or oral surgeons in collaboration with orthodontists and other dental and medical specialists. Procedures involving the mandible are preferred whenever possible, because the mandible has fewer important interconnections with other bones of the skull than has the maxilla.

There is considerable controversy about the

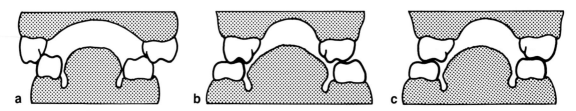

a   b   c

Figure 5.6   Posterior crossbite. a. Mandibular teeth lingual to normal position. b. Mandibular teeth buccal to normal position. c. Unilateral crossbite: right side normal; left side, mandibular teeth buccal to normal position. (From Wilkins EM, McCullough PA. Clinical practice of the dental hygienist. 2nd ed. Philadelphia: Lea & Febiger, 1964.)

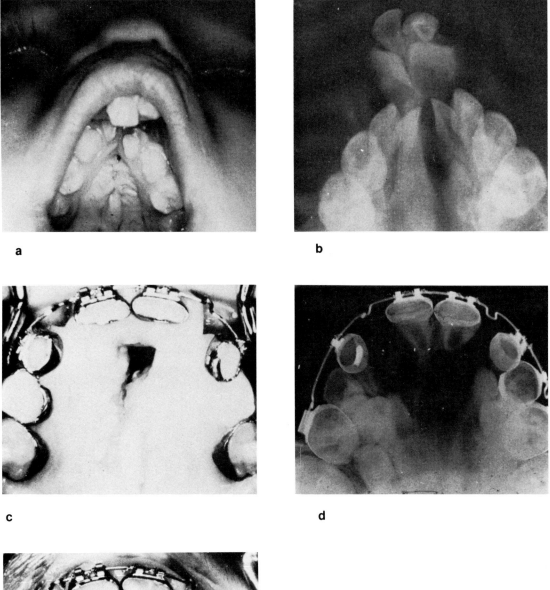

a

b

c

d

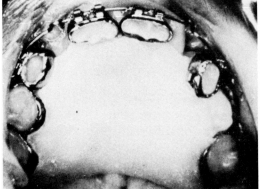

e

Figure 5.7 Photographs and radiographic palatal views of a patient with severe constriction and deformity of palate and dental arch a. and b. before, c. and d. after orthodontic treatment; e. a palatal appliance used to maintain the expansion and to obturate the palatal fistula. (From Coccaro PJ, Valuri AJ. Orthodontics in cleft lip and palate children. In: Converse JM, ed. Reconstructive plastic surgery, 2nd ed. Vol. 4, Philadelphia: WB Saunders, 1977.)

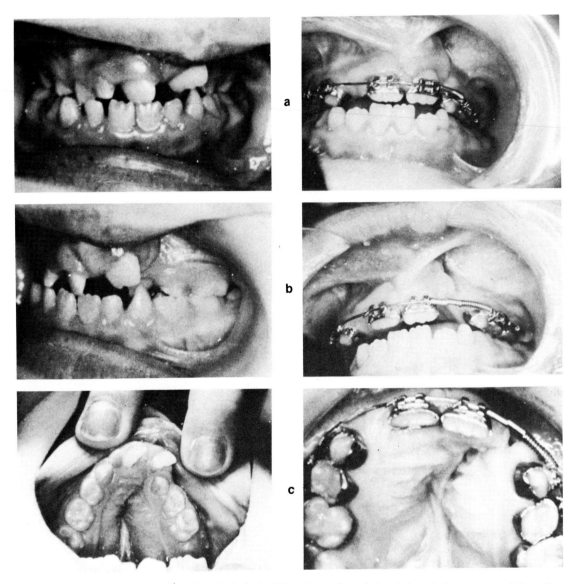

Figure 5.8 Orthodontic therapy during the period of mixed dentition. a. frontal view, b. lateral view, c. a palatal view of a patient with a unilateral cleft lip and palate before and after orthodontic treatment. (From Coccaro PJ, Valuri AJ. Orthodontics in cleft lip and palate children. In: Converse JM, ed. Reconstructive plastic surgery, 2nd ed. Vol 4. Philadelphia: WB Saunders, 1977.)

appropriate timing of surgical orthodontics. Surgery is often delayed until the major portion of growth is completed. Sometimes, however, there are indications for surgery at an earlier age. The field of surgical orthodontics is relatively new, so the number of descriptive texts or the amount of evaluational data is in short supply. The best reference text available is that of Bell et al. (1980).

Evaluation data are especially needed for information about the effects of these procedures on cosmesis, growth, deglutition, and, of course, speech (see Garber et al., 1981, for a recent report about the effects on speech of surgical premaxillary osteotomy). In the case of maxillary surgery, there is a particular need for further investigation as to whether the gains outweigh the risks. Clinical

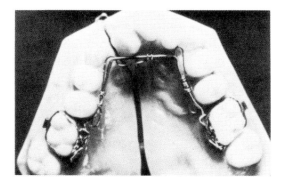

a

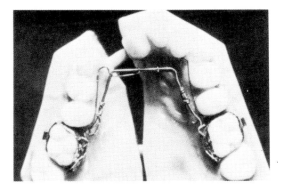

b

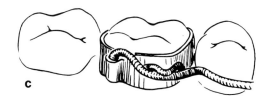

c

Figure 5.9 Expansion arch: (a) activated; (b) result; (c) detail of molar attachment. (From Ross RB, Johnston MC. Cleft lip and palate. Baltimore: Williams & Wilkins, 1972.)

experience, however, suggests that such procedures as maxillary advancements are quite successful.

ORTHODONTICS FOR THE CLEFT LIP AND PALATE PATIENT

The orthodontist is a vital member of the cleft palate team and must participate in the care

of the patient from infancy to adulthood (Ross and Johnston, 1972). The premises and procedures outlined above for diagnosing and treating malocclusion in general are the same as those for managing the malocclusion associated with cleft lip and palate. However, a complicating factor in these patients is the complex interaction between cleft lip and palate surgery and malocclusion and orthodontic treatment. For example, in our discussion of cleft palate surgery, we learned that timing of surgery is frequently decided on the basis of dental considerations. Some of those considerations are related to midfacial growth and development, which is discussed later in this chapter. There is the assumption that preoperative dental status is an important factor to consider in surgical planning and that, in turn, the surgery influences arch growth so that the type, timing, and extent of the orthodontic treatment needed for malocclusion and related disorders is also affected (Vig and Turvey, 1985).

A particularly bothersome problem in planning orthodontic treatment for cleft lip and palate patients is the lack of alveolar bone at the site of the cleft. If the deficit is considerable, the options for alignment of individual teeth are seriously reduced. For some patients and under some circumstances, a bone graft is placed at the site of the alveolar cleft. This is usually done after major growth has been completed, although such procedures have been carried out in infancy with questionable results. The theory is that the bone graft provides a base that will satisfactorily support the teeth (Ross and Johnston, 1972; Bergland et al, 1986). An alternative procedure is a fixed or removable dental prosthesis that restores the arch and replaces the missing teeth. These prosthetic devices are designed and constructed by a prosthodontist.

The patient with a bilateral cleft lip and palate poses special problems to the orthodontist as well as to the surgeon. Not only may there be serious bony deficits on both sides of the cleft, but the prolabium, or midportion of the upper lip, and the premaxilla, or prepalate, may be anteriorly displaced to a marked extent. This displacement results in a malocclusion that is usually difficult to treat and requires careful study over time, with close coordination between the orthodontist and the surgeon. Formerly, the premaxilla was surgically removed in many of these patients, but that course of action is seldom followed now. Although surgical removal solved the problem, at least partially, while the child was young, it resulted in interference with subsequent growth of the midface so that, at an older age, there were severe cosmetic and functional deficits.

MAXILLOFACIAL DEFICIENCIES

We have already referred to the importance of the growth and development of the midface. Essentially, tissue deficits in the midface or maxillofacial complex result in a facial profile more concave in appearance than is normal. Typically, these bony deficits contribute to malocclusion in which the maxillary arch is foreshortened relative to the mandibular arch. There may be a narrowing of the maxillary arch, sometimes referred to as arch collapse, or the two arches' may be in a crossbite relationship. These abnormalities have adverse affects on appearance, speech production, and, in severe cases, mastication.

There is considerable controversy about whether these deficiencies are the result of the cleft, the palatal surgery, or a combination of the two. Both factors are probably important, with the surgery contributing relatively more than the cleft (Bishara, 1973; Bishara et al., 1976). It may also be that cleft lip surgery has some deleterious effects on subsequent midface development (Bardach et al., 1980).

The mechanisms by which surgery may impair arch growth and development are not yet clearly understood. One mechanism suggested a number of years ago (Graber, 1950), and still accepted by many surgeons, is that the surgery either damages the blood or nerve supplies to the growth sites of the maxillofacial complex or injures the growth sites directly. Surgeons usually attempt to preserve the integrity of the posterior neurovascular bundle during palatal surgery, even though the attachments of the bundles, one on each side, may limit the amount of repositioning of elevated soft tissue flaps in such procedures as the V-Y pushback technique. There are some data, however, that indicate that the neurovascular bundles can be severed without causing severe midfacial deformities (Morris, 1978).

In recent years, the concern about palatal surgery and maxillofacial growth and development appears to have shifted away from growth interference and toward the importance of maxillary arch collapse as a result of factors that might be regarded as mechanical. There are probably several reasons for the change in emphasis. The major reason may be that growth sites are now thought to be less specific in location than was formerly thought, so the relationship between surgical procedures and subsequent growth may not be as direct or as strong as it was previously believed to be. Certainly the data about severance of the neurovascular bundle indicate the strong possibility that the systems for nerve and blood supply to the region are more redundant than is postulated by such a simplistic model.

Present emphasis, then, seems to be on the importance of arch collapse rather than growth deficit. The theory is that scar tissue that forms as a result of palatal surgery, primarily from the denudation of bone during surgery, both contracts with maturity and fails to expand with growth. In this way, the scar tissue serves to prevent normal palatal growth and, in the extreme situation, to reduce maxillary dimensions, especially arch width. The results may be a smaller-than-normal maxillary arch, an arch which does not have a normal configuration, or one that is in a crossbite relationship with the mandibular arch.

This is a reasonable point of view based on present knowledge about the composition of scar tissue, maxillofacial growth patterns in the normal range, and the several factors that are possible hazards to those growth patterns. There are indications from animal data that the larger the denuded area and the closer it is to the alveolar ridge, the greater the collapse (Kremenak and Searls, 1971).

Unfortunately, current procedures for palatoplasty result in denudation of the palatal bone in order that the soft tissue flap may be elevated and retropositioned. Since such denudation is always followed by granulation and scar tissue, some contraction is unavoidable in present-day cleft palate treatment. The relevant questions are: How much collapse can be expected? Can it be prevented? If it cannot be prevented, how can it be treated? Of what consequence is it, and, for our purposes, to what extent does it adversely affect the speech mechanism? The answers to these questions are probably similar for both unilateral and bilateral clefts, but patients with bilateral clefts present unusual orthodontic problems and require special cooperation between the orthodontist and the surgeon from birth.

DENTAL MALOCCLUSION AND SPEECH PRODUCTION

Our primary discussion of speech patterns associated with cleft lip and palate and associated disorders is presented in Chapters 13 through 23. However, certain statements should be made here about the effects of malocclusions on speech. Reports by Fricke (1970), Morris (1971) and Wertz (1972 and 1973) cover a wide range of topics about speech production and dentition and represent the state of the science for the early 1970s. Little has been published since.

Understanding of the relationships between dental and occlusal factors and speech production in normals is far from complete. However, there is a satisfactory basis for several general statements. For example, dentition and occlusion play a crucial role in establishing the size and configuration of the oral cavity. A severe occlusion defect such as an overbite or underjet can affect tongue carriage during rest and speech. While the tongue appears to be highly adaptable to the size and shape of the oral cavity, there are undoubtedly limits to that adaptability. Examples of this adaptability are children who are in the process of losing deciduous teeth and gaining permanent teeth and older adults who have full-mouth dental extractions and then are fitted with dentures. Many people seem to accommodate well to the temporary loss of teeth, even the incisors. Perhaps the accommodation is so easily made because the speaker originally had normal structures and so had developed normal speech articulation patterns. Those patterns are less affected by the temporary loss of dental structures and are easily reestablished once the dental structures are regained. In contrast, our clinical impression is that dental anomalies that are congenital are less easily compensated for. Patients with congenital abnormal oral structures and structural relationships have never had the opportunity of obtaining a normal baseline of speech production. Although we have little supporting evidence for the premise, it seems probable that children with clefts may experience different difficulties in speech production with, for example, missing incisors than do children whose oral structures are normal.

In addition, these children probably experience more changes in oral structural relationships because of surgery and orthodontic treatment than do children without clefts. That process of more or less continual change could be expected to make it difficult for the child with a cleft to seek and maintain articulatory behaviors that are maximally efficient in producing speech. Certain orthodontic appliances cause sufficient change in the size and shape of the oral cavity to hamper that articulation. Extraoral appliances may restrict jaw movements for speech; however, such restrictions on speech production are not usually clinically significant.

Surgical orthodontics is a different matter in terms of possible aftereffects on speech production. As we have indicated earlier, the relationship between oral structures and speech production movements is by no means clear. However, it seems reasonable to expect that movement patterns of the articulators are monitored and perhaps maintained by sensory feedback from the oral structures. For example, the child who is losing deciduous teeth and gaining permanent teeth may have temporary difficulty with sibilants because of some crucial changes in landmarks. The same is probably true in the case of the older adult who loses teeth by extraction and subsequently is fitted with dentures (Zimmermann et al., 1980). According to clinical observations, the majority of patients in both groups eventually accommodate to the new oral environment. However, it is equally true that some people find the process of accommodation to be very difficult, and they need assistance in adjusting to their altered oral environments.

In the same way, some patients who have surgical orthodontics or some form of orthognathic surgery demonstrate considerable difficulty with speech production following the surgery. For others, the new relationships facilitate rather than hamper speech production (Vallino et al., 1988). The major point is that we have not yet enough data about the process for making predictions either about the nature or bases of any changes that might occur. Data are badly needed, but because of the nature of the problem they will be difficult to obtain.

DENTAL MALOCCLUSION AND ORAL FUNCTION

We indicated earlier that there are suggestions that patterns of oral function may cause malocclusion. Most commonly, behaviors such as thumb-sucking and maladaptive swallowing are cited as major suspects. The theory is that these behaviors subject the incisors and perhaps the supporting alveolar tissues to abnormal pressures of sufficient magnitude that arch shape and tooth position are substantially altered toward malocclusion. Furthermore, the theory holds that, in the presence of these functional forces, orthodontic treatment will be successful only so long as proper appliances are in place. Once the appliances are removed, presumably when normal occlusion has been restored, these forces, if not corrected, will cause recurrence of the malocclusion. Whether these relationships, if they exist, are common in patients with cleft lip and palate is as yet unclear. However, discussion of the topic seems warranted here because the speech pathologist interested in cleft palate is also likely to be consulted about other aspects of oral structure and function.

Thumb-Sucking

In our opinion, thumb-sucking and other finger habits may disrupt normal occlusion, but only if during the sucking behavior the child pushes the thumb outward with considerable force over an extended period of time. There is no clear evidence that normal, passive, sucking behavior, whether on the thumb or a pacifier, results in malocclusion. The position can be taken that the child who sucks his or her thumb has not yet filled some natural need for such behavior and ought to be allowed to do so. Besides, it is very difficult to correct such habits. Typically the behavior is self-limiting and generally is not observed after the age of 3 or 4 years. As a consequence of all these considerations, it seems unlikely that thumb-sucking is a major cause of dental malocclusion. Even malocclusions associated with prolonged thumb-sucking seem to self correct when the habit is discontinued.

Tongue-Thrusting

During normal swallowing, the tongue tip seals against the hard palate in the initial stages of moving the bolus down the pharynx toward the esophagus, and there is little protrusive force by the tongue against the incisors and anterior aspects of the alveolar ridge (Ardran and Kemp, 1955; Best and Taylor, 1961). In contrast, the theory about deviant swallowing is that the tongue pushes against the incisors and anterior alveolar ridge during these initial stages of swallowing instead of making the seal superiorly. Mason (1988) suggested that resting postures are equally important, etiologically. Over time, this pressure is presumed to force the occlusion into openbite with vertical space between the upper and lower incisors. The relationship between tongue-tip position during swallowing and the presence of openbite is considered circular: the larger the interdental space, the more protrusion of the tongue in swallowing, and the more protrusion, the larger the space becomes. In addition, claims have been made that patients who show tongue-thrust swallowing also exhibit unusual weakness in the muscles that encircle the mouth, mainly the orbicularis oris. Mason (1988) refers specifically to lip incompetence (failure to meet normally). This weakness is presumed to be a significant factor in the origin and maintenance of the deviant swallowing pattern. The assumption is also made that this deviant pattern was acquired in early childhood, perhaps as a result of faulty sucking behavior. Some orthodontists maintain that malocclusion that seems to result from abnormal swallowing patterns cannot be satisfactorily treated so long as the patterns persist.

There has been considerable interest in the question of whether this disorder is a clinical entity and, if so, what etiological factors are important and what treatment methods are effective. For example, Moyers (1988) endorses the validity of the general description provided above, with some differences in classification, and describes methods for treatment that include both orthodontic and behavior therapy. This is a controversial subject and will probably continue to be so ("Position Statement on Tongue Thrust," 1975). The relationships between oral function and oral structure are difficult to study. It seems likely that longitudinal data are needed to address some of the important questions. Although some advances have been made, (Proffit and Norton, 1970; Mason and Proffit, 1974), there continues to be a need for better methods for assessing such things as lingual pressure against the dentition during swallow, the normal swallowing process, and the variations that exist within normal populations. In addition, more definitive information is necessary about the natural history of both swallowing patterns and openbites.

Without question there are occasional patients who fit the tongue-thrust description. They typically have openbite and, significantly, both upper and lower incisors are bucally tipped. Furthermore, during swallowing, they may show signs of unusual lip protrusion with the tongue in an interdental position. Certainly many of these patients produce oral distortions of sibilants because of the malocclusion. These patients usually can be treated successfully with standard orthodontic techniques, but there may be reversion to malocclusion when the appliances are removed. On the other hand, there is also spontaneous improvement in many of these patients at or around puberty.

We have had personal experience with attempting to change swallowing patterns. Our clinical impressions coincide with our interpretation of existing data to the effect that it seems unlikely that therapy will yield significant, lasting results. The swallowing act is a reflexive, complex behavior that is very difficult to change. A more reasonable measure, in our opinion, is the use of a long-term orthodontic maintainer appliance to prevent movement of the dentition back toward malocclusion. To our knowledge there are no supportive data for this method in the literature, but clinical experience indicates that it is frequently effective.

THE ROLE OF THE SPEECH PATHOLOGIST

The speech pathologist is primarily interested in malocclusion as a possible factor in the etiology of speech disorders. If occlusion is important in speech production, it will be so in the production of fricatives, mainly sibilants. We emphasize that the decision about how occlusion is etiologically related to errors in speech production is to be made by the speech pathologist. In the same way, the decision about whether or not there is a malocclusion and, if so, whether it merits orthodontic treatment is to be made by a dental specialist.

Discussions about diagnosis and treatment of speech and language disorders of patients with orofacial anomalies, including malocclusion, are presented in the last two sections of this book. We have indicated that speech therapy is frequently (but not always) delayed during orthodontic treatment because both the structure and the appliance may interfere with speech articulation. Some-

times, even though the malocclusion is clearly hazardous to speech production, treatment may be less than optimal because of limited financial or dental resources, or health or other problems. In such cases, the speech pathologist must set realistic goals for treatment and must be careful to share, with parents, patient, and other interested professionals, information about these goals and, if relevant, the reasons for terminating therapy in the presence of a continuing speech disorder. In some patients there may be the potential for compensation for structural deviations. However, there are limits to the amount of compensation it is reasonable to expect. These decisions are seldom clear-cut. Many times consultation with a fellow speech pathologist who is experienced in orofacial anomalies is very useful.

PROSTHETIC DENTISTRY

The general mission of prosthodontics is the replacement of missing dental or other oral structures in the maxillofacial complex by means of various appliances. For cleft lip and palate management, that includes dental replacements such as bridges, partial or full dentures, obturators or speech aids, and palatal lifts.

Dental Replacements

We indicated earlier that patients with clefts that extend through the alveolar ridge frequently have missing teeth, primarily the lateral incisor or the first cuspid. The resulting space in the maxillary arch interferes with a pleasing appearance and may also create difficulties in speech production, mainly with sibilants. Occasionally, if the alveolar cleft is not large or can be treated by a bone graft and if the general dental arrangement in the maxillary arch is suitable, the space usually occupied by the missing tooth can be closed by orthodontic treatment. On the other hand, a fixed or removable bridge may be required. In the majority of patients, the latter is the more satisfactory approach.

Managing the Palatal Cleft by Obturation

In contemporary practice, the majority of cleft palate defects are corrected surgically. However, management by obturation is used sufficiently often to merit discussion here.

The obturator (Adisman, 1971) is a special kind of dental prosthesis designed and constructed by the prosthetic dentist (Fig. 5.10). It occludes the palatal cleft so that the palate can serve as an effective partition between the oral and nasal cavities during speech. Typically, it consists of an anterior portion on which dental clasps are placed for securing the obturator to the teeth and a posterior portion or speech bulb. The palatal portion covers the cleft if there has been no previous cleft palate surgery on the hard palate. The appliance then extends posteriorly into the velopharyngeal space, which is filled by the speech bulb. Velopharyngeal competence is obtained by mesial movement of the lateral and posterior pharyngeal walls and, in some patients, posterior and superior movement of the palatal tags. The obturator may be used as a primary management procedure or, in some cases, as a secondary procedure following unsuccessful palatal surgery. Many prosthodontists consider construction of an obturator for secondary management to be technically more difficult than it is for primary management.

Management by obturation has several distinct advantages. The prosthesis is designed and constructed in the dental chair and requires no surgery or general anesthesia. That fact alone makes it attractive for patients with other health problems: for whom surgery requiring general anesthesia should be avoided, for children whose families have religious beliefs that contraindicate surgery, and for patients who wish to avoid cleft surgery for other reasons.

Modification of a poorly fitting prosthesis also can be accomplished without surgery. In contrast, further management for velopharyngeal incompetence following unsuccessful cleft palate repair usually means another surgical procedure.

Another primary advantage of the obturator is that it is a satisfactory method of compensating for tissue deficiency. Consequently, it is considered by some to be an acceptable alternative to palatal surgery for patients with very wide clefts. In these patients, there frequently appears to be insufficient palatal tissue on either side of the cleft to be

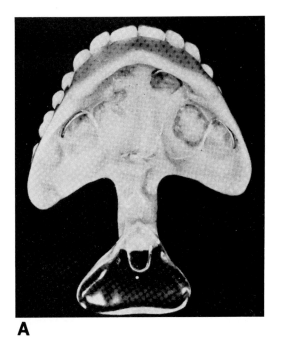
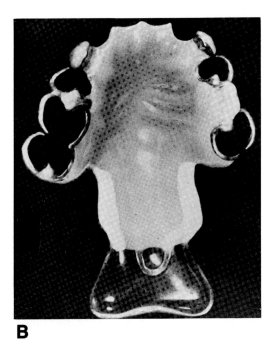

A   **B**

Figure 5.10   A. A prosthetic speech aid incorporating dentures. B. A prosthetic speech aid showing the clasps used for retention. (From Harkins CS. Principles of cleft palate prosthesis. New York: Temple University Publications by Columbia University Press, 1960.)

used in preparation of the soft-tissue flaps for the repair of the cleft. Not all surgeons and not all cleft palate teams agree with this point of view, and many prefer to close the palate surgically when there are no clear medical contraindications.

The obturator has several disadvantages. Like other dental prostheses, it requires good dental hygiene, periodic observation, maintenance, and replacement. In addition, it is subject to damage from careless handling. Wearing an obturator is also a more "unnatural" condition than is the case when there has been successful palatal surgery. It may be also that wearing an obturator contributes to the patient's feeling of being different, since it is a constant reminder of the cleft palate.

Few patients with obturators report difficulties in swallowing or in any other oral activities. A hyperactive gag reflex can be a problem initially, but patients usually adapt to the appliance, particularly if the palatal extension is increased over time.

Construction of an obturator requires great skill. The prosthodontist usually constructs the palatal portion first, adapting it to the patient's dental status to ensure suitable retention of the appliance. The impression for the speech bulb is then prepared. As indicated earlier, the objective is to construct the speech bulb so that criteria for both velopharyngeal opening (normal nasal breathing, normal nasalization of speech) and velopharyngeal closure (normal oralization of speech) are met. We recommend that it be constructed and tested with the speech pathologist in attendance and that particular attention be given to leakage around the edges of the appliance.

In summary, management by obturator is a highly satisfactory and effective approach and may be the procedure of choice for certain patients. Clinical observations lead to the conclusion that, to be successful, an obturator must be constructed taking into account the same speech physiology that is relevant to palatal surgery. Considerable movement of the pharyngeal walls during speech is a prerequisite to success. The requirements that the velopharyngeal port be closed during non-nasal speech and open during nasal breathing and the production of nasals are the same whether surgery or an obturator is used to close the palatal cleft. In the case of surgery, the opening-closing activity is provided at least in part by the repaired palate. The obturator is not

capable of such movement, however, so the need for pharyngeal wall activity during speech is even greater.

Finally, programs of obturator-reduction have been described as a treatment procedure for velopharyngeal incompetence in Chapter 23. The prosthodontist will be directly involved in this system of treatment whenever it is applied.

The Palatal Lift

In recent years, prosthodontists have made an important contribution to the management of many other types of palatal problems through the use of the palatal lift (Gibbons and Bloomer, 1958; Gonzales and Aronson, 1970; Mazaheri and Mazaheri, 1976; LaVelle and Hardy, 1979; McGrath and Anderson, in press).

The palatal lift (Figs. 5.11 and 5.12) is not an obturator since it is not designed to substitute for missing tissue. Rather, it is a prosthetic device for mechanically lifting an intact palate into a position in which the velum approximates the pharyngeal walls. It is used when palatal length is

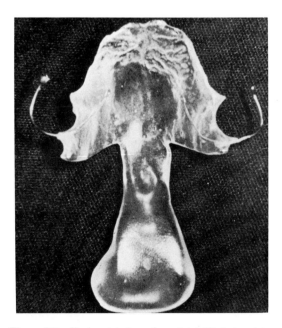

Figure 5.11 Horizontal view of a palatal lift designed to elevate the soft palate. (From LaVelle WE, Hardy JC. Palatal lift prostheses for treatment of palatopharyngeal incompetence. J Prosth Dent 1979; 42:308.)

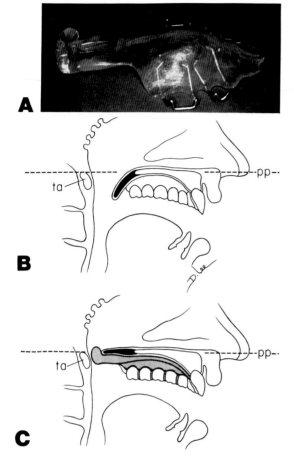

Figure 5.12 A. modified palatal lift with an obturator; B. congenital anatomic insufficiency of palatopharyngeal region; C. palatal lift-obturator in place, elevating the soft palate and obturating the palatopharyngeal space (pp, palatal plane; ta, median tubercle of the atlas). (From Gonzalez JB, Aronson AE. Palatal lift prosthesis for treatment of anatomic and neurologic palatopharyngeal insufficiency. Cleft Palate J 1970; 8:96.)

adequate, but palatal movement is not. The palatal lift is a useful nonsurgical technique in the patient with palatal paresis, either congenital or acquired (Hardy et al., 1969; Marshall and Jones, 1971). It is seldom used in patients with cleft palate because they often have insufficient palatal length.

SUMMARY

The frequent and sometimes severe dental and occlusal disorders shown by patients with clefts of the lip and palate require considerable attention by dental and other cleft palate specialists. Some of these disorders directly affect speech production. The orthodontist, pediatric dentist, and prosthetic dentist are important members of the cleft palate team, and make valuable contributions to the overall treatment results.

REFERENCES

Adisman IK. Cleft palate prosthetics. In: Grabb WC, Rosenstein SW, Bzoch KR, eds. Cleft lip and palate: surgical, dental, and speech aspects. Boston: Little, Brown, 1971; 617.

Angle EH. Treatment of malocclusion of the teeth. 7th ed. Philadelphia: SS White, 1907.

Ardran GM, Kemp FH. Radiographic study of movements of the tongue in swallowing. Dent Pract 1955; 5:252.

Bardach J, Morris HL, eds. Multidisciplinary management of cleft lip and palate. Philadelphia: WB Saunders, in press.

Bardach J, Roberts DM, Yale R, Rosewall D, Mooney M. The influence of simultaneous cleft lip and palate repair on facial growth in rabbits. Cleft Palate J 1980; 17:309.

Bell W, Profitt WR, White RP. Surgical correction of dentofacial deformities. Vol. I, II. Philadelphia: WB Saunders, 1980.

Bergland O, Semb G, Abyholm FE. Elimination of residual alveolar cleft by secondary bone grafting and subsequent orthodontic treatment. Cleft Palate J 1986; 23:175.

Best CH, Taylor NB. Physiological basis of medical practice. A text in applied physiology. 7th ed. Baltimore: Williams & Wilkins, 1961:685.

Bishara SE. Cephalometric evaluation of facial growth in operated and non-operated individuals with isolated clefts of the palate. Cleft Palate J 1973; 10:239.

Bishara SE, Orth D, Krause CJ, et al. Facial and dental relationships of individuals with unoperated clefts of the lip and/or palate. Cleft Palate J 1976; 13:238.

Bloomer HH. Speech defects associated with dental malocclusions and related abnormalities. In: Travis LE, ed. Handbook of speech pathology and audiology. Englewood Cliffs, NJ: Prentice-Hall, 1971:715.

Bohn A. Dental anomalies in harelip and cleft palate. Acta Odont Scand 1963; 21 (Suppl 38):1.

Burdi AR, Moyers RE. Development of the dentition and the occlusion. In: Moyers RE, ed. Handbook of orthodontics. 4th ed. Chicago: Year Book, 1988:99.

Coccaro PJ, Valauri AJ. Orthodontics in cleft lip and palate children. In: Converse JM, ed. Reconstructive plastic surgery: principles and procedures in correction, reconstruction and transplantation. Vol 4. 2nd ed. Philadelphia: WB Saunders, 1977:2213.

Foster TD. A textbook of orthodontics. Oxford: Blackwell, 1975.

Fricke JE, ed. Speech and the dentofacial complex: the state of the art. ASHA Reports No 5, 1970.

Garber SR, Speidel TM, Marse G. The effects on speech of surgical premaxillary osteotomy. Am J Orthod 1981; 79:54.

Gibbons R, Bloomer HH. A supportive-type speech prosthetic aid. J Prosth Dent 1958; 8:362.

Gonzalez JB, Aronson AE. Palatal lift prosthesis for treatment of anatomic and neurologic palatopharyngeal insufficiency. Cleft Palate J 1970; 7:91.

Graber TM. Changing philosophies in cleft palate management. J Pediatr 1950; 37:400.

Graber TM, ed. Orthodontics; principles and practice. 2nd ed. Philadelphia: WB Saunders, 1966.

Graber TM, Swain BF. Orthodontics, current principles and techniques. St Louis: CV Mosby, 1985.

Hardy JC, Netsell R, Schweigert JW, Morris HL. Management of velopharyngeal dysfunction in cerebral palsy. J Speech Hear Dis 1969; 34:123.

Harkins CS. Principles of cleft palate prosthesis. New York: Temple University Publications, Columbia University Press, 1960.

Jordon RE, Kraus BSD, Neptune CM. Dental abnormalities associated with cleft lip and/or palate. Cleft Palate J 1966; 3:22.

Kremenak CR Jr, Searls JC. Experimental manipulation of midfacial growth: a synthesis of five years of research at the Iowa Maxillofacial Growth Laboratory. J Dent Res 1971; 50:488.

LaVelle WE, Hardy JC. Palatal lift prostheses for treatment of palatopharyngeal incompetence. J Prosth Dent 1979; 41:308.

Loevy HT, Aduss H. Tooth maturation in cleft lip, cleft palate, or both. Cleft Palate J 1988; 25:343.

Marshall RC, Jones RN. Effects of a palatal lift prosthesis upon the speech intelligibility of a dysarthric patient. J Prosth Dent 1971; 25:327.

Mason RM. Orofacial myology: current trends. Intern J Orofacial Myology. 1988;

Mason RM, Profitt WR. The tongue thrust controversy: background and recommendations. J Speech Hear Dis 1974; 39:115.

Mazaheri M. Prosthodontic care. In: Cooper HK, Harding RL, Krogman WM, Mazaheri M, Millard RT, eds. Cleft palate and cleft lip: a team approach to clinical management and rehabilitation of the patient. Philadelphia: WB Saunders, 1979; 269.

Mazaheri M, Mazaheri EH. Prosthodontic aspects of palatal elevation and palatopharyngeal stimulation. J Prosth Dent 1976; 35:319.

McGrath CO, Anderson NW. Prosthetic treatment of velopharyngeal incompetence. In: Bardach J, Morris HL, eds. Multidisciplinary management of cleft lip and palate. Philadelphia: WB Saunders, in press.

Morris HL, ed. Patterns of orofacial growth and development. ASHA Reports No 6, 1971.

Morris HL, ed. The Bratislava project: some cleft palate surgical results. Iowa City: University of Iowa Press, 1978.

Moyers RE. Handbook of orthodontics. 4th ed. Chicago: Year Book, 1988.

Position statement on tongue thrust. Asha 1975; 17:331.

Prahl-Andersen B. The dental development in patients with cleft lip and palate. Eur Orthod Soc Trans. 52nd Congress 1976; 155.

Proffit WR, Norton LA. The tongue and oral morphology: influences of tongue activity during speech and swallowing. ASHA Reports No 5, 1970.106.

Ranta R. Eruption of the premolars and canines and factors affecting it in unilateral cleft lip and palate cases. An orthopantomographic study. Suom Hammaslaak Toim 1971; 67:350.

Ranta R. A comparative study of tooth formation in the permanent dentition of Finnish children with cleft lip and palate. An orthopantomographic study. Suom Hammaslaak Toim 1972; 68:58.

Ross RB, Johnston MC, eds. Cleft lip and palate. Baltimore: Williams & Wilkins, 1972.

Starr CD. Dental and occlusal hazards to normal speech production. In: Bzoch KR, ed. Communicative disorders related to cleft lip and palate. 2nd ed. Boston: Little, Brown, 1979:90.

Vallino LD, Pierre J, Andrews J. Speech and hearing before and after orthoquathic surgery. Annual Convention of the American Cleft Palate Association, Williamsburg, 1988.

Vig KW, Turvey TA. Orthodontic-surgical interaction in the management of cleft lip and palate. Clin Plastic Surg 1985; 12:735.

Wertz RT, ed. Orofacial function: clinical research in dentistry and speech pathology. ASHA Reports No 7, 1972.

Wertz RT, ed. Orofacial anomalies: clinical and research implications. ASHA Reports No 8, 1973.

Wilkins EM, McCullough PA. Clinical practice of the dental hygienist. 2nd ed. Philadelphia: Lea and Febiger 1964.

Zimmermann G, Kelson JAS, Lander L. Articulatory behavior pre- and post full-mouth tooth extraction and alveoloplasty: cinefluorographic study. J Speech Hear Res 1980; 23:630.

6 | OTOLOGICAL AND AUDIOLOGICAL DISORDERS

One characteristic of the cleft palate population about which there is widespread agreement is the prevalence of middle ear disease, universal in infancy, and the resulting conductive hearing impairment which persists in some older children and adults. This problem is one of the major complications of palatal clefts and should be well understood by speech pathologists.

THE NORMAL MIDDLE EAR

The normal ear is an air-filled cavity without fluid. Drainage from the middle ear presumably takes place through the eustachian tube, but fluid may also be absorbed. The eustachian tube also serves to equilibrate air pressure behind the tympanic membrane to atmospheric pressure and, at the same time, to replenish oxygen that has been absorbed. A third function of this important tube is to protect the middle ear from nasopharyngeal secretions. Bluestone and Klein (1983a) referred to these three major functions as clearance, ventilation, and protection (Fig. 6.1). Ventilation appears to be the most important function. The process of equalization of air pressure within the middle ear makes it possible for the tympanic membrane to respond in a highly sensitive manner to subtle variations in sound pressure levels.

The eustachian tube leads from the middle ear to the nasopharynx. In its rest position, the tube is closed, but it opens frequently during such activities as swallowing and yawning and in response to other changes in air pressure. The tensor veli palatini muscle appears to have the primary responsibility for opening the eustachian

tube. In fact, Cantekin et al. (1979) and Honjo et al. (1979) said that it is the only muscle active in the opening process. Closure of the tube is usually attributed to the passive return of the tubal walls to a position of rest, although Cantekin et al. suggested that the internal pterygoid muscle may serve as a constrictor. The tensor veli palatini muscle is made up of two bundles of fibers, which are divided by a layer of fibroelastic tissue. The inferior bundle, referred to by Bluestone and Klein (1983a) as the *dilatator tubae*, attaches to the fibroelastic layer and runs to a supermedial attachment on the lateral wall of the eustachian tube. Figure 6.2 illustrates the important relationship between these fibers and the eustachian tube.

Theoretically, in order for the eustachian tube to open, the tensor must contract and it must be properly related to the tubal wall or it cannot operate efficiently. Thus, the integrity of the soft palate is important to normal middle ear function. Other factors that may be involved are the stiffness of the tube, its angle, and its configuration.

OTITIS MEDIA

DeWeese and Saunders (1968), Payne and Paparella (1976), Bluestone (1982), and Bluestone and Klein (1983a) presented excellent descriptions of otitis media as a disease process. It is hypothesized but not proven that dysfunction of the eustachian tube results in faulty ventilation of the middle ear cavity, and this, in turn, leads to inflammation and fluid accumulation. Secondary bacterial infection may also occur. The tympanic membrane may become retracted, thickened, and

104

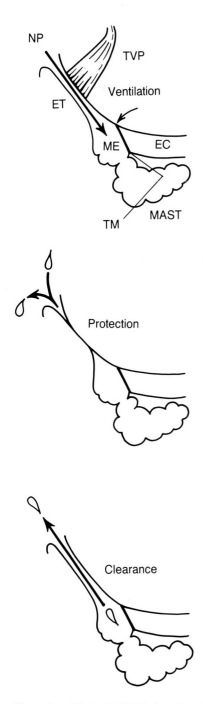

discolored. The sound conduction mechanism of the middle ear is thus impaired, and mild to moderate hearing loss occurs.

Paradise (1980) indicated that there is a question as to whether middle-ear infection, as distinct from sterile inflammation, can develop in the absence of eustachian tube obstruction. He speculated that if that is possible, the infection would probably very quickly result in tubal obstruction as a consequence of both inflammatory edema and the accumulation of middle-ear secretions. If the disease becomes chronic, especially when infection is present and untreated, permanent damage to the middle ear and adjacent regions of the temporal bone may result. Paradise (1980) and Bluestone and Klein (1983a), summarized their own work and that of others, saying that otitis media is the most frequent diagnosis made when children visit physicians because of illness. They pointed out, however, that the children so diagnosed do not all suffer from the same clinical

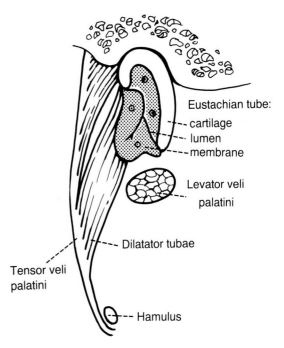

Figure 6.1 Three physiologic functions of the eustachian tube in relation to the middle ear. NP. nasopharynx. ET. eustachian tube; TVP. tensor veli palatini muscle; ME. middle ear; MAST. mastoid; TM. tympanic membrane; EC. external canal. (From Bluestone CD, Klein JO. Otitis media with effusion, atelectasis and eustachian tube dysfunction. In: Bluestone CD, Stool SE, eds. Pediatric otolaryngology. Vol 1. Philadelphia: WB Saunders, 1983.)

Figure 6.2 Diagrammatic representation of the relationship between the superficial muscle bundle (tensor veli palatini) and the deep bundle (dilatator tubae) to the lateral wall of the eustachian tube. (From Bluestone CD, Klein JO. Otitis media with effusion, atelectasis, and eustachian tube dysfunction. In: Bluestone CD, Stool SE, eds. Pediatric otolaryngology. Vol 1. Philadelphia: WB Saunders. 1983.)

entity. Otitis media means only that there is an inflammation of the middle ear and is not specific as to etiology or pathogenesis.

Otitis media with *effusion* is inflammation accompanied by a collection of liquid with no perforation of the tympanic membrane. When the effusion is *serous*, the liquid is thin and watery. If it is *mucoid*, it is thick and mucus-like. It is pus-like when it is *purulent*. When the ear disease is accompanied by discharge, the condition is called *otorrhea*. Many combinations of these conditions may occur.

As noted earlier, otitis media may be accompanied by changes in the tympanic membrane. Commonly found conditions are bulging, collapse or retraction, color changes, thickening, changes from translucent to opaque, scarring, and reduction in mobility.

It is thought that eustachian tube dysfunction may arise from different causes related to abnormal patency and to obstruction (Fig. 6.3). Paradise (1980) commented that the causes of eustachian tube obstruction have not been well substantiated but that it probably comes from a number of factors or combinations of factors. Even the functions of protection and clearance may be involved in some unknown way. It is clear that additional research is needed to prove or disprove the hypotheses about eustachian function and its relationship to otitis media.

The prevalence of otitis media varies with age. Young children are more prone to develop the disease than are older children and adults, but it occurs in all age groups. It also varies from one racial group to another; it is common among American Indians (Beery et al., 1980). Thus, there may be genetic factors that predispose individuals or races to otitis media. It is also seen more frequently in white than in black children despite the possibility that low socioeconomic status may be associated with an increase in this disease. Cambon et al. (1965) went so far as to say that "the running ear is the heritage of the poor." Many possible reasons exist for the apparent increase in otitis media among poor children, but the real explanation is unknown. Another group of children at high risk for otitis media are those born with clefts of the palate.

Otitis Media Associated with Cleft Palate

Heller (1979) and Bluestone and Klein (1983a) presented historical information about ear disease associated with palatal clefts. The first references to the problem appeared in the literature in 1878 and 1879 when Alt reported improvement in hearing following treatment of otorrhea occurring together with cleft palate. Gutzmann was apparently the first to recognize the increased prevalence of middle-ear disease in patients with clefts in 1893. Brunck, in 1906, observed middle ear pathology in patients with clefts and emphasized their need for otologic examination.

In the years that have followed, many studies have been carried out showing the prevalence of

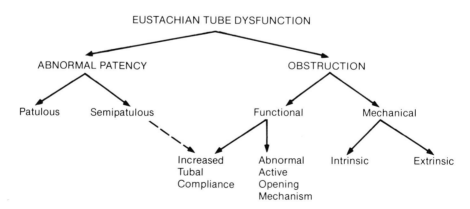

Figure 6.3 Various types of eustachian tube dysfunction. (From Bluestone CD, Klein JO. Otitis media with effusion, atelectasis, and eustachian tube dysfunction. In: Bluestone CD, Stool SE, eds. Pediatric otolaryngology. Vol 1. Philadelphia: WB Saunders. 1983.)

hearing impairment in this population. Unfortunately, these have frequently not specified what was meant by "hearing loss," how the measurements were derived, what the ages of the subjects were, what ear care the subjects had had, what their otological status was, or the conditions under which the data were gathered. Criteria for establishing hearing loss differed from study to study. It would obviously be desirable to report exact thresholds so that data from one study could be compared with those from another. In spite of the shortcomings of the research that has been done, there is general agreement that the losses are overwhelmingly conductive and that they tend to range from mild to moderate, with most being in the mild range.

Infant Studies

Although it was recognized for many years that individuals with cleft palates were at increased risk for ear disease, it was thought that the disease occurred primarily in early or middle childhood (Skolnick, 1958), and very little was done about the problem unless the symptoms became acute. Babies' ears were only infrequently examined, and even older children often received only cursory otological attention. Some clinics did not even have audiometers, and referrals for ear care were made as various members of the team thought it was necessary.

In the mid-1960s, Stool and Randall (1967) and Paradise et al. (1969) independently began to observe infant ears. Stool and Randall made their observations in the operating room at the time of lip or palate repair. Using an operating microscope, they examined the tympanic membranes of 25 babies ranging in age from 9 days to 12 months. Forty-seven of the 50 ears contained mucoid material of varying degrees of viscosity. Only three of ten infants with clefts of the prepalate showed evidence of ear disease. Children with clefts of the prepalate, those structures anterior to the incisive foramen, are not at increased risk for ear disease.

Paradise et al. (1969) reported their otological findings in 50 infants with cleft palate. Forty were a year of age or younger; eight were examined within the first month of life; and ten were between 13 and 20 months of age. Standard otoscopic techniques were used. Ninety-six percent of the 100 infant ear drums were abnormal;

the most frequent findings were opacification and impaired mobility followed by fullness or bulging and, finally, by color changes. While these conditions occurred in infants with cleft lip only, the prevalence rate was only 22%, the exact percentage shown in the same study for 100 infants without clefts—although the normal babies may not have been typical of the general population. Myringotomies were performed on 86 of the 96 diseased ears (the cleft group), and the presence of fluid was confirmed in all. In another study, otitis media was found in all 21 infants examined in the first 3 months of life. Those observations have since been reconfirmed.

Paradise and Bluestone (1974) reported that the occurrence of otitis media is less frequent in infants after palatal repair, and other studies have shown that hearing losses are less apparent in older children than in younger ones (Goetzinger, 1960; Spriestersbach et al., 1962 and Graham, 1964). Because hearing improves in children with clefts as they get older just as it does in noncleft children, it is not clear whether the palatal repair is responsible for the change, whether the improvement is a function of age, or whether both factors are important.

Stool and Randall (1967) studied 10 specimens of the material removed from the ears of the patients they treated for otological disease and found it to consist primarily of poorly organized granulation tissue. Lupovich et al. (1971) found sterile, inflammatory effusions of varying viscosity. Left untreated, however, the nature of the liquid changes, and it may become purulent.

Recently, Paradise (in press) reports that middle ear effusion is not necessarily invariable in babies with cleft palate. He also infers from the available data that impaired eustachian tube function is not the sole etiological factor but that there may be also nutritional factors. Specifically, he reports indications that babies with cleft palate who are fed breast milk (usually expressed manually) have fewer episodes of otitis media than those who receive other milk or infant formula.

The Origins of Otitis Media in Children with Clefts

Many theories have been advanced about the causes of otitis media in children with clefts. An old idea was that milk seeped into the middle ear and caused contamination. That now seems a simplistic explanation. Another explanation that has been offered is that the unrepaired cleft palate permits bacterial contamination of the middle ear from the nasopharynx. This seems unlikely because the fluid has been shown to be sterile. However, the open palate is implicated in other ways. Doyle et al. (1980) found otitis media in laboratory animals in whom they had surgically created palatal clefts.

We indicated earlier that the majority of people who have otitis media probably have impaired functioning of the eustachian tube. This holds for cleft patients as well when the cleft is unrepaired and, for many, after it has been closed. The theory of eustachian tube malfunction was advanced by Holborow in 1962. Prior to surgery, the problem seems to result from functional obstruction of the eustachian tube, which leads to an abnormal opening mechanism (Fig. 6.4). Otitis media that persists after palatal closure may be related to unusual distensibility of the eustachian tube (Paradise and Bluestone, 1974), to a defective opening mechanism, or to both (Bluestone, 1971; 1972a, Bluestone et al., 1972b, 1972c).

The variations in tubal function described here are associated with high negative pressures in the middle ear and with effusion. However, hypotheses about the mechanisms by which otitis media occurs, while generally agreed upon, are far from being proved.

One idea that merits additional exploration was advanced by Holborow (1962). He thought that the malfunction of the eustachian tube might

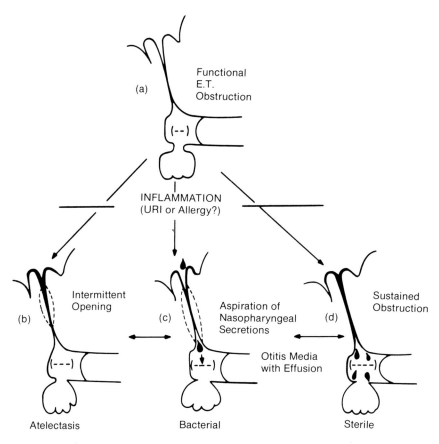

Figure 6.4 Mechanism by which functional obstruction of the eustachian tube results in otitis media with effusion. (From Bluestone CD, Klein JO. Otitis media with effusion, atelectasis and eustachian tube dysfunction. In: Bluestone CD, Stool SE, eds. Pediatric Otolaryngology. Vol 1. Philadelphia: WB Saunders, 1983.)

be attributed to poor development of the tensor veli palatini muscles "in conformity with general hypoplasia of the muscles of the soft palate" in patients with clefts. He also cited the absence of a firm midline anchorage for the tensor when a cleft is present. This theory is not unreasonable since surgeons often report difficulties with muscle dissection when the tissue is thin and sparse. Holborow also speculated about possible damage to the tensors during palatoplasty.

Calderelli (1975) and Paradise (1980) have questioned the role of faulty velopharyngeal valving in otitis media. Such valving deficits may result in disturbances of the aerodynamic and hydrodynamic relationships in the nasopharynx and the eustachian tubes. If that were occurring, one would expect to find improved ear status following secondary surgery to correct velopharyngeal valving deficits. Data on this relationship vary from no change following the flap (Graham and Lierle, 1962; Bennett, 1972) to some slight improvement (Aschan, 1966; and Yules, 1970). Additional well controlled investigation is warranted on this question. Of special interest would be the possible changes in ear status with reconstruction of the levator sling. Another way to evaluate this relationship is to compare children with velopharyngeal competence following surgical repair with those who have velopharyngeal incompetence. Yules (1970) reported that the latter group had poorer hearing; however, these data are not conclusive. Another relevant consideration is the sometime practice of fracturing the hamulus of the pterygoid plate to obtain greater relaxation of the tensor muscle (Millard, 1980; Bardach and Salyer, 1987).

EXTENT OF HEARING LOSS

Because otitis media is capricious, accompanying hearing loss is also inconsistent. The hearing impairment may be unilateral or bilateral, the involvement may shift from one ear to the other, and the degree of loss may fluctuate. These variable characteristics account in part for the divergent test results reported in the literature and for the differences observed in the same patient even over a short period of time.

If the hearing loss is related only to otitis media, it will range in severity from 5 dB to 55 dB, and bone thresholds will be normal. Table 6.1 presents a probable distribution (Fria 1983). Hearing loss appears to be unquestionably related

to the cleft but to be influenced by other variables such as surgery as well.

Musgrave et al. (1975) completed a longitudinal investigation of 11 children who had had the von Langenbeck straight-line surgical procedure and eight who had had the V-Y retroposition. The children were evaluated first at about 4 years, 9 months of age. Sixty percent of the von Langenbeck group had pure tone hearing thresholds that averaged no higher than 20 dB in the better ear, but this was true for 75 percent of the children who had had the V-Y procedure. Two years later, the von Langenbeck group averaged 17.8 dB in the left ear and 16.2 dB in the right. This compared to 8.33 dB for the left ear and 12.92 dB for the right in the V-Y group. This finding confirms that of Masters et al. (1960). The V-Y procedure seems to result in slightly better hearing than does the von Langenbeck.

In another study, McWilliams and Matthews (1979) examined 226 children at a mean age of 10 years. One hundred and eleven subjects had unilateral complete clefts of the lip and palate; 16 of these had associated abnormalities. One hundred and fifteen subjects had palatal clefts posterior to the incisive foramen; 76 of these had no other congenital malformations, and 39 had associated defects. *All* of the children in this study had air-bone gaps of mild degree. However, mean discrimination scores ranged between 95% and 99% for both ears, indicating that they probably had no serious auditory handicaps. Most of the children in all of the groups demonstrated pure tone averages no worse than 20 dB in the better ear. However, when that criterion was not met, the child usually had an isolated cleft. Overall, the children who had no other congenital malformations had better hearing than did those who had additional birth defects, regardless of cleft type. However, information about the influence of cleft type on the prevalence of hearing loss conflicts with this.

Masters et al. (1960), Spriestersbach et al. (1962), and Heller et al. (1975) reported that hearing losses are more prevalent in those with clefts of the palate only, but Pannbacker (1969) reported that hearing impairment is more prominent among those with clefts of the lip and palate. Holmes and Reed (1955) and Swigert (1976) found no differences.

Since everyone who has a palatal cleft starts life with otitis media, it is important for us to understand the natural history of the disease and

TABLE 6.1   Probable Handicapping Conditions Associated with Hearing Loss

Conductive Hearing Loss

Condition	Degree of Loss at Present	Probable Effect on Function
Evidence of past ear disease 1. Perforation 2. Scarring	5–20 dB	1. Subtle auditory dysfunction 2. Infantile speech 3. Articulation problems 4. Language retardation
Serous otitis	10–30 dB	1. Inattention 2. Speech and language retardation if persistent
Chronic otitis	15–55 dB	1. Inattention 2. Speech and language retardation if persistent
Middle ear anomaly	30–65 dB	1. Marked articulation problems 2.. Serious language retardation

Sensorineural Hearing Loss

Condition	Degree of Loss	Probable Effect on Function	
Congenital loss	25–40 dB	Mild speech and language retardation	
	40–65 dB	Moderate to severe speech and language retardation	
	70–85 dB	Severe speech and language retardation	If habilitation is not started very early
	85 dB +	No speech or language	
Acquired loss	25–100 dB	If acquired after 2 years of age, speech and language need not be retarded if rehabilitation begins promptly. Speech deterioration if loss is profound.	

From Fria TJ. The assessment of hearing and middle ear function in children. In: Bluestone CD, Stool SE, eds. Pediatric otolaryngology. Vol 1. Philadelphia: WB Saunders, 1983.

what ultimately happens to hearing as it relates to cleft type, other complicating abnormalities, aggressiveness of ear care, and the nature of treatment. At present, there are few answers to these questions, and careful prospective studies are needed.

HEARING LOSS ASSOCIATED WITH OTHER PALATOPHARYNGEAL ABNORMALITIES

Some information is available about ear disease or hearing loss in individuals who have velopharyngeal incompetence as the result of structural or functional deficits other than overt palatal clefts. These include submucous cleft palate, occult submucous cleft palate, structural disproportion, and palatal paresis. In general, these abnormalities are accompanied by an increased risk for both middle ear disease and

hearing impairment (Smith, 1968; Bergstrom and Hemenway, 1971; Beeden, 1972; Morgan et al., 1972; Taylor, 1972; Heller, 1975; Saad, 1975; Swigert, 1976). In these studies combined, approximately 50% of the patients had ear disease, and 45% had hearing losses, about what would be expected in subjects with cleft palate. As Heller (1979) suggested, subjects with velopharyngeal incompetence (including submucous cleft palate) "differ appreciably from the normal and more closely resemble a cleft palate population."

EFFECTS OF OTITIS MEDIA AND HEARING LOSS

There is considerable disagreement about effects of chronic otitis media in childhood. In 1982, a conference was held for the purpose of addressing the issue of the effects of otitis media on the child (Bluestone et al., 1983). The conferees concluded that:

Little doubt exists that at least temporary developmental impairments result from hearing loss of moderate or severe degree that is long-standing and unremitting, but no convincing evidence exists at present to relate developmental impairments to single and multiple episodes of short-term hearing loss or to mild hearing loss irrespective of duration. Future studies directed toward better understanding of the effects of otitis media, and of the variable hearing loss that accompanies it, will require the participation of investigators from varied disciplines and the application of rigorous principles of research design.

Some specific findings about the question come from a major study conducted at the University of Pittsburgh (Hubbard et al., 1985). They studied two closely matched groups of children with cleft palate, one with continuous monitoring and treatment for middle-ear disease and one without. Both groups showed eardrum scarring, depressed hearing levels, and impaired consonant articulation, but the treated group showed better hearing and consonant articulation than the untreated group. Mean verbal, performance, and fullscale IQs were normal for both groups, as were psychosocial indices, and there were no differences between the two groups in these regards.

We agree with the conferees of the 1982 workshop in their recommendation that all children have careful otoscopic examinations *whenever* they see physicians. Those with acute symptomatic otitis media should receive appropriate antimicrobial medication for an adequate period of time, should be reexamined until the condition has cleared, and should be treated rigorously. This is certainly true for infants and children with clefts. It may well be that otitis that exists as a single entity is different in its outcome from what it is when it is one of several disabilities. That issue must also be addressed. In the meantime, speech pathologists should be zealous in their attention to patients' hearing and should work closely with audiologists.

It is obvious that children who have chronic conductive hearing losses may require preferential seating in the classroom and in other group situations. If the hearing impairment is significant, it may interfere with educational and social

functioning. The exact degree of loss associated with disabilities of these types probably depends somewhat upon the compensatory abilities of the person with the loss. However, that is true only up to a certain point. If the loss is moderate and bilateral, the use of a hearing aid could be considered. The audiologist and the otolaryngologist will make that decision but will certainly consider relevant information provided by the speech pathologist.

COMPLICATIONS OF OTITIS MEDIA

If otitis media is untreated and fails to resolve spontaneously, there is the possibility that more serious pathologies will develop (Bellucci, 1972). This is important information in the management of children with clefts because their ear disease is persistent. Among the complications are perforation of the tympanic membrane, chronic otitis media, cholesteatoma, ossicular discontinuity and fixation, mastoiditis, labyrinthitis, and infections in the external auditory canal (Severeid, 1977; Bluestone and Klein, 1983b). In severe involvement, sensorineural components in the hearing loss may develop as the result of invasion of the inner ear. Complications such as these are rare in children with clefts who are treated and monitored from birth. For example, Dominguez and Harker (1988) found evidence of cholesteatoma in only four of 153 cleft patients treated between 1969 and 1977. Generally, children with clefts who are treated, and monitored from birth retain only minimal residual evidence of otitis media, including mild air-bone gaps, and demonstrate hearing that is functionally normal. There are exceptions to this, of course, even with careful management.

AUDIOLOGICAL ASSESSMENT

The audiologist is a vital member of the cleft palate team and is an important source of information and support to the speech pathologist. Audiological assessment is made by the use of standard procedures (Northern, 1976; Martin, 1978; Anderson and Davis, 1978; Hodgson, 1981; and Fria, 1983). The speech pathologist should be aware that audiological evaluations are necessary for children with clefts and that hearing cannot ever be ignored when treatment for communications problems is being considered. Audiological techniques will not be considered in depth here, but speech pathologists should understand the basic examination protocol so they will appreciate what the audiologist is doing and why.

Tympanometry

Tympanometry is helpful and can be introduced at about 7 months of age (Paradise et al., 1976). Prior to that age, babies with middle ear effusion often show normal tympanograms probably because the walls of the infant auditory canal tend to be distendible. After 7 months, the tympanogram becomes a much better predictor of ear disease. Paradise et al. identified five different tympanometric patterns that are commonly encountered and related them to middle-ear effusion. Bess et al. (1975, 1976) discussed impedance measurements in children with clefts.

Behavioral Observation Audiometry

Hearing testing is undertaken as early as it is feasible. One way to begin is to use behavioral observation audiometry. The basic method can be used as an informal screening technique, which speech pathologists are encouraged to learn in order that they may make observations that will assist them in communicating with audiologists in planning early intervention strategies and in making responsible referrals. The audiologist will do any definitive testing that is required, as it invariably is in children with clefts.

Behavioral observation involves the use of various noise-makers, which are presented to each ear. Music boxes, toys that make different noises such as animal sounds, and other things may be used. Fria (1983) mentioned crinkling onion-skin paper, which we consider to be one of the more valuable techniques for this purpose because infants seem to enjoy it. We suggest that a range of intensities and frequencies be introduced if possible. As the sounds are presented, the examiner watches for and records any evidence of auditory response.

Obviously, this is a screening technique. A very severely retarded infant or young child may fail to respond or may respond only to sounds that, for some reason, capture his or her attention. In addition, children with mild conductive hear-

ing losses are likely to respond because the noise levels are above their thresholds. High-frequency losses are likely to be missed completely. Parents cannot be assured that their child has no hearing loss on the basis of this crude testing. Speech pathologists who want to use this informal approach should work with it under the supervision of an audiologist, so they can learn what to look for. For more information about the technique, see Northern and Downs (1974).

In most cleft palate centers or audiology clinics to which referrals are made, the audiologist has the equipment and the training necessary to perform precise behavioral audiometry using stimuli of known intensity presented through loudspeakers in an audiometric test booth. This may require two examiners, although the mother can often hold the child on her lap while the audiologist presents stimuli and observes from an adjoining booth. At 6 weeks of age, infants respond at between 40 and 60 dB relative to audiometric zero. The thresholds for normal babies drop dramatically to 21 dB by 4 to 7 months and very gradually thereafter to 5 dB by 13 to 16 months.

Traditional audiometric testing is difficult with young children, and play audiometry has long been used instead. The child is conditioned to respond to a pure tone or to speech by engaging in some play activity. The child may be asked to put objects into a box, point to pictures, repeat words, place rings on a peg, or engage in some other activity of interest. The same approach can be used as a means of eliciting responses to pure tones and speech using earphones. It is sometimes possible to get a complete audiogram, including both air and bone thresholds, at least for some frequencies. The approach used will depend upon the cooperation and maturity of the child as well as upon the skill of the examiner.

Pure-tone audiometric testing can often be accomplished in quite young children using traditional techniques. Some children, however, because of associated problems including mental retardation, may never be able to cooperate in such testing. Others can do so as early as 3 years of age. The examiner must be sensitive to the capabilities of the child and not make demands that are beyond his developmental level. After that, the goal is to get air-and bone-conduction thresholds, speech-reception thresholds, and discrimination scores. The importance of bone-conduction thresholds cannot be overemphasized. Eagles et al. (1963) found that children who hear normally may respond at from -10 to 0 dB, so that children responding at zero on air-conduction tests, may actually have air-bone gaps. Fria (1983) and Heller (1979) discussed this problem

Hearing tests are a means for determining the extent and nature of hearing impairment but are not a method of diagnosing the presence or absence of middle-ear effusions. Bluestone et al. (1973) found that only half of the ear effusions present in a group of children evaluated by them were detected by audiometric screening techniques. Acoustic-reflex testing may also be used (Harford et al., 1978).

It is important to remember that some children with clefts have sensorineural hearing impairment, and some may have complex structural variations in the middle ear as the result of, or in addition to, otitis media. These are overlooked occasionally because of the middle-ear disease. If the loss is purely conductive, it will not be greater than 55 dB. Testing bone conduction in addition to air conduction will make it possible to determine whether the loss is conductive, sensorineural, or mixed.

Frequency of Audiological Testing

Hearing testing is usually done routinely every 3 to 6 months for as long as there is any indication that hearing has not stabilized. During episodes of active ear disease, hearing testing may be more frequent because it will always be done following any type of treatment. Once the hearing has reached a plateau and ear disease is no longer apparent, the child should be followed at least annually until all other treatment has been completed. In addition, parents and children should be carefully instructed so that they will recognize the signs of hearing loss and of otitis media and understand the importance of seeking medical attention. It will usually be the otolaryngologist and the audiologist who will be responsible for this part of the program, but the speech pathologist should be well informed of the ear status of any child enrolled in speech therapy.

MEDICAL AND SURGICAL TREATMENT OF OTITIS MEDIA

In many instances, when the problem is not severe, the otolaryngologist may place the patient under observation, using antibiotics to treat any infection. When the problem is recurrent, a myringotomy is indicated with insertion of a

ventilating tube. This idea was first suggested by Politzer in the mid-1860s but was not widely used until Armstrong revived the method in 1954. It is now the most common surgical procedure requiring anesthetic performed on children (Bluestone and Klein, 1983a).

Myringotomy is the surgical puncture of the tympanic membrane which permits drainage and removal, usually by suction, of fluid in the middle ear cavity. The ventilating tubes provide for pressure equalization. Figure 6.5 shows the steps in a myringotomy with tube insertion.

The tympanic membrane heals rapidly, and the surgical incision would be closed in a matter of days if a ventilating tube were not used (Donaldson, 1966). Fluid reaccumulates if aeration is not maintained. As a result, ventilating tubes are commonly used and appear to be highly effective as temporary substitutes for malfunctioning eustachian tubes.

Paradise (1976) noted, however, that children with tubes require frequent examinations to determine whether or not the tubes are in place and patent and that they often need repeat myringotomies when the tubes have been extruded. In addition, purulent otorrhea may occur along with eardrum scarring. The patient may also be limited in certain activities. Swimming is particularly hazardous because of the direct communication between the external auditory canal and the middle ear provided by the tube. In addition, Paradise (in press) concludes in a review paper that some of the late otological findings may be the result of treatment measures such as repeated myringotomies.

In spite of the drawbacks to aggressive treatment of otitis media in cleft children, Paradise (1976, 1983) recommended that, until further data are available from longitudinal studies, it is reasonable to provide for myringotomy with tympanostomy-tube insertion within the first 6 months of life. For children with cleft lips as well as cleft palates, it seems logical to do the myringotomy at the time of lip repair. When the tubes are extruded, he felt that treatment should be repeated as long as there is evidence of persistent middle-ear effusion.

Antibiotic therapy should be used when indicated and may help to stave off repeated myringotomies. Bluestone and Klein (1983a) believed, however, that middle-ear effusion that persists for 3 months should probably be interpreted as chronic and that active treatment should be at least considered to avoid serious sequelae.

Even then, if the hearing loss is mild and there is no evidence of serious secondary changes in the tympanic membrane, watchful waiting may be the preferred procedure. Regardless of the treatment philosophy, children with clefts require close monitoring of their ear and hearing status.

Of special significance to speech pathologists is the fact that all children with clefts will require attention to their ear health. However, treatment protocols will vary from one child to another. The speech pathologist can be helpful in this regard by working cooperatively with the otolaryngologist and the audiologist to see that the child remains under active care for as long as it is necessary.

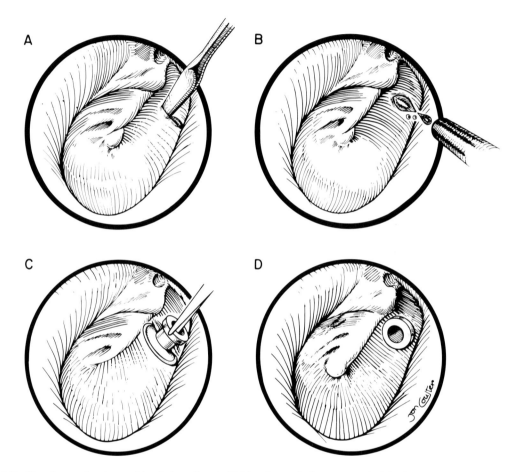

Figure 6.5 Steps in a myringotomy with tube insertion. A. Making the surgical puncture or incision in the drum membrane. B. Removal of middle ear fluid. C. Placing a ventilating tube. D. The ventilating tube in place. (From Bluestone CD, Klein JO. Otitis media with effusion, atelectasis, and eustachian tube dysfunction. In: Bluestone CD, Stool SE, eds. Pediatric otolaryngology. Vol 1. Philadelphia: WB Saunders, 1983.)

REFERENCES

Anderson CV, Davis JM. Differential diagnosis of hearing disorder. In: Darley FL, Spriestersbach DC, eds. Diagnostic methods in speech pathology. 2nd ed. New York: Harper & Row, 1978;445.

Aschan G. Hearing and nasal function correlated to postoperative speech in cleft palate patients with velopharyngoplasty. Acta Otolaryngol 1966;61:371.

Bardach J, Salyer K. Surgical techniques in cleft lip and palate. Chicago: Year Book, 1987.

Beeden AG. The bifid uvula. Laryngoscope 1972;86:815.

Beery QC, Doyle WJ, Cantekin EI, Bluestone CD, Wiet RJ. Eustachian tube function in an American Indian population. Ann Otol Rhinol Laryngol 1980;89:28.

Bellucci RJ. Fundamental principles in treatment of otitis media. In: Glorig A, Gerwin KS, eds. Otitis media. Springfield, IL: CC Thomas, 1972:210.

Bennett M. Symposium on ear diseases. III. The older cleft palate patient (a clinical otologic audiology study). Laryngoscope 1972;82:1217.

Bergstrom L, Hemenway WG. Otologic problems in submucous cleft palate. South Med J 1971;64:1172.

Bess FH, Lewis HD, Cierliczka DJ. Acoustic impedance measurement in cleft palate children. J Speech Hear Dis 1975;40:13.

Bess FH, Schwartz DM, Redfield NP. Audiometric, impedance, and otoscopic findings in children with cleft palates. Arch Otolaryngol 1976;102:465.

Bluestone CD. Eustachian tube obstruction in the infant with cleft palate. Ann Otol Rhinol Laryngol 1971;80(Suppl 2):1.

Bluestone CD. Otitis media. In: Gates GA, ed. Current therapy in otolaryngology-head and neck surgery. Toronto: BC Decker, 1982:1.

Bluestone CD, Beery QC, Paradise JL. Audiometry and tympanometry in relation to middle ear effusions in children. Laryngoscope 1973;83:594.

Bluestone CD, Klein JO. Otitis media with effusion, atelectasis and eustachian tube dysfunction. In: Bluestone CD, Stool SE, eds. Pediatric otolaryngology. Vol 1. Philadelphia: WB Saunders, 1983a:356.

Bluestone CD, Klein JO. Intratemporal complication and sequelae of otitis media. In: Bluestone CD, Stool SE, eds. Pediatric otolaryngology. Vol 1. Philadelphia: WB Saunders, 1983b;513.

Bluestone CD, Klein JO, Paradise JL, et al. Workshop on effects of otitis media on the child. Pediatrics 1983;71:639.

Bluestone CD, Paradise JL, Beery QC. Symposium on prophylaxis and treatment of middle ear effusions: IV. Physiology of the eustachian tube in the pathogenesis and management of middle-ear effusions. Laryngoscope 1972a;82:1654.

Bluestone CD, Paradise JL, Beery QC, Wittel R. Certain effects of cleft palate repair on eustachian tube function. Cleft Palate J 1972b;9:183.

Bluestone CD, Wittel RA, Paradise JL. Roentgenographic evaluation of eustachian tube function in infants with cleft and normal palates (with special reference to the occurrence of otitis media). Cleft Palate J 1972c;9:93.

Cambon K, Galbraith JD, Kong G. Middle-ear disease in Indians of the Mount Currie reservation. British Columbia. Can Med Assoc J 1965;93:1301.

Cantekin EI, Doyle WJ, Reichert TJ, Phillips DC, Bluestone CD. Dilation of the eustachian tube by electrical stimulation of the mandibular nerve. Ann Otol Rhinol Laryngol 1979;88:40.

Calderelli DD. Incidence and type of otologic disease in the older cleft palate patient. Cleft Palate J 1975;12:311.

DeWeese DD, Saunders WH. Textbook of otolaryngology, 3rd ed. St Louis: CV Mosby, 1968.

Dominguez S, Harker LA. Incidence of cholesteatoma with cleft palate. Annals Otol Rhinol Laryngol 1988;97:659.

Donaldson JA. The role of artificial eustachian tube in cleft palate patients. Cleft Palate J 1966;3:61.

Doyle WJ, Cantekin EI, Bluestone CD, Phillips DC, Kimes KK, Siegel MI. Nonhuman primate model of cleft palate and its implications for middle-ear pathology. Ann Otol Rhinol Laryngol 1980;89(Suppl 68):41.

Eagles EL, Wishik SM, Doerfler LG, Melnick W, Levine HS. Hearing sensitivity and related factors in children. Laryngoscope Monograph, 1963.

Fria TJ. The assessment of hearing and middle-ear function in children. In: Bluestone CD, Stool SE, eds. Pediatric otolaryngology. Vol 2. Philadelphia: WB Saunders, 1983:152.

Goetzinger CP, Embrey JE, Brooks R, Proud GO. Auditory assessment of cleft palate adults. Acta Otolaryngol 1960;52:551.

Graham MD. A longitudinal study of ear disease and hearing loss in patients with cleft lips and palates. Ann Otol Rhinol Laryngol 1964;73:34.

Graham MD, Lierle D. Posterior pharyngeal flap: palatoplasty and its relationship to ear disease and hearing loss. Laryngoscope 1962;72:1750.

Harford ER, Ross FH, Bluestone CD, Klein JO, eds. Impedance screening for middle ear disease in children: proceedings of a symposium held in Nashville, Tennessee, June 20-22, 1977. New York: Grune and Stratton, 1978.

Heller JC, Gens GW, Moe D, Croft CB. Conductive hearing loss in patients with velopharyngeal insufficiency. Annual Meeting of the American Cleft Palate Association, New Orleans, 1975.

Heller JC. Hearing loss in patients with cleft palate. In: Bzoch KR, ed. Communicative disorders related to cleft lip and palate. 2nd ed. Boston: Little, Brown, 1979:100.

Hodgson WR. Basic audiologic evaluation. Baltimore: William & Wilkins, 1981.

Holborow CA. Deafness associated with cleft palate. J Laryngol Otol 1962;76:762.

Holmes EM, Reed GF. Hearing and deafness in cleft palate patients. Arch Otolaryngol 1955;62:620.

Honjo I, Okazaki N, Kumazawa T. Experimental study of the eustachian tube function with regard to its related muscle. Acta Otolaryngol 1979;87:84.

Hubbard TW, Paradise JL, McWilliams BJ, Elster BA, Taylor FH. Consequences of unremitting middle-ear disease in early life. Otologic, audiologic, and developmental findings in children with cleft palate. N Engl J Med 1985;312:1529.

Lupovich P, Bluestone CD, Paradise JL, Harkins M. Middle ear effusions: preliminary viscometric, histologic and biochemical studies. Ann Otol Rhinol Laryngol 1971;80:342.

McWilliams BJ, Matthews HP. A comparison of intelligence and social maturity in children with unilateral complete clefts and those with isolated cleft palates. Cleft Palate J 1979;16:363.

Martin FN, ed. Pediatric audiology. Englewood Cliffs, NJ: Prentice-Hall, 1978.

Masters FW, Bingham HG, Robinson DW. The prevention and treatment of hearing loss in the cleft palate child. Plast Reconstr Surg 1960;25:502.

Millard DR. Cleft craft: alveolar and palatal deformities. Vol III. Boston: Little, Brown, 1980.

Morgan A, Dumolard P, Laurent M, Armand P, Arnaud H. Les problemes de paudition dans Pinsuffisance velaire. J Francais d'otorhinolaryngol 1972;21:891.

Musgrave RH, McWilliams BJ, Matthews HP. A review of the results of two different surgical procedures for the repair of clefts of the soft palate only. Cleft Palate J 1975;12:281.

Northern JL, ed. Hearing disorders. Boston: Little, Brown, 1976.

Northern JL, Downs MP. Hearing in children. Baltimore: Williams & Wilkins, 1974.

Pannbacker M. Hearing loss and cleft palate. Cleft Palate J 1969;6:50.

Paradise JL. Management of middle ear effusions in infants with cleft palate. Ann Otol Rhinol Laryngol 1976;85(Suppl 25):285.

Paradise JL. Otitis media in infants and children. Pediatrics 1980;65:917.

Paradise JL. Otitis media in infants and children with cleft palate: current epidemiological issues. Ann Otol Rhinol Laryngol, in press.

Paradise JL. Primary care of infants and children with cleft palate. In: Bluestone CD, Stool SE, eds. Pediatric otolaryngology. Vol 2. Philadelphia: WB Saunders, 1983:924.

Paradise JL, Bluestone CD. Early treatment of the universal otitis media of infants with cleft palate. Pediatrics 1974;53:48.

Paradise JL, Bluestone CD, Felder H. The universality of otitis media in 50 infants with cleft palate. Pediatrics 1969;44:35.

tional Conference on Cholesteatoma. Birmingham: Aesculapius Publishing, 1977.

Skolnick EM. Otologic evaluation in cleft palate patients. Laryngoscope 1958;68:1908.

Smith JL. Cleft palate: auditory and otologic findings. Tex Med 1968;64:69.

Spriestersbach DC, Lierle DM, Moll KL, Prather WF. Hearing loss in children with cleft palates. Plast Reconstr Surg 1962;30:336.

Stool SE, Randall P. Unexpected ear disease in infants with cleft palate. Cleft Palate J 1967;4:99.

Swigert E. Hearing sensitivity of adults with a cleft lip and or palate or VPI. Annual Meeting of the American Cleft Palate Association. San Francisco, 1976.

Taylor GD. The bifid uvula. Laryngoscope 1972;82:771.

Yules RB. Hearing in cleft palate patients. Arch Otolaryngol 1970;91:319.

Paradise JL, Smith CG, Bluestone CD. Tympanometric detection of middle ear effusion in infants and young children. Pediatrics 1976;58:198.

Payne EE, Paparella MM. Otitis media. In: Northern JL, ed. Hearing disorders. Boston: Little, Brown, 1976:119.

Saad EF. The bifid uvula in ear, nose, and throat practice. Laryngoscope 1975;85:734.

Severeid LR. Development of cholesteatoma in children with cleft palate: A longitudinal study. In: McCabe BF, Sade J, Abramson M, eds. Transactions of the First Interna-

7 | TONSILS AND ADENOIDS

Some detailed discussion of the tonsillar and adenoidal masses is warranted because of their special relevance to the velopharyngeal mechanism, and hence oral/nasal regulation of speech, as well as to the otolaryngologic status of the patient. Tonsils and adenoids are surgically removed less frequently today than was formerly the case. These lymphoid masses were once seen as an important seat of infection, but the emphasis now is on their protective role. However, tonsillectomy and adenoidectomy continue to be necessary in selected cases, including an occasional patient with a palatal cleft or some other related condition affecting velopharyngeal valving. When the potential for velopharyngeal valving deficits is present, adenoidectomy may have adverse effects on speech. Tonsils may also be important, but their role is less clearly defined.

There are also questions about normal decrease in size, usually referred to as involution or atrophy, of these lymphoid masses and specifically the effect of adenoidal atrophy on velopharyngeal status.

ADENOIDS

The adenoids influence the size and configuration of the pharynx (Morris, 1975; Paradise and Bluestone, 1976). Adenoids are usually located in the concavity of the nasopharynx, the most common site of contact between the soft palate and the pharyngeal wall during velopharyngeal function. When oral structures are intact and are of normal size and innervation, the adenoids apparently have no effect on speech production unless the tissue mass is greatly enlarged, in which case the nasal airway may be partially or totally occluded with the result that speech is either hyponasal or denasal.

Adenoidal Atrophy

As Figure 7.1 demonstrates, the adenoids gradually increase in size until puberty, when they very gradually begin to atrophy. At the same time there is an increase in vertical distance between the soft palate and the adenoidal pad because of vertical growth (Fig. 7.2). In adulthood, it is unusual to find a marked adenoid pad. As the atrophy takes place, the dimensions of the pharyngeal space increase, and the velum and pharyngeal walls must adapt to the new relationships if the velopharyngeal port is to be closed during speech (see Fig. 7.2). Since velopharyngeal dimensions increase with age in small increments (Subtelny and Koepp-Baker, 1956), most people apparently make the necessary adjustments in velopharyngeal activity with little difficulty.

However, these accommodations are not possible for some individuals, particularly those with repaired cleft palate or other related structural or functional deficits.

When they are unable to drive their velopharyngeal valving mechanisms enough to span the space or when the tissues are simply inadequate to do so, the result is excessive nasalization of speech and surgical reduction of the velopharyngeal valve may be required. If the individual has no history suggestive of velopharyngeal deficiency, the onset of this distressing speech deterioration can be traumatic. For an individual who has a cleft, the loss of capabilities thought to be permanently mastered can be devastating.

There has been interest in discovering ways to predict that velopharyngeal incompetence is likely to occur. Mason and Warren (1980) used aerodynamics, cephalometrics, and clinical examination to study 122 patients whom they considered to be at risk for developing velopharyngeal

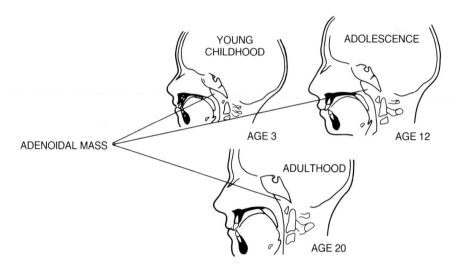

Figure 7.1 Tracings of cephalometric x-ray films of the same individual depicting the full cycle of adenoid growth. (From: Subtelny JD, Koepp-Baker H. The significance of adenoid tissue in velopharyngeal function. Plast Reconstr Surg 1956; 17:235.)

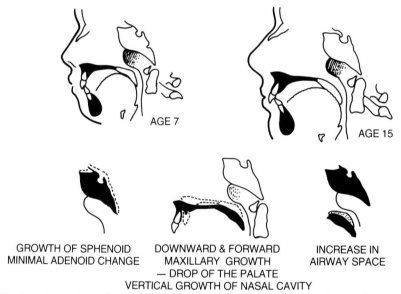

Figure 7.2 Tracings of cephalometric x-ray films of the same individual at two age levels, revealing the changed relationships between the adenoids and the surrounding structures (From: Subtelny JD, Koepp-Baker H. The significance of adenoid tissue in velopharyngeal function. Plast Reconstr Surg 1956; 17:235.)

incompetence as a result of adenoid involution. They reported that 40 of the 122 required surgery for incompetence in association with adenoid involution. Specific findings for two patients with clefts were included. One of the two clearly had

marginal velopharyngeal dysfunction before adenoidal involution.

Siegel-Sadewitz and Shprintzen (1986) used nasopharyngoscopy and multiple view videofluoroscopy to observe changes in velopharyngeal valving with age in 20 children with structurally normal palates, five with surgically repaired cleft palate, and five with unrepaired submucous clefts. None of the latter two groups showed any signs of velopharyngeal insufficiency. For all children, initial examination was conducted from 4 to 8 years, and follow-up examination from 14 to 18 years. They reported that none of the members in any of the three groups developed velopharyngeal insufficiency as shown by their examination procedures. They suggest that "structural changes which occurred in the pharynx with time compensated for the gradual involution of the adenoids."

Morris et al., (in press) followed 39 children with clefts longitudinally from the age of 6 to 16 years. These particular children were selected because at age 6 they showed velar contact in midline against hypertrophied adenoids. Lateral x-ray films were taken at yearly intervals to determine the relative size of the adenoids and the status of velopharyngeal closure. Analysis of variance of group findings indicated that adenoidal size did indeed decrease with age and that velar-pharyngeal contact was not lost as the subjects got older. However, three of the 39 subjects showed loss of midline velar-pharyngeal contact with adenoidal atrophy during the period of study. In addition, four more of the 39 had secondary palatal surgery after the study was completed, indicating the development of velopharyngeal incompetence even after the age of 16.

These available findings indicate that while the velopharyngeal status of many patients with structurally abnormal palates is not adversely affected by adenoidal atrophy, in some it is. The problem deserves continued attention, particularly with focus on identification of those who may eventually have problems. It is an important clinical mission.

Adenoidectomy

Normals

Although most children gradually lose the bulk of their adenoids through the normal developmental process and are able to make the necessary compensations, the removal of the adenoid mass by surgery brings about an abrupt structural change that demands sudden readjustments in velopharyngeal behavior. Individuals who have normal structures and function can usually compensate for this loss of tissue very

quickly. Temporary hypernasality may be heard immediately after the surgery, especially until the soreness subsides, but it usually does not persist for longer than a few days or weeks at the most.

Some interesting data about the problem were reported by Neiman and Simpson (1975) who used lateral x-ray films to describe physiological relationships before and after adenoidectomy on 15 normal children, 4 to 7 years of age. They reported that none of the 15 developed indications of velopharyngeal incompetence after adenoidectomy even though the physiological dimensions after surgery were similar to those reported earlier by other investigators for patients with congenital palatal incompetence. They attributed the successful adaptation by their normal subjects to adenoidal surgery to increased velar mobility, increased height of velopharyngeal closure, increased velar stretch, and anterior movement of the posterior pharyngeal wall. They concluded that the normal velopharyngeal mechanism has the capacity to overcome the imbalance between pharyngeal dimensions and velar length caused by adenoid removal and that the compensations used are often typical of those seen in adequate mechanisms.

Their findings are generally consistent with those reported earlier by Subtelny and Koepp-Baker (1956), Simpson and Austin (1972), Mourino and Weinberg (1975), Simpson and Colton (1980), and Simpson and Chin (1981). The notion of velar stretch is an interesting one, as applied in this context, and deserves further study.

At-Risk patients

When there is a deficit in the velopharyngeal valving mechanism and adenoidectomy is performed, the sudden increase in velopharyngeal depth may be too great for the palate and the pharyngeal walls to span even with the increased effort, which is characteristic of postadenoidectomy behavior. Under these circumstances, the velopharyngeal orifice remains open during speech, the nasal and oral cavities are coupled, and hypernasality results. People with clefts of the palate, submucous clefts, congenital palatal incompetence, and motor deficits are at risk for this outcome. The hypernasality is likely to be permanent and to respond poorly to speech therapy. Treatment is usually the same as that for patients with clefts who have hypernasality after surgery (Goode and Ross, 1972; Bradley, 1979).

Attempts are now being made to identify

those patients who are likely to experience speech deterioration (excessive nasalization) after adenoidectomy. Such predictions help the surgeon, the patients, the parents, and the speech pathologist to plan wisely (Lubit, 1967; Mason, 1973; and Morris et al., 1982). Unfortunately, there is not yet any way of making reliable and valid predictions about valving status following adenoidectomy. Certain procedures are helpful, however, and they will be reviewed here.

Croft et al. (1978) indicated the possibility that a deficiency in the musculus uvulae can be detected before adenoidectomy by nasoendoscopy. They suggested that a V-shaped defect on the nasal surface of the velum represents either absence or hypoplasia of the musculus uvulae, a condition suggestive of occult submucous cleft palate. Defects of this type can also be seen when

multiview videofluoroscopy is used (Fig. 7.3). Other evidence from videofluoroscopy considered to be suggestive of velopharyngeal valving problems includes any sign of borderline valving. In lateral projection, this is seen as touch closure or light, short contacts of the soft palate against the posterior pharyngeal wall, the adenoids, or both. It is also sometimes associated with loss of closure when the neck is extended. A Passavant's ridge may also be seen. In frontal projection, the lateral pharyngeal walls may be marked by extensive movement. These two latter findings suggest a borderline mechanism. In base view, a small, central, pin-hole opening indicates a borderline mechanism, as does absence of the uvular bulge or barium reflux. This system of analysis is consistent with the research described in Chapter 11. These characteristics are sometimes seen in asso-

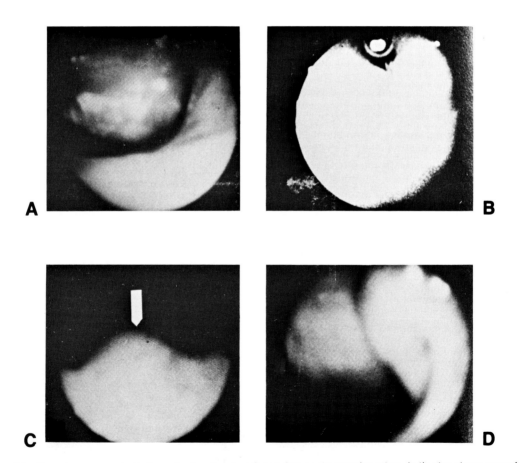

Figure 7.3 Nasopharyngoscopic photographs showing: A. a flat surface on the superior velum, indicating absent musculus uvulae; B. a small central gap in the velopharyngeal sphincter with air bubble in the mucous; C. a prominent musculus uvulae bulge in a normal subject; and D. eustachian tube orifice in a normal subject. (From: Croft CR, Shprintzen RJ, Daniller A, Lewin ML. The occult submucous cleft palate and the musculus uvulae. Cleft Palate J 1978; 15:150.)

ciation with essentially normal speech but are also typical of patients with mild symptoms of velopharyngeal incompetence. Patients who demonstrate these variations in valving with or without nasal escape—visible, audible, or both—are likely to show nasalized speech after adenoidectomy. More data are needed about this important problem.

Paradise (1983) recommended that *all* children who are potential candidates for adenoidectomy be carefully examined for bifid uvula, widening and attenuation of the median raphe of the soft palate, and notching of the hard palate— the traditional triad of symptoms associated with submucous cleft palate. If there is any sign of these abnormalities or if hypernasality is present in the absence of these findings, adenoidectomy is contraindicated in his view. Such children, he suggested, should be referred to a cleft palate team or to some individual who is experienced in in-depth evaluations. This philosophy expressed in clinical practice would undoubtedly prevent some of the unexpected results of adenoidectomy.

Only under very specific circumstances is adenoidectomy sometimes unavoidable. Occasionally, massive hypertrophy of the tonsils, the adenoids, or both results in dysphagia, in marked discomfort in breathing, or in alveolar hypoventilation or cor pulmonale. Even then, microbial treatment should be tried before resorting to adenoidectomy (Paradise, 1983).

Morris et al. (1982) reviewed previously published findings and reported new data on the early symptoms of congenital palatal incompetence (CPI) in 28 patients. Since the study was retrospective and depended on parental recall, these may have been under- rather than over-reporting of relevant signs. Significant differences between the CPI patients and the normal control subjects were found in early speech patterns, as might be expected. More parents of CPI children remembered that speech was difficult to understand, and more CPI than normal children were thought to have had nasalized speech during early childhood. Birth weight for the CPI group was significantly lower, but no differences were found in prenatal maternal health, complications during delivery, language development as opposed to speech production, feeding problems, physical development, or general health. The information about feeding problems is of particular interest because our clinical impression has been that CPI patients have a high frequency of nasal leakage in early infancy.

On the basis of their and other findings, particularly the report of Mason (1973), Morris et al. listed several symptoms that may predict CPI before adenoidectomy. Evidence of any structural or neurological abnormality of the velopharyngeal structures, family history of cleft lip, cleft palate, CPI, or related disorders, indications of neurologic impairment of other body functions, history of early speech disorders, especially nasalization, and nasal leakage during feeding in infancy all appear to be relevant. The authors suggested that, if any of these signs is present, the surgeon (and the speech pathologist) should inform the parents of the likelihood that hypernasality will occur following the adenoidectomy. This matter is usually also discussed with the child, who is, after all, most intimately concerned.

Adenoidectomy should probably be rigorously avoided whenever possible in patients with cleft palate, submucous clefts, CPI, motor deficits, or any other suspicious signs of potential valving problems. If, for any of the reasons previously mentioned, the procedure must be performed and hypernasality results, the patient will usually be a candidate for velopharyngeal valve correction if normal speech or even significantly improved speech is the goal.

TONSILS

Most of the published information about the role of the tonsils in speech production is based on clinical experience (Subtelny and Koepp-Baker, 1956; Morris, 1975; Trost-Cardamone, 1986; Henningsson, 1988; Shprintzen, 1989), and generalizations are difficult. It seems likely that tonsils that are markedly hypertrophied may be obstructive, decreasing the size and configuration of the oropharyngeal cavity. The tonsillary mass might also obstruct velopharyngeal activity, particularly if the mass extends upward to a position within the velopharyngeal port. Radiographic study by Subtelny and Koepp-Baker (1956) showed that tonsils move upward, backward, and mesially in concert with soft palate movement (Fig. 7.4 and 7.5).

On the other hand, enlarged tonsils might assist in velopharyngeal closure, especially in patients with a pharyngeal flap.

MESIAL AND UPWARD MOVEMENT
REST AND PHONATION OF [a]

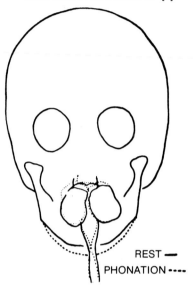

REST —
PHONATION ····

Figure 7.4 Frontal laminagraph tracing showing the movement of the tonsil masses in the frontal plane. (From: Subtelny JD, Koepp-Baker H. The significance of adenoid tissue in velopharyngeal function. Plast Reconstr Surg 1956; 17:235.)

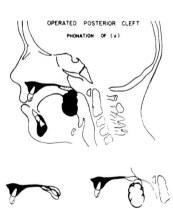

OPERATED POSTERIOR CLEFT
PHONATION OF (u)

Figure 7.5 Position of the tonsil masses (black) during sustained phonation. Lower left: movement of the soft palate from rest to phonation, at which time it contacts the adenoid tissue. Lower right: position of the tonsil mass at rest and during phonation (stippled). (From: Subtelny JD, Koepp-Baker H. The significance of adenoid tissue in velopharyngeal function. Plast Reconstr Surg 1956; 17:235.)

In view of the limited information about tonsils, the best approach is a careful examination of the individual patient. If the tonsils are diminishing the efficiency of the speech mechanism, to clinical significance, tonsillectomy, preferably without adenoidectomy, may be recommended. The converse is true if the tonsils appear facilitating. More data are needed.

REFERENCES

Bradley DP. Congenital and acquired palatopharyngeal insufficiency. In: Bzoch KR, ed. Communicative disorders related to cleft lip and palate, 2nd ed. Boston: Little, Brown, 1979:77.

Croft CB, Shprintzen RJ, Daniller A, Lewin ML. The occult submucous cleft palate and the musculus uvulae. Cleft Palate J 1978;15:150.

Goode RJ, Ross J. Velopharyngeal insufficiency after adenoidectomy. Arch Otolaryngol 1972;96:223.

Henningsson G. Impairment of velopharyngeal function in patients with hypernasal speech. Dissertation, Karolinska Institutet: Stockholm, 1988.

Lubit EC. Before an adenoidectomy—stop!, look!, and listen!. New York State J Med 1967;67:681.

Mason RM. Preventing speech disorders following adenoidectomy by preoperative examination. Clin Pediatr 1973;12:405.

Mason RM, Warren DW. Adenoid involution and developing hypernasality in cleft palate. J Speech Hear Dis 1980;45:469.

Morris HL. The speech pathologist looks at the tonsils and the adenoids. Ann Otol Rhinol Laryngol 1975;84:63.

Morris HL, Krueger LJ, Bumsted RM. Indications of congenital palatal incompetence before diagnosis. Ann Otol Rhinol Laryngol 1982;91:115.

Morris HL, Wroblewski S, Brown CK, Van Demark DR. Velar-pharyngeal status in cleft palate patients with expected adenoidal involution. Ann Otol Rhinol Laryngol, in press.

Mourino AP, Weinberg B. A cephalometric study of velar stretch in 8 and 10 year-old children. Cleft Palate J 1975;12:417.

Neiman GS, Simpson RK. A roentgencephalometric investigation of the effect of adenoid removal upon selected measures of velopharyngeal function. Cleft Palate J 1975;12:377.

Paradise JL. Tonsillectomy and adenoidectomy. In: Bluestone CD, Stool SE, eds. Pediatric otolaryngology. Vol 2. Philadelphia: WB Saunders, 1983:992.

Paradise JL, Bluestone CD. Toward rational indications for tonsil and adenoid surgery. Hosp Pract 1976;11:79.

Shprintzen RJ. Nasopharyngoscopy. In: Bzoch KR, ed. Communicative disorders related to cleft lip and palate, 3rd ed. Boston: Little, Brown, 1989:211.

Siegel-Sadewitz VL, Shprintzen RJ. Changes in velopharyngeal valving with age. Intern J Pediatr Otorhinolaryngol 1986;11:171.

Simpson RK, Austin AA. A cephalometric investigation of velar stretch. Cleft Palate J 1972;9:341.

Simpson RK, Chin L. Velar stretch as a function of task. Cleft Palate J 1981;18:1.

Simpson RK, Colton J. A cephalometric study of velar stretch in adolescent subjects. Cleft Palate J 1980;17:40.

Subtelny JD, Koepp-Baker H. The significance of adenoid tissue in velopharyngeal function. Plastic Reconstr Surg 1956;17:235.

Trost-Cardamone JE. Effects of velopharyngeal incompetence on speech. J Child Commun Dis 1986;10:31.

8 | CHILD

The purpose of this chapter is to discuss, from a developmental perspective, the cleft problem as it affects children from infancy through the school years. Children with clefts have special needs that cannot be denied and must be managed but that do not clearly differentiate them from other children. With insightful nurture and clinical care, prognosis is usually excellent when the cleft is uncomplicated by other conditions.

SPECIAL PROBLEMS OF INFANCY

A baby with some form of cleft is likely to have a number of hurdles to overcome early in life, and these may serve to retard initial development. Problems exist as well for the parents, whose responsibility for providing the early assistance to the infant is essential to successful outcome. Aside from their special requirements, children with clefts are like other infants in that they are not alike but are growing, developing, unique people with personalities of their own. It is not possible, nor is it desirable, to make the assumption that babies with clefts share similar life experiences and that their parents are alike. In spite of this, certain problems occur more frequently in such infants than in other children, and they are likely to encounter certain hazards that relate to the cleft.

Diagnosis

The first need is obviously for diagnosis of the child's condition. Only rarely are clefts detected prenatally by ultrasound. Thus, parents usually learn of the defect when the baby is born. The physician in attendance at the birth is the first person to face the question of diagnosis. Depending on familiarity with the defect and the available facilities, the examination may range from super-

ficial to complete, including the face and oral structures. If a cleft is found, the physician may ask for the assistance of a pediatrician, a plastic surgeon, or a specialized management team.

As with all infants, it is mandatory that the child's general status also be assessed. In this regard, this baby's needs are the same as those of any other baby, and they will remain so throughout life. However, as is mentioned in Chapters 1 and 10, the child with a cleft, particularly if it is a cleft of the palate only, is at increased risk for other birth defects, including syndromes with major life implications. Thus, the initial assessment must be thorough, and the child must be carefully watched during the first several weeks so that other birth defects, if they exist, can be discovered and appropriately treated. Some of these may be minor, but others, such as congenital heart malformations, deformities of the gastrointestinal tract, or neurological disorders may be life-threatening. Treatment necessary to preserve life will have a higher priority than the cleft. In short, the general health of the infant will dominate treatment needs, and that will not change throughout the span of life.

Informing Parents of the Cleft

Of major importance after diagnosis are informing the parents about the cleft and any other conditions that may exist, providing initial counseling, developing a feeding program, and arranging for special treatment. Parental needs are discussed in Chapter 10, but we note here that parents require compassion, understanding, patience, and information from well-informed professional people. Parents are likely to be shocked and grief-stricken when they learn of the cleft, and they deserve the best information available, delivered in the most compassionate, supportive manner possible. What and how the new parents

124

are told about the cleft has an impact on their later feelings and on the coping mechanisms they develop (Spriestersbach, 1973).

Regardless of who does the early counseling, the purpose is, first of all to listen and give the parents an opportunity to express their feelings and ask their most pressing questions. That precedes information giving, although that too is important, and acquainting them with available treatment programs. In this early interaction, the counselor, who may be a speech pathologist or from some other related profession, strives to be comforting, matter-of-fact, and optimistic, without making promises that may be impossible to keep. Ideally, this early phase of counseling extends over several sessions because new parents cannot deal with everything at once or even remember what they have heard.

Some speech pathologists believe that information about the speech and language consequences of cleft lip and palate should be discussed early, probably after the immediate concerns about survival, feeding, and plans for repairing the cleft lip have been addressed. Others are somewhat more indirect and answer questions as they arise, provide counseling when appropriate, and gently guide the parents to be good language and speech stimulators. The latter group want to avoid creating undue anxiety, which may be a negative outcome of the more direct approach. Wisely handled, either method can be successful, and both require that the speech pathologist be among those specialists who examine the baby and see the parents during the first month or so following birth.

Feeding

Feeding is a common problem and one of potential concern to parents. The baby with cleft lip only may have only minor difficulties or, often, none at all. At greatest risk is the infant with cleft palate, especially isolated cleft palate (Jones, 1988). The baby, although able to make appropriate sucking movements, cannot impound the negative intraoral pressure necessary to extract fluids from a bottle. Both blowing and successful sucking are dependent upon separation of the nasal and oral cavities. When there is an open cleft, the cavities are coupled, and it is difficult to

create both positive and negative pressures. For this reason, these babies may have feeding problems that require special attention. The pediatric nurse has usually had extensive experience with feeding young babies and can be helpful. If this is not the case, the baby and parents may leave the hospital without resolution of the feeding problems. The cleft palate team then provides feeding counseling. Any one of several specialists may assume that responsibility—the pediatrician, a nurse, a surgeon, a social worker, or, in some clinics, the speech pathologist.

Breast feeding is generally difficult for most babies with cleft palates. However, a highly motivated mother of a baby with a partial cleft palate can sometimes be successful with breast feeding. Mothers who want to breast-feed may compromise by extracting milk using a breast pump. They can then feed their infants by bottle but have the satisfaction of giving them breast milk.

Some specialists recommend that infants with clefts be fed with lamb's nipples, duckbill nipples, syringes, or other such devices. Clarren et al. (1987) review a number of feeding methods. Others suggest the construction of a small plastic prosthetic appliance designed to close the cleft in the hard palate to permit better suction and a variety of other approaches are also suggested (Jones, 1988). In our experience, such special procedures usually are not necessary, and most parents, given proper instruction, can learn to feed their babies successfully by adaptations of more conventional techniques described below.

Paradise et al. (1974) have shown that the weight gain in babies whose parents are left to resolve feeding problems on their own is extremely slow. Providing feeding instruction is one way to reduce this hazard. When parents are taught to hold their babies in a sitting position during feedings, to use a cross-cut nipple, and to adapt a plastic bottle with slotted sides so that the feeder can compress the plastic insert and assist with the flow of formula, feeding problems decrease in intensity, and weight gain is remarkably improved (Paradise and McWilliams, 1974). The soft Mead-Johnson nurser is an acceptable alternative and works on the same general principle but is more expensive.

Even with feeding instructions, Seth and McWilliams (1988) found that children with clefts showed a drop in weight percentile from birth to 20 months of 35% for males and 29% for females. At least 71% of all children had lower relative weights at 20 to 24 months than at birth. Duncan et al. (1983) questioned the ultimate outcome so far as height is concerned as well. These authors studied 65 children with clefts over a period of 11 years. Startlingly, height percentiles decreased as the children got older. Eight of 31 patients with isolated palatal clefts were consistently below the fifth percentile in height. In the 34 patients with clefts of the lip and palate, height percentiles were bimodal after the age of 4. The "short" group (65% of the subjects) included those who fell below the 50th percentile; the "tall" group (35% of the subjects) included those who were at or above the 70th percentile. This finding may reflect some genetic interference, since the parents were of normal height. This growth pattern approached that of individuals with isolated growth-hormone deficiency. The possibility of such a deficiency had been previously suggested (Laron et al., 1969; Gouny et al., 1978; and Roggazzeni et al., 1978). Studies are currently in progress to explore the possibility of growth-hormone deficiency in some children with clefts.

Although there are certainly exceptions, clinical experience and some data (Spriestersbach, 1973; Paradise and McWilliams, 1974; Jones, 1988) indicate that, with proper counseling and help with feeding, most infants and parents cope relatively well. This positive note should not be interpreted to mean that the situation can be taken lightly, however. A constantly hungry baby who must be fed often and for extended periods of time creates anxiety for parents, particularly if they have not had other children.

In spite of the hopeful outlook, feeding is handled in different ways by different people, and it remains a major concern of parents (Spriestersbach, 1973). Norval et al. (1964) reported that 35 of the 51 mothers they studied recalled feeding problems, and 31 said that their cleft babies had been harder to care for than their other children. They did not provide information as to whether the mothers who remembered fewer early problems fell into the low- or high-stress classifications that they described, how the children may have differed from each other, or what, if any, feeding help was provided. Those data would be useful in planning counseling and are relevant in view of

the work of Rintala and Gylling (1967), who reported that Finnish babies with clefts had decreased birth weights and an increase in prematurity. These factors might well influence the results of feeding studies. The infants studied by Seth and McWilliams (1988) had normal birth weights and no increase in prematurity.

Spriestersbach (1973) noted that feeding difficulties resulted in maternal anxiety. This view is supported in a poignant article by a mother (Gibbs, 1973). On the other hand, early feeding disturbances usually had no far-reaching effects on the growth and development of the children in the Spriestersbach study.

At least a part of the concern about feeding is its relationship to early psychosocial growth and development. An underfed baby is not as responsive as one who is gaining well, and parents are bound to feel anxious and frustrated. In addition, parents are undoubtedly nurtured when their infant is progressing well. The longer feeding difficulties persist and the farther behind the baby falls, at least temporarily, the harder the parents must try to overcome the problems. Since success or failure is reflected objectively in the baby's weight gain, parents may use this information as a measure of their own effectiveness.

These early feeding experiences may be highly relevant to both psychosocial and speech and language abilities later. It is difficult for the mother to look at her baby and talk gently during feeding if the baby is having episodes that are frightening to her. These very early interactional aspects of development must surely be influential in the infant's emerging social awareness. Those working in speech and language pathology know that communicative interests and skills begin long before the infant uses actual words with a communicative intent.

We take the position, certainly shared by many other speech and language pathologists, that sucking is a part of normal oropharyngeal development and that the behavior is importantly related to the development of normal speech and language, even though we cannot specify the exact relationship. It follows that the speech pathologist has a special concern about feeding and that solving feeding problems early and simply is essential to creating a firm foundation for future language and speech development. The speech pathologist must often assume the role of feeding specialist if attention is to be given to this important need, which is still too often neglected.

EARLY DEVELOPMENT OF CHILDREN WITH CLEFTS

Speech pathologists and other clinicians have voiced concerns about the developmental, psychological, and social handicaps that may be associated with cleft lip and palate. They believe that these aspects of development warrant routine consideration in diagnosis and treatment. Although research findings have been equivocal and have often not supported the hypothesis that psychological differences are any more prevalent in individuals with clefts than in those without, the conviction persists that there are psychosocial variations and that better methodologies will eventually reveal them.

Comprehensive reviews of the literature have appeared regularly over the years (Phipps, 1965; Matthews and Ohsberg, 1966; Goodstein, 1968; McWilliams, 1970; Wirls, 1971; McWilliams and Smith, 1973; Clifford, 1973; Richman and Eliason, 1986; Tobiason, in press). They have all noted the disparity between what the clinician senses and what researchers find. Thus, each review has begun by recognizing that there is a certain logic in the belief that children who have marked facial disfigurement, feeding problems, frequent hospitalizations, early and late surgery, speech problems, and exposure to a possibly hostile world are candidates for psychosocial disorders.

The output of behavioral research has increased since the early 1960s, and, as might be expected, research designs have become increasingly better adapted to answering questions. In spite of this, with few exceptions, descriptive data are still too scant and predictors of future outcome still too poorly defined to permit us to modify the environment to prevent undesirable behavior, even if such behavior could be agreed upon. Yet, in small steps, we move toward the goal of understanding the problems of this relatively large group of people, some of whom are significantly handicapped. We recognize that the "cleft- palate child" does not exist. Each child with a cleft is first of all a child with personal strengths and weaknesses, a family, a genetic make-up, and special mental and physical attributes. This is a unique person who is called upon to deal with certain stresses associated with clefts. This does not necessarily imply fundamental differences from peers, who also have stresses by which they too might be categorized. It is impossible to control all of the variations that influence a child, but we can strive to understand what part the cleft plays under certain circumstances and what can be done clinically to make alterations where they are required. Hackbush (1951) said essentially the same thing more than 35 years ago.

Developmental and psychosocial research in cleft problems has necessarily been carried out in many ways and has focused on limited rather than broad aspects of development. Clifford (1988) suggested that our observations thus far have been rudimentary with little attention to how the defect is incorporated into the development of interpersonal and communication skills, self esteem, and cognition. Although that is partially true, it is worthwhile to consider the work that has been done because it provides information about psychosocial issues useful to the clinician and to the researcher in charting future directions.

It is logical to assume that the early problems of children with clefts may influence the ages at which significant developmental landmarks are reached. Several investigators have explored this important area.

Plotkin et al. (1970) administered the Cattell Infant Intelligence Scale (Cattell, 1940) to 33 subjects at 6 months of age, 55 at 12 months, 48 at 18 months, and 31 at 24 months. No control group was used. All of the children in this study developed normally through the first 2 years of life with the possible exception of language, which was questionable.

Starr et al. (1977) used the Bayley Scales of Infant Development (Bayley, 1969) to evaluate the development of 82 children with various types of clefts uncomplicated by other defects. These children did not differ from the normative data on either the Mental Development Index (MDI) or the Psychomotor Development Index (PDI) at 6 or 12 months. After 12 months, the developmental profiles varied widely on the two scales, but overall the children were functioning normally.

Of special interest in this study is the finding that at 12 and 24 months the children with clefts were less responsive to their mothers than the normative babies. By 24 months, children with palatal clefts with or without clefts of the lip were also significantly reduced in imaginative play, a result consistent with the depressed creativity reported by Smith and McWilliams (1966). Starr et al. (1977) concluded that the children, although developing normally in many ways, were, when compared to children without clefts, more passive and more likely to avoid sensorimotor stimuli. Passivity is a description that occurs in the literature again and again.

Fox et al. (1978) compared 24 children at a mean age of 17.7 months and with various types of palatal clefts with a matched control group. The subjects were given the Denver Developmental Screening Scale (Frankenburg and Dodds, 1969), the Expressive Emergent Language Scale (Bzoch and League, 1971), and the Birth-to-3 Scale (Bangs and Garrett, 1973). When the subtests from the three instruments were considered together, there was a significant difference between groups in favor of the control subjects, and it was possible to group 79% of the subjects accurately, based solely on the developmental tests.

It is clear that, early in life, children with clefts are not seriously impaired but that their development shows irregularities and some lags not typically found in children who have no birth defects. Although those developmental characteristics must be recognized and carefully evaluated, there is danger that clinicians will be too zealous in their interpretations of early tests results and will intervene actively and relentlessly so that they may increase the infant's developmental risk by creating an environment that responds to subtle differences rather than to developmental potential.

Since the results obtained from infant assessments are not very reliable even for unimpaired children, all we can say at this time is that infants with clefts are likely to place at the low end of normal on developmental scales, that there are many exceptions to this in both directions, that it is irresponsible to alarm parents unduly, and that caution is the key word. On the other hand, awareness of the possibility of developmental lags should help clinicians understand the importance of making more precise observations of infants, improving parent counseling, and devising nonintrusive intervention techniques to minimize potential problems—especially with regard to language and social skills.

INTELLIGENCE

The foregoing discussion alerts us to the possibility of developmental variations in children with clefts but does little to answer questions unequivocally. The confusion is compounded when the literature regarding mental development in preschool and older children is reviewed.

A number of studies (Billig, 1951; Means and Irwin, 1954; Munson and May, 1955; Illingsworth and Bush, 1956; Goodstein, 1961; Lewis, 1961; Ruess, 1965) over the past third of a century have shown that children with clefts, particularly those with palatal clefts only, have mean IQs that place them in the low average classification rather than at the population mean.

As long ago as 1932, however, Wolstad expressed the opinion that children with clefts were not subnormal in any way. In addition, a study of 27 children by Rattner et al. (1958) reported normal IQs for the 17 children examined. Cervanka and Drabkova (1965) found normal intelligence in 42 subjects with unilateral complete clefts and isolated palatal clefts, whereas 19 children with bilateral complete clefts had a mean IQ of only 87. It is difficult to have confidence in these latter findings since 5 of the 19 subjects had IQs below 68, a high proportion, and no child in the other cleft groups had an IQ that low. While the conflict in the literature is obvious, the prevailing view historically was that there was a mild reduction in mean IQ.

Goodstein's analysis by cleft type revealed that children with cleft palate only had significantly lower IQs than children with clefts of both the lip and the palate. He suggested, as had Lewis in 1961, that this could be related to the higher incidence of other congenital abnormalities in the group with isolated palatal clefts.

Ruess (1965) compared 49 cleft children, aged 7 to 12 years, with their siblings closest in age. The Wechsler Intelligence Scale for Children showed that the subjects with cleft and their siblings were similar on performance and full-scale IQs, but the children with clefts were inferior to their siblings on verbal IQ. Sex, age, severity of cleft, and the degree of speech impairment did not affect the magnitude of the relationships. It is important to note that, as in most studies, the means of the children with clefts fell within the average range but were below the sibling means.

Goodstein (1968) later summarized research done to establish the functional level of children with clefts and concluded with these words:

The probability of intellectual impairment in children with cleft palate strongly suggests the importance of including a rather complete intellectual assessment in the planning of any total habilitative program for them, particularly in view of the tendency for some of their parents to have unrealistically high academic or professional goals for these children.

Goodstein's view about testing continues to be sound even though additional information has come to light casting doubt on the wisdom of pooling children with clefts and describing them as if they were a homogeneous group.

McWilliams (1970) referred to "intellectual depression" rather than "impairment" and suggested that many factors may contribute to a functional level that does not reflect ability in the true sense. Other studies have confirmed that position.

In 1973, Lamb et al. published material based on an evaluation of 26 children with clefts of the palate or lip and palate and 26 of their siblings. The children were given the Peabody Picture Vocabulary Test (PPVT) (Dunn, 1959), the Wechsler Intelligence Scale for Children (WISC), Cohen's Verbal Comprehension Factor (VC), and Cohen's Perceptual Organization Factor (POF) (Cohen, 1959). Both of the Cohen "factors" are derived from averaging certain subtests scores from the WISC. The subjects with clefts were divided into two groups—one with poor hearing (average loss in the better ear of 20 dB or more for the speech frequencies) and one with normal hearing (average loss of less than 20 dB in the better ear). The cleft subjects scored lower than their siblings on the PPVT, WISC verbal tests, and the VC factor. They did not differ in performance, full-scale IQ, or perceptual organizational abilities. Overall, the reported IQs were at or above normal. This probably resulted from eliminating children with IQs below 80.

When Lamb et al. analyzed the data according to normal or poor hearing in the cleft subjects, the PPVT scores for children with clefts associat-ed with poor hearing were significantly lower than they were for their siblings, but subjects with clefts with normal hearing showed no such differences. However, both groups of children with clefts showed a significant reduction in verbal IQ as measured by the WISC when compared to their siblings. Hearing status bore no relationship to performance IQ or to the POF.

Of interest in this study was the finding of visual-perceptual-motor deficits, as suggested by Smith and McWilliams (1968a and b) and Tisza et al. (1958). These differences were intrafamilial and occurred more frequently in subjects with clefts with poor hearing. Poor hearing emerges as a possible partial explanation for variations in IQ in children with clefts in spite of the fact that hearing levels at the time of testing may not have been representative of "usual and customary" auditory sensitivity. Studies like this are therefore indicators of possible differences in IQ, but results should be interpreted cautiously.

Also in 1972, McWilliams and Musgrave published the results of a study of 170 children with clefts divided into three groups based on speech. Thirty-two children in Group I had normal speech; 77 in Group II had articulation errors but no evidences of hypernasality; 61 in Group III had velopharyngeal incompetence. Groups I and II were similar on both the WISC and the Stanford-Binet, Form L-M (Terman and Merrill, 1960) and showed no impairment in comparison to normative data. Group III, however, fared less well and was inferior to the other two groups on the WISC. Differences approached significance for the Stanford-Binet. This study did not, for any of the groups, find higher performance than verbal IQs. In fact, even the poor speakers often had higher verbal than performance IQs.

This study, like the previous one, suggests that the presence of a cleft per se is not a sufficient foundation upon which to draw conclusions about intelligence. Paradise et al. (1972) further strengthened this observation when they found that children who had had aggressive ear care from birth showed no reduction in intelligence as measured by the Stanford-Binet Form L-M. A number of variables are related to measurements of mental functioning, and this increases the difficulty of designing investigations that control adequately for cogent factors. It also makes generalization unwise.

Another study (Musgrave et al., 1975) involved 19 children with clefts of the palate only. These subjects were evaluated longitudinally from the preschool years through age 10 for the purpose of assessing the efficacy of two different surgical procedures. An unexpected finding was the change in IQ over time. During the preschool years, the children tested at low average, with 70% falling in that range. By 10 years of age, they tested in the high-average range, with about half the group a little above the population mean and ranging into the superior areas. It is important to note that two-thirds of the children at initial testing and all but one at final examination had hearing losses averaging no greater than 20 dB in the better ear.

This study, while small, raises questions about the effect of maturation on children with clefts. It would surely be unwise to examine a preschooler with a cleft and accept the results as valid evidence of his capabilities. He may score much higher a few years later. Tests given to preschoolers are always less reliable than those administered later. At these early ages, errors occur in both directions so that some children are overestimated and others are underestimated. For children with clefts, however, the tendency was to underestimate their abilities in the preschool years.

McWilliams and Matthews (1979) shed additional light on this issue. One hundred and ten children with unilateral complete clefts of the lip and palate and 108 with clefts of the palate only were evaluated. The children were divided into four groups on the basis of the presence or absence of other congenital abnormalities. While there were both retarded and gifted children in all groups as assessed by the appropriate form of the Wechsler (Wechsler, 1955, 1967, 1974), children with unilateral complete clefts performed better overall than did any of the other groups. Those with palatal clefts only were somewhat less able but were superior to children who had other congenital malformations.

The unilateral and isolated groups were alike on verbal IQ, with means of 105 and 101 respectively but differed on performance IQ. The unilateral group had a mean of 104 while those with isolated clefts had a mean of 97, similar to the 96 achieved by those with unilateral clefts and other anomalies. Verbal IQ was not inferior to performance IQ in any of the groups.

The distribution of full-scale IQs is of interest. Fifty-one per cent of the children with isolated clefts associated with other anomalies had full-scale IQs of 89 or below, and 37% had IQs of 69 or below. This group is at higher risk for mental retardation than are any of the other groups. In comparison, 21% of subjects with unilateral clefts associated with other abnormalities had IQs of 69 or lower. This was true for only 5% of the isolated group with no additional problems and for only 3% of the unilateral group.

Goodstein (1961) reported that 40% of the children with clefts in his study had full-scale IQs of less than 90 as opposed to the expected 25%. These results differ from those of the investigation just described. About 34% of the children in that study had IQs of 89 or below. However, the percentages differed from one group to the other in dramatic fashion. In the unilateral group, 16% were at IQ 89 or below. In the isolated group, the percentage was twice that. The unilateral group with other anomalies rose to 37% and the isolated group with other anomalies to 51%. Thirteen per cent of the isolated group and 21% of the unilateral group had IQs over 120. When other anomalies were present, only 6% of the unilaterals and 6% of the isolated groups had IQs over 120.

The children reported here do not conform to previously published data in that those with unilateral clefts and no other congenital abnormalities appear to be at no higher risk for intellectual impairment than do other children. However, if other anomalies are a part of the clinical picture, the children are, as a group, more likely to show some evidence of mild to moderate reduction in mental abilities. While isolated cleft palate is associated with increased risk for some intellectual deficit, there is also a very good chance that mental abilities will not be impaired. When isolated cleft palate is associated with other anomalies, the occurrence of serious deficits in intelligence greatly increases. This is a finding of some magnitude when it is remembered that associated abnormalities are much more frequent in the isolated group.

It is possible that the results of the study by McWilliams and Matthews show the bias introduced by treatment having been carried out in one center with a specific philosophy of management. For example, the type of cleft did not influence the degree of hypernasality, and most of the subjects either had no abnormal nasality or were only very mildly hypernasal. The highest nasality rating attained by any child was 4 on a 7-point scale. Thus, none of these children had severe velopharyngeal incompetence. In addition, hearing had been carefully monitored.

The findings of the previous study are supported by data on psychiatric diagnoses reported by Simonds and Heimberger (1978). They found a much higher occurrence of both mental retardation and psychiatric problems in children with clefts and second anomalies. A 1972 study by Gall et al. reported that even minor dysmorphology in association with palatal clefts is accompanied by an increased risk of school-handicapping conditions. Tobiason et al. (1987), in a study of 78 cleft subjects with and without associated congenital anomalies, reported that parents more frequently identified deficits in following instructions, learning, paying attention, and finishing work when other abnormalities were present.

These data support other similar investigations. Stone et al. (1969) found, as might be expected, different behavior patterns in cleft children enrolled in special-education programs. Richman and Eliason (1988) investigated reading skills in children with no other congenital abnormalities and found that 35% of 272 subjects with clefts had moderate reading disabilities and that 17% had severe reading disorders. However, only 9% of the children with clefts of the lip and palate had reading problems, a rate similar to that found in the general population, while 33% of those with cleft palate only were similarly affected. Since there is considerable variation in the rigor with which coexisting malformations are explored and in the criteria used for determining what will and will not be so defined, this work should be repeated in another center. Reading is considered further in the chapter on language.

Richman (1978b) used the WISC to examine 87 children with cleft palate, cleft lip, or both. His purpose was to discover the influence of facial appearance on teachers' perceptions of mental abilities. Thus, he reported his test data merely to provide comparisons for teacher ratings and made no point of the test results *per se*. However, it is relevant to consider them here. Children who were rated as having normal facial appearance had a mean verbal IQ of 103.6 and a mean performance IQ of 105.8. Those with significant facial disfigurement had means of 104.0 and 106.1. Thus, facial appearance was not a factor in results obtained on intelligence tests. Of interest also is the similarity between verbal and performance IQs in these children, all of whom were enrolled in regular classrooms.

It appears that children with clefts and no other anomalies are not at increased risk for developmental problems. Children with isolated palatal clefts, however, may fare somewhat less well than do those with clefts of the lip and palate. The presence of additional anomalies, regardless of cleft type, signals the high probability of significant developmental deficits and the need for complete assessment so that appropriate treatment planning can occur.

The results of intelligence testing in the past have been related to a number of variables other than clefting. It has long been recognized that children with clefts are not a homogeneous group (Spriestersbach et al., 1964) simply because they share a general type of birth defect. Recent data attest to that and strongly argue against studies, regardless of topic, which use populations "with clefts." Illingsworth and Bush (1956) found the general depression in IQ typical of the time in which their work was carried out, but they concluded with a prophetic statement:

It will be interesting to repeat this survey in, say, 15 years to see whether the lessening of the handicap by modern surgical techniques will have caused the mean IQ of cleft palate and hare lip[1] patients to have moved nearer to the mean of the general population.

Certainly some changes are being noted. Discrepancies between verbal and performance IQ are now not typically found at later ages. This probably represents generally improved speech, hearing, and life status as compared to what was common a number of years ago. However, it is still obvious that certain groups of children with clefts, particularly those with other congenital abnormalities, are at increased risk for developmental variations as indicated by intelligence tests to extents great enough to warrant consideration in treatment planning.

Richman and Eliason (1982) and Eliason (in press) stress the obvious need to study the different patterns of cognitive abilities seen even within groups of verbally deficient cleft children in order to learn more about the neuropsychological as-

---

[1] a term now discarded

pects of language functioning and their relationship to measures of intelligence. Yet, most treatment programs do not yet make any form of developmental testing a routine part of the clinical protocol. More investment in this aspect of treatment is needed as is more definitive research.

SOCIAL MATURITY

Social maturity is considered independently because it has often been studied as a single set of attributes without reference to its relationship to measures of mental and language development. The reader is reminded, however, that these developmental phenomena are not independent of each other and that they, in turn, interact with a variety of other influential variables.

Goodstein (1961) studied social competence by interviewing 139 mothers of children with clefts and 174 mothers of children with no known health problems and rating them according to the Vineland Social Maturity Scales (Doll, 1965). The children were well matched for age, sex, birth order, and social class. The control children were more socially competent than were the children with clefts. However, the mean social quotient for children with clefts through age 5 was 11.8 points lower than the mean for the control subjects, whereas it was only 3.7 points lower after age 5. In short, as in the case of intelligence, the younger children appeared to be less competent than the older ones. Although this was not a longitudinal study, it does strongly suggest that deficits early in life are minimized as the children grow older, and it explains the similarity between subjects with clefts and controls found by Sidney and Matthews (1956). Why this occurs is not clear. It may be that the habilitation process, which is concentrated in important ways in the early years, is too demanding to permit the child to develop apace with noncleft peers. Energies are perhaps needed elsewhere, and a period of "recovery" is both reasonable and necessary.

McWilliams and Matthews (1979) also investigated social maturity. They used the Vineland scales to study 226 children with clefts. Children with unilateral clefts and no other anomalies had a mean social quotient of 107.33 and those with isolated palatal clefts a mean of 102.09. When other anomalies were present, the unilateral group mean dropped to 96.69 and the isolated

group mean to 84.49. Large standard deviations attested to wide scatter, particularly when other congenital anomalies were present. In this study, measures of social competence mirrored those of intelligence.

The results of these two studies of social competence suggest that social development may be somewhat slower in the preschool years, that many at-risk children will later overcome these early deficits, but that, if other congenital problems are present, the overall outlook is less optimistic, especially in children with clefts of the palate only.

It would be of value to examine the effects of environmental manipulation on the social development of children with clefts. Of special interest would be the assessment of the influence of preschool and parent counseling. Clinically, no attempt should be made to prejudge any child or parent. Instead, careful assessment should form the foundation for any intervention that is necessary.

Adjustment to School

Speech pathologists and other clinicians have suspected that children with clefts may have less than ideal school experiences, both academically and socially. This would be expected for children with below-average mental or social abilities or both, but might not necessarily be true for children developing normally. Only a few studies have been reported in this area, and they present conflicting results.

Early information about school experience was provided by Birch (1952). He reviewed the literature up to that time and found no direct studies of "the personalities of cleft palate patients." He reviewed the records of the 600 "most severely maladjusted" children in the Pittsburgh Public Schools and found no children with clefts in the group. Although this does not prove or disprove the contention that individuals with clefts are damaged emotionally, it does point out that, more than 35 years ago, the Pittsburgh schools, at least, were not sufficiently troubled about the school adjustment of children with clefts to include any in their population of severely disturbed children. The problems of the 600 "most severely maladjusted" are not described, but it is safe to assume that many represented disruptive behavior in the classroom and so were readily identified. Perhaps the children with clefts, if they had problems, did not have the high visibility of the children whose records were reviewed. Birch concluded that there was need for extensive, shared research, since any point of view then held was purely tentative.

Sidney and Matthews (1956) evaluated school adjustment by utilizing five instruments: a sociometric questionnaire; the California Personality Test (Thorpe et al., 1953); the Thematic Apperception Test (Murray, 1935); the Vineland Social Maturity Scale (Doll, 1965); and a rating system designed by the authors and used by the teachers. Twenty-one children with various types of palatal clefts were in the experimental group and were matched with children in two control groups on sex, age, race, intelligence, and grade. The authors concluded that the adjustment of the children with clefts was not markedly inferior to that of the normal children.

Richman (1976) investigated school behavior and achievement in 44 children with clefts ranging in age from 9 to 14 in grades 4 through 8. The sample contained almost twice as many children (29) with cleft palate only as with cleft lip and palate (15). Each child with a cleft was individually matched with a control subject on the basis of sex, age, grade, socioeconomic status, and intelligence. The Behavior Problem Checklist (Quay and Patterson, 1967) was used for teachers' ratings of behavior, and achievement data were derived from the Iowa Tests of Basic Skills (1979). The Behavior Problem Checklist yields two independent factorial dimensions: conduct disorder, which implies externalization of behavior or the excessive expression of impulses, and personality disorder, which implies internalization of behavior or the excessive inhibition of impulses.

Both boys and girls with clefts were rated by their teachers as having significantly more internalizing behavior and more inhibition (personality disorder) than their controls and than the children in the published test norms. Subjects with clefts did not differ from their controls on conduct disorder.

On measurements of achievement, both boys and girls with clefts had significantly lower composite scores than had their peers, but this was especially marked in boys.

Richman concluded that the findings in no way pointed to emotional maladjustment. Rather, the children with clefts may have been demonstrating adaptive behaviors in order to avoid negative responses from others even though impulse inhibition could be counterproductive academically. Learning more about the possible negative social influences leading to variations in school behavior should help in the search for improved methods of management. It is also necessary to view information of this type in relation to possible differences in intelligence, hearing, communication skills, and environment outside of school.

In a later study, Richman (1978a) again used the Behavior Problem Checklist, to which parents and teachers responded, with reference to 136 7- to 12-year-old children with clefts. There were no significant differences between the ratings of mothers and fathers for any of the comparisons. However, the teachers evaluated the males with clefts as having significantly less acting-out behavior and significantly greater inhibition than did either the mothers or fathers. Teachers rated girls with clefts as more inhibited than did their parents. The author suggested that "different expectations at home and school may contribute to the different perceptions of behavior in those environments." Inhibition emerges once again in regard to children with clefts in the broader social milieu of the classroom and may explain why Birch (1952) found no children with clefts among school children identified as having significant problems.

In a more recent paper, Harper et al. (1980) compared 62 cleft subjects, 10 through 18 years of age, matched with 62 subjects with cerebral palsy in the same age range. Thirty-four subjects in each group were rated as having mild impairment and 28 as having severe involvement. The Behavior Problem Checklist was again employed. The females with mild clefts were rated higher on the conduct-disorder dimension than did those with mild cerebral palsy. The females in the severe cleft group were rated higher than those in the group with severe cerebral palsy, and males with severe clefts were rated higher than males with severe cerebral palsy. Males with mild clefts and those with mild cerebral palsy had similar ratings. Analysis of personality disorder (excessive inhibition of impulses) revealed that the children with clefts expressed their impulses significantly more often than did the cerebral-palsied subjects.

Harper et al. concluded that disability types and degree of impairment have different effects on different modes of behavioral expression. It should perhaps be added that these evaluations were made by classroom teachers, who undoubtedly set the tone of teacher-student interaction whether their perceptions are accurate or inaccurate.

In another study, Richman and Harper (1978) compared a sample of 39 mildly impaired 10- to 15-year-old children with clefts, a group of mildly involved cerebral-palsied children of similar age, and a matched control group on the Behavior Problem Checklist and the Iowa Tests of Basic Skills. The groups were similar on measures of conduct disorder. However, the two disability groups both demonstrated significantly greater inhibition of impulse and lower educational achievement than their matched controls. The evidence did not support the contention that the children were maladjusted but did indicate that, in the classroom, behavior was modified by a handicap, even a mild one. This hypothesis is worthy of additional investigation, since theoretically it should be possible to make positive environmental alterations.

Richman (1978b) also explored the influence of facial disfigurement on teachers' perceptions of ability in children with clefts. The work was undertaken because of the persistent finding in a number of studies (Berscheid and Walster, 1974) to the effect that teachers generally view physically attractive children as having more socially desirable behaviors and higher mental abilities than less attractive children. In this study, there were 87 subjects from 8 to 14 years of age, 48 with clefts of both the lip and palate and 41 with clefts of the palate only. All of the children had relatively normal speech and hearing. Forty-three were rated as essentially normal in facial appearance, and 44 had significant facial disfigurement.

Each classroom teacher completed the Behavior Problem Checklist. The two groups of children did not differ from each other on these behavioral indices. Achievement test scores were obtained from the Iowa Tests for Basic Skills. Each child's teacher rated the child on intellectual ability using a 6-point scale, later collapsed to represent above-average, average, and below-average intellectual ability. Wechsler IQs, unknown to the teachers, were similarly grouped.

Teachers rated the children with minimal facial disfigurement more accurately than they did those with more severe deficits. Children with noticeable facial disfigurement and above-average intelligence were underestimated, whereas children with noticeable facial disfigurement and below-average ability were overestimated. Since these children were similar in behavior profiles,

intelligence, and achievement, it is unlikely that the teachers were influenced by variables other than appearance.

School experience is obviously influenced by a variety of factors over which children have little or no control. Another of these is speech. Although many children with clefts now under care do not develop the serious speech problems that were once almost inevitable, the record is not yet perfect. For this reason, the study of Blood and Hyman (1977) is important. They had 120 normal children in kindergarten and first and second grades listen to four recorded speech samples of girls with normal speech and mild, moderate, and severe nasal resonance. After each sample, the children were asked 5 questions: (1) Did you like the person telling the story? (2) Did you like the way the person talked? (3) Do you think she had trouble talking? (4) Would you like to talk like that person? (5) Do you think she needs some help with her talking?

At all grade levels, the percentages of negative responses increased as the hypernasality increased. There were no positive or neutral responses to the speaker with the most severe hypernasality. Since all questions about the speaker tended to be answered in the same way, the children apparently responded globally and made up their minds about a speaker rather than about the speaker in relationship to the question asked. If this did indeed occur, it could mean that a hypernasal speaker experiences problems in peer relationships that transcend the actual speech deficit. This possibility is of real concern because the children in this study showed a marked negative response to hypernasality as early as kindergarten. We do not know how early such judgments are made, nor do we know how they influence the social milieu of children with clefts. More importantly, we do not known whether children learn to evaluate hypernasal speech from influential adults or whether they simply listen and decide what they do and do not like.

Schneiderman and Harding (1984) asked 78 students in second, third, and fourth grades to rate color slides of 3 children with bilateral cleft lips, 3 with unilateral cleft lips, and 3 with normal facial features. Of the 15 variables studied, the children with clefts were rated more negatively than were children without facial scars, and children with bilateral clefts were rated less favorably than those with unilateral clefts on 7 of the variables.

These findings are supported by Tobiason

(1987), who had 317 school-aged children respond to photographs of children with clefts and then to photographs of the same children with the evidences of facial disfigurement removed. The faces with clefts were rated as less friendly, less popular, less likely to be chosen as friends, less intelligent, and less good looking than the corrected faces, regardless of age or gender. Tobiason suggests that facial deformity may be a central cue for social stereotyping, since facial deformity may be seen as ugly and ugly as bad.

In a later study, Tobiason and Hicbert (1988) found children to be reliable raters of photographs and to show greater agreement with each other as they got older. They consistently preferred unimpaired faces, faces that were moderately attractive, or both.

Studies examining real-life experiences of children with clefts are badly needed since interactions among children involve many more factors than can be measured from tape recordings or photographs, valuable though they are in directing our attention to relevant life issues.

A sizable segment of the child's experience occurs in the school setting, where teachers often have little understanding of cleft problems (Mitchell et al., 1984). Piecing together the few shreds of information available about prevailing attitudes leads to the tentative conclusion that education may be less than nurturing for children with clefts, especially if they have both facial disfigurement and speech problems, and that the children probably respond by withdrawing and inhibiting impulses somewhat more than their peers. This behavior may be reasonable in the presence of aversive stimuli and does not mean that these children are emotionally disturbed or suffer from personality disorders. However, it points to the probability that the educational and social milieu of the school makes it necessary for many children with clefts to cope with stresses that are less common in the lives of their peers. They must discover the means of dealing with these pressures if they are to survive without damage. The fact that they are able to find mechanisms that work is at the same time their salvation and their undoing. In the trade-off, they sacrifice something of their freedom to express themselves fully. This would account in part for the earlier findings of Smith and McWilliams (1966) relative to reduced creativity and to the clinical impression that children with clefts are often underachievers. It also sheds light on the findings of Spriestersbach (1973) that fewer subjects with clefts than controls liked school, volunteered for class recitation, liked their schoolmates, or wanted education after high school. Mothers of the clinical subjects were aware that their children's classroom participation was below average. It is notable, however, that fewer mothers of children with clefts indicated that school problems had been discussed with them by their children's teachers.

These findings in combination reinforce the conclusion that school adjustment is probably marginal for many children with clefts. Thus, it is clear that successful "team" treatment must include the school as a full partner and must reach out to enlist the aid and understanding of both teachers and peers.

PERSONALITY

The studies discussed in the previous section on school experience failed to reveal gross differences between subjects with clefts and those without but did present evidence of behavioral variations that may represent coping strategies adopted by children who encounter unusual environmental pressures. The same general conclusion may be drawn about studies of personality. Data available from different sources using a variety of methodologies require cautious interpretation and recognition of the tentative state of our knowledge.

Goodstein (1968) concluded his discussion of the personality and adjustment of children with clefts with the words:

The only evidence that these children are emotionally maladjusted or disturbed appears to be rather impressionistic and nonsystematic. Until more convincing evidence is provided, it appears safe to conclude that as a group children with cleft palate are not typically maladjusted or seriously disturbed emotionally, although they may have some problems of social acceptance.

Wirls (1971) concurred:

In spite of the compelling theoretical basis of social and psychological maladjustment in children with cleft palate, the research results have been inconclusive. If the results tend in any direction, it is toward the absences rather than the existences of maladjustments.

As we shall find, we are still plagued with unanswered questions and with disagreement among findings from one study to another. In addition, clinical impressions of psychological problems persist with a tenacity that is difficult to understand in the face of contrary data. Many clinicians today would undoubtedly find little to fault in the 1943 statement of Backus et al. that "symptoms of personal and social maladjustment are usually present, both because of defective speech and real or fancied facial deformity."

The "feeling" that there are personality differences was noted by Hackbush (1951), who concluded that, although there is probably no such thing as a cleft-palate personality, results of projective testing pointed to "limited personalities with little emotional content."

McWilliams and Smith (1973) indicated that we should perhaps worry less about such illusive constructs as self-image, attitudes, and feelings, which are difficult to assess, and, instead, observe behavior that can be quantified and compared within and among groups. We need also to explore the manner in which personality develops in the presence of different types of clefts, some resulting in little or no handicap.

Human-Figure Drawings

Drawings of the human figure have been used frequently to assess self image. Abel (1953) explored the same-sex drawings of 74 adults with facial disfigurement, not necessarily clefting. Some of the subjects completely rejected the task, and 21 with mild disfigurement, which they expressed verbally, showed no distortions in their drawings. Over half of 19 subjects with severe disfigurement showed body distortions in their drawings, but the rest did not. Thus, it is clear that the degree of facial disfigurement is relevant to expression through drawings but that specific representations of disfiguring conditions are very often rejected. Denial is a possible explanation. It is not apparent from this study how responses might differ for subjects with congenital disfigurement as opposed to those with acquired defects.

Palmer and Adams (1962) administered the Draw-a-Person (Machover, 1951) and the Draw-a-Face tests to 20 children with palatal clefts with or without clefts of the lip. Two matched control groups were used. The authors found no differences between drawings of children with clefts and those without, regardless or age.

Corah and Corah (1963) compared the human-figure drawings of 12 children with clefts of the lip and palate with the drawings of 12 control subjects. The drawings of the children with clefts were inferior to those of their peers without clefts, although none portrayed the specific cleft deformity or otherwise distorted the face. This was a small sample, and the children who participated were enrolled in a special class for physically handicapped children, which could have influenced their performance.

Wirls and Plotkin (1971) asked 66 children with clefts and 66 of their siblings to draw a picture of a person, a picture of a person of the opposite sex, and a picture of themselves. The group with cleft palate only drew the head larger in proportion to the rest of the body than did the sibling group. Since so many other comparisons were not significant, that difference could have occurred by chance, and no significance can be attached to it.

In the larger study referred to earlier (McWilliams and Matthews, 1979), unreported data on children with unilateral clefts and isolated clefts showed that the children, even when subdivided into groups with and without additional abnormalities, were similar in their human-figure drawings. However, there was remarkable variability in all of the groups, and group means tended to fall below the 50th percentile. The two exceptions were for the drawing of a man by subjects with unilateral clefts (mean percentile, 52.86) and by those with isolated clefts (mean percentile, 49.31). However, the unilateral group with other anomalies had a mean percentile of only 38.15. On the drawing of a woman, all groups were below the 50th percentile. These data suggest immaturity, especially in children of normal intelligence.

Overall, studies that have explored self concept through human-figure drawings have been inconclusive, but they do indicate that, for whatever reason, children with clefts are less skillful on this task than are their peers. Although there is little, if any, direct evidence to support the contention that the lowered scores reflect poor self image—a position that has face validity, findings are sufficiently consistent to warrant further investigation using different methodologies.

Other Drawing Tasks

Teenagers were asked to create drawings reflecting their feelings about having clefts (Cleft Palate Center, University of Pittsburgh, 1973). The children then described the feelings behind their drawings as sadness, the wish to be treated just like others, concern about limitations placed upon them by other people, and a sense of loneliness and rejection. Figure 8.1 shows one of the drawings. The artist, a highly creative and gifted child, explained that she was struggling to rise above the horizon but was constantly being pushed down by society.

Semantic Differential Approaches

Clifford (1967) examined 20 subjects with clefts utilizing a semantic-differential technique in order to discover the meaning of certain concepts

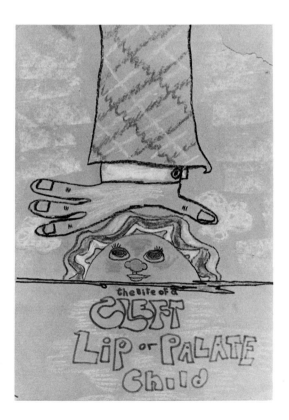

Figure 8.1 Drawing depicting what it feels like to have a cleft. The desire is to rise and live a full life, but the world keeps pushing the person with a cleft back below the horizon.

related to cleft lip and palate. Results indicated that the children, who had a mean age of 12.54 years, an IQ range of 89 through 128, and defective speech, rated cleft palate alone slightly more positively than cleft lip. This is not an unexpected outcome since cleft palate alone is not a visible deformity. However, both cleft lip and cleft palate were rated more positively than asthma, amputation, or crippling; both were seen to be in the range of mild illness, slightly less undesirable than headache. Whether this comparison is meaningful is questionable. As the author pointed out, children are perhaps more accepting of known than of unknown problems. The children valued body parts distal to the defect more highly than they did mouth, nose, or face. Since no controls were used, it is difficult to know how normal children or those with other handicaps would respond to such questions.

Clifford (1968, 1969) then used self-report, interview schedules to assess the impact of symptoms, perceptions of parental acceptance at birth, and self concepts. He compared data for 39 subjects with clefts and 68 with asthma. The subjects with clefts had an average age of 13.07 years as opposed to 12.32 years for the asthmatic subjects. They were similar in school placement in spite of the fact that the subjects with clefts were somewhat older.

There were no differences between the groups in their feelings about having their particular conditions, and both groups had mean scores skewed toward the positive end of the scale. When questioned about how they would feel if their symptoms were lost, there were again no significant differences. Slightly more than 50% of the children in both groups thought that life would be neither better nor worse if symptoms were eliminated. The children with asthma perceived a significantly higher degree of parental acceptance at birth than did the children with clefts, and children with cleft palates perceived their parents as being more accepting than did those with clefts of both the lip and palate. There were no differences between the subjects with clefts and those with asthma in self-concept as it was measured in this study.

The meaning of this study is unclear. Given the common assumption that asthma is at least in part a psychosomatic illness, one might have expected children with clefts to fare somewhat better than they did. Thus, it may be that both groups had problems. All that can be inferred from these findings is that the children with clefts and those with asthma were much alike except that the children with clefts felt less acceptable at birth than did their asthmatic cohorts, whose problems were probably not obvious at birth.

Brantley and Clifford (1979) used discriminant function analyses "to establish linear combinations of variables that would identify group membership correctly" for 100 normal adolescents, 51 with cleft palates, and 22 who were obese, all between the ages of 10 and 18. They looked at a number of variables including cognition, body image, and self-concept. Measures of body image were clearly discriminative for obese subjects but not for the normal group and the group with clefts. The linear combination of self-concept measures differentiated subjects with clefts from normals. Subjects with clefts, on these measures, had higher self-esteem than normals, and this poses a credibility problem. Denial or some other mechanism might explain this finding. Another possibility is the racial make-up of the normal and cleft groups. Only 9% of the group with clefts were black as compared to 29% of the obese subjects. Data were not analyzed to determine the possible influence of race on self concept.

Clifford (1971) concluded from his studies of adolescents with clefts that their self esteem was almost uniformly high. However, similar results obtained in a study at the University of Pittsburgh were never submitted for publication because the investigators questioned the validity of the subjects' responses. Discrepancies were frequently noted between verbal and nonverbal behaviors and between known and described problems. Subjects often responded that they talked "just like everybody else" when they had marked speech defects.

Personality Scales

Sidney and Matthews (1956) used the California Test of Personality (Thorpe et al., 1953) and the Thematic Apperception Test (Murray, 1935) in a study of school-aged subjects with and without clefts and found no differences between groups.

Watson (1964) evaluated 93 boys between 8 and 14 years of age divided into normal, cleft, and handicapped groups. The children were compared on the basis of the Rogers Personal Adjustment Scale (Rogers, 1961). The groups were similar on the five adjustment scales included, and the responses of the children with clefts were not influenced either by speech characteristics or by facial disfigurement. Watson concluded that his results cast doubt on the popular assumption that cleft palate is associated with personality disturbances. Little has changed in 25 years.

Kapp (1979) published a study of self-concept in 34 11- to 13-year-old children with clefts. The subjects with clefts were heterogeneous relative to cleft type, speech, hearing, and physical appearance, all variables that could influence the outcome of an assessment of self-concept. They were matched with 34 control subjects. The Piers-Harris Children's Self-Concept Scale (Piers, 1969) was administered. Since there were no significant differences among the cleft types, the data were pooled for comparison with the control subjects. There were no significant differences between the group with clefts and the control group on global self-concept scores. The subjects with clefts did not see themselves as any less socially acceptable than did the controls. However, the children with clefts reported significantly less "global happiness and satisfaction" than did their peers. There were differences also for three cluster scores—anxiety, intellectual and school status, and happiness and satisfaction. Males, regardless of group, were similar, but females with clefts rated themselves significantly lower than girls without clefts. There were no differences between groups on the physical-attributes subscore.

As a group, both males and females with clefts expressed greater dissatisfaction with personal appearance than did those without clefts. Overall, the study suggests that both males and females with clefts were less satisfied with physical appearance than were their matched controls but that the females were significantly more anxious, less successful in school, and more unhappy and dissatisfied. The author hypothesized that girls may be more adversely affected by the stigma of physical disability, perhaps because of the importance society attaches to physical attractiveness in females.

Kapp-Simon (1986) further explored self-concept when she compared the responses of 50 children with clefts to those of unimpaired children between the ages of 5 and 9 on the Primary Self-Concept Inventory (Muller and Leonetti, 1974). There were no significant differences by sex or cleft type, but significantly more children with clefts than control subjects had scores which placed them in an "at-risk" category. The children with clefts saw themselves as less acceptable than their peers, more likely to require assistance, and more frequently sad and angry. They tended to identify with passive and isolated children, a finding that is consistent with other evidence of social inhibition.

Richman (1983) examined 30 adolescents with clefts divided into two groups. One group of 16 was considered to have adequate personality adjustment as reflected by normal MMPI scores on all scales, whereas the second was composed of 14 adolescents who had one or more elevated MMPI scores. In this study, elevated scores occurred most frequently on Scale 0 indicating social introversion. Scale 2, suggesting lack of self worth, and Scale 7, reflecting excessive rumination and worry, were the only other elevated scales.

Subjects with clefts and control subjects were given structured interviews to determine self-perceived educational and social participation. For this part of the study only, a control group was used since there were no normative data on the interview questions. The adolescents with clefts also answered questions concerning the extent of their concerns about speech and facial appearance.

There were no significant differences between the cleft and control subjects in educational or social satisfaction. However, when adolescents with clefts showed elevations on the MMPI, they also expressed less satisfaction with their educational and social functioning than did their peers who were thought to demonstrate good adjustment. It is probable that similar attitudes might be found in poorly adjusted adolescents without clefts. Of special interest, however, is the finding that adolescents with clefts with marked concerns about facial appearance also demonstrated significantly higher scores on the Social-Introversion Scale. Concerns about speech showed no such relationship.

Richman et al. (1985) divided 36 adolescents with unilateral or bilateral cleft lips and palates into two groups on the basis of behavioral ratings by their parents on the Behavior Problem Checklist. The group considered to be well adjusted rated both their facial appearance and their behavior in a manner similar to the ratings provided by their parents and teachers. The poorly adjusted group, on the other hand, rated themselves as having significantly less social inhibition and better appearance than did parents or teachers. In short, the better adjusted group

appeared to have more realistic self-perceptions than did the more poorly adjusted subjects.

These studies provide evidence of the need for clinical intervention when adolescents express dissatisfaction with school and social adjustment and when they have marked concern about facial appearance. They also suggest that adolescents should be given the opportunity to talk about their feelings and that these feelings should become a part of the formula when deciding about the timing of secondary surgical procedures to improve appearance.

For some young people, more than how they look may be at stake. Of special concern is the probability that children's perceptions of their deformities are incorporated into their personalities and persist there long after the deformity itself has been minimized (Schwartz and Landwirth, 1968). It is improbable that children with clefts would be more satisfied with themselves than are children who do not have such physical problems, as some studies have suggested. Since few life experiences can be described as neutral, it is unlikely that a cleft would not be responded to in some way. This is not to suggest that children with clefts are "mentally disturbed," only that the cleft has an impact, probably in a variety of ways, and that that becomes a matter of clinical significance, particularly when inhibition and social distancing are present.

Projective Techniques

As noted earlier, Sidney and Matthews (1956) failed to find differences in the responses of children with clefts and control children to the Thematic Apperception Test (TAT), which is a projective instrument. Later, Wirls and Plotkin (1971) compared 66 children with clefts and 66 sibling controls using the TAT, the Rorschach (Klopfer and Davidson, 1960), the Kahn Test of Symbol Arrangement (Kahn, 1956), and the Draw-a-Person Test. Data from the latter test were presented earlier in this chapter. On the TAT, only three of the many comparisons were statistically significant, but they all occurred when children with clefts of the palate only were compared with their siblings. The children with clefts of the palate only significantly more often projected themselves into the story, suggesting a tendency to refer events to themselves. In addition, they more often perceived characters as neglectful, rejecting, or hateful, and they were more negative in the stories they told than were their siblings. It is possible but not probable that these differences could have come from sources other than the clefts in this group of subjects.

Rorschach responses were compared using 316 tests of significance. Of these, only three were significant at the 0.05 level of confidence. Since chance would have yielded 16 differences significant at this level, we must conclude that children with clefts were similar to their siblings in their responses to the Rorschach—as they were on the Kahn Test of Symbol Arrangement.

A relevant issue in the interpretation of this study is the extent to which siblings may be affected by each other. The authors noted also that children from 7 to 14 were lumped together and that this might have influenced the results. This is a cogent point because we know nothing of how closely the siblings were matched in age.

Wirls and Plotkin concluded that their study did not support the commonly held assumption that specific forms of somatic disorders are associated with specific personality types and that a disability is necessarily sufficient cause for psychological maladjustment.

In a more recent study, Richman and Harper (1969) administered the Missouri Children's Picture Series (Sines et al., 1971) to 45 children with clefts of the lip and palate and to 45 children with orthopedic impairment matched for sex, age, and intelligence. Males with cleft lips and palates scored significantly higher on the maturity scale but showed greater inhibition than did boys with orthopedic impairment, who had higher scores on measures of aggression, activity level, and somatization.

Like males with clefts, females were significantly higher on the scales of maturity and inhibition than were their female counterparts, who were higher on the masculinity-femininity scale. The authors suggested that there were probably different personality adaptations for different types of physical impairments and that girls with clefts appeared to adapt well socially in the early years (the mean age for this group was 9.5) but that, based on data not included, had less social success than males during adolescence, although both males and females showed inhibition.

Since no control group of unaffected children was used, this study is limited in the conclusions that can be drawn. Both groups of children

were impaired but in different ways and might be expected to respond differently because their life situations imposed different restrictions.

Harper and Richman (1978) administered the Minnesota Multiphasic Inventory (Hathaway and McKinley, 1951) to 46 adolescents with orthopedic problems and to 52 with cleft lip and palate and mild-to-severe facial disfigurement. The two groups differed, and it was concluded that type of disability has differential effects on adolescent personality characteristics. Although both groups were within normal limits for adolescents, indicating that neither suffered from severe personality deviations, both showed inhibition as one of their outstanding characteristics. Adolescents with clefts were involved in social activities, but they experienced anxiety, self-doubt, and discomfort regarding interpersonal relationships. The orthopedically handicapped, on the other hand, were physically and psychologically isolated from peer interaction.

These last two studies show no evidence of pathological personality characteristics, but they point to areas of stress that should be considered in planning treatment and in assessing individual children.

Observed and Reported Behaviors

Interviews

In one of the earlier landmark studies of personality, MacGregor (1951) described 115 patients with varying degrees of facial disfigurement. From data from in-depth interviews, she concluded that "the majority" were dismayed by their own mirror images and "saw their handicaps reflected in the reaction of others toward them." They reported "staring, remarks, curiosity, questioning, pity, rejection, ridicule, whispering, nicknames, and discrimination," responses that made them "self-conscious" and "unhappy." The majority of patients suffered from feelings of inferiority, self-consciousness, frustration, preoccupation with the deformity, hypersensitivity, anxiety, hostility, paranoia, and wanting to withdraw from social activities that varied from partial to complete "antisocial behavior and psychotic states." MacGregor ended her report with these words:

It should be recognized that the problems associated with facial deformities and the problems of adjustment are not those of the handicapped individuals alone, but are of equal importance for the nonhandicapped, who by their negative attitudes and prejudices help to create or perpetuate the difficulties.

These insights, gleaned from interviews as opposed to various formal and informal tests, must be taken seriously even though subjective interpretations are obviously involved. It may be that people do not readily admit to personal concerns when faced with specific questions about themselves. However, given time and opportunity to explore and discuss their feelings, they reveal their true attitudes and heartaches. Preteen and teenage groups (Cleft Palate Center, University of Pittsburgh, 1973, 1977) met for many months before they were willing to discuss their feelings. While that program was going on, a similar one, with similar behavioral observations, was being carried out by Peter at the Lancaster Cleft Palate Center (personal conversation). The problems that eventually emerged had to do with being treated as "special" people, concern for parents, fear for any children who might be born to them, resentment about lack of understanding at school, and teasing by other children. These feelings were worked into two films created by the children to inform others of the meaning of clefts in their lives. The conclusions drawn from this experience were subjective but were based on what the children said when they were sufficiently comfortable to engage in such discussions. This is not to say that all children feel this way, only that some do and that strong defense mechanisms may prevent the easy expression of these underlying concerns.

A partial explanation for this seeming reluctance to discuss problems may relate in part to the observations of Tisza et al. (1958). They conducted psychiatric evaluations of 20 children with clefts and their mothers as a routine part of the clinical procedure. They noted that the mothers' descriptions of their children rarely incorporated the characteristics that the child presented. The mothers minimized speech problems and emphasized their children's brightness. After the mothers were reassured about intelligence following psychological testing, they began to express prior fears that their children might also have been somehow damaged "inside their heads." This attitude is well expressed by Schwartz and Landwirth (1968): "The belief that a warped body

means a warped mind is deeply rooted in the public unconscious." Most of the parents in the study by Tisza et al. had not discussed the nature of the deformity with their children or even the reasons for the surgery that had been required. As might be expected, the children collaborated in the denial by refraining from asking questions. Although these mothers expressed concern about their children's separation anxieties, they were often unaware of any other special sensitivities. "Nothing bothers him," was a frequent comment. The examiners were impressed with the apparent self-sufficiency of the children but also with their postural tension and muscular rigidity. In addition, the children were described as an "activity-oriented" group, always busy.

Tisza et al. reported no data to support these impressions gleaned during psychiatric interviews, but they cannot, nonetheless, be dismissed. The observations suggest that children under the rigid control exhibited in these interviews would not be likely to reveal themselves in more formal testing situations if they could avoid it. They might well resort to denial and report that they were average or better in such things as popularity. The study by Tisza et al. was published more than 30 years ago, but the problems apparent then are with us still. Indirect support for these findings is provided by the work of Walesky-Rainbow and Morris (1978). Interviews can often identify areas in need of future research. One of these that emerges from the observations of Tisza et al. is nonverbal communication and what it can reveal about the status of children whether they have clefts or not.

Schwartz and Landwirth (1968) hypothesized that, in late childhood, the personality responses to a deformity may be incorporated as an integral part of personality so that, even after the defect is repaired, the child may continue to behave as if it were present. In support of this contention, they presented the history of Tony, an 8-year-old boy with cleft palate. This child was described as aggressive and provocative and the victim of teasing at school, where he was often addressed as "you with a hole in your face." After the cleft was repaired, the family moved to a new neighborhood, where Tony attended a different school with new classmates who did not speak to him or of him in derogatory terms. In spite of this, his old defenses went with him into the new situation as a protection against his fear of rejection. He would not permit others to like him, and his poor self-esteem was reinforced. No claim is made that all children with clefts have problems similar to Tony's, but when they occur, they affect the course and nature of treatment.

Tisza et al. (1973) evaluated the content of stories emerging from 32 2-hour creative dramatics sessions with 11 cleft children aged 3.5 to 6, all of whom were below-average on the Illinois Test of Psycholinguistic Abilities in spite of normal intelligence. The psychodynamics that finally emerged were not at first apparent. The children showed intense interest in alligators, crocodiles, dinosaurs, dragons, snakes, monsters, and gorillas. The animals were used to represent "attacking, tearing, biting, and devouring." Although animals of this type are common in the play of preschool children, these children chose them to the exclusion of more common domestic animals, which they in fact rejected. A second recurring theme was hurting and being hurt, and it took a long time for the children to introduce a hospital as a source of help. The commitment to and the depth of such themes is not usually found in the creative-dramatics expressions of children who are not impaired. These children, however, were mutually supportive and eventually expressed their feelings in the presence of an accepting leader who helped them keep their aggressions under control.

Tisza et al. submitted material from these protocols to seven child psychiatrists and 11 experienced pediatric nurses who had had broadly based courses in child development.

All of the child psychiatrists suspected that the children had had life experiences different from the average child, and they wondered what traumatic events might explain the preoccupation with medical topics. Four of the seven volunteered that the play was different from that of preschool children generally. All agreed that the children showed an unusual amount of oral aggression in words rather than oral behavior and noted the relationship of the aggression to preoccupation with pregnancy and death. Other prominent comments related to castration and separation anxieties and to the children's perception of themselves as "bad," unacceptable even after having undergone treatment.

The nurses also noted the oral aggression and the preoccupation with pregnancy and death. Most suggested that the stories reflected oedipal conflict, castration anxiety, and fear of parental rejection.

Although these play themes are found in preschool children who do not have clefts, the intensity of these concerns for this group of children was remarkable. These children, according to Tisza et al., "played out their most painful conflicts, but when the play was 'finished,' they crossed the bridge back to reality and went about the business of life as usual." The ability to return to reality was a tribute to their ego strength. We cannot ignore the evidence that children with clefts have problems with which they must learn to cope and that they experience pain and anxiety even though they are not necessarily mentally ill.

Behavioral Reports

Gluck et al. (1965) compared the behavioral characteristics of 50 children with clefts with those of 292 children who had been seen in a child-guidance center. More children with clefts were reported to be shy and enuretic than were the children seen in the guidance center. When children with clefts were enuretic, they also had a greater number of other behavioral problems, 7 as compared to 4 for other children with clefts. In the child-guidance group, children without speech problems had a mean of almost 7 symptoms, whereas those with speech problems had a mean of 8. It is possible that enuretic children with clefts have more significant problems than those who do not have clefts. Once again, shyness and inhibition were noteworthy.

McWilliams and Musgrave (1972) studied 170 children with clefts to determine whether there were behavioral differences among those with normal speech, those with normal resonance associated with articulation disorders, and those with hypernasality and consonant articulation disorders at least partially related to velopharyngeal incompetence. The three groups differed from each other in major ways. The normal speakers had a mean of 1.97 behavioral symptoms, significantly fewer than in the other two groups. The most frequently occurring symptoms included nervousness, excitability, restlessness, enuresis, difficulty in disciplining, fearfulness, moodiness, preferring to be alone, and nail biting. The group with normal speech had no one symptom that occurred more often than in either of the other groups. However, 45% of the group with articulation disorders were described as having bad tempers as opposed to 18% and 15% in the other two groups. These children were also enuretic and preferred to be alone more frequently than subjects in either of the other two groups.

The symptom "bad temper" was always an indication that there would be other behavioral problems. Six normal speakers with bad tempers had a mean of 3.66 symptoms as opposed to 1.97 for the entire group and 1.57 for the 26 children without bad tempers. In the group with articulation errors, bad temper was associated with a mean of 5.61 symptoms compared to the group mean of 3.76 and of 2.12 for the children who did not have bad tempers. The same pattern held for the group with poor speech, and all the differences were significant beyond the 1% level of confidence. When bad temper was not a factor, the groups were similar relative to the numbers of behavior problems.

This study showed that children with clefts are not all alike. While more are inhibited, some act out. Speech attributes, perhaps in association with other variables that were not explored, seem to have an influence. Other studies that have described children with clefts as inhibited may have used populations with speech problems, particularly those associated with faulty velopharyngeal valving. As methods of care and patient outcomes improve, other developmental factors may change as well.

Tobiasen and Hiebert (1984) also studied behavior problems in 41 children with clefts and found them to be similar to the 512 children who provided the standardization data for the Eyberg Child Behavior Inventory (Robinson et al., 1980). However, significantly fewer parents of children with clefts rated existing behaviors as problems. Thus, they appeared to be more tolerant of behavioral deviations than did the parents in the standardization sample. This was especially true of their acceptance of socially aggressive behaviors, which may signal other problems as well. Tobiasen and Hiebert did not analyze their data from that perspective.

These studies offer insights into the behaviors of cleft children and their interpretation by parents, who may lower their expectations and demands for conformity as they are unwilling to do for so-called normal children. If this is indeed the case, it is a strong argument for early counseling of parents to help them provide nurture and support for their children without, at the same time, communicating the devastating message of inferiority and incapacity necessitating lowered standards for living.

Irwin and McWilliams (1974) alluded to the unresolved feelings of the children with whom they undertook various types of play therapy. They found, however, as had Tisza et al., that the children were capable of expressing feelings, of revealing through play unconscious conflicts or inappropriate behaviors requiring further attention, and of experiencing a make-believe control of life events about which they had previously felt a sense of helplessness. These creative-play activities are viewed as helpful techniques for enriching the psychological growth of young children, especially those with burdens greater than average. They are techniques that speech pathologists can safely use after appropriate training.

Walesky-Rainbow and Morris (1978) investigated what information about clefts was available to children with clefts. The children in their study did not know as much about their clefts as their mothers or professional people thought they did. Children require information about their complex problems and should be given the opportunity to ask questions and to talk out their concerns with appropriate professional people. This need was expressed strongly as well by the children preparing the films discussed earlier (Cleft Palate Center, University of Pittsburgh, 1973, 1977). Clinical recognition of the possible psychodynamics operating in the lives of these children should help to ensure that this important part of team management is not ignored and that extra support and therapy are provided when they are needed. Currently, that is occurring infrequently (Broder and Richman, 1987).

METHODOLOGICAL PROBLEMS

There are serious problems with any research that attempts to describe personality or personal attributes. Formal measurement techniques are limited, are often too gross to pick up any but marked differences, are sometimes poorly standardized, may be of questionable validity, and may fail to elicit accurate responses from subjects.

Various psychiatric and play interviews and other types of subjective evaluations appear to be more valid than any formal tests that have yet been devised. However, these approaches are considerably more prone to problems of reliability because they are unstructured. In addition, we have little or no information about their predictive value. It is apparent that research of this type must, in the future, use larger populations than have been customary and that control groups are mandatory unless the goal is to seek differences among various cleft types. Even then, it eventually becomes necessary to relate findings to comparable populations if generalizations are to be drawn. The difficulties inherent in this type of behavioral and personality research have discouraged many investigators.

McWilliams and Smith (1973) concluded their review with a statement that is still applicable:

It is crucial that future research in the psychology and sociology of cleft palate be directed toward (1) determining the behavioral characteristics of the various populations of cleft palate children, adolescents, and adults and (2) providing a detailed portrait of the environmental correlates of whatever unique behavior may be discovered. This latter point is important because it focuses upon phenomena that are observable. Information of this type would help to dispel our present dilemma of having many possible explanations which defy empirical validation and which in no way lead to the development or rearrangement of medical and behavioral programs of management.

SUMMARY

Children with clefts and no additional abnormalities begin life with developmental irregularities that seem to even out with the passage of time, and they fall generally within the normal range of mental development. Developmental problems often persist when cleft palate without cleft lip is present, particularly if there are also other congenital abnormalities. In spite of usually average intelligence, many children achieve less than would be expected academically.

Although we do not yet have complete understanding of the educational problems that are often found, data suggest that social discrimination may well be operative and that these children must learn to cope with teacher and peer evaluations that overemphasize the importance of the residual evidences of the cleft condition and underestimate capabilities and talents. The social isolation that may result leads to reduced spontaneity; decreased levels of participation; somewhat inhibited behaviors or, in some cases, acting out;

lowered expectations on the part of parents, teachers, and peers; and, often, restricted life patterns.

There is no evidence to support the conclusion that children with clefts are seriously emotionally disturbed or that they have classifiable personality deviations. Rather, they encounter unusual social pressures to which they must accommodate, and they do so at a distinct cost in social freedom and comfort. It is not surprising that many retain concerns about appearance and speech even though they are usually accepting of the efforts to correct their birth defects.

Children with clefts are not alike in their adjustment strategies; there is considerable overlap in these regards with their noncleft peers. In spite of this, there is constant need for concern for the psychological well-being of children whose requirements for physical restoration may well overwhelm their parents and their treatment teams to the point that no attention is paid to the psychological aspects of development. Failure to treat the *person* may render all other work futile. The speech pathologist must be alert to the psychological requirements of patients and should carefully follow, document, and provide treatment or referral as required in individual cases.

REFERENCES

Abel TM. Figure drawings and facial disfigurement. Am J Orthopsychiatry 1953; 23:253.

Backus O, Clancy J, Henry LD, Kemper J. The child with a cleft palate. Ann Arbor: University of Michigan, 1943.

Bangs TE, Garrett SB. Birth to three scale (Experimental Edition). Houston: Speech and Hearing Institute, 1973.

Bayley N. Bayley scales of infant development. New York: The Psychological Corporation, 1969.

Berscheid E, Walster E. Physical attractiveness. In: Berkowitz S, ed. Advances in experimental psychology. Vol 7. New York: Academic Press, 1974.

Billig A. A psychological appraisal of cleft palate patients. Proc PA Acad Sci 1951; 25:29.

Birch JD. Personality characteristics of individuals with cleft palate: research needs. Newsletter Bull Am Assoc Cleft Pal Rehab 1952; 2:5.

Blood G, Hyman M. Children's perception of nasal resonance. J Speech Hear Dis 1977; 42:446.

Brantley H, Clifford E. Cognitive, self-concept and body image measures of normal, cleft palate, and obese adolescents. Cleft Palate J 1979; 16:177.

Broder H, Richman L. An examination of mental health services offered by cleft/craniofacial teams. Cleft Palate J 1987; 24:158.

Bzoch K, League R. Assessing language skills in infancy. Gainesville, FL: Tree of Life Press, 1971.

Cattell P. The measurement of intelligence of infants and young children. New York: Psychological Corporation, 1940.

Cervenka J, Drabkova H. The intelligence quotient in cleft lip and palate. Acta Chir Plast 1965; 7:58.

Clarren SK, Anderson B, Wolf LS. Feeding infants with cleft lip, cleft palate, or cleft lip and palate. Cleft Palate J 1987; 24:244.

Cleft Palate Center, University of Pittsburgh. Everything you've always wanted to know about clefts and were afraid to ask. 16 mm motion picture. 1973.

Cleft Palate Center, University of Pittsburgh. We're all different somehow. 16 mm motion picture. 1977.

Clifford E. Connotative meaning of concepts related to cleft lip and palate. Cleft Palate J 1967; 4:165.

Clifford E. The impact of symptom in the child: comparative studies of clinical populations. J School Health 1968; 6:342.

Clifford E. Cleft palate and the person: psychologic studies of its impact. J South Med Assoc 1971; 64:1516.

Clifford E. Psychosocial aspects of orofacial anomalies: speculations in search of data. ASHA Reports No. 8, 1973:2.

Clifford E. The state of what art? Cleft Palate J 1988; 25:174.

Cohen J. The factorial structure of the WISC at ages 7 1/2, 10 1/2, and 13 1/2. J Consult Psych 1959; 23:285.

Corah N, Corah P. Study of body image in children with cleft palate and cleft lip. J Genet Psych 1963; 103:133.

Doll E. Vineland social maturity scale. Circle Pines, MN: American Guidance Service, 1965.

Duncan PA, Shapiro LR, Soley RL, Turet SE. Linear growth patterns in patients with cleft lip or palate or both. Am J Dis Child 1983; 137:159.

Dunn LM. Manual for the Peabody picture vocabulary test. Philadelphia: American Guidance Service, 1959.

Eliason MJ. Neuropsychological perspectives of cleft lip and/or palate. In: Bardach J, Morris HL, eds. Multidisciplinary management of cleft lip and palate. Philadelphia: WB Saunders, in press.

Fox D, Lynch D, Brookshire B. Selected developmental factors of cleft palate children between two and thirty-three months of age. Cleft Palate J 1978; 15:239.

Frankenburg WK, Dodds JB. Denver developmental screening test. Mead Johnson Laboratories, 1969.

Gall JC, Hayward JR, Harper ML, Garn SM. Studies of dysmorphogenesis in children with oral clefts: 1. Relationship between clinical findings and school performances. Cleft Palate J 1972; 9:326.

Gibbs JM. Cleft palate babies: one mother's experience. Nursing Care 1973; 6:19.

Gluck MR, Wylie HL, McWilliams BJ, Conkwright EA. Comparison of clinical characteristics of children with cleft palates and children in a child guidance clinic. Percept Mot Skills 1965; 21:806.

Goodstein LD. Intellectual impairment in children with cleft palates. J Speech Hear Res 1961; 4:287.

Goodstein LD. Psychosocial aspects of cleft palate. In: Spriestersbach DC, Sherman D, eds. Cleft palate and communication. New York: Academic Press, 1968; 201.

Gouny F, Dalens B, Malpuch G. Association d'une dysrophia de la ligne mediane et d'une insuffisance antehypophysaire congenitale avec micropenis et hypoglycemie neonate. Pediatrie 1978; 33:551.

Hackbush F. Psychological studies of cleft palate patients. Cleft Palate Bull 1951; 1:7.

Harper DC, Richman LC. Personality profiles of physically impaired adolescents. J Clin Psychol 1978; 34:636.

Harper DC, Richman LC, Snider W. School adjustment and degree of physical impairment. J Pediatr Psychol 1980; 5:377.

Hathaway S, McKinley J. Minnesota multiphasic personality inventory. New York: Psychological Corporation, 1951.

Illingsworth RS, Bush LB. The intelligence of children with cleft palate. Arch Dis Child 1956; 31:300.

Iowa tests of basic skills. Boston: Houghton Mifflin, 1979.

Irwin E, McWilliams BJ. Play therapy for children with cleft palates. Child Today 1974; 3:18.

Jones WB. Weight gain and feeding in the neonate with cleft: a three-center study. Cleft Palate J 1988; 25:379.

Kahn T. Kahn test of symbol arrangement: administration and scoring. Percep Mot Skills 1956; 6:4.

Kapp K. Self concept of the child with cleft lip and/or palate. Cleft Palate J 1979; 16:171.

Kapp-Simon K. Self concept of primary-school-age children with cleft lip, cleft palate, or both. Cleft Palate J 1986; 23:24.

Klopfer B, Davidson H. Rorschach technique and development. Rorschach, 1942, New York: Harcourt, Brace and World, 1960.

Lamb M, Wilson F, Leeper H. The intellectual function of cleft palate children compared on the basis of cleft type and sex. Cleft Palate J 1973; 10:367.

Laron Z, Taube E, Kaplan I. Pituitary growth hormone insufficiency associated with cleft lip and palate. An embryonal developmental defect. Helv Paediatr Acta 1969; 24:576.

Lewis R. A survey of intelligence of cleft lip and cleft palate children in Ontario. Presented at the 19th Annual Meeting of the American Association of Cleft Palate Rehabilitation Montreal, 1961.

MacGregor FC. Some psycho-social problems associated with facial deformities. Am Soc Rev 1951; 16:629.

Machover K. Drawing of the human figure. In: Anderson HH, Anderson GL, eds. An introduction to projective techniques. Englewood Cliffs, NJ: Prentice-Hall, 1951.

Matthews J, Ohsberg O. Survey of research in psychosocial aspects of cleft palate for the period 1940-1965. American Cleft Palate Association Mexico City, April, 1966.

McWilliams BJ. Psychosocial development and modification. ASHA Reports, No. 5, 1970:165.

McWilliams BJ, Matthews HP. A comparison of intelligence and social maturity in children with unilateral complete clefts and those with isolated cleft palates. Cleft Palate J 1979; 16:363.

McWilliams BJ, Musgrave R. Psychological implications of articulation disorders in cleft palate children. Cleft Palate J 1972; 9:294.

McWilliams BJ, Smith RM. Psychological considerations. ASHA Reports, No. 9, 1973:43.

Means B, Irwin J. An analysis of certain measures of intelligence and hearing in a sample of the Wisconsin cleft palate population. Cleft Palate Newsl 1954; 2:4.

Mitchell C, Lott R, Pannbacker M. Perceptions about cleft palate held by school personnel: suggestions for in-service training development. Cleft Palate J 1984; 21:308.

Muller DG, Leonetti R. Primary self-concept inventory test manual. Austin, TX: Learning Concepts, 1974.

Munson S, May A. Are cleft palate persons of subnormal

intelligence? J Educ Res 1955; 48:617.

Murray HA. Thematic apperception test. New York: Psychological Corporation, 1935.

Musgrave R, McWilliams BJ, Matthews H. A review of the results of two different surgical procedures for the repair of clefts of the soft palate only. Cleft Palate J 1975; 12:281.

Norval M, Larson T, Parshall P. The impact of the cleft lip and palate child on the family: a preliminary survey. Crippled Children Services, State of Minnesota, 1964.

Palmer J, Adams M. The oral image of children with cleft lips and palates. Cleft Palate Bull 1962; 12:72.

Paradise JL, McWilliams BJ, Bluestone CD, Dickinson P. Ears, hearing and speech in cleft palate children receiving surgical management of middle ear disease. Presented at the 30th Annual Meeting of the American Cleft Palate Association, Phoenix, 1972.

Paradise JL, McWilliams BJ. Simplified feeder for infants with cleft palate. Pediatrics 1974; 53:566.

Paradise JL, Mangubat V, Josefczyk P. Undernutrition in infants with cleft palate. Presented at the 32nd Annual Meeting of the American Cleft Palate Association, Boston, 1974.

Phipps GT. Psychosocial aspects of cleft palate. ASHA Reports, No. 1, 1965:103.

Piers EV. Manual for the Piers-Harris children's self-concept scale. Nashville, TN: Counselor Recordings and Tests, 1969.

Plotkin RR, Wirls CJ, Finney BJ. Developmental evaluation of the cleft infant. Presented at the Annual Meeting of the American Cleft Palate Association, Portland, Oregon, 1970.

Quay H, Patterson D. Manual for the behavior problem checklist. Champaign, IL: University of Illinois, 1967.

Rattner LJ, Carter NJ, Pelkey L. Intelligence quotient of children with congenital cleft palate. J Dent Res 1958; 37:79.

Richman LC. Behavior and achievement of cleft palate children. Cleft Palate J 1976; 13:4.

Richman LC. Parents and teachers: differing views of behavior of cleft palate children. Cleft Palate J 1978a; 15:360.

Richman LC. The effects of facial disfigurement on teachers' perception of ability in cleft palate children. Cleft Palate J 1978b; 15:155.

Richman LC. Self-reported social, speech, and facial concerns and personality adjustment of adolescents with cleft lip and palate. Cleft Palate J 1983, 20:108.

Richman LC, Eliason MJ. Psychological characteristics of children with cleft lip and palate: Intellectual, achievement, behavioral and personality variables. Cleft Palate J 1982; 19:249.

Richman LC, Eliason MJ. Development in children with cleft lip and/or palate; intellectual, cognitive personality, and parenteral factors. Sem Speech Language 1986; 7:225.

Richman LC, Eliason MJ, Lindgren SD. Reading disability in children with clefts. Cleft Palate J 1988; 25:21.

Richman LC, Harper D. School adjustment of children with observable disabilities. J Abnorm Child Psychol 1978; 6:11.

Richman LC, Harper D. Self-identified personality patterns in children with facial or orthopedic disfigurement. Cleft Palate J 1979; 16:2.

Richman LC, Holmes CS, Eliason MJ. Adolescents with cleft lip and palate: self-perceptions of appearance and behavior related to personality adjustment. Cleft Palate J 1985; 22:93.

Rintala AE, Gylling UO. Birth weight of infants with cleft lip and palate. Scand J Plastic Reconstr Surg 1967; 1:109.

Robinson E, Eyberg S, Ross A. The standardization of an inventory of child conduct problem behaviors. J Clin Child Psychol 1980; 9:22.

Rogers CR. Personal adjustment inventory. Manual of directions. New York: Association Press, 1961.

Roggazzeni F, La Causa C, Marianalli L. Il Nanisimo Ipofisario da labiognato-palatochisi. Minerva Pediat 1978; 30:1163.

Ruess AL. A comparative study of cleft palate children and their siblings. J Clin Psychol 1965; 21:354.

Schneiderman CR, Harding JB. Social ratings of children with cleft lip by school peers. Cleft Palate J 1984; 21:219.

Schwartz AH, Landwirth J. Birth defects and the psychosocial development of the child: some implications for management. Conn Med J 1968; 32:457.

Seth AK, McWilliams BJ. Weight gain in children with cleft palate from birth to two years. Cleft Palate J 1988; 25:146.

Sidney R, Matthews J. An evaluation of the social adjustment of a group of cleft palate children. Cleft Palate Bull 1956; 6:10.

Simonds JF, Heimburger RE. Psychiatric evaluation of youth with cleft lip-palate matched with a control group. Cleft Palate J 1978; 15:193.

Sines JO, Pauker JD, Sines LK. The Missouri children's picture series test manual. Iowa City: University of Iowa Press, 1971.

Smith RM, McWilliams BJ. Creative thinking abilities of cleft palate children. Cleft Palate J 1966; 3:275.

Smith RM, McWilliams BJ. Psycholinguistic abilities of children with clefts. Cleft Palate J 1968a; 5:238.

Smith RM, McWilliams BJ. Psycholinguistic considerations in the management of children with cleft palate. J Speech Hear Dis 1968b; 33:27.

Spriestersbach DC. Psychosocial aspects of the cleft palate problem. Vol 1. Iowa City: University of Iowa Press, 1973.

Spriestersbach DC, Moll KL, Morris HL. Heterogeneity of the cleft palate population and research designs. Cleft Palate J 1964; 1:210.

Starr P, Chinsky R, Canter H, Meier J. Mental, motor, and social behavior of infants with cleft lip and/or cleft palate. Cleft Palate J 1977; 14:140.

Stone FB, Wilson MA, Spencer ME, Gibson RC. A survey of elementary school children's behavior problems. Am J Orthopsychiatry 1969; 39:389.

Terman LM, Merrill MA. Stanford-Binet intelligence scale, Form L-M. Boston: Houghton Mifflin, 1960.

Thorpe LP, Clark WW, Tiegs EW. California test of personality. Monterey, CA: CTB, McGraw Hill, 1953.

Tisza VB, Silvertone B, Rosenbloom G, Hanlon N. Psychiatric observations of children with cleft palate. Am J Orthopsychiatry 1958; 28:416.

Tisza VB, Irwin E, Scheide E. Children with oral-facial clefts: a study of the psychological development of handicapped children. J Am Acad Child Psychiatry 1973; 12:292.

Tobiason JM. Social judgments of facial deformity. Cleft Palate J 1987; 24:323.

Tobiason JM. Psychosocial adjustment to cleft lip and

palate. In: Bardach J, Morris HL eds. Multidisciplinary management of cleft lip and palate. Philadelphia: WB Saunders, in press.

Tobiason JM, Hiebert JM. Parents' tolerance for the conduct problems of the child with cleft lip and palate. Cleft Palate J 1984; 21:82.

Tobiason JM, Hiebert JM. Reliability of esthetic ratings of cleft impairment. Cleft Palate J 1988; 25:313.

Tobiason JM, Levy J, Carpenter MA, Hiebert JM. Type of facial cleft, associated congenital malformations, and parents' ratings of school and conduct problems. Cleft Palate J 1987; 24:209.

Walesky-Rainbow M, Morris H. An assessment of informative-counseling procedures for cleft palate children. Cleft Palate J 1978; 15:20.

Watson CG. Personality adjustment in boys with cleft lips and palates. Cleft Palate J 1964; 1:130.

Wechsler D. Wechsler intelligence scale for children. New York: Psychological Corporation, 1949.

Wechsler D. Wechsler adult intelligence scale. New York: Psychological Corporation, 1955.

Wechsler D. Wechsler preschool and primary scale of intelligence. New York: Psychological Corporation, 1967.

Wechsler D. Wechsler intelligence scales for children—revised. New York: Psychological Corporation, 1974.

Wirls CJ. Psychosocial aspects of cleft lip and palate. In: Grabb WC, Rosenstein SW, Bzoch KR, eds. Cleft lip and palate. Boston: Little, Brown, 1971:119–129.

Wirls CJ, Plotkin RR. A comparison of children with cleft palate and their siblings on projective test personality factors. Cleft Palate J 1971; 8:399.

Wolstad DM. The handicap of cleft palate speech. Ment Hyg 1932; 16:281.

9 | ADULT

The goal of treatment for children with clefts is to accomplish results compatible with a satisfying life in the adult years. In spite of this, there is almost no information about the status of adults with clefts, and what little is available is not clear.

The assumption has been that, if appearance is as good as possible, speech is intelligible, hearing is within or close to normal limits, and teeth are properly placed and restored, the outcome is excellent. In a sense this is true. The quality of life would not be as satisfactory if these results were not achieved. On the other hand, some of the most beautiful, talented people have miserable lives because of psychological and social scars that cannot be eradicated. This is also the case for people with clefts, and they may have the added burdens of facial scarring, dental replacements, midface deficiencies, hearing deficits, and speech problems, none of which society rewards or even accepts.

It is surprising that so little effort has been directed toward learning about adults with clefts and how their lives finally evolve. We know these patients well, since their treatment continues for a period of 18 to 20 years. Yet, we often lose touch with them after treatment is terminated.

It seems logical that major centers should develop means for keeping in contact with their patients even after their care has been completed. Perhaps there are cleft-related needs that have not yet been identified, and there is surely a gold mine of information that could be gleaned from these adults.

Although we know far less than we ought to know, we shall discuss the limited number of adult studies that are found in the literature.

EDUCATION

Demb and Ruess (1967) investigated the educational experience of Illinois adults with clefts. They examined by questionnaire the high-school drop-out rate of 64 cleft subjects with no other serious problems as compared to 98 of their siblings. The drop-out rate was 25% for the cleft subjects and 42% for the sibling group. Neither cleft type nor severity of speech and hearing disorders was related to drop-out rate. The cleft group and their sibling controls did not differ with respect to school achievement. The drop-out rates for these two groups, compared to United States and Illinois high-school drop-out rates of 30% indicated that the group with clefts left school less frequently than their siblings or than normative populations. More males with clefts (31%) than females (20%) dropped out of school. While the authors hypothesized that family patterns rather than clefting form the primary basis for whether or not a child with a cleft will ultimately complete high school, this does not explain the difference they found between the group with clefts and their siblings. Could parents perhaps feel that completion of high school is more important for their children with clefts than it is for their sons and daughters who do not begin life with special differences?

McWilliams and Paradise (1973), also using a questionnaire, analyzed data on 115 subjects with clefts and their 97 siblings somewhat more extensively than did Demb and Ruess. In the later study, both subjects with clefts and the sibling subjects achieved significantly higher levels of education than had their parents. However, unlike the findings of Demb and Ruess, 23% of the cleft subjects as opposed to only 13% of their siblings dropped out of high school. Twenty-four of the 26 subjects with clefts who left high school before completion had siblings, and only 42% of those siblings also dropped out of school. This was a significant difference between the two groups. When the upper end of the educational scale was evaluated, subjects with clefts attended college and graduated from college with the same frequency as did their siblings. These findings supported the conclusion of Demb and Ruess (1967) that family patterns are influential in determining whether subjects with clefts will complete high school or not. They suggest, however, that, when family members tend not to finish high school, those with clefts will drop out more often than will their siblings who do not have clefts. Thus, the fact of the cleft appears to be more influential in families who do not stress education than in families who do.

Clifford et al. (1972) interviewed 98 subjects with clefts in order to gather descriptive information about their adult lives, including education. The average subject completed 11.8 years of school. Twenty percent had completed at least 9 years of education; 49% 10 to 12 years; and 31% some education beyond high school. However, no actual information was given about high-school drop-out rate. The subjects were asked to rate their educational satisfaction on a scale of 1 (low) to 5 (high). The mean rating was 3.25, an expression of mild satisfaction. How this finding would compare with similar data on people in general is not known.

A study of educational level among subjects with clefts was conducted in Finland by Lahti et al. (1974). Their data are difficult to interpret because of the differences in the Finnish school system and culture as compared to the United States. They began with a group of 514 subjects with cleft lips and palates or cleft palates alone. Mail questionnaires were answered by 296. The information about educational levels was compared to normative information available for Finland. At the "lower and middle" levels of education, the subjects with clefts matched or slightly exceeded national norms. At the higher end of the educational scale, they did not reach the national norms. For example, 99.7% of the respondents with clefts completed "primary school" as compared to 99.9% for the country as a whole. Thirty-two percent completed "junior secondary school" as opposed to only 22.2% reported in the national averages. At the university level, the pattern is reversed, 8.6% for the respondents with clefts and 15.2% for the entire country. On the other hand, 31.5% of the subjects with clefts completed "vocational school" as compared to 19.5% for the nation as a whole. Thus, Finnish individuals with clefts attend college less frequently but graduate from some type of vocational school more frequently than do their noncleft peers. These data must be interpreted cautiously but kept available for future consideration.

Peter and Chinsky (1974b) used a 62-area questionnaire to study educational achievement in 195 cleft subjects, 190 of their siblings, and 209 nationally-drawn random control subjects. Cleft subjects had a 27% drop-out rate, not greatly different from the rate reported by Demb and Ruess (1967) and McWilliams and Paradise (1973). The drop-out rate for siblings was 25% and for random controls, 31%. The differences among these groups were not significant. The mean educational level attained by all groups was just over 12 years, suggesting high-school graduation. Males with clefts in this study left school prior to graduation at a rate of 29%, whereas the male siblings left at a rate of 23% and the control males at a rate of 26%. For females with clefts and their siblings, the dropout rate was 26% as opposed to the control rate of 35%. There were no differences attributable to cleft type.

Just as many subjects with clefts (26%) attended college as did their siblings (29%), and these rates did not differ significantly from the national control group (34%). There was a significant difference between subjects with cleft lip and palate and those with cleft palate only relative to frequency of college attendance. A significantly higher proportion of those with cleft lip and palate had education at the college level. This is a reasonable finding when it is remembered that there is a greater prevalence of developmental problems in subjects with isolated clefts than in those with both cleft lip and palate. Peter and Chinsky concluded that "cleft palate subjects" achieved educational levels similar to those of their siblings and random control subjects. Although this conclusion is accurate based on these data, we cannot generalize from any of the studies discussed, since there may be differences between subjects who live in cities and those who live in rural and small communities; there was no assurance that the subjects with clefts and their siblings were or were not similar in mental capacities; and many other variables such as speech, appearance, and hearing were not controlled, as they have not been in other studies.

It is undoubtedly true that the percentages of people who complete high school and go to college is a reflection of the times in which they live, their cultural mores, economic conditions both national and local, family patterns, and many other possible variables. The studies reported here all came from different types of communities and, therefore, cannot be readily compared. The most that can be said is that there is not strong evidence to support the conclusion that children with clefts are either more or less likely to drop out of high school than are their peers. This issue should be explored further with more rigid control of a multitude of variables than has yet been undertaken. Such work can probably best be approached through collaborative research. Until the research is done, those working with children with clefts should help in every way possible to motivate them to seek the highest level of education of which they are capable.

MARRIAGE

Van Demark and Van Demark (1970) indicated that their subjects with clefts appeared to date less frequently than their noncleft peers, and this observation is often made in clinics where teenagers and young adults with clefts are treated. This finding leads naturally to an interest in the marriage patterns of these young people.

Peter and Chinsky (1974a) reported that subjects with clefts married people of equal or higher educational attainment, as did their siblings and the random control subjects. This educational equality in marriage was only minimally affected by cleft type. Those with both cleft lip and palate, thus those with facial scarring, showed a slight tendency to marry downward on the educational scale. Females with clefts married slightly downward, whereas sibling and control females married slightly upward. These were only trends, since significant statistical differences were not found.

Another interesting finding in their study is the relationship between college attendance and the frequency of marriage. Five percent of the male and female control subjects who did not attend college remained single, whereas 15% of those subjects with clefts who attended college had not married at the time of the study. However, female cleft subjects who had attended college married as frequently as the noncleft females who had not attended college. Forty-five percent of the cleft males who attended but did not complete college remained single, as compared to 14% of their male siblings and 12% of the male controls. On the other hand, cleft males who completed college married significantly more frequently than did their siblings or the noncleft controls. This latter group of males with clefts may be composed of individuals who have made a better overall accommodation to their problems and thus are generally ambitious and aggressive.

McWilliams and Paradise (1973) also studied marriage in 115 cleft subjects and their 97 sibling controls. The subjects with clefts were or had been married much less frequently than had their siblings. This may mean only that individuals with clefts marry later than do their siblings, particularly if they are males who graduate from college. However, since the mean age of the cleft group was 24 years and of the sibling group 27 years, it is difficult to know whether or not most of the cleft subjects eventually did marry. This is a topic that should be pursued in greater depth in the future.

Peter and Chinsky (1974a) found that cleft subjects who married did so 4 years later than did their sibling and random controls and that subjects with both cleft lip and palate married later than did those with palatal clefts only. Subjects with palatal clefts only, especially males, also married more frequently. The group with clefts, as a whole, showed significantly fewer marriages than the control groups, a finding similar to that of McWilliams and Paradise (1973). Heller et al. (1981) reported that only 18% of the young adults they studied (mean age 22.5) were married as compared to 39% in the same age group in Montreal, where the study was done.

In the Peter and Chinsky study, childless marriages were more often reported in the groups with clefts than in the control groups, and subjects with clefts had significantly fewer children and fewer children per year of marriage.

Bjornsson and Agustsdottir (1987) analyzed responses to questionnaires of 63 adults with clefts of the palate or lip or both. The authors, working in Iceland, had a total pool of 79 adult former patients, only 10 of whom could not be located. For the remaining 69, the compliance rate was 91%, almost unheard of in research of this type. They learned that only 50% of the males and 60.9% of the females were married or living with a partner as opposed to 87.9% of the males and 89% of the females in the comparison group.

The studies of McWilliams and Paradise (1973), Peter and Chinsky (1974a), Heller et al. (1981), and Bjornsson and Agustsdottir (1987), all suggest that marriage is another area of adult life that differs for subjects with clefts as compared to those not similarly affected. This may be especially true when there is visible facial scarring. Although these data are not conclusive and represent clinical results achieved more than 20 years ago, they do cast some doubt on the conclusion often seen in the literature that people with clefts are "just like everyone else." That is obviously an oversimplification that does not hold up when actual behavior is studied. It is to be remembered, however, that marriage is not the index of social acceptability that it once was and that future research designs must take these changing mores into account.

It is notable that few treatment programs offer counseling to teenagers and young adults about relationships with the opposite sex, dating, marriage, parenting, and feelings related thereto. Yet, clinical experience tells us that these young people are often bursting with concern about these aspects of their lives. At the very least, we should be open to discussing these issues with them and to offering discussion groups whenever possible, recognizing the real difficulty that many of our patients have in focusing on these sometimes painful issues. Speech pathologists should be available for such interactions but should also know when to refer to other specialists.

APPEARANCE

Crocker et al. (1973) examined body satisfaction as expressed by a group of 98 adults with cleft lip and palate. Satisfaction levels were high in comparison to a control sample. This is another study that fails to explain why subjects with clefts should be better satisfied with themselves than are people in general. It seems, on the surface at least, that an element of denial must be present. It is therefore, reassuring that the cleft subjects in this study recognized the relative flaws in themselves when they expressed least satisfaction with the mouth, teeth, lips, voice, talking, and speech.

Bjornsson and Agustsdottir (1987) found their subjects to be relatively satisfied with the treatment they had received, but their expectations regarding the outcome of surgery exceeded what had actually been realized. Yet, these subjects did not express dissatisfaction with outcome or feel that the clefts had greatly influenced their

lives. Females, however, were more self conscious than males, particularly with respect to how other people saw them.

Since an objective view of oneself usually includes recognition of variations that make one less than perfect and since a subjective self appraisal will often result in the overemphasis of even minor flaws, it is obviously necessary to carry out additional studies that are directed toward learning more about the relevance of clefts and their sequelae in adult life. It is possible of course that progress toward improved appearance and better speech may be a source of satisfaction that is reflected in increased self acceptance. However, this theoretical explanation is not completely supported by the work of Heller et al. (1981). Half of their subjects considered to be "adequate" in psychological functioning were dissatisfied with appearance, as were 59% of those described as "possibly inadequate" and all of those thought to be "inadequate."

Although Richman et al. (1985), as reported in Chapter 8, found that better adjusted adolescents had more realistic perceptions of their life conditions than had those who were less well adjusted, acceptance of reality and refusal to use denial as a coping mechanism may not always mean lack of concern. Caring about appearance is understandable, given social attitudes toward physical beauty. However, perceptions of physical beauty may be influenced by other factors. Glass and Starr (1979) found that ratings of attractiveness decreased as ratings of hypernasality increased. Sinko and Hedrick (1982) reported that untrained observers were somewhat more lenient in their ratings of appearance than they were of speech patterns in adolescents with clefts. Although adolescents and young adults may be more concerned about appearance than they are about speech, it may well be that decreasing nasality will help to enhance physical attractiveness as it is perceived by others and aid in reducing the social penalties that contribute to elevated concerns about appearance.

OCCUPATION

McWilliams and Paradise (1973) reported that adults with clefts and their sibling controls achieved higher educational levels than had their fathers but that neither group surpassed their fathers in occupational levels. This may be related both to clefting and to the influence of the cleft on the nearest-aged sibling. In fact, many mothers, when asked if they had questions about the interview, expressed concern that the care, time, and energy expended on the child with the cleft may have resulted in neglect of their other children. If this were the case, it is probable that the sibling closest in age would be the one most likely to feel the effects. However, we do not have the answers to this question, and other interpretations are possible.

Berg (1970) has pointed to a number of factors that work together to determine occupational status. These include the influence of family and associates, personal ambition, intelligence, character, and physique. We would add that graduation from high school is also a more common occurrence than was once true, so that people who achieve educational levels beyond those of their parents may do so because of changing social mores. Improved occupational status may not necessarily follow.

Peter et al. (1975a) also studied occupation in subjects with clefts, their siblings, and a randomly selected control sample. Males with clefts were not upwardly mobile, but their siblings and random controls were. Thus, income was lower for the subjects with clefts.

For the most part, subjects with clefts remained with the same employer as frequently as their noncleft peers. The only exception to this was males with cleft palate only, a group likely to suffer from other developmental difficulties. Clifford et al. (1972) reported that males with clefts had held significantly more jobs than females. The meaning of this finding is not clear, since greater job mobility may well be true of males in general. In the study by Peter et al. (1975a), when unemployment was part of the history, subjects with clefts were without jobs more often and for longer periods of time than were the random controls. However, with the exception of males with cleft palates, the subjects with clefts were not unemployed more frequently than their siblings. Females with clefts had the highest rate of unemployment. In spite of their employment histories, however, subjects with clefts, particularly males with cleft lips and palates, reported more feelings of insecurity about their jobs than did their siblings or random controls.

Subjects with clefts, especially males with cleft lips and palates, felt that their jobs were unsuitable more often than did the control subjects but not more often than their siblings, another finding suggestive of family patterns that may differ from the norm. It is perhaps significant that subjects with clefts had higher job aspirations than either their siblings or random controls, an outcome that supports Van Demark and Van Demark (1970) in their conclusion that subjects with clefts had somewhat unrealistic vocational goals. On the other hand Peter et al. (1975a) found that subjects with clefts and their siblings had lower income aspirations than did the random controls. Thus, the subjects with clefts aspired to better jobs but lower incomes than did the controls, a finding that is contradictory to the mores of a society that equates achievement with financial gain.

The studies by Peter et al. and the one by McWilliams and Paradise (1973) both suggest that individuals with clefts may fail to find job satisfaction and that, to a lesser extent, this also applies to their siblings. These results are in sharp contrast to those of Clifford et al. (1972). The cleft group in their study was compared to the normative data for the Minnesota Scale for Parental Occupations, and the cleft subjects were found more frequently in the professional, managerial, and skilled trades groups. Interestingly enough, only 4% of Clifford's subjects were dissatisfied with appearance. Given the presence of facial scarring in individuals with both cleft lips and palates, one wonders again how much denial might have been involved. Clifford pointed out, however, that denial that helps the individual to achieve personal growth and mastery can be healthy. This interpretation of denial is undoubtedly true in some cases. In others, it represents defensiveness that can have a marked negative impact on satisfaction.

We still have much to learn about the employment of people with clefts and their siblings. The best evidence to date is indicative of a less than ideal outcome for both groups. Treatment programs should probably be concerned with family dynamics and with the noncleft siblings as well as with the social and economic structure into which the person with a cleft must eventually move. Such programming is expensive, and it is improbable that the current economy can support such an ideal. Additional studies must now be done to determine whether or not the cleft adult who successfully completes higher education is also limited in job outlook. We have only anecdotal information on that question.

SOCIAL INTEGRATION

A few studies have investigated the social integration of adults with clefts. These studies point to life patterns that differ in some important respects from those of individuals who do not have clefts.

Van Demark and Van Demark (1970) interviewed 39 subjects aged 18 or 19 years. The subjects with clefts were not grossly different from others in their families, but they reported that they had experienced less teasing within their family groups than would have been expected in the average family. This might be indicative of subtle differences in the interactions of cleft and noncleft family members that could act to make the member with the cleft feel "different." Van Demark and Van Demark also concluded that their subjects were often observers of life rather than participants and that they were uncertain about their social abilities. Thus, they preferred individual rather than group activities and were not likely to join organizations.

Peter et al. (1975b), from their study of 195 cleft subjects, 190 sibling controls, and 209 random controls from a national pool, drew conclusions similar to those of Van Demark and Van Demark (1970). Subjects with clefts more frequently lived with other family members than did their siblings or random controls. If they did not live with relatives, they visited in the "extended family" more often. Subjects with clefts and their siblings remained close to their parental homes after completion of school more frequently than did the controls. The reason for this is unclear. It could be a geographical characteristic, but the same general trend was reported by Heller et al. (1981).

In the study by Peter et al., subjects with clefts more frequently chose passive activities to fill their leisure time than did either siblings or controls. High levels of passivity were characteristic among patients with all types of clefts with the exception of males with cleft palate only. This latter group, however, showed greater dependence upon family than did any of the other subgroups. Making initial social contacts was often more difficult for the group with clefts than for noncleft subjects. The differences reached significance, however, only for females with cleft lip and palate.

Data concerning friendship patterns were not definitive with one exception. Both sibling and control groups reported that most of their friends knew each other. This was not true for subjects with clefts regardless of cleft type or sex. Significance at the 0.001 level of confidence is substantial evidence that the cleft subjects were not experiencing group identification and integrated friendships.

Subjects with clefts in this study, as in the study by Van Demark and Van Demark (1970), joined organizations less frequently than did their controls, but the differences were significant only for females with clefts of both the lip and palate. Peter et al. wisely pointed out that answers to any questionnaire may not reflect actual behavior. However, this criticism cannot be applied to such things as living with other family members.

Thought must be given to the possible influence of geography upon the results. Where there were no differences between cleft and sibling groups, conclusions would have been more robust had a local rather than a national control group been used. However, in those important matters where the subjects with clefts and their siblings differed from each other, it seems clear that there is some limitation in adulthood associated with having a cleft. This interpretation was strengthened by Heller et al. (1981). Over half (56%) of their subjects expressed dissatisfaction with their social lives, and nearly half had few leisure activities. Evidence of mild social problems in adulthood continues to mount as does the obvious clinical need to include social planning from the preschool years forward (Bjornsson and Agustsdottir, 1987). Speech pathologists working in public schools can be alert to early social differences and, as a specific part of communicative therapy, strive to minimize them.

SUMMARY

Although information about adults with various types of clefts is too sparse to justify strong, conclusive statements about their psychosocial attributes in adult life, one cannot ignore the probability that these individuals do not have life experiences equivalent to those of others. Although there is no support for the conclusion that they are severely disturbed, they do appear to have increased difficulty with peer relationships, marriage, occupational fulfillment, and the realization of their stated goals. Part of the explanation for these perhaps marginal positions in life may lie with the individual, but part may also reside in social attitudes (McWilliams, 1970). It was apparent then, as it is now, that society "creates pressures, which it then minimizes and denies so that the person with a cleft . . . experiences the subtle . . . forms of discrimination which majorities practice against minorities."

REFERENCES

Berg I. Education and jobs: the great training robbery. New York: Praeger, 1970.

Bjornsson A, Agustsdottir S. A psychological study of Icelandic individuals with cleft lip or cleft lip and palate. Cleft Palate J 1987; 24:152.

Clifford E, Crocker E, Pope B. Psychological findings in the adulthood of 98 cleft lip-palate children. Plast Reconstr Surg 1972; 50;234.

Crocker E, Clifford E, Pope B. The cleft palate child grows up: an analysis of the adulthood of former patients. In: Clifford E, ed. Psychosocial aspects of orofacial anomalies: speculations in search of data. ASHA Reports No 8, 1973:2.

Demb N, Ruess A. High-school drop-out rate for cleft palate patients. Cleft Palate J 1967; 4:327.

Glass L, Starr C. A study of the relationships between judgment of speech and appearance of patients with orofacial clefts. Cleft Palate J 1978; 16:436.

Heller A, Tidmarsh W, Pless IB. The psychological functioning of young adults born with cleft lip or palate. Pediatrics 1981; 20;459.

Lahti A, Rintala A, Soivio A. Educational level of patients with cleft lip and palate. Cleft Palate J 1974; 11:36.

McWilliams BJ. Psychosocial development and modification. ASHA Reports No. 5, 1970:165.

McWilliams BJ, Paradise L. Educational, occupational, and marital status of cleft palate adults. Cleft Palate J 1973; 10:223.

Peter J, Chinsky R. Sociological aspects of cleft palate adults: I. Marriage. Cleft Palate J 1974a; 11:295.

Peter J, Chinsky R. Sociological aspects of cleft palate adults: II Education. Cleft Palate J 1974b, 11:443.

Peter J, Chinsky R, Fisher M. Sociological aspects of cleft palate adults: III Vocational and economic aspects. Cleft Palate J 1975a; 12:193.

Peter J, Chinsky R, Fisher M. Sociological aspects of cleft palate adults: IV Social integration. Cleft Palate J 1975b; 12:304.

Richman LC, Holmes CS, Eliason M. Adolescents with cleft lip and palate: self perception of appearance and behavior related to personality adjustment. Cleft Palate J 1985; 22:93.

Sinko GR, Hedrick DL. The interrelationships between ratings of speech and facial acceptability in persons with cleft palate. J Speech Hear Res 1982; 25:402.

Van Demark D, Van Demark A. Speech and socio-vocational aspects of individuals with cleft palate. Cleft Palate J 1970; 7:284.

10 | PARENTS

Since parents are responsible for the early nurture of their babies, it is assumed that infants, especially those with clefts, born to loving and accepting parents who are free from unusual stresses, capable of coping with the day-to-day problems of living including management of their families, consistent in their behavior, and honest with themselves and others will fare better than infants born to unstable parents. To this end, parents have been the subject of study. This does not mean that competent, well-adjusted parents are guaranteed competent, well-adjusted children, but that they may have a better chance of such an outcome than parents who bring to the parenting experience numerous unresolved problems of their own.

It is also logical to assume that parents who do well with a normal baby will also be successful with an infant with a cleft. Things will not be as easy; there will be times of sorrow and concern; yet they will do what they have to do. Their child will be loved, nurtured, and accepted by two parents who have a good, strong marriage. The child will learn to value himself as a human being and to cope successfully with the stresses of life, including the cleft.

Less well integrated parents may do a fairly good job of parenting a normal baby but be less able to handle the added problems of an infant with a cleft. It may take them longer to accept the defect; they may be less consistent in the love and care they provide; and a few may have feelings of rejection toward their baby. The infant may develop marginally well but may ultimately be less certain of personal worth than are his normal siblings and less secure in interaction with others. If parental uncertainties find expression in over-protection, the outcome may be even more disastrous for the child.

Other parents may be inadequate to deal with either a normal or a cleft infant. Although their child with a cleft may not do well, the cleft is not the major contributing factor.

Still another possibility is inadequacy relative to any child, coupled with an inability to accept the defective child. Sometimes this child becomes the family scapegoat or is abused or battered. The possible combinations are infinite—the mother who is supportive combined with the father who is not or vice versa. The marriage, poor at the outset, sometimes cannot survive the added burden that the infant with a cleft presents. It is clear that the baby is born into a family that existed before he or she joined it. The baby did not create the parents' difficulties and is not responsible for the "impact" that his birth may have upon them. The baby is, however, the product of their union in the emotional as well as in the physical sense.

IMPACT OF THE CLEFT

The impact of the cleft will depend upon the parents—how much their egos are threatened by a congenital anomaly in their baby and to what extent they have access to and can use various psychological coping mechanisms (McWilliams, 1970). These vast individual differences may explain why studies directed toward the measurement of impact have yielded inconsistent and inconclusive information. It could not be otherwise. Nevertheless, it would be ridiculous to assert that a baby born with a cleft does not affect his parents in some way (Adler, 1987). It is unlikely that an infant with birth defects is ever a pure expression of the parents' dreams. In reality, all parents experience emotions akin to grief over the loss of the perfect baby and must mourn for the child who is not to be (Solnit, 1961; Tisza and Gumpertz, 1962; Slutsky, 1969). Spriestersbach (1973) concluded from his structured retrospective interviews with 713 mothers and 455 fathers of children with clefts that shock is a universal response among parents and that shock and mourning are also common responses among the professional persons involved in the delivery. Others have alluded to the feelings that are typical of parents in "crisis" (Green and Durocher, 1965).

This attitude is reinforced by a recent study (Salazar, 1988) in which maternal behavior in rats was studied. The mothers retrieved all of the noncleft animals and took them to the nest as they did 14 of 18 rats with repaired cleft lips, but only four of 18 with unrepaired lips were retrieved. However, the extent to which these emotions are experienced and the manner in which they are resolved depends upon several factors yet to be specified. The major one, of course, is the strength the parents themselves bring to the experience. Slutsky (1969) wrote that 79% of the 66 mothers he interviewed reported that their own strength and ability were the most effective factors in the successful management of their children. However, other factors are of importance as well, although we have few data to guide us in addressing these clinically. On the other hand, we know that most parents work through their grief, recover from the initial impact quickly and overcome their pain so that they can love and show compassion for their infants (Tisza and Gumpertz, 1962).

Clifford (1968), in a study of 60 pairs of parents, reported that the effects of the initial shock had usually been dissipated before the mother and child were discharged from the hospital. Although this points to human resilience, it does not permit us to ignore potential problems. Tobiason (1984) makes a strong case for possible long-term effects on parent-child relationships.

FACTORS AFFECTING PARENTAL ATTITUDES

Extent of Deformity

First, the infant who has only some form of cleft presents a different problem from that of the child who has a cleft combined with other congenital abnormalities, and less extensive clefts are probably easier for most parents to accept than are more complex ones. As early as 1956, Hill, from his interviews and "objective tests" of 70 parents, reported that parents of children with clefts of the lip alone gave significantly fewer responses suggestive of rejection than did parents of children with more extensive defects. In contrast, when facial disfigurement was present, parents expressed significantly more personal guilt than when only the palate was involved.

Spriestersbach (1973) pointed out that parents of children with clefts of the palate with no lip involvement had fewer profound concerns than parents of children with clefts of both lip and palate.

Norval et al. (1964) reported no "high-stress" families when children had cleft lips only. Clifford (1969), in a study of 60 pairs of parents and 60 cleft children below the age of 2 years found that infants with clefts of both the lip and palate received higher severity ratings than did infants with clefts of the lip or palate alone. Husbands and wives agreed with each other significantly on their ratings, and the extent of the deformity influenced their other ratings of their children. For example, infants with more extensive clefts were seen as more active-irritable and as having less pleasant personality characteristics. This, of course, may have been reality-based. However, these observations fit with those from a later study in which Clifford and Crocker (1971) found that the degree of "shock" a mother experiences at the birth of her child with a cleft is related to the extent of the deformity.

These data suggest that the extent of the deformity will influence how parents view their children and points to the need to study subgroups in future research. We must recognize, therefore, that infants born with more complex clefts, and perhaps with other congenital malformations, and their parents constitute different populations from those born with clefts involving only the lip or palate. Counseling needs of the different parental groups may also be different, although there will be strong and weak parents in all groups and, thus, much overlapping.

This is no small problem when it is understood that malformations in addition to clefts are relatively common, especially in association with isolated palatal clefts (Spriestersbach et al., 1962). As diagnostic techniques have become more sophisticated, higher occurrence rates of associated anomalies have been found. Fogh-Anderson (1942) reported an occurrence rate of 10%. Loretz et al. (1961) reported a rate of 18%. Pannbacker (1968) examined the records of 100 cleft patients at the University of Oklahoma Medical Center and found that 31% had congenital malformations in addition to the cleft. Fifteen of these (49%) had two or more associated birth defects. Almost twice as many males as females had additional malformations. McWilliams and Matthews (1979) reported that 14% of children with unilateral cleft lips and palates had associated birth defects, and 34% of those with isolated palatal clefts had other birth defects. In the latter group, more than 50% had developmental disorders involving mental abilities. Thus, the parent who views the isolated cleft as a minor disorder early on may be unaware that the child is at high risk for later complications.

Rollnick and Pruzansky (1981) found that 35% of patients with clefts of the lip with or without palatal clefts had multiple anomalies as compared to 54% of those with isolated palatal clefts and 55% of those with submucous clefts. Shprintzen et al. (1985) reported that associated malformations occurred in 63.4% of their cleft subjects. These authors looked carefully at both major and minor deformities.

More recently, Jones (1988) wrote that additional anomalies were present in 14% of her patients with cleft lip with or without cleft palate, 55% with cleft palate, 76% with velopharyngeal insufficiency, and 83% with unusual forms of clefting.

As improved methods of discernment become available and as the importance of even minor malformations is recognized, the figures on occurrence continue to increase. However, in spite of that, there is never any disagreement about the increased risk in infants with isolated palatal clefts. The data reflect the need for in-depth pediatric evaluations for all infants with clefts and the desirability of careful follow-up with developmental testing incorporated into routine clinical procedures. Only in that way is it possible to provide the required support to parents, who too often are left to cope alone as best they can.

Uncertainty is a fertile ground for the growth of parental anxieties, and troubled parents are less able to provide a positive emotional climate for their child. Counseling is often needed, and it must address the issues that are perceived by the parent as relevant and important rather than theoretical issues that may not apply in a particular case.

Familiarity with Clefts

A second area of concern is the parents' familiarity with clefts. Since 76% of parents interviewed by Slutsky (1969) and more than half of those surveyed by Middleton et al. (1986) had

never even heard of clefts, it is clear that many parents come to this experience with no prior knowledge of the condition and no idea of what to do about it. In general, the more familiar the family is with the defect, the more easily they can be expected to adjust, but there are notable exceptions. Parents who already have a child with a severe cleft and other problems as well might be deeply upset by the birth of a second child with a cleft, even if it is less complex. Familiarity is often an issue in families who have several members with clefts and in racial groups in which clefting is either frequent or rare. For example, the incidence of cleft lip with or without cleft palate among the Japanese is approximately 2.13 per 1000 live births, among Caucasians, 1.34, and among Blacks, 0.41 (Fraser, 1971). One might assume that the "impact" of the cleft on parents would differ as a function of the frequency of the defect and as well as in relationship to the social attitudes toward birth defects in given cultures. External pressures encountered by both child and parents also differ from one culture to another (Strauss, 1985). To our knowledge, there are no data on how parents are influenced by these factors, but it warrants investigation.

Age of the Parents

MacMahon and McKeown (1953), Fraser and Calnan (1961), Woolf et al. (1963), and Green et al. (1965) have all reported a significant positive relationship between parental age, particularly paternal age, and cleft lip with or without cleft palate. Green et al. found that increasing age of both parents was related to the frequency of cleft lip with cleft palate and of isolated cleft palate.

Hay (1967), working with records for the years 1962 and 1964 from 29 states and two large cities, studied all birth certificates on which any congenital defect was noted, and 1% of the records of babies for whom no malformations were recorded. For the 6000 cases of cleft lip and palate, the occurrence of cleft palate and of cleft lip and palate was increased among older fathers, especially for those over 40. When the clefts occurred in conjunction with other birth defects, the relationship to greater paternal age held for all forms of clefts. Thus, paternal age is identified as a factor in etiology, and it may be as influential in increased stress, although the only available data on this issue suggest that younger parents experience greater stress than older parents (Norval et al. 1964). While it is conceivable that less experienced parents might feel greater stress and be in need of more support than more experienced parents, it is also not improbable to suppose that older parents, weary of the tasks associated with child rearing, might also, at least in some instances, be in need of special nurture. Research directed to the age question would be of help.

How Parents are Informed of the Cleft

Another element that affects how parents respond to having a child with a cleft is the manner in which they are informed about the defect and the kind of counseling and support they receive. We know too little about this subject, and most of the information is retrospectively reported by parents. Slutsky (1969) noted that an overwhelming 99% of mothers questioned said that they would have preferred hearing of the cleft from their attending physicians, but this actually occurred in only 71% of the cases and in approximately 75% of those interviewed by Spriestersbach (1973). Actually, it is often reported that the father is the one to inform the mother or, surprisingly, the mother who must tell the father. Spriestersbach (1973) concluded that parents retain negative feelings about this matter for years after their children are born.

Spriestersbach (1973) also found that about one-fourth of the parents whose infants had clefts involving the lip were not told of the defect on the day of birth. This implies that they also did not see their babies on that first day. A few were not told until at least 3 days post-partum. When there was cleft palate only, 32% of parents learned of the defect from 3 to 6 days post-partum, and 27% received no information for at least 1 week. The delay is even greater in cases of submucous clefts.

Knowing when information was provided is vital in understanding both parent and child responses. Clifford (1971) and Clifford and Crocker (1971) point out that the degree of "shock" that a mother feels is related to both the extent of deformity and the time that elapses before she sees her baby. A similar observation was made by Dar et al. (1974) on the basis of a retrospective study in northern Israel. Since the early hours after birth are crucial in the mother-child bonding process, it would be desirable to investigate how such delays relate to later parental and child attitudes and to child development, particularly speech and language development.

CONCERNS OF PARENTS

Weachter (1959) asked parents to list their major concerns about their children with clefts. In order of frequency, they named: (1) appearance, (2) immediacy of surgery, (3) speech, (4) feeding, (5) reactions of the other parent, (6) responses of brothers and sisters, (7) reactions of other family members and friends, (8) mental development, (9) finances, and (10) the possibility of recurrence in future children.

Clinically, these 10 concerns are common to most parents at some point in the life of a child with a cleft, but the priority for a given parent probably depends upon the age of the child and the particular problem that is paramount at that stage of development. Parents' concerns are not static. They change as the child grows and develops (Spriestersbach, 1973). In fact, Hill (1956) reported that parents generally have more positive attitudes as their children enter the later stages of treatment.

Regardless of the age of the child, family stresses are variable. Norval et al. (1964) found that the 51 mothers whom they studied showed higher indices of stress when: (1) either parent felt guilt, (2) the child was perceived as different, (3) the parents thought treatment was taking too long, (4) the parents were not satisfied with explanations about the child's condition, (5) the mother thought there were a lot of feeding problems, or (6) the parents were unusually worried about having more children. Knowing how parents may be feeling is useful in seeking direction in planning appropriate counseling, which most parents require at some stage in the life of their child.

There is evidence that parents want and need more information about clefting and related problems than they often are given, especially in the first year of their child's life when confusion and misunderstanding are likely to be at a peak (Bradley, 1960). Spriestersbach (1961) found that, even after counseling, the parents of children with clefts were often poorly informed. Arbeitel (1985), assessing the effectiveness of genetic counseling, learned that the parents were satisfied with the experience but retained very little of what had been presented.

Walesky-Rainbow and Morris (1978) reported that professional people were somewhat inconsistent in what they expected parents to know. This is serious because misinformation and confusion lead to unnecessary anxiety and poor parental cooperation with treatment programs. Clearly, more written reports should be provided to parents.

This sense of confusion may account in part for the success of certain parent groups and for the support that new parents find through association with more experienced parents who have faced and surmounted similar problems (Irwin and McWilliams, 1973). This seeking of mutual support varies from parent to parent, and not all are comforted and helped by the same procedures. Nevertheless, the Cleft Palate Foundation[1] (formerly the American Cleft Palate Educational Foundation), in recognition of unmet needs of parents, provides referral information through its toll-free cleft line, answers letters of inquiry from parents, publishes informational materials and a newsletter for parents, and serves in a parent advocacy role. In addition, the Foundation has published a manual (1978) to assist in the formation of parent groups, which are gradually growing in numbers and beginning to interact with each other on state and national levels. This movement has led to the formation of the National Cleft Palate Association,[2] which is primarily a parent organization.

PARENTAL PERSONALITY

No one has shown that parents of children with clefts are different in important ways from the parents of children who do not have clefts. Goodstein (1960a, b) compared the responses to the Minnesota Multiphasic Inventory (MMPI) (Hathaway and McKinley, 1942) of 170 mothers and 157 fathers of children with clefts and those of 100 control parents. There were no outstanding differences between the two groups, and both

---

[1]Additional information may be obtained from the Cleft Palate Foundation, 1218 Grandview Avenue, Pittsburgh, Pa. 15211.
[2]National Cleft Palate Association
2485 D South Xanader Way
Aurora, Colorado 80014

were well within normal limits. Since the MMPI was designed to identify people with serious psychopathologies, it is perhaps not surprising that the groups were similar. The parents of children with clefts, however, seemed to be somewhat more anxious than their counterparts in the control group. There was evidence to suggest that parents, particularly fathers of older children with clefts, were somewhat less well adjusted than were the parents of younger children. This may relate to the children's continuing need for care, to less than hoped-for results, or to the child's broadening world with its increased social demands. MMPI scores did not relate positively to type of cleft, to the children's social adjustment, or to adequacy of child management as rated on a 9-point scale. In summary, the parents of children with clefts appear to represent a cross-section of parents generally and to be no different from other parents in their MMPI responses.

Goodstein (1960a) made the point that there can be personality and adjustment differences among the parents of children with clefts and that these are theoretically and practically important, despite the fact that the experimental and control groups did not differ in important ways. The clinical implication of this is clear. If parental problems are influential in the management of a particular case, those problems become key elements in treatment planning.

ATTITUDES TOWARD CHILD REARING

Richman and Harper (1978), from a review of the literature about the effects of physical disfigurement on attitudes toward child rearing, concluded that data on child-rearing practices and the role of parental attitudes in outcome are insufficient and equivocal. They explored this issue by studying the perceptions of maternal child-rearing tactics of 68 children with palatal clefts, 68 with cerebral palsy, and 68 with no physical impairments. The children, between 9 and 18 years of age, were individually matched for age, intelligence, grade, and socioeconomic status.

The Child's Report of Parental Behavior Inventory (Schaefer, 1965), as modified by Burger and Armentrout (1971), was administered to each child. The inventory yields scores for three behavioral factors including (1) acceptance-rejection, (2) psychological control-psychological autonomy, and (3) firm control-lax control. The three groups were similar on Factors 1 and 3. On Factor 2, however, the children with clefts, primarily the males, perceived their mothers as exerting greater psychological control or intrusiveness than did either the children with cerebral palsy or the normal children. Richman and Harper speculated that mothers may have a tendency to nurture their handicapped offspring and to foster a dependency that is unacceptable to the male child with a cleft when he reaches the age when he is capable of independence, as the cerebral palsied male is not. Girls, on the other hand, appear to maintain relatively stable dependency patterns into adulthood, a condition that is likely to change as cultural mores for the sexes change.

Brantley and Clifford (1979) studied 44 mothers and their cleft children between 9 and 18 years of age. These subjects were compared to 61 unimpaired children of similar age on measures of locus of control (Rotter, 1960, 1966), field articulation (Witkin et al., 1954, 1962), feelings of parental acceptance, and teacher ratings. The mothers were also examined to determine their loci of control and their personal perceptions about the births of their children.

The mothers of the subjects with clefts reported significantly more concern about their babies and more negative feelings about showing their babies to others and about child care than did the mothers of children with no birth defects. The two groups were similar on locus of control or the extent to which they felt that their lives were controlled by fate, destiny, or outside forces (external locus of control) or by self-determination (internal locus of control).

The children with clefts, on the other hand, thought that their births had caused more negative feelings and greater worry for their parents than did the unimpaired subjects. However, they did not translate these perceived negative parental feelings into lack of caring.

The subjects with clefts, not unexpectedly, felt more external controls in their lives than did the normal subjects, and they more often relied on the context in which events occurred than they did on their own internal cues in relationship to context. The controls were described as more "field-independent" in that the context of events was mediated by personal feelings. This is an important finding, since families who encourage their children to mature and become independent seem to have children who are "field-independ-

ent." In view of this, it is not surprising that the teachers in this study rated the subjects with clefts as having more academic problems than the controls. Brantley and Clifford concluded with the admonition that it may be wise:

. . . to intensify efforts to engage and involve them (parents and children) as active collaborators in the treatment and decision-making process in management rather than to allow them to feel that the experience is beyond their control.

SUMMARY

Much has been written in the past about the parents of children with various types of clefts, but the picture remains cloudy largely because of limitations in research design and because methodologies for exploring "feelings" and "attitudes" are inadequate. In spite of these shortcomings, the research indicates, overall, that parents are distressed about their children's birth defects but that most come to terms with the situation and do about as well as parents in general. McWilliams (1973) wrote that:

. . . facial disfigurement becomes a condition of stress with which they (parents) deal as effectively or ineffectively as they handle stress in general. . . Perhaps studies of child rearing practices, parent-child interaction, and child-sibling relationships viewed from a behavioral stance would help to answer today's questions, which are not basically different from those posed 10 years ago.

That holds true today, and little has happened to assess the parent in a behavioral sense. However, the evidence is overwhelming that no general description of parents of children with clefts should be drawn and acted upon in individual cases. Parents are undoubtedly weary of the vast and costly efforts to characterize them as a group when, individually, they are capable of discussing matters of concern and are in need of treatment and counseling that recognizes their uniqueness, their special requirements, and, often, their great reservoirs of personal integrity and strength.

Counseling should be available during times of crisis—and these are bound to occur—and should be an ongoing part of the child's treatment. Obviously, not all parental needs can be met in the period immediately following the child's birth. In that important period, however, the groundwork for the future will be laid. Speech pathologists will find that recognizing the need for counseling, understanding the nature of parental concerns, and developing the ability to provide appropriate help, either personally or through referral, will significantly influence the outcome for children with clefts.

REFERENCES

Adler J. Every parent's nightmare, Newsweek, March 16, 1987:57.

American Cleft Palate Educational Foundation. Considerations in establishing a group for parents of children with cleft palate. Pittsburgh, 1978.

Arbeitel B. The effectiveness of genetic counseling at the University of Pittsburgh Cleft Palate Center, Master's Thesis, University of Pittsburgh, 1985.

Bradley D. A study of parental counseling regarding cleft palate problems. Cleft Palate Bull 1960; 10, 71.

Brantley H, Clifford E. Maternal and child locus of control and field-dependence in cleft palate children. Cleft Palate J 1979; 16:183.

Burger GK, Armentrout JA. A comparative study of methods to estimate factor scores for report of parental behavior. Procedures of the 79th Annual Convention of American Psychology Association 1971; 6:149.

Clifford E. The impact of symptom on the child: comparative studies of clinical populations. J School Health 1968; 38:342.

Clifford E. Parental ratings of cleft palate infants. Cleft Palate J 1969; 6:235.

Clifford E. Cleft palate and the person: psychologic studies of its impact. J South Med Assoc 1971; 64:1516.

Clifford E, Crocker E. Maternal responses: the birth of a normal child as compared to the birth of a child with cleft palate. Cleft Palate J 1971; 8:298.

Dar H, Winter ST, Tol Y. Families of children with cleft lips and palates: concerns and counseling. Develop Med Child Neurol 1974; 16:513.

Fogh-Anderson P. Inheritance of cleft lip and cleft palate. Copenhagen: Nyt Nordisk Forlag-Arnold Busck, 1942.

Fraser FC. Etiology of cleft lip and palate. In: Grabb WC, Rosenstein SW, Bzoch KR, eds. Cleft lip and palate: Boston: Little, Brown, 1971:54.

Fraser GR, Calnan JS. Cleft lip and palate: seasonal incidence, birth weight, birth rank, sex, site, associated malformations and paternal age. a statistical survey. Arch Dis Child 1961; 36:420.

Goodstein LD. MMPI differences between parents of children with cleft palate and parents of physically normal children. J Speech Hear Res 1960a; 3:31.

Goodstein LD. Personality test differences in parents of children with cleft palates. J Speech Hear Res 1960b; 3:39.

Green M, Durocher MA. Improving parent care of handicapped children. Children 1965; 12:185.

Green JC, Vermillion JR, Hay S. Utilization of birth certificates in epidemiologic studies of cleft lip and palate. Cleft Palate J 1965; 2:141.

Hathaway S, McKinley J. Minnesota multiphasic personality inventory. New York: The Psychological Corporation 1942; Rev Ed, 1951.

Hay S. Incidence of clefts and parental age. Cleft Palate J 1967; 4:205.

Hill MJ. An investigation of the attitudes and information possessed by parents of children with clefts of the lip and palate. Cleft Palate Bull 1956; 6:3.

Irwin E, McWilliams BJ. Parents working with parents: the cleft palate program. Cleft Palate J 1973; 10:360.

Jones MC. Etiology of facial clefts: prospective evaluation of 428 patients. Cleft Palate J 1988; 25:16.

Loretz W, Westmoreland WW, Richards LF. A study of cleft lip and cleft palate births in California. Am J Pub Health 1961; 31:873.

MacMahon B, McKeown T. The incidence of harelip and cleft palate related to birth rank and maternal age. Am J Hum Genet 1953; 5:176.

McWilliams BJ. Psychosocial development and modification. ASHA Reports No. 5, 1970:165.

McWilliams BJ, Matthews H. A comparison of intelligence and social maturity in children with unilateral complete clefts and those with isolated cleft palates. Cleft Palate J 1979; 16:363.

McWilliams BJ, Smith RM. Psychological considerations. ASHA Reports No. 9, 1973:43.

Middleton G, Lass N, Starr P, Pannbacker M. Survey of public awareness and knowledge of cleft palate. Cleft Palate J 1986; 23:58.

Norval M, Larson T, Parshall P. The impact of the cleft lip and palate child on the family: a preliminary survey. State of Minnesota: Crippled Children Services, 1964.

Pannbacker M. Congenital malformations and cleft lip and palate. Cleft Palate J 1968; 5:334.

Richman L, Harper D. Observable stigmata and perceived maternal behavior. Cleft Palate J 1978; 15:215.

Rollnick BR, Pruzansky S. Genetic services at a center for craniofacial anomalies. Cleft Palate J 1981; 18:304.

Rotter JB. Some implications of a social learning theory for the prediction of goal directed behavior from testing procedures. Psych Rev 1960; 67:301.

Rotter JB. Generalized expectancies for internal versus external control of reinforcement. Psych Monogr 1966; 80:1.

Salazar A. Intrauterine repair of a lesion resembling cleft lip and its effect on maternal behavior in rats. Cleft Palate J 1988; 25:38.

Schaefer ES. Childrens' report of parental behavior: an inventory. Child Develop 1965; 36:413.

Shprintzen RJ, Siegel-Sadewitz VL, Amato J, Goldberg RB. Anomalies associated with cleft lip, cleft palate, or both. Am J Med Genet 1985; 20:585.

Slutsky H. Maternal reaction and adjustment to birth and care of the cleft palate child. Cleft Palate J 1969; 6:425.

Solnit AJ, Stark MH. Mourning and the birth of a defective child. Psychoanal study of the child 1961; 16:523.

Spriestersbach DC. Evaluation of a technique for investigating the psychosocial aspects of the "cleft palate problem." In: Pruzansky S, ed. Congenital anomalies of the face and associated structures. Springfield, IL: CC Thomas, 1961:345.

Spriestersbach DC. Psychosocial aspects of the cleft palate problem. Vol. 1. Iowa City: University of Iowa Press, 1973.

Spriestersbach DC, Spriestersbach BR, Moll KL. Incidence of clefts of the lip and palate in families with children with clefts and families with children without clefts. Plast Reconstr Surg 1962; 29:392.

Strauss R. Culture, rehabilitation, and facial birth defects: international case studies. Cleft Palate J 1985; 22:56.

Tisza V, Gumpertz E. The parents' reaction to the birth and early case of children with cleft palates. Pediatrics 1962; 30:86.

Tobiason JM. Psychosocial correlates of congenital facial clefts: a conceptualization and model. Cleft Palate J 1984; 21:131.

Walesky-Rainbow PA, Morris H. An assessment of informative-counseling procedures for cleft palate children. Cleft Palate J 1978; 15:20.

Weachter EH. Concerns of parents related to the birth of a child with a cleft of the lip and palate with implications for nurses. Master's Thesis, University of Chicago, 1959.

Witkin HA, Dyk RB, Faterson HF, Goodenough DR, Karp SS. Psychological differentiation: studies of development. New York: Wiley, 1962.

Witkin HA, Lewis HC, Hertz M, Machover K, Meissner PB, Wapner S. Personality through perception: an experimental and clinical study. New York: Harper, 1954.

Woolf CM. Paternal age effect for cleft lip and palate. Am J Hum Genet 1963; 15:389.

11 | INSTRUMENTATION FOR ASSESSING THE VELOPHARYNGEAL MECHANISM

Use of instruments is essential in the evaluation of velopharyngeal function and of treatments addressed to that function. Many advancements in speech pathology have rested on new instrumentation. Instruments for assessing velopharyngeal valving and selected related variables are described here because of their importance to research and clinical practices considered later in the book. Relationships among measures obtained with different instruments are also considered. Emphasis is placed on radiographic, aeromechanical, and endoscopic devices. Historical perspective is provided in a review by Hirschberg (1986).

RADIOGRAPHY

Radiography permits the imaging of internal body parts. The roentgen ray (x-ray) is projected through the body directly to film which it exposes or to a fluoroscopic screen. The screen converts photons to light which may be photographed or videorecorded. There are a number of different radiographic methods from which the researcher or clinician may choose. Certain procedural and measurement problems are shared among them, whereas others are unique to a particular technique. Scheier reported radiographic studies of speech in 1909, and over the years radiography has contributed much to understanding of the function of the speech mechanism—especially the

velopharyngeal valve. It continues to be used in diagnosis and treatment planning.

GENERAL BACKGROUND

Regardless of whether static or motion radiographic techniques are selected, ionizing radiation is used. The radiation dosage differs from one technique to another, but radiation is always potentially hazardous. Kuehn and Dalston (1988) stated that a typical multiview work-up requires from 1.5 to 3 rad. To reduce radiation hazard, exposure time is kept to the minimum required to obtain needed information, lead shielding is used, and the roentgen ray beam is filtered and coned down to the target area. Isberg et al. (1989) stated that use of a head fixation device permits the radiologist to cone the field of exposure, thus protecting eyes and thyroid gland while permitting study of the velopharyngeal mechanism. They described speech study sequences as requiring 5 seconds for coning the field, 3 seconds for setting of the automatic exposure control, and 40 seconds for recording speech. This was repeated for additional views. They found that videofluoroscopy required only one-tenth the radiation of cinefluorography. Pulsing of the radiation beam in synchrony with film frame exposure during cinefluorography reduces the radiation required for use of that technique. Lead shields should be worn by the patient, the radiologist, and the participating speech pathologist during the examination. Radiation exposure is reduced as equipment is improved and well maintained. Stringer and Witzel (1989) described the minimization of radiation risk to patient and clinicians through "...the use of new remote imaging systems with overtable x-ray tubes and rare earth filtration (e.g., ytterbium)..." Staff exposure must be monitored closely by radiation experts, and equipment must be checked for safe function. Landa (1967) suggested the establishment of a radiation exposure registry to record for each patient the nature of each study performed, the dosage, and the place and date of the examination.

Speech pathologists and others in need of information about velopharyngeal valving can derive much information from radiographic study. However, this tool should only be used to answer important clinical questions that are not answered by other procedures. Fletcher et al. (1960) noted that as new information about a disability is accumulated, the need for radiography declines. Knowledge of strong correlations between radiographic data and other measures should decrease the frequency with which fluoroscopy is needed in the evaluation of patients with clefts. The use of radiographic procedures in research is closely monitored by institutional committees concerned with the rights and well-being of human subjects.

CEPHALOMETRICS

Orthodontists and specialists in facial growth developed cephalometrics as a radiographic procedure for measurement of craniofacial bones and soft tissue. In lateral or sagittal views, still radiographs are taken with the patient stabilized in a headholder; the head is secured by earposts relative to a landmark called the Frankfort horizontal line, which runs from the inferior margin of the left ocular orbit through the superior margin of the left external auditory meatus (Keller, 1987). The patient's midline is positioned at a constant distance from the x-ray source (Subtelny et al., 1957; Bateman and Mason, 1984). The use of a constant source-to-patient midline distance permits the measurement of change in structure over time. Without the constant distance, measures would be confounded by enlargement associated

A

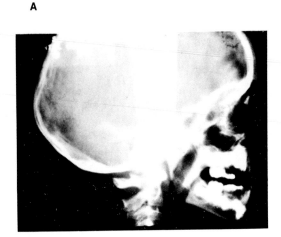

B

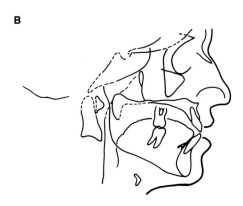

C

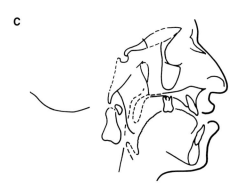

Figure 11.1 *A.* shows a cephalometric radiograph; *B.* is a tracing of a cephalometric film taken during normal /s/ production, and *C.* shows a tracing of a cephalometric film taken during production of /s/ associated with a velopharyngeal opening and tongue protrusion. (From McWilliams BJ. Cleft palate. In: Shames GH, Wiig EH, eds. Human communication disorders. Columbus: CE Merrill, 1982.)

with change in the subject-radiation source relationship. Use of the constant relationship permits the superimposition of radiographs (or the comparison of measurements) from one examination to another for the purpose of identifying change.

The interpretation of radiographs involves meticulous tracing of the structures and measurement of the distances and angles between landmarks. This tracing is time-consuming and requires special training, along with the development of tracer reliability. However, all orthodontists have the ability to do these evaluations as do some speech pathologists. Although computer technology is now available for certain kinds of assessments, tracing is still commonly used.

Studies such as that of Hixon (1949) adapted orthodontic cephalometric techniques to real-size measurements of the velopharyngeal structures and their spatial relationships. Figure 11.1 shows a cephalometric radiograph and two tracings, one taken during the production of a normal /s/ and the other during a defective /s/. It should be understood that a radiograph provides an image that is a summation of the tissue through which the x-ray beam has passed. If a person had palatal closure on one side but not on the other, the midsagittal view would show velopharyngeal closure, because the beam would pass through the tissue on the closed side, and the resulting image might not yield information about the opening. The velopharyngeal valve is three-dimensional, and its attributes cannot all be captured in the midsagittal view alone. This limitation is discussed in the next section of this chapter. Another problem with still cephalometric films is that they capture only a moment in speech production. Connected discourse cannot be studied by this means, nor is it possible to specify precisely what event will be filmed in the course of production of a single sound. We shall discuss this matter further in Chapter 19.

CINE- AND VIDEOFLUOROSCOPY

The use of cinefluoroscopy (radiographs recorded on motion picture film) in the study of speech of patients with cleft palate was introduced at the Lancaster Cleft Palate Clinic in the 1950s. Use of videofluoroscopy (radiographic images recorded on videotape) in the study of patients with clefts was reported by McWilliams and Girdany (1964). Videorecording had the advantage of instant playback; and avoided the delay previously required to process and develop film. Also, radiation exposure was reduced with use of videorecording. Figure 11.2 shows a person in position for midsagittal cine- or videofluorography and the equipment used.

When motion techniques for speech study first became available, only midsagittal and occasionally frontal studies were done. The midsagittal view provides information about movement of the velum and posterior pharyngeal wall and about height of the velum and velar relationship to adenoids and posterior pharyngeal wall, but it doesn't provide information about the velum off midline nor about movement of the lateral pharyngeal walls. Frontal films or recordings provide information about movement of the lateral pharyngeal walls but do not show clearly their relationship to the velum. The two views supplement each other but leave unanswered the question of whether a velopharyngeal opening during speech exists, and if so where it is in the vertical plane.

In order to extract more information from videofluoroscopy, Skolnick (1970) introduced

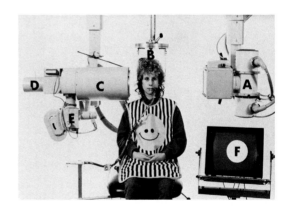

Figure 11.2 The radiographic equipment. *A*. X-ray tube; *B*. cephalostat; *C*. image intensifier; *D*. Vidicon camera; *E*. cinecamera; *F*. TV-monitor. (From Isberg A, Julin P, Kraepelien T, Henrikson CO. Absorbed doses and energy imparted from radiographic examination of velopharyngeal function during speech. Cleft Palate J 1989; 26:106.)

multiview videofluoroscopy, a technique that adds a base view to the traditional lateral and frontal projections. This series of three views provides a more complete picture of the velopharyngeal valve. For base-view videofluoroscopy, the patient is placed in a sphinx-like position, with the neck extended as shown in Figure 11.3. In this way, the x-ray beam can be directed upward, from under the chin through the velopharyngeal portal. Figure 11.4 shows the radiographic positioning required for all three views. These views are usually obtained sequentially.

Skolnick (1975) wrote that the multiview system allows the clinician to estimate the location of the base view within the vocal tract. This is done by putting together information from all three views. The frontal view shows the vertical location of major pharyngeal wall movement; the midsagittal view shows the soft palate and the posterior pharyngeal wall relative to each other; and the base view shows all of these except vertical location. What is observed on the base view must be consistent with what is seen on the other views. For example, the study is improperly done if the lateral view shows closure but the base view shows a large midline opening or vice versa. It is possible, however, to see a small central opening on base view—or a unilateral opening—that could not be seen on lateral projection. The three views com-

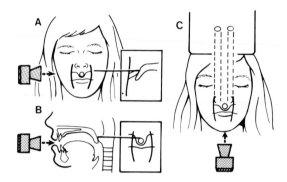

Figure 11.4 Radiographic positioning of a patient for (a) lateral, (b) frontal, and (c) base views of velopharyngeal portal. (From Skolnick ML, McCall GN. Velopharyngeal competence and incompetence following pharyngeal flap surgery: videofluoroscopic study in multiple projections. Cleft Palate J 1972; 9:1.)

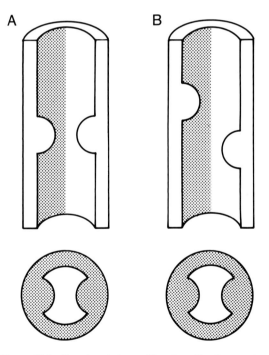

Figure 11.5 Drawing *A* shows ridges intruding into a tube at two different levels; drawing *B* shows comparable ridges intruding at the same level. The relationships in *A* and *B* would be indistinguishable in base view. (After a suggestion by Skolnick.)

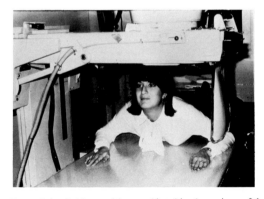

Figure 11.3 Sphinx position used in taking base views of the velopharyngeal valve. (From McWilliams BJ. Communication problems associated with cleft palate. In: Van Hattum RJ, ed. Communication disorders. New York: Macmillan, 1980.)

plement each other, and are interpreted together. Kuehn and Dolan (1975) and Schwartz (1975) questioned the accuracy of the base view. Skolnick (1982), however, reiterated his position that the vertical location of the sphincter visualized in base view can be satisfactorily estimated by comparing the cross-sectional dimensions with those measured from frontal and sagittal views. He noted that, in base views, bulges into the vocal tract that occur at two different levels will appear to be located at the same level (Fig. 11.5). However, reference to sagittal and frontal views will protect against erroneous interpretations.

Other views of the velopharyngeal valve have been devised and recommended for clinical use as alternatives to the base view. Zwitman et al. (1973, p. 474) studied a submentovertical projection in which the upright patient is turned to face the image amplifier. "...he is asked to step forward and to tilt his head back until it rests against the upright x-ray table." The patient is then standing with the neck extended and the face directed to the ceiling. Stringer and Witzel (1986, 1989) described the Towne view in which the radiographic beam is perpendicular to the velopharyngeal sphincter, thus resembling the base view. In the Towne view, the patient lies supine on the x-ray table with the head, neck, and shoulders flexed upward from the table and supported by a wedge. This permits recording of the velopharyngeal sphincter. The authors noted that in the Towne view, the main radiographic beam is not directed to the thyroid gland and that the eyes can be protected by careful coning of the beam. As shown in Figure 11.6, with some equipment it is possible to obtain Towne views by adjusting equipment to the patient rather than the reverse. That is, the patient can be studied in an upright posture, thus avoiding the narrowing of the velopharyngeal port that is associated with cervical flexion.

Stringer and Witzel (1985) described the Waters projection as an alternative to the frontal view for study of the lateral pharyngeal walls. The patient faces the camera with the head and neck extended. This posture displaces bony structures that would otherwise make it difficult to visualize the lateral walls. The authors report that the Waters projection permits visualization of the lateral walls in a fashion equal or superior to that associated with the frontal view. The authors note

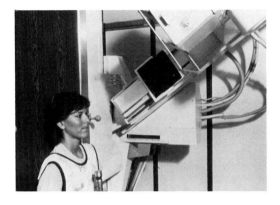

Figure 11.6 Patient in the upright position for the Towne view with overtable x-ray equipment. (From Stringer DA, Witzel MA. Comparison of multi-view videofluoroscopy and nasopharyngoscopy in the assessment of velopharyngeal insufficiency. Cleft Palate J 1989; 26:91.)

that head extension may unmask marginal velopharyngeal disfunction.

Rotation of the cineradiographic camera around the patient provides a three-dimensional image of the velopharyngeal mechanism (Massengill, 1966). A similar effect can be achieved by rotating the patient as he or she is positioned relative to a standard cineradiographic unit (Skolnick, 1982).

Procedural Issues in the Use of Cine- and Videofluoroscopy

In cephalometrics, an important aspect of the procedure is the use of a headholder. The need for careful head stabilization in a known position carries over into cine- and videofluoroscopy. Early lateral studies routinely used some type of cephalostat. The use of such devices is still common, but it is certainly not universal. Since it is not, there is no real assurance that evaluations are of consistent quality from one institution to another. In addition, there may not be consistency in the obtained views. Cephalometrics, standardized as they are, speak a common language to all who use them, and measurements derived in one situation are comparable with those generated in another.

Additional thought should be given to this issue as it affects the standardization of motion radiography.

Videotapes do not have the quality problems that occur with film, but cinefluoroscopy, especially when it was first used for speech research, did have variations caused by the nature of the film selected for use. Moll (1960) discussed film types and equipment settings necessary to assure the greatest contrast and resolution.

Moll and others have also considered methods of outlining soft tissues that otherwise may be difficult to see on radiographs. Metal chains were once used to mark the midline of the tongue; metal markers are now sometimes glued to the tongue, velum, and pharyngeal walls so that they will show up clearly on the radiograph, whereas the soft tissue alone would not. The Skolnick system requires instillation of a radiopaque material that clearly outlines the structures of interest. Care must be taken, because instilling too much of the liquid may obscure rather than clarify. Placing a marker of known size in the subject's midline is a technique that has been used often, particularly in research. This marker permits the projection of the image at life size or the correction of measurements to life size.

Measurement Techniques

Clinical descriptions and ratings of motion x-ray images provide the information needed to answer certain specific questions. However, for many research and some clinical purposes, frame-by-frame measurement is necessary (Moll, 1964). Frame-by-frame analysis has been highly productive in studies of the speech of both normal and pathologic subjects. Frame-by-frame tracings and measurement of different structures combined with use of a sound track to identify acoustical phenomena allows identification of movement relationships among different speech organs and specification of the timing relationships among structures and contexts.

Frame-by-frame measurement requires a stop-frame projector and a tracing device. Moll (1960) demonstrated that measurements made from the projected image or from tracings of the image are usually highly reliable. Mean discrepancies between repeated measurements are small. Moll measured the distance between the velum and the posterior pharyngeal wall, the distance from tongue to alveolus, the size of the incisal opening, and the extent of contact between the velum and the posterior pharyngeal wall. The later measurement was less reliable than the others.

For many purposes, the standard camera film frame advancement rate of 24 frames per second is satisfactory. However, articulatory movements can occur between frames exposed at that speed. Bjork (1961) found the velum to move as much as 3 mm between frames at 50 frames per second. For research purposes, camera frame advancement rates as high as 150 frames per second have been used. Video recordings of the radiographic image are usually made at a speed equivalent to a film speed of 30 frames per second (Shelton and Trier, 1976). Videofluoroscopic tapes do not lend themselves readily to frame-by-frame measurement unless they are first converted to film and then traced or some other special procedure is used such as stopping the tape, a procedure that may or may not provide images of sufficient quality for measurement purposes. When the tapes are transferred to film, there is sometimes a loss of quality (McWilliams and Girdany, 1964; and McWilliams-Neely and Bradley, 1964). Glaser (1980) took 35-mm photographs of selected images from the television screen, enlarged them to 8×10 prints, and then traced the structures of interest. For some purposes, this method is effective and reliable.

McWilliams-Neely and Bradley (1964) prepared psychophysical rating scales to establish standard procedures for the analysis of videofluorographic images. Variables to be rated included approximation or contact between the velum and the posterior pharyngeal wall, thickness of the soft palate, length of the soft palate, extent of vertical contact between velum and posterior pharyngeal wall, location of velopharyngeal closure relative to the anteriormost projection of the tubercle of the first cervical vertebra, and location of closure relative to the hard palate. Timing factors were later added. Ratings made by two observers of 16 subjects were analyzed in terms of the percentages of agreement between the two ratings and in terms of Pearson correlations between the pairs of ratings. Most of the correlations were in the 0.70s and 0.80s, and the percentages of agreement ranged from 38 to 81 with a mean of 65. Only five of 288 paired observations

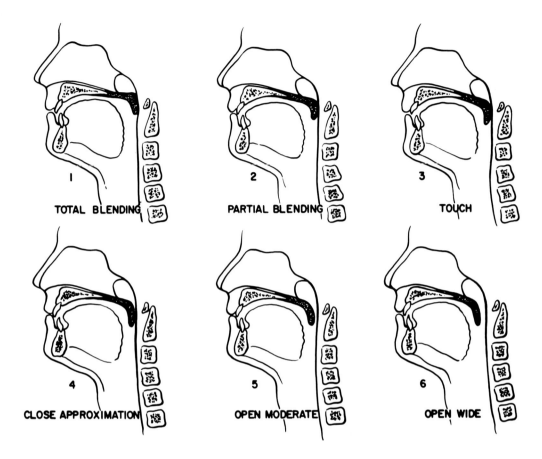

Figure 11.7   Six different relationships between the soft palate and the posterior pharyngeal wall. (From McWilliams BJ, Bradley DP. Ratings of velopharyngeal closure during blowing and speech. Cleft Palate J 1965; 2:46.)

differed by more than one scale value. The authors noted that rating scales provide consistency in reporting and that the ratings take much less time to perform than do other methods. They stressed that those doing the ratings must be trained for the task. Such training would be facilitated by demonstration tapes serving as standards against which to compare ratings made by clinicians in training.

McWilliams and Bradley (1965) illustrated the rating scale for velopharyngeal closure and used it later in a study that compared connected speech, blowing with the nares open, and blowing with the nares closed. Figure 11.7 shows the ratings used. Reliability coefficients for repeated ratings of three performances by 37 cleft palate patients ranged from 0.84 to 0.96, indicating that high levels of agreement can be developed using this system. Their procedure was later adapted for use in evaluating still radiographs by Van Demark et al. (1975).

Lewis and Pashayan (1980) illustrated a scale for use in rating medial movement of the lateral pharyngeal walls in frontal motion radiographic views (Fig. 11.8).

TOMOGRAPHY

Tomography permits the filming of body sections that are off midline. It can be used to obtain frontal views of the velum and lateral

FRONTAL

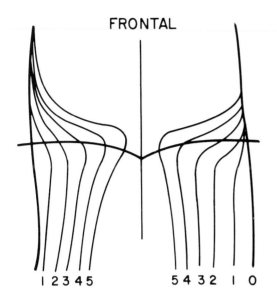

| 2 3 4 5   5 4 3 2 | 0

Figure 11.8 Diagrammatic scheme for the grading of lateral pharyngeal wall motion as seen on frontal view. (From Lewis MB, Pashayan HM. The effects of pharyngeal flap surgery on lateral pharyngeal wall motion: a video radiographic evaluation. Cleft Palate J 1980; 17:302.)

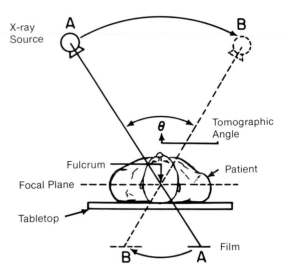

Figure 11.9 An example of a tomographic system. (From Kuehn D, Dolan K. A tomographic technique of assessing lateral pharyngeal wall displacement. Cleft Palate J 1975; 12:200.)

pharyngeal walls (Kuehn and Dolan, 1975; Iglesias et al., 1980). As shown in Figure 11.9, the x-ray source and the film are displaced in opposite directions and in an orientation perpendicular to the desired focal plane as the film is exposed. As a result, the images of structures above and below the focal plane are blurred, but the images at the focal plane are well delineated on the film. Kuehn and Dolan reported that simultaneous exposure of anterior-posterior tomograms and sagittal radiographs allowed them to identify the location of the lateral pharyngeal walls relative to the anterior-posterior relationship between the velum and the posterior pharyngeal wall.

Dickson and Maue-Dickson (1980) presented different types of midsagittal tomograms of an adult cadaver head. They anticipated research into normal and abnormal velopharyngeal structures utilizing computerized tomography. Weiss and Blackley (1981) described a computerized tomographic (CT) body scanner in the study of the velopharyngeal mechanism. This device employs a rotating x-ray beam and computer processing of the exit beam as collected in a series of scintillation counters. The image is displayed on a cathode-ray tube, and the operator has some ability to highlight portions of the image. Images are in the axial plane, which is comparable to the base view described in connection with cine- and videofluoroscopy. X-ray dosage was reported as 2 to 4 roentgens per examination.

In a demonstration project, Moon and Smith (1987) described and illustrated (Figs. 11.10, 11.11) use of cine computed tomography to obtain serial sections at different levels of the velopharyngeal region. The sections were taken at 650-millisecond intervals (more than 2 frames per second). This is too slow for definitive study of speech movements, so the method is more useful for the study of structure than of movement. However, as the authors indicated this instrument is capable of displaying the velopharyngeal mechanism in three dimensions. Future development of this instrument may make higher speeds available.

Computed tomographic (CT) imaging is being used in many creative ways, one of which is to plan craniofacial surgery. Cutting et al. (1986) described an application that utilized cephalometric data from the patient and from tables of norms plus patient CT data. The surgeon was able to interact with the computer in such a fashion as to

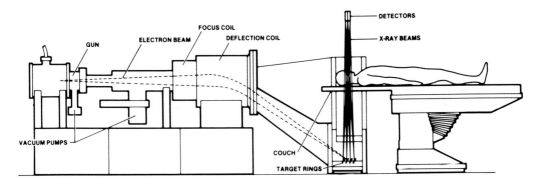

Figure 11.10 Cine computed tomography (Imatron) system. (From Moon JB, Smith WL. Application of cine computed tomography to the assessment of velopharyngeal form and function. Cleft Palate J 1987; 24:228.)

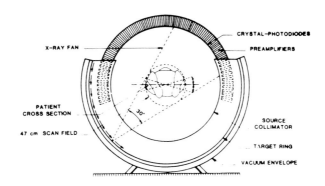

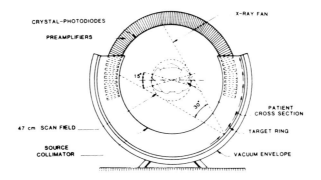

Figure 11.11 Orientation of electron beam in cine computed tomography system. (From Moon JB, Smith WL. Application of cine computed tomography to the assessment of velopharyngeal form and function. Cleft Palate J 1987; 24:228.)

simulate the operation being planned. This application of computed tomography is new and as such subject to discussion and debate. CT scans were used in the evaluation of the effects on the pharyngeal skeleton of early closure of the soft palate (Oesch et al., 1987). Lowe et al. (1986) used three-dimensional CT to reconstruct tongue volume and airway in the evaluation of persons with obstructive sleep apnea. A group of investigators at the University of Pittsburgh has used three-dimensional computer graphics in anatomical research. For example, they reconstructed histological preparations of the nasal capsules of normal and cleft palate fetal specimens (Kimes et al., 1988). This capsule is located above the palatal plane, which extends from the anterior to the posterior nasal spines. In this application of computer imaging, photomicrographs were used. The nasal capsules of the cleft specimens were deficient relative to the comparison specimens. For example, capsule volume was small and septum volume large. Mean airway volume was small.

X-RAY MICROBEAM

A recent development in radiologic instrumentation is the microbeam, which uses computer-generated pulses to track lead pellets attached to articulators. Two-dimensional plots over time may be related to acoustical information. Descriptions of this instrument and its use were provided recently by Kuehn and Dalston (1988) and Hardcastle et al. (1989). Since the radiation level is low, this instrument seems appropriate for certain types of speech research, including studies of velopharyngeal function. Microbeam facilities are located at the University of Tokyo and the University of Wisconsin-Madison. The Wisconsin installation constitutes a national shared laboratory. Investigators from other institutions may make application for use of this facility (ASHA Research Bulletin July 1, 1988, page 4).

ULTRASOUND

Ultrasound is another device that has been employed in the evaluation of velopharyngeal function, or at least of movements of the lateral pharyngeal walls. It is not suitable for displaying motions of the velum because of problems in transmitting ultrasound through bone overlying the palate (Hawkins and Swisher, 1978). Parush and Ostry (1986) interpreted their ultrasound observations of the lateral pharyngeal walls relative to the literature regarding velar movement because they could not study the latter by means of ultrasound.

Theory, instrumentation, and technique for the use of ultrasound in speech-related research were described by Kelsey et al. (1969). So far as we know, ultrasound equipment is free of hazard to either patient or operator. Shawker et al. (1984) imply safety when they state that ultrasound may be used for biofeedback of information about tongue position in articulation therapy. However, Keller (1987) keeps the amplitude of the emitting crystal at a minimal level and directs the beam only to muscular tissue.

In studies of the lateral pharyngeal walls, a transducer placed on the patient's neck pulses an ultrasound beam toward the pharyngeal wall, and the beam is deflected back to the transducer when it reaches the interface between the mucosa of the pharyngeal wall and the air in the pharynx (Skolnick et al., 1975). The signal is monitored on an oscilloscope. The position of the probe is changed until a satisfactory signal is seen and its identity determined by having the subject speak and swallow as the signal is monitored. A dot on the screen of the oscilloscope reflects motion in the pharyngeal wall contacted by the ultrasound pulses. With suitable equipment, the motion of the wall can be displayed, videorecorded, photographed, and measured. Kelsey et al. (1969) noted that the time and motion method of displaying ultrasound data shows the distance between the transducer and the pharyngeal wall. Consequently, any movement of the neck wall against which the transducer is placed, as well as motion of the lateral pharyngeal wall, will be reflected in the measurement obtained. Minifie et al. (1970) calibrated ultrasound equipment for depth of measurement by moving a submerged transducer in 1-cm steps away from the bottom of a water-filled container. Time calibration was determined from the time base of the oscilloscope.

Early applications of ultrasound used a single transducer and recorded the motion of only a single point on one lateral pharyngeal wall. Later, multitransducer equipment was built that permits visualization of the vertical length of the lateral pharyngeal wall from nasal to oral pharynx (Skolnick et al., 1975) (Fig. 11.12). Two sets of equipment are required if both lateral walls are to be measured simultaneously.

Another development is the computerization of ultrasound. Microelectronics and computers can be used in conjunction with ultrasound to achieve information of higher quality. Although not directly related to the assessment of velopharyngeal closure, the work of Ewanowski et al. (1981) is of interest. They applied ultrasound technology to the study of tongue function in the production of glottal stops and pharyngeal fricatives. Their equipment involved pulsed echo ultrasound and employed a rotor-driven scanner with three transducers. The image was videorecorded. The scanner was placed under the mandible and could be positioned to display either the midsagittal surface of the tongue by longitudinal scan or the groove of the tongue by lateral scan. The authors made a number of points relative to their use of ultrasound in the study of tongue function in articulation. They obtained reliable data; the displays differentiated among tongue postures for different vowels, and they were able to describe

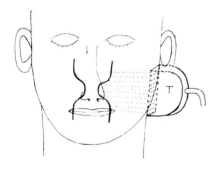

Figure 11.12 Schematic drawing illustrating multi-element transducer placement along left side of neck oriented perpendicular to lateral pharyngeal walls. Dotted lines indicate paths of ultrasound beams between the multiple elements of transducer and the lateral pharyngeal walls. (From Skolnick ML, Zagzebski JA, Watkin KL. Two-dimensional ultrasonic demonstration of lateral phryngeal wall movement in real time—a preliminary report. Cleft Palate J 1975; 17: 299–303.)

tongue posture during glottal stops and pharyngeal fricatives. Generally, the longitudinal scans gave better information than the lateral scans. The latter provided information about tongue groove, but these displays were impaired by air located beneath the tongue's lateral margins. In the longitudinal scans, the tongue tip was difficult to visualize because of the air space between the floor of the mouth and the underside of the tongue. The researchers noted that ultrasonic equipment of the sort they employed is available in many medical settings. They stated that it should be possible to visualize two or more structures simultaneously.

Shawker et al. (1984) wrote that after an initial flurry of interest by speech investigators, use of ultrasound in speech research declined. They reported that equipment has improved and that real-time scanners are in use. They anticipate future advancement in the use of this instrument for studies of speech and deglutition. However, their discussion focused on the tongue. The authors noted that palate and teeth aren't visible in ultrasonic studies; consequently, the tongue can't be studied relative to them. Keller (1987) described use of a computerized ultrasound system for differentiation of tongue motion in patients with various types of nonstructural speech impairment. The ultrasonic transducer was placed in a vertical posture under the mandible–initially at a 90-degree angle to the Frankfurt horizontal line. The syllable /ka/ was studied in different contexts and at different rates. Syllables with more anterior consonants could not be recorded because of an air pocket beneath the tongue.

Although ultrasound is apparently not being used to study the velopharyngeal mechanism, it is being used to identify birth defects in fetuses. Strauss and Davis (1989) stated that images of lip and nares can be obtained in over 50% of diagnostic ultrasound studies of unborn fetuses. They addressed the ethics of surgery for unborn fetuses.

ENDOSCOPY

Endoscopes are optical instruments consisting of viewing lens, shaft or body, and an eye piece that can be attached to a camera. They require a light source and proper grounding. Both rigid and flexible endoscopes are in use. Endoscopes can be passed through body openings and pathways to reach internal organs that cannot otherwise be directly visualized. These instruments have wide application in medicine and are especially useful in viewing the velopharyngeal valve and the larynx. Endoscopic examination of the velopharyngeal port provides a view similar to the base view obtained in motion fluorographic studies. The endoscope permits observation of the velum and pharyngeal walls as they move in relationship to one another. The examiner may visualize, photograph, or record structures in the field of view.

In 1966, Taub introduced a rigid endoscope, which he called the "panendoscope", to study the velopharyngeal mechanism. This scope, too large for passage through the nasal cavities, was introduced through the mouth. It included a light bulb at the side of the lens, a feature that created troublesome heat and electrical hazard in the patient's mouth. This instrument, even though it was cumbersome and interfered somewhat with speech production, represented a breakthrough in assessment of velopharyngeal function. Later rigid endoscopes utilized fiberoptic bundles to transmit light from a remote source to target structures; the scopes themselves resemble telescopes and have excellent optics and fields of view (Shprintzen, 1989). With the fiberoptic feature, no heat is introduced into the patient's mouth. The diameter of rigid scopes now in use is considerably smaller than that of the panendoscope, and some can be inserted transnasally.

An examiner inspecting an open port through an oral endoscope will see the posterior segment of the nasal septum at the top of the image. The lateral and posterior pharyngeal walls will appear at the middle and bottom of the image respectively. When the velum is elevated, it will occupy the top portion of the image, and the posterior segments of the lateral walls and the posterior wall will appear below it. When the portion of the velopharyngeal port nearest the lens is almost closed, it is not possible to tell whether closure occurs at a higher level that is out of view. This problem may also exist when the examiner looks down on the velopharyngeal port through a nasally placed scope, since only the superior surface of the valve can be seen. Figure 11.13 shows several views of the mechanism ob-

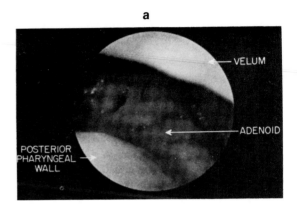

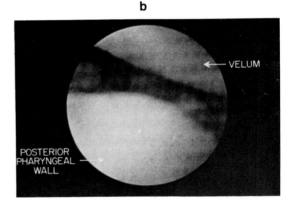

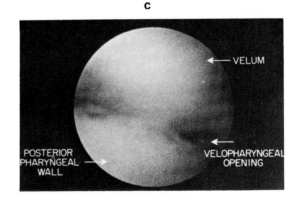

Figure 11.13 Oral videoendoscopic photographs: *A.* subject at rest; *B.* during blowing; *C.* during /pa/. The bulge on the posterior wall of the pharynx, particularly evident in *B*, is presumed to reflect a vertebral defect. (From Shelton RL, Beaumont K, Trier WC, Furr ML. Videoendoscopic feedback in training velopharyngeal closure. Cleft Palate J 1978; 15:6.)

tained with an oral endoscope. With nasendoscopy, the velum is at the bottom of the picture.

Various problems arise when oral endoscopy is used for the study of velopharyngeal valving. Placement of the scope in the mouth restricts speech to bilabial stops and fricatives combined with low vowels and sequenced with varied prosody. Gagging is a problem for some patients, and even it it is not, time is needed to teach the patient to accept the scope and to assume a position that permits viewing of the velopharyngeal port.

Use of nasendoscopy avoids the problems just described, and flexible nasendoscopes are now commonly preferred for use in assessment of velopharyngeal function. The term, flexible fiberoptic nasopharyngoscopy (FFN), is now commonly used in reference to use of flexible scopes. There are two types of flexible scopes: end-viewing and side-viewing. The first may be directed into the velopharyngeal port whereas the second must be positioned above it (Shprintzen, 1986, 1989). The angle formed by the lens end of flexible fiberscopes and the remainder of the cable can be altered by a control easily accessible to the examiner. Use of this feature enhances visualization of selected structures.

Wilson et al. (1986) described videoendoscopic equipment (scope, light source, camera, videorecorder, and television monitor) and procedures for its use including patient preparation. These authors conducted three to five examinations of velopharyngeal mechanism, larynx, or both within a period of 1 hour. The authors used a short-arc zenon light with a rating of 6,000 Kelvin. They state that home video cameras will produce reasonable images but that studio quality three-tube plumbicon cameras will do much better. Small cameras designed and constructed for use with endoscopes are available. Increasing use is being made of "chip-type" solid state camera (Yanagisawa, Godley, and Muta, 1987; Wilson, 1988). Shprintzen (1989) reported that some home videorecorders record images in low light. Another consideration in the selection of equipment is the resolution of camera, recorder, and monitor, which is indicated by the number of lines in each field (frame). Consideration should also be given to fields per second and to camera signal-to-noise ratio. It should be possible to attach the scope to the camera without loss of light.

Lens choice is important. Wilson et al. (1986) demonstrated the relationship between lens focal length and image clarity. Depth of field is important; it should be possible to conduct the endoscopic examination without need to refocus the camera. They reported that with a suitable mounting adaptor, the endoscope can be attached to a camera without use of a camera lens—the endoscope lens is all that is needed. A second lens absorbs light and reduces picture quality. In assembling equipment for videonasendoscopy, one should pay particular attention to lens mounting and light requirements, since they relate to quality of picture including field of view. The adaptor used to attach an endoscope to a camera lens may act as a tunnel and narrow the field of view.

The examiner must decide whether to hold the camera and endoscope by hand or to use a tripod. Wilson et al. (1986) positioned the endoscope in the patient and then attached it to a tripod-mounted camera. This eliminates movement of the scope within the vocal tract by the examiner and may contribute to the reliability and safety of the examination.

Issues in the use of videoendoscopy were summarized for this chapter by David L. Jones as follows:

Video-endoscopy requires the use of a rigid (Fig. 11.14) or flexible (Fig. 11.15) endoscope, a light source (Fig. 11.16), and any one of many videocameras that are available for recording the endoscopic image (Figs. 11.17 and 11.18). Transnasal insertion of the flexible fiberscope is used most commonly to examine the velopharyngeal mechanism, although some prefer to use the rigid endoscope via the transnasal or transoral approach. There are several models of light source that are available. Light sources vary with regard to the source of illumination (halogen lamp versus xenon lamp) and the degree to which the light intensity can be controlled. In general, the xenon light source is more expensive than the halogen light source, but it provides greater illumination.

There are a number of video cameras that are available for recording the ensocopic image. The cameras vary in terms of the image pickup device used, resolution, sensitivity to light, and cost. For years, the vacuum tube pickup device was standard. However, solid state pickup devices are now equally (if not more) common. Whereas the tube camera currently provides superior resolution and light sensitivity, solid state cameras are less fragile and easier to handle due to their smaller size. As the current video technology is improved, it is likely that the solid state camera will eventually be equal to the tube camera in image quality. For more information on the characteristics of video

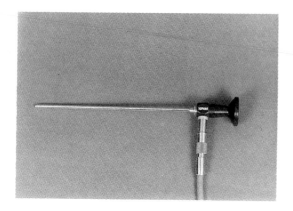

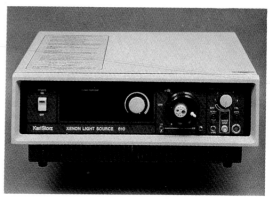

Figure 11.14 A rigid endoscope (Hopkins). The light from the light source enters the system through the cable; the lens is at the tip, left; the eyepiece is on the right, where a video camera might be attached. (Photos for Figures 11.14 to 11.18 provided by Ruben Barreras and Dr. David L. Jones, University of Iowa.)

Figure 11.16 Endoscopic light source (Storz Xenon, Model 610).

cameras, the reader should refer to Yanagisawa et al. (1987), who provide a detailed description of the types of cameras that are commonly used for endoscopy and a comprehensive comparison of nine different cameras.

The video-endoscopic image is usually recorded on videotape to allow the examiner the opportunity to review the structures of interest and to keep a permanent record for comparison with future examinations.

Most conventional videotape cassette recorders will suffice, but some features are worthy of mention. For instance, assuming that the quality of the video monitor is above average, a videotape machine that uses 3/4 inch videotape will provide greater resolution than a standard VHS machine (1/2 inch videotape). Also, a playback speed control and frame advance control can enhance analysis of the examination.

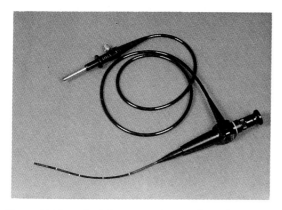

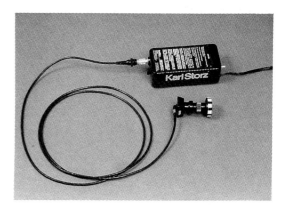

Figure 11.15 A flexible endoscope, sometimes called nasendoscope or nasopharyngofiberscope (Olympus ENF P2, enviewing). The light from the light source enters the system through the cable; the lens is at the tip, left; the eyepiece is on the right, where a video camera might be attached.

Figure 11.17 Video camera for recording endoscopic examination (Storz Charge Couple Device). The camera is coupled with a video cassette recorder.

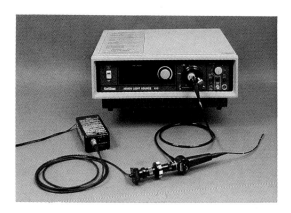

Figure 11.18 Equipment assembled for examination flexible endoscope, to be video recorded.

D'Antonio et al. (1986) described use of videonasendoscopy with children. They recommended explaining the endoscopic procedure to the child as a part of the speech evaluation that precedes it. They tell the child that the camera tube may be felt in the nose but that it won't hurt.

As with other instruments, questions arise relative to the quality of information derived from nasendoscopy. Comparisons drawn across repeated examinations of the velopharyngeal port are ·confounded to the extent that differences in scope placement in repeated examinations probably introduce different perspectives. Ibuki et al. (1983) and Karnell et al. (1983) attempted to control that variable in their studies of the reliability of nasendoscopy by requiring that the endoscopic image included all four "boundaries" of the velopharyngeal mechanism—the velum, the posterior pharyngeal wall, and the two lateral pharyngeal walls. Nasendoscopy usually involves administration of a topical anesthetic by a physician, and that may influence subject compliance and performance. Use of nasal scopes is contraindicated when there is significant nasal obstruction. Neither endoscopy nor motion fluoroscopy can be counted on for the identification of velopharyngeal closure that is not air tight. Examiners fall back on the identification of air

bubbles in either barium or mucous to detect nasal air escape.

Dickson and Maue-Dickson (1980) noted that a nasally placed endoscope with a lens at a right angle to the long axis of the scope looks directly downward and may miss movement of the superolateral walls of the nasopharynx. Paradoxically, a view directly into the velopharyngeal port is not always achieved with an end-viewing nasendoscope. Rather, the view is sometimes analogous to that obtained when attempting to look over the edge of a precipice without getting too close to the edge. Experienced endoscopists can usually avoid this problem. Pigott (1980) described and compared several rigid and flexible endoscopes in terms of their ease of introduction into the nose, clarity of image, field of view, and maneuverability. He also discussed several problems that can occur in endoscopy, including underestimation of the area of an open port, underestimation of structural movement, and a wide-angle effect whereby structures near the periphery of the field of view are distorted. Pigott utilized a split screen technique for simultaneous recording of endoscopic and videofluoroscopic images. Convergence problems in fiberoptic nasendoscopes were discussed by Schwartz (1975).

The extraction of information from videoendoscopic recordings is often a matter of clinical judgment, which is especially vulnerable to bias. Shelton et al. (1978) reported good agreement among observers rating velopharyngeal performance from oral videoendoscopic taped images. Ibuki et al. (1983) and Karnell et al. (1983) in a study of normal adults, found that velar movement and the size of the velopharyngeal opening can be reliably assessed by both measurements and judgments made from photographs of nasal endoscopic views. Ratings of these variables agreed relatively well with lateral radiographic data.

Lateral wall movement was not reliably assessed by either measurements or judgments of nasendoscopic images. A major reason for using an endoscopic procedure is to learn about the contribution of the lateral pharyngeal walls to velopharyngeal function. The data of Ibuki et al. showed that movement of the wall opposite the nostril in which the fiberscope was inserted was assessed reliably. Some investigators have assumed symmetry of lateral wall movement in making their judgments, but this assumption is questionable. Posterior pharyngeal wall movement was not investigated in these studies. Further data relative to the reliability and validity of endoscopic measurements are needed. In the meantime, the technique is quite commonly used clinically and has much to offer in the hands of trained examiners.

Karnell et al. (1988) devised a means of measuring velar displacement field by field from a videonasendoscopic recording made at a rate of 60 fields per second (Figs. 11.19, 11.20, 11.21, 11.22). Movements of the subject's head and of the nasendoscope were controlled by placing the subject in a cephalostat and by clamping the scope to the cephalostat. A millimeter scale was placed on the video screen and positioned along the axis

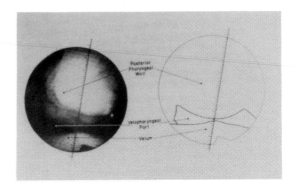

Figure 11.20 Videoendoscopic image of the velopharyngeal area (left) with tracing (right) provided to facilitate interpretation for the reader. A linear scale placed along the line of velar movement trajectory was used to track small changes in velar position.

of movement of the soft palate midline. This scale was interpreted to reflect arbitrary rather than millimeter units because of enlargement and distortion associated with videonasendoscopic recording units. The authors stated that comparison of movement patterns or contours across subjects is justified but that differences in absolute values would be influenced by positioning of the scope and by image distortion. This procedure is too time-consuming for clinical use and would not

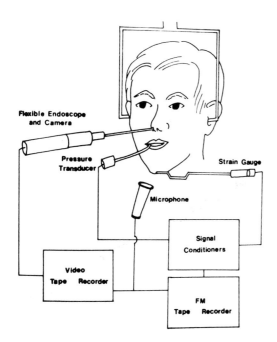

Figure 11.19 Schematic representation of data collection and recording system. (Figures 11.19–11.22 are from Karnell MP, Linville RN, Edwards BA. Variations in velar position over time: a nasal videoendoscopic study. J Speech Hear Res 1988; 31:417–424.)

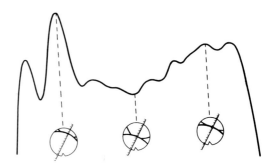

Figure 11.21 Relationship of the velar tracking technique to a displacement by time plot of velar movement during oral speech production.

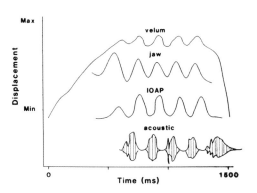

Figure 11.22 Example of temporal relationships among velar displacement, jaw movement, intraoral air pressure (IOAP) and the acoustic waveform.

answer many clinical questions. Rating routines or other measurement procedures for use with videoendoscopy are needed.

D'Antonio et al. (1989) devised and tested rating forms for use in analyzing videorecordings of flexible fiberoptic nasopharyngoscopic examinations. Ninety-five of 160 consecutive FFN evaluation recordings met criteria for inclusion in the study. Experience influenced the consistency of ratings, and the sound track influenced results, especially those reported by speech pathologists.

AERODYNAMICS

Aerodynamics is a branch of mechanics that deals with the motion of air and other gases and with the effects of that motion on bodies in the air (Flexner, 1987). In this section we review instrumentation for the aerodynamic estimation of the narrowest cross-sectional areas of the velopharyngeal port and of the nasal pathway. Data collected for those measures may also be used to quantify the resistance of each passage to airflow. Attention is given to precautions to be observed in using aerodynamic equipment. Devices and procedures for screening velopharyngeal competence are described in Chapter 19. Estimation of velopharyngeal area and other applications of aerodynamics in the study of velopharyngeal function is commonly discussed in reference to the expression, *pressure-flow technique.*

Measurement of the Area of Velopharyngeal Opening at Its Narrowest Cross Section

The area of an orifice can be determined by measuring the air flow through and air pressure drop across that orifice. The narrowest constriction of the velopharyngeal port during /p/ may be determined by measuring the nasal airflow through one naris and the difference in air pressure between pressure-sensing tubes placed in the mouth and in the second naris. The data can also be used to calculate the resistance of the velopharyngeal pathway (Warren and Du Bois, 1964; Warren, 1984 and 1989).

Dalston and Warren (1986, page 110) summarized their use of aeromechanical instrumentation for estimation of velopharyngeal area: "Briefly, the adequacy of the velopharyngeal port was assessed by simultaneously measuring the airflow through it and the pressure drop across it. Nasal airflow ($\dot{V}n$) was recorded by means of a heated pneumotachograph connected to plastic tubing of sufficient size to fit snugly in the subject's more patent nostril. The pressure drop across the velopharyngeal orifice (ΔP) was obtained by placing one catheter within the mouth and a second catheter in the subject's other nostril. The nasal catheter was secured by a cork stopper that occluded the nostril, thereby creating a stagnant air column." Their placement of pressure and flow sensing tubing and use of transducers, pneumotachograph, and computer are shown in Figures 11.23 and 11.24.

The area of the velopharyngeal opening is obtained by multiplying the differential air pressure by 980, which converts to dynes, and entering that value and nasal airflow in the following equation provided by Warren and DuBois (1964):

$$A = \frac{\dot{V}n}{k\sqrt{\dfrac{2\,(P_1 - P_3)}{D}}}$$

where:
A is area in cm^2
$\dot{V}n$ is nasal air flow in liters per second
P_1 and P_3 are oral and nasal air pressures in dynes
D is density of air (0.001 g/cm^3)
k is a correction factor (0.65)

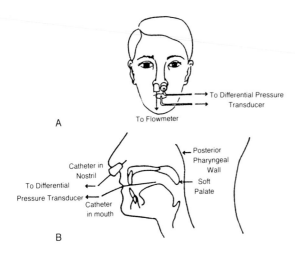

Figure 11.23 Catheters are placed above and below the orifice to measure the differential pressure. The catheter placed in the left nostril is secured by a cork, which plugs the nostril and creates a stagnant air column above the orifice (*A*). The second catheter is placed in the mouth (*B*). Both catheters are connected to a differential pressure transducer. The pneumotachygraph is connected to the right nostril and collects orifice airflow through the nose. (From Warren DW. Aerodynamics of speech production. In: Lass NJ, ed. Contemporary issues in experimental phonetics. New York: Academic Press, 1976.)

The correction factor of 0.65 was obtained by Warren and DuBois through use of a model of the vocal tract with known velopharyngeal orifices. Their model—and others—and the correction factor have been studied by many investigators (Lubker, 1969; Smith and Weinberg, 1980, 1982; Smith et al., 1985; Selley et al., 1987; Guyette and Carpenter, 1988).

As an alternative to use of the formula, the clinician can enter oral-nasal differential air pressure and nasal air flow into a chart devised by Moon and Weinberg (1985) (Fig. 11.25) and derive velopharyngeal area.

The resistance of the passage between two pressure-sensing tubes is calculated by dividing oral-nasal differential air pressure by nasal airflow. The resistance is expressed in centimeters of water per liter per second:

$$R = \frac{\Delta P}{\dot{V}_n}$$

where:
R is resistance expressed in centimeters of water/liter/second
ΔP is oral-nasal differential air pressure
$\dot{V}_n$ is nasal airflow in liters per second

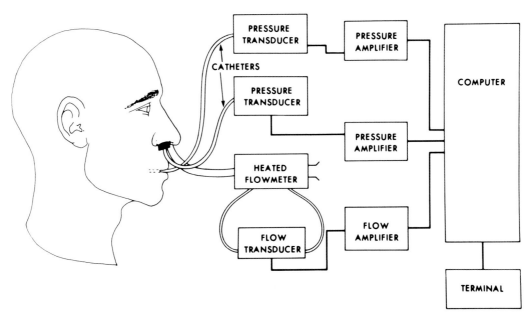

Figure 11.24 Equipment used to record intraoral pressures. (From Dalston RM, Warren DW, Morr KE, Smith LR. Intraoral pressure and its relationship to velopharyngeal inadequacy. Cleft Palate J 1988; 25:212.)

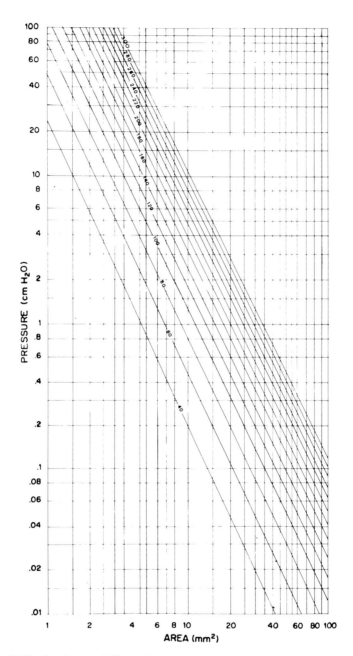

Figure 11.25 Log-log graph illustrating relationship between orifice differential pressure and orifice area as a function of nasal airflow rate. (From Moon JB, Weinberg B. Two simplified methods for estimating velopharyngeal orifice area. Cleft Palate J 1985; 22:5.)

Although this formula is used to measure laminar flows, which we do not have in velopharyngeal assessment, it provides adequate estimates of resistance if the measurement is always obtained at a given rate of nasal air flow. Commonly, resistance is measured at 0.25 or 0.5 L/sec/cm H_2O. If one of the pressure-sensing tubes used to measure oral-nasal differential air pressure is placed at the nares, the resistance measured reflects the influence of the velopharyngeal port and the nasal pathways combined. Isshiki et al. (1968) wrote that any resistance calculated is the sum of the resistances present—those of the velopharyngeal port, the nasal pathways, and the pneumotachometer itself. Hixon et al. (1976) discussed the matter of differentiating between velopharyngeal and nasal pathway resistance to nasal air flow. We assume that during /p/, the resistance measured reflects primarily the influence of the velopharyngeal port and that during nasal breathing the nasal passages have the greatest influence on the resistance measure.

Pressure-flow assessment of velopharyngeal function requires pressure transducers, a pneumotachograph, a recorder, and calibration equipment. An aerodynamic system called PERCI II is available that includes the needed equipment. As described by Campbell et al. (in process), it is a personal computer-based system for the assessment of speech aerodynamics. It permits measurement and storage of air pressure, air flow, and voicing data during speech, and it calculates velopharyngeal cross-sectional areas. Nasal pathway resistance and cross-sectional area during breathing, airflow volume during speech, and laryngeal resistance may also be quantified through use of PERCI II. An example of a computer printout of pressure-flow data and their computer analysis from Warren's laboratory is shown in Figure 11.26. Comparable analyses may be obtained with use of PERCI II. The pressure channel is calibrated against a water manometer and the flow channel against a rotameter.

Warren (1989) and colleagues at the University of North Carolina use pressure-flow instrumentation to measure velopharyngeal opening during /p/ in various contexts. Production of /mp/ as in *hamper* requires the velopharyngeal mechanism to open and close quickly. Performance during that word is contrasted with performance in less demanding non-nasal contexts such as *papa*. Velopharyngeal area is measured during /p/ because during that sound the air in the oral and nasal passages is stagnant or still, and the pressure detected at the mouth is the same as that just below the velopharyngeal port and that detected at one naris is the same as that just above the velopharyngeal port. Thus the pressure-drop that is recorded is across the velopharyngeal port. Warren (1989, p. 244) wrote that application of the orifice equation is most accurate when measurements are made at the flow peak where the rate of change of flow is zero. However, oral air pressure and nasal air-flow peaks during /p/ coincide when the velopharyngeal port is not closed, and

the area estimate is commonly described as being made at the moment of peak oral air pressure or oral-nasal differential air pressure.

For sounds other than /p/ or /b/, the pressure drop might be across a constriction other than the one formed by the velopharyngeal valve. The production of /b/ is not used because of the reduction in air pressure associated with voicing. The PERCI manual (p. 18) indicates that during /p/ produced with a velopharyngeal opening, change in respiratory effort influences oral and nasal pressures equally.

Velopharyngeal Closure Categories and Variables that May Confound Measurement

Warren and colleagues use pressure-flow assessment to categorize patients with clefts into three categories of velopharyngeal competence: adequate, borderline, and inadequate or incompetent (Warren 1979). Dalston and Warren (1986, p. 113) indicated that their terms *adequate, borderline,* and *inadequate* pertain to "...velopharyngeal function in terms of the respiratory requirements of speech. The pressure-flow technique does not evaluate speech performance... When velopharyngeal closure is less than total, [its influence on speech] depends upon the anatomic configuration of the oral and nasal cavities as well as the extent to which other speech structures adapt to the incompetency" (p. 113). They go on to indicate that oral closure may shunt acoustic energy into the nasal passages, and that timing of speech events contributes to the quality of speech in individuals within a given closure category.

That resistance associated with tongue posture and the nasal pathways influences nasal airflow at a constant velopharyngeal opening was confirmed by Selley et al. (1987) who utilized CT scans in construction of a "fully anatomical" model of the vocal tract. The model was constructed so that oral port size and tongue posture as well as velopharyngeal opening could be varied. Data obtained with the model indicated that nasal air flow was similar with velopharyngeal openings of 55 and 16 mm^2 respectively if the larger opening were associated with a flat tongue and the smaller opening with a humped tongue. Tongue posture and velopharyngeal opening also interact with oral port opening. Tongue posture had no influence on airflow through a velopharyngeal opening if the anterior oral port opening was small, but

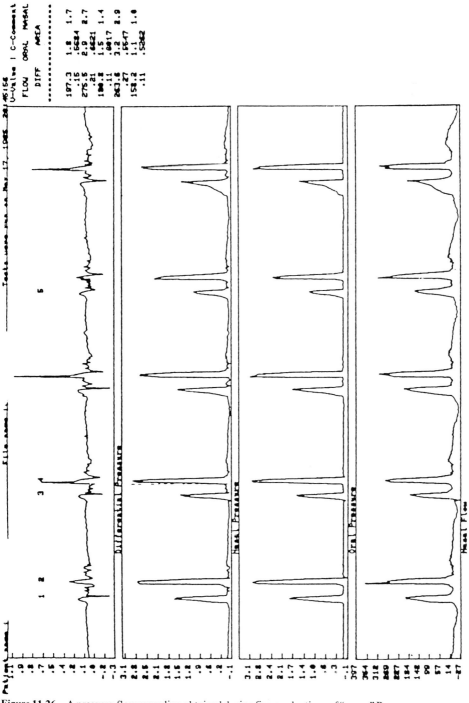

Figure 11.26 A pressure-flow recording obtained during five productions of "papa." Pressures are measured in centimeters of water and flows in cubic centimeters per second. The upper right hand corner reports nasal air flow, oral air pressure, nasal air pressure, oral-nasal differential air pressure, and velopharyngeal area. These data are for the moments in time associated with electronic cursors descending vertically from each of the numbers 1 through 5 in the differential pressure box. For the first entry, the values are as follows: nasal flow 197.3, oral air pressure 1.2, nasal pressure 1.7, oral-nasal differential pressure 0.15, and velopharyngeal area 0.56 cm². (Courtesy Dr. Donald W. Warren, University of North Carolina).

tongue humping "...caused...[an] increase in nasal airflow with both small and large velopharyngeal ports when the anterior oral port was large..." (p. 379). Velopharyngeal areas from 40 to 60 mm^2 were interpreted as sort of a threshold value beyond which "the nose controls the flow." The nasal pathway resistance to airflow in this model differed from that of the Warren model, which offered resistance comparable to that observed in normal persons. To the extent that the resistance does not correspond to that of the human, findings may be in error (Warren 1984 and personal communication).

Precautions Relative to Pressure-Flow Measurements

Pressure-flow measurements provide information about the coupling of the oral and the nasal cavities during speech and about resistance in the system. They describe neither the movement of particular structures, such as the velum and lateral pharyngeal walls, nor the location and configuration of any opening that is present. Radiography or endoscopy must be used to obtain that information.

Hardy (1965) wrote that transducers used in air pressure studies involving speech should be linear over the pressure range of interest. Frequency response characteristics are also important. Hardy suggested 200 Hz as an upper limit for the frequency response needed to study intraoral air pressures. He noted that the frequency response of the weakest component in a pressure-flow measurement system will determine the response of the entire system. Temperature variations may also influence output from a transducer.

Measurement of high-frequency oscillations is influenced by certain characteristics of the pressure-sensing tube. Tubes should be straight, short, and as large in internal diameter as possible. Very small tubes are easily clogged by mucus, whereas very large tubes do not allow tight lip closure. Pressure-sensing tubes should be positioned *perpendicular* to the air stream; false readings occur when air flow travels directly into the tube.

A concise description of several problems in aeromechanical assessment was presented by Müller and Brown (1980). They indicated that calculations of orifice areas for ports of the same size but of different geometric configurations may

differ slightly from one another. Müller and Brown also indicated that an area estimate is influenced by the shape of the entry and exit to the port, the presence or absence of a distinct periodic component to the flow, and the nature of the flow, that is, whether it is turbulent, laminar, or transitional. Other variables that may influence estimates of velopharyngeal area and nasal pathway resistance include the biomechanics of the tissues of the pertinent structures and changes in those tissues.

Warren (1989) responded to Müller and Brown by saying that the correction factor he uses works satisfactorily for the port configurations and air flows associated with speech and breathing. He agreed with them, however, that the hydrokinetic equation has limitations. He emphasized the importance of attention to detail in aerodynamic assessment of velopharyngeal area.

Warren (1989) recommended balancing transducers and calibration of equipment at the beginning of work with each patient. He would also calibrate the equipment against a tube with a known orifice. Kinks in tubing and leaks in the system—including the juncture of cork with nose—will invalidate findings. Both nostrils should be patent. Riski and Warren (1988) said that if one side is more open than the other, the more open side should be used for measuring flow. The catheter tubing selected for measurement of nasal air flow should fit the naris snugly. If one side is obstructed, area may not be estimated. However, oral-nasal differential air pressure may be measured using the open side and velopharyngeal competence estimated as discussed in Chapter 19 under the topic of screening. Placement of the oral catheter is not critical so long as it taps the stagnant air column and lip closure is airtight. Riski and Warren mentioned use of relief wax and rope wax to seal tubing connections, and they stated that the pressure-flow system is forgiving in the sense that speech intensity is not a variable that requires control.

Bumping a pressure-sensing tube will result in measurement of a pressure increase. Tubing may be obstructed by contact with tissue as well as by the accumulation of mucus. During strings of /pV/ syllables, the oral pressure trace should return to baseline each time the lips open. If it fails short of the baseline, something is wrong (Anne H.B. Rochet, personal communication). Nasal air flow during utterance offset, nasal consonants, and respiration between test passages is normal.

Alternative Aeromechanical Procedures

Various sorts of aeromechanical equipment have been used in the study and evaluation of velopharyngeal and nasal pathway structure and function (Hardy, 1965; Subtelny et al., 1966; Hixon et al., 1967, and Hixon et al., 1976). Stuffins (1989) described the clinical use of nasal anemometry in Great Britain. The Exeter Nasal Anemometry equipment, which includes an anesthetist's nasal mask and a microphone, is used to record nasal air flow and speech. The recording is sent to a processing center where nasal flow and oscillographic traces are prepared.

Sandham and Solow (1987) described the use of anterior and posterior rhinomanometry (rhinometry) in measuring nasal respiratory resistance and reported results obtained. Anterior and posterior rhinomanometry differ in placement of tubing used to measure differential air pressure across the nasal pathway. The anterior method is used to measure unilateral nasal respiratory resistance, and the posterior method is used to measure bilateral nasal respiratory resistance (see also Riski, 1988). The measurement of nasal pathway area and of mouthbreathing is considered further in the next section.

Measurement of Nasal Pathway Area and Mouthbreathing

Patients with clefts are at risk for an inability to close the velopharyngeal port adequately for speech. Furthermore, beyond the velopharyngeal port the nasal airway may be reduced in area with resulting high resistance to airflow. Interpretation of the influence of the velopharyngeal valve on a patient's speech depends upon information about nasal pathway patency. Hairfield et al. (1987) referred to the nasal valve which they located "...in the region between the upper and lower lateral cartilages [of the nose] and the pyriform aperture just beyond the anterior ends of the inferior turbinates" (p. 184). We understand the nasal valve to include the liminal valve, which is the most constricted portion of the nostril. It is located about 1 cm posterior to the nostril opening (Bateman and Mason, 1984).

Warren (1984) described the application of pressure flow technique to the estimation of the cross-sectional area of the nasal passage. Hairfield et al. (1987) used posterior rhinomanometry to measure nasal valve area during nasal breathing. During nasal breathing, the velopharyngeal port is open, and the narrowest constriction between

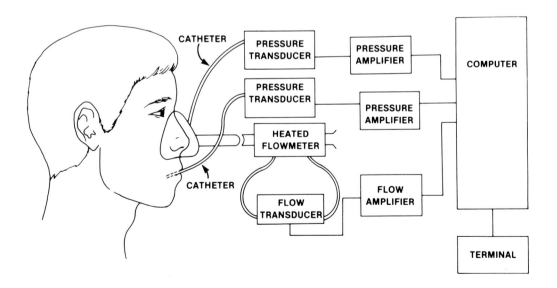

Figure 11.27 Schematic diagram of method used for measurement of nasal cross-sectional areas. (From Hairfield WM, Warren DW, Hinton VA, Seaton DL. Inspiratory and expiratory effects of nasal breathing. Cleft Palate J 1987; 24:185.)

an oral pressure-sensing tube and a nose cap is at the nasal valve. As shown in Figure 11.27, to measure the smallest nasal cross sectional area, Hairfield et al. placed a cap over the nose and measured differential air pressure between the cap and the mouth and flow through the nose. Area was again calculated by use of the hydrokinetic equation. A patient study is shown in Figure 11.28.

Hairfield et al. (1988) studied the prevalence of mouthbreathing in patients with cleft palate. Mouthbreathing was defined in terms of the ratio of nasal-to-tidal volume during respiration. Tidal volume was measured by means of inductive plethysmography, which senses movements of ribcage and abdomen; nasal volume was measured by use of a nose cap and pneumotachograph (Fig. 11.29).

Hairfield et al. wrote:

Each [plethysmography] transducer measures changes in inductance that are proportional to changes in thoracic cage and abdominal volumes. Breathing changes the cross-sectional area of the transducer coils and the resulting inductance changes are converted to proportional voltages. The rib cage and abdominal signals are then calibrated against a known volume by having the subjects breathe into a spirometer. The sum of the calibrated signals (i.e., thoracic and abdominal) is equivalent to tidal volume (p. 136).

Breathing mode was defined by using the following classifications of percent nasal breathing: 80 to 100 percent, nasal; 60 to 79 percent, predominantly nasal; 40 to 59 percent, mixed oral-nasal; 20 to 39 percent, predominantly oral; 0 to 19 percent, oral (p. 135).

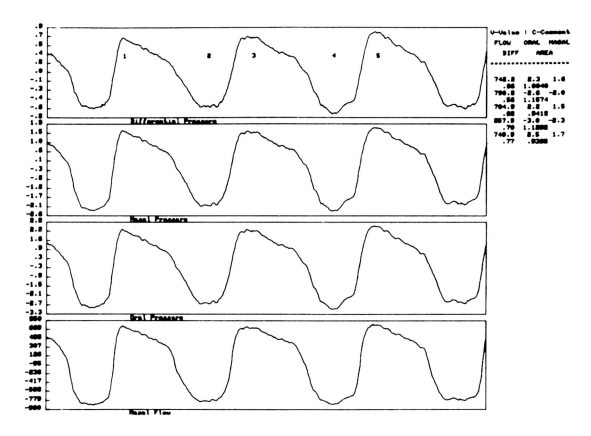

Figure 11.28 Hard copy of inspiratory and expiratory waveforms. Numerals 1 through 5 indicate the position of the electronic cursors where values were selected for analysis. (From Hairfield WM, Warren DW, Hinton VA, Seaton DL. Inspiratory and expiratory effects of nasal breathing. Cleft Palate J 1987; 24:186.)

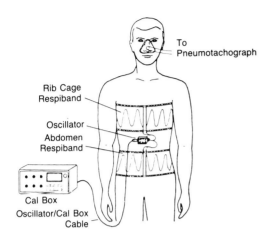

Figure 11.29 Schematic diagram of nasal cap placement and configuration of induction coils used for plethysmography. (From Hairfield WM, Warren DW, Seaton DL. Prevalence of mouthbreathing in cleft lip and palate. Cleft Palate J 1988; 25:136.)

Clinical use of pressure-flow technique and other instruments is discussed in Chapter 19.

PHOTODETECTION

Velopharyngeal function has been studied by measuring light introduced into the velopharyngeal mechanism. Kunzel (1979) described a velograph to be used in that fashion. Another instrument, the photodetector (Dalston, 1982), measures the amount of light introduced into the mouth that can be detected above the velopharyngeal port. The photodetector (Fig. 11.30) includes a light source and a light detector (Dalston, 1982; Dalston and Keefe, 1987). Each is attached to a light-transmitting fiber. The fibers are coated for optical isolation and cemented together. The distal end of the transmitting fiber extends 30mm beyond the end of the detecting fiber. They are passed through a naris and positioned so that the emitting fiber is in the oral cavity and the detector is in the nasal cavity. The two fibers are a constant distance from one another, and the light source doesn't vary in luminescence. Dalston (1982) reported a correlation coefficient of 0.91 between endoscopic and aeromechanical measurement of velopharyngeal port size at the moment of peak oral-nasal differential air pressure for /p/ in syllable context. Dalston and Keefe (1987) described use of the photodetector with a personal

computer and a means for its possible use in biofeedback therapy. It has been used to study timing of movement onset and offset.

Moon and Lagu (1987) described a second generation phototransducer. Data collected through use of a test box indicated that there is a strong linear relationship between aperture area and light output (r = 0.998). Jones and Moon (1989) noted that photodetection readings will vary with the proximity of the light source to orifice or cavity walls. Movement of photodetector fibers may confound timing studies. The phototransducers used by Dalston and by Moon and Lagu have response times more than adequate for study of speech movements.

The photodetector is more intrusive than aeromechanical probes and doesn't show structural movement as does endoscopy. However, Dalston and Keefe (1987) state that the photodetector has a capability for quantitative, real-time measurement of moment-to-moment changes in the velopharyngeal port opening area that spectrography, aeromechanics, and nasopharyngoscopy lack.

NASOMETER

The nasometer is a micro-computer based acoustical instrument designed for use in assessment and treatment of patients with nasality problems (Instruction Manual. Kay Elemetrics Corp. 12 Maple Ave. Pine Brook, NJ). The nasometer computes the ratio between acoustic energy detected by microphones positioned at the nose and the mouth. This variable is termed *nasalance*. The result of this computation may be displayed in several ways including statistical table, time history display, or nasogram that shows nasalance for time periods from 2 through 100 seconds, and bar graph showing moment to moment nasalance peaks for feedback purposes. The nasometer (Fig. 11.30) includes an input device consisting of headgear, a sound separator baffle, oral and nasal microphones, a nasometer unit, a printed circuit board for use with Apple or IBM personal computers, computer software, and a calibration stand. The nasometer unit amplifies and filters signals from each microphone and converts them from analog to digital form. It also serves a calibration function. The nasometer replaces Tonar (the oral nasal acoustic ratio), which was a similar acoustic device for

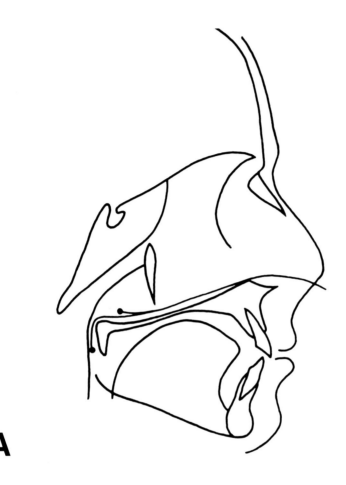

A

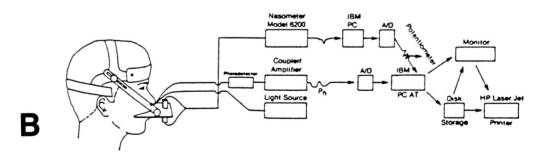

B

Figure 11.30 The photodetector: *A*. Placement of the photodetector probe. *B*. Schematic diagram of the photodetector system and nasometer employed in this study. (From Dalston RM. Using simultaneous photodetection and nasometry to monitor velopharyngeal behavior during speech. J Speech Hear Res 1989; 32:195–202.)

the measurement of nasalance. Tonar data have been shown to correlate highly with psychophysical ratings of hypernasality, and some research has been published relative to the effectiveness of Tonar as a biofeedback device for the reduction of hypernasality (Fletcher et al., 1989). Few data collected with the nasometer have been published, but the device seems to be well received within the professional community. Dalston (1989, p. 196) wrote that the nasometer is being field tested at the University of Alabama at Birmingham and at the University of North Carolina at Chapel Hill. We see the nasometer as a promising instrument for study of nasalance-hypernasality. Nasalance correlates with indices to velopharyngeal function, but we would not use it as a preferred instrument for study of velopharyngeal function. In a later section, we review information regarding relationships between nasalance measures and other variables.

Karling et al. (1985) described a device called a nasal-oral-ratio-meter that uses contact microphones placed at nose and thyroid cartilage to study the relationship between total speech time and duration of nasalized portions. The authors noted that normal speakers producing passages free from nasal consonants may show nasalization at word boundaries and at the end of phrases.

ACCELEROMETERS

Accelerometers have also been used in the study and treatment of nasalance (Stevens et al., 1975), and an extensive literature regarding their use has been published. Horii (1983) has been prominent in this research. Accelerometers are sensitive to vibrations, and have been placed on naris and larynx in order to study sound energy at the nose relative to that at the larynx. Vibrations picked up at a naris are amplified, filtered, rectified, and smoothed (Stevens et al., 1975). For sentences free from nasal consonants, Reich and Redenbaugh (1985) found statistically significant correlations from 0.85 to 0.92 between nasalance measured with accelerometers and ratings of hypernasality. Larson and Hamlet (1987) interpreted nasalance to reflect oral-nasal acoustical coupling but not necessarily physiological opening of the velopharyngeal port: the lower the frequency of the first formant of vowels the greater the nasalance will be. Because of this acoustical relationship, nasalance varies with vowel height.

High vowels have greater nasalance than do low vowels.

SPECTROGRAPHY

The spectrograph provides a visual display of changes in the frequency and intensity of speech over time. It has been used to identify the acoustical characteristics of hypernasality and of other forms of speech nasalization. The work of Philips and Kent (1984) and Ericsson (1987) in the acoustical description of nasalized speech is cited elsewhere in this book. Kent et al. (1989) recommended spectrographic analysis for use in planning and evaluating therapy for velopharyngeal disability. Spectrographic analysis may help the clinician understand the nature of nasalized speech samples that puzzle the ear.

ELECTROMYOGRAPHY

Electromyography (EMG) is an instrumental technique for displaying electrical activity that accompanies muscle contraction (Cooper, 1965). When a neural impulse triggers muscle contraction, a depolarization wave passes along the muscle fibers as they contract. This wave is termed the *action potential* (Harris, 1970). The instrument has been used in the study of skilled movements to determine which muscles are moving, when they move, and the strength of contraction.

Minimal equipment for EMG studies includes electrodes to detect electrical activity, preamplifiers and amplifiers to allow display of electrical activity, and a display device. The signals may be displayed on an oscilloscope or chart recorder, or broadcast through a loud speaker.

Different sorts of electrodes have been used to detect action potentials in EMG studies. Surface electrodes have been positioned over muscles, and needle electrodes have been inserted into muscles. The needle electrodes offer greater opportunity to identify the muscle that is being studied. However, needle electrodes may be dislodged during an examination. In order to solve that problem, some investigators have used hooked-wire electrodes inserted into the muscle by means of a hypodermic needle. The electrode remains in place when the needle is removed. These electrodes are difficult to adjust for position once they have been placed (Harris, 1970).

It is desirable to study several muscles simultaneously, since this affords information about interaction among muscles in the performance of skilled movements. A common practice in speech research is to have the subject repeat speech gestures several times and to average the EMG traces associated with those gestures. This may be done by computer.

Warren (1973) noted that in electromyography it is difficult to know exactly what muscle is being sampled, particularly in patients with cleft palate whose muscles have been affected by birth defect and surgery. Warren also noted that it is difficult to establish the relationship between observed electrical activity in a muscle and the actual muscle contraction. This issue has been addressed by investigators who have performed simultaneous electromyographic and cinefluorographic examinations (Lubker, 1968; Fritzell, 1969).

There is a wide body of research literature involving EMG, and the studies have contributed greatly to our understanding of the velopharyngeal valving mechanism (Kuehn et al, 1982; Kuehn et al., 1988). It is a laboratory technique whose invasiveness, discomfort, and complexity make it more appropriate for research than for clinical use in the study of cleft palate.

ELECTROPALATOGRAPHY

Laboratories in Great Britain, Japan, and the United States are using electropalatography in the study and treatment of articulatory disorders in patients with speech disorders including cleft palate (Fletcher, 1985; Hardcastle et al., 1989; Michi et al., 1986; Ohkiba and Hanada, 1989). To use this procedure, each subject is custom fitted with a palatal plate, and electrodes are positioned and embedded into the plate. Contacts between tongue and electrodes are fed into the computer. They may be displayed to the subject and compared with displays showing wanted articulatory patterns.

RELATIONSHIPS AMONG MEASUREMENTS FROM DIFFERENT INSTRUMENTS

Of the instruments considered here, radiography, endoscopy, and pressure-flow are regularly used to evaluate velopharyngeal competence,

and the photodetector is under development for that application. The nasometer measures nasalance that is influenced by velopharyngeal competence. Knowledge of relationships among measures made with these devices is clinically important. Instruments differ in their strengths and weaknesses and consequently supplement one another in helping the clinician arrive at a valid understanding of the patient's velopharyngeal function. Orderly patterns in findings obtained with different instruments support confidence in our understanding of velopharyngeal function for speech. In this section we review research that reported relationships among measures made with these instruments.

Even findings obtained with the same instrument and the same subject will not always agree. Where observations are made sequentially rather than simultaneously, the differences may reflect variability in subject performance or differences attributable to the instrument or its application. When findings between two measures of the same variable differ, regardless of whether the measures are instrumental, it is difficult to know which if either measure is valid. This is a recurring problem in the evaluation of velopharyngeal function for speech because we have no single measure of velopharyngeal competence that can be used with confidence as a valid criterion for answering all clinical questions. Stringer and Witzel (1986) provided an example of the kinds of differences in findings that are frequently reported among measures. They compared lateral, Towne, and basal videofluorographic views for effectiveness in identifying velopharyngeal insufficiency. The lateral view missed openings identified with basal and Towne views, and the Towne view identified openings that were missed with the basal view when large adenoids were present.

Radiography and Aeromechanics

McWilliams et al. (1981) studied agreement among speech observations, videofluoroscopy, and pressure-flow data in the classification of patients' velopharyngeal adequacy. The pressure-flow data tended to classify as competent patients who were considered incompetent on the basis of fluorographic findings. This may have resulted because the aeromechanical observations were based on study of /p/ sounds, and some individuals who closed the velopharyngeal port during those sounds did not close it during all other sounds. Such openings could be identified but not quantified for area by measuring nasal air flow as other obstruents are sampled.

Radiography and Nasendoscopy

Clinicians have reported disagreements in findings obtained with nasendoscopic and videofluorographic assessment of velopharyngeal function. Stringer and Witzel (1989) compared lateral, Towne, and base views and nasopharyngoscopy for effectiveness in identifying velopharyngeal insufficiency in subjects who ranged in age from 4 to 41 years and who presented hypernasal speech. The authors concluded that the Towne view usually agreed with nasopharyngoscopy. However, there were enough disagreements to warrant further study and identification of reasons for the disagreements. The Towne view was said to be superior to the base view when adenoids were a problem. Skolnick (1989) in commenting on the Stringer and Witzel report said that while the Towne oblique view may substitute for the base view, a frontal view is still needed for study of movement of the lateral walls in their full vertical extent.

Shprintzen (1983) reported that nasendoscopy performed with a side-viewing endoscope missed lateral wall movement in one-third of a group of patients in whom movement was seen fluoroscopically. He attributed this to the use of a side-viewing endoscope that required placement high in the nasopharynx. Shprintzen (1989) prefers to use an end-viewing scope that he can position within the velopharyngeal passage. Henningsson and Isberg (1988) reported that their use of an end-viewing endoscope failed to identify movements of the lateral walls in one-third of a group of patients in whom such movement was seen in frontal videofluorography. They attributed the failure to the influence of adenoids or Passavant's ridge on the configuration of the nasopharynx. That is, in some patients the small angle formed by the palatal plane and a line tangent to the posterior nasopharyngeal wall was not conducive to positioning the endoscope for a satisfactory nasendoscopic examination of the velopharyngeal mechanism.

Radiography and Photodetector

Zimmerman et al. (1987) addressed relationships among photodetector and lateral cineradiographic indices to "opening and closing movements of the velum" and correspondence between the two indices over time. Cineradiography was done at 100 frames per second. Dependent variables were the times of occurrence of onset of velopharyngeal opening, maximum velopharyngeal opening, onset of velopharyngeal closure, and velopharyngeal contact. The authors concluded that output of the photodetector varied with opening and closing movements of the velopharyngeal port as observed in lateral cineradiography. "The majority of photodetector output changes occurred within 30 ms of corresponding changes in velar position measured by cineradiography" (p. 569). For 68 measures analyzed, photodetector output and velar displacement correlated 0.89 for subject one and 0.78 for subject two. These results were statistically significant.

Photodetector and Nasendoscopy

Karnell et al. (1988) attached a photodetection fiber to a flexible nasendoscope to permit their simultaneous insertion and use to study velopharyngeal function. The authors wished to learn if signals from the two instruments "change in a similar fashion over time" and if there is "temporal agreement between the two procedures when used to determine onsets and offsets of velopharyngeal opening and closing." The nasendoscope was positioned to observe the velopharyngeal mechanism, and the light detector fiber was passed through the velopharyngeal port into the oral cavity. This arrangement permitted the recording of endoscopic image and of light from the endoscope as detected in the oral cavity. Two normal adults served as subjects. The speech samples studied were "Come to my house tonight for ice cream cake" and "nap nap nap." These samples were selected to elicit changes in velopharyngeal movement. Reliability for repeated judgments by two observers was reported in terms of standard error of measurement for time of occurrence of onset and offset of velopharyngeal opening and closing. Temporal measurement errors were usually within 16.67 ms which was the time associated with one television visual field or frame. Agreement varied for subject, type of gesture, and "premovement state of the velopharyngeal mechanism"—open or closed. Photodetector reliability was not influenced by the size of the opening.

Findings obtained with the two instruments tended to agree within 2 visual fields. However, again agreement differed with the two subjects and with the part of a gesture under study. For example, agreement tended to be better for studying minimal as contrasted with maximal openings. The latter involved movement outside the view of the endoscope. Under some circumstances, agreement was better for opening onsets than for closing offsets. A display of photodetector voltage over time for the sentence corresponded well in form (peaks and valleys) with plots reflecting velar displacement as measured by the technique of Karnell et al. (1988) which was cited earlier in the endoscopy section of this chapter. Slight variations in closure identified by nasendoscopy were missed by the photodetector. We may see small movements endoscopically that don't influence port size. Some light may be photodetected because of tissue translucency.

Aeromechanics and Tonar

Dalston and Warren (1986) used aeromechanical assessment to sort 124 consecutive patients into adequate, borderline, and inadequate velopharyngeal function categories. Subjects' speech was rated for hypernasality, and nasalance was measured with Tonar. Nasalance and hypernasality increased across velopharyngeal function categories. Area measures taken aeromechanically at the moment of peak oral-nasal differential air pressure during the /p/ in *hamper* correlated 0.80 (Spearman) with listener judgments. Other correlations were 0.76 for Tonar and listener judgments and 0.74 for Tonar and area. Twenty-two of 30 subjects in the adequate closure category presented some hypernasality. Variables such as degree of mouth opening may account for this. Nonetheless, the three measures tend to lead to the same treatment recommendations.

Photodetector and Nasometer

Dalston (1989) obtained photodetector and nasometric data simultaneously in study of 6 normal adult subjects. Data were stored and processed in the same computer; this permitted display of data on the same time line. The nasometer data served as an index to voice onset and offset as well as to nasalance (ratio of nasal energy to oral-plus-nasal energy), and the photodetector data provided an index to velopharyngeal opening. Voice onset and offset data were compatible with older research findings, which indicated that velopharyngeal closure is achieved ahead of voice onset and maintained until voicing has ended. Closure led voicing and was maintained after voicing more strongly when sentences studied begin with obstruents rather than sonorants. Energy peaks associated with nasal consonants as measured by the two instruments were located closely together in time. That is, the data indicate that the maximum for nasal consonants obtained through the two instruments agreed within a mean of 1 ms (SD = 16.4 ms).

DISCUSSION AND SUMMARY

There are several instrumental procedures for assessing the velopharyngeal mechanism and its function and each has advantages and disadvantages. Radiography and endoscopy are relatively direct in that they provide a means for visual inspection of the mechanism at rest and during activities such as speech. Still radiographs can be used only for evaluating structures at rest or in production of a sustained sound in isolation. Radiographic measures of any kind require a radiologist, preferably one familiar with the velopharyngeal mechanism and its role in speech production.

Endoscopy is vulnerable to failure to position the scope for adequate viewing of the velopharyngeal port and to impressionistic and perhaps unreliable or invalid interpretation of recordings. Oral endoscopy interferes with articulation, and topical anesthesia is usually needed for nasendoscopy.

Aerodynamic measures give data about the area of the velopharyngeal opening and nasal pathway resistance. They also provide data about nasal air leakage and about intraoral air pressure during speech. They do not provide information about the relative contributions of the velum and the pharyngeal walls to velopharyngeal function.

The appraisal of velopharyngeal function of patients and of research subjects is influenced by the examiner's conceptualization of velopharyngeal function. The act of evaluating a patient's velopharyngeal function may influence that function, and it is always possible that the performance observed is not representative of the patient's usual performance—let alone capability. There is little evidence that the instruments reviewed here offer precise prediction of future velopharyngeal or speech behavior of individuals. We are more successful anticipating group trends. For clinical decision making, we rely on—we are dependent upon—the identification of patterns of velopharyngeal function across tasks, time, and various instruments (Shelton and Trier, 1976). As indicated by Dalston and Warren (1986) listener judgment findings are better understood as the patient is evaluated with more than one additional measure. The measures considered in this chapter are somewhat independent of one another in terms of how they relate to velopharyngeal function conceptually. That is, velopharyngeal function as studied radiographically is a different thing than velopharyngeal function studied aerodynamically. In a statistical sense, different measures may account for different portions of velopharyngeal function variance. From either perspective, different measures of velopharyngeal function supplement rather than replace one another.

Research is continuing into the identification of variables that influence clinically relevant interpretation of instrumental measures. New insights into velopharyngeal function contribute to use of instruments in patient evaluation. Chapter 12 cites the observation that some individuals maintain velopharyngeal closure during nasal consonants. Karnell et al. (1988a) noted that in individuals with marginal velopharyngeal mechanisms the velopharyngeal port may open and close with the normal small upward and downward displacements of the velum associated with tongue height in running speech. This may constitute the best performance of which those patients are capable, and they may not be candidates for therapy to improve their velopharyngeal function. At this time, we are not sure of the predictive interpretation to be drawn from identification of this pattern in an individual. Instrumentation is used in evaluation to characterize individual patients, and treatment is then organized to meet the needs of the individual within the potential and limitations of the professions serving the patients.

In conclusion, we note that the use of instrumentation in the study of velopharyngeal structure and function is not necessarily more objective than is study of speech by ear. If *objective* means freedom from observer bias, objectivity is not assured simply because an instrument is used. Rather objectivity depends on evidence that qualified observers working independently of one another arrive at similar findings (Guilford, 1954). The avoidance of observer bias in the interpretation of psychophysical or instrumental measures is enhanced when procedures for analysis of images or other stimuli are established and followed by clinicians using the instruments. For some instruments satisfactory analysis protocols have not been developed.

REFERENCES

Bateman HE, Mason RM. Applied anatomy and physiology of the speech and hearing mechanism. Springfield: CC Thomas, 1984.

Björk L. Velopharyngeal function in connected speech. Acta Radiol 1961; Suppl 202.

Campbell TF, Linville RN, Yates C. Aerodynamic assessment of speech using the PERCI-PC: assessment and reliability. In process.

Cooper FS. Research techniques and instrumentation: EMG. ASHA Reports No. 1, 1965.

Cutting C, Bookstein FL, Grayson B, Fellingham L, McCarthy JG. Three-dimensional computer-assisted design of craniofacial surgical procedures: optimization and interaction with cephalometric and CT-based models. Plast Reconstr Surg 1986; 77:877.

Dalston RM. 1982 Photodetector assessment of velopharyngeal activity. Cleft Palate J 1982; 19:1.

Dalston RM. Using simultaneous photodetection and nasometry to monitor velopharyngeal behavior during speech. J Speech Hear Res 1989; 32:195.

Dalston RM, Keefe MJ. The use of a microcomputer in monitoring and modifying velopharyngeal movements. J Computer Users Speech Hear 1987; 3:159.

Dalston RM, Warren DW. Comparison of Tonar II, pressure flow, and listener judgments of hypernasality in the assessment of velopharyngeal function. Cleft Palate J 1986; 23:108.

D'Antonio L, Chiat D, Lotz W, Netsell R. Pediatric videonasendoscopy for speech and voice evaluation. Otolaryngol Head Neck Surg 1986; 94:578.

D'Antonio LL, Marsh JL, Province MA, Muntz HR, Phillips CJ. Reliability of flexible fiberoptic nasopharyngoscopy for evaluation of velopharyngeal function in a clinical population. Cleft Palate J 1989; 26:217.

Dickson DR, Maue-Dickson W. Velopharyngeal structure and function: A model for biomechanical analysis. In: Lass NJ, ed. Speech and language: advances in basic research and practice. Vol 3. New York: Academic Press, 1980.

Ericsson G. Analysis and treatment of cleft palate speech: some acoustic-phonetic observations. Linkoping, Sweden: Linkoping University Medical Dissertations No. 254, 1987.

Ewanowski SJ, Bless DM, Zagzebski JA. Ultrasound assessment of tongue posturing in glottal stop and pharyngeal fricative misarticulation. Presented at 4th International Congress of Cleft Palate and Related Craniofacial Anomalies, Acapulco, 1981.

Fletcher SG. Speech production and oral motor skill in an adult with an unrepaired palatal cleft. J Speech Hear Dis 1985; 50:254.

Fletcher SG, Adams LE, McCutcheon MJ. Cleft palate speech assessment through oral-nasal acoustic measures. In: Bzoch KR, ed. Communicative Disorders Related to Cleft Lip and Palate. 3rd ed. Boston: College-Hill, 1989.

Fletcher SG, Shelton RL, Smith CC, Bosma JF. Radiography in speech pathology. J Speech Hear Dis 1960; 25:135.

Flexner SB. The Random House dictionary of the English language. 2nd ed. New York: Random House, 1987.

Fritzell B. The velopharyngeal muscles in speech. Göteborg: Orstadius Boktryckeri Aktiebolag, 1969.

Glaser ER. A multiview videofluoroscopic study of Passavant's ridge in patients with and without velopharyngeal insufficiency. Unpublished Doctoral dissertation. University of Pittsburgh, 1980.

Guilford JP. Psychometric methods. 2nd ed. New York: McGraw- Hill, 1954.

Guyette TW, Carpenter MA. Accuracy of pressure-flow estimates of velopharyngeal orifice size in an analog model and human subjects. J Speech Hear Res 1988; 31:537.

Hairfield WM, Warren DW, Hinton VA, Seaton DL. Inspiratory and expiratory effects of nasal breathing. Cleft Palate J 1987; 24:183.

Hairfield WM, Warren DW, Seaton DL. Prevalence of mouthbreathing in cleft lip and palate. Cleft Palate J 1988; 25:135.

Hardcastle W, Morgan Barry R, Nunn M. Instrumental articulatory phonetics in assessment and remediation: case studies with the electropalatograph. In: Stengelhofen J, ed. Cleft palate the nature and remediation of communication problems. Edinburgh: Churchill-Livingstone, 1989.

Hardy JC. Air flow and air pressure studies. ASHA Reports No. 1, 1965:41.

Harris KS. Physiological measures of speech movements: EMG and fiberoptic studies. ASHA Reports No. 5, 1970:271.

Hawkins CF, Swisher WE. Evaluation of a real-time ultrasound scanner in assessing lateral pharyngeal wall motion during speech. Cleft Palate J 1978; 15:161.

Henningsson G, Isberg A. A comparison between videofluoroscopic and nasopharyngoscopic registrations of velopharyngeal movements in hypernasal patients. In: Henningsson G, ed. Impairment of velopharyngeal function in patients with hypernasal speech. Stockholm: Department of Logopedics and Phoniatrics and the Department of Oral Radiology, Karolinska Institutet, 1988.

Hirschberg J. Velopharyngeal insufficiency. Folia Phoniatr 1986; 38:221.

Hixon EG. An x-ray study comparing oral and pharyngeal structures of individuals with nasal voices and individuals with superior voices. Unpublished Masters thesis. University of Iowa, 1949.

Hixon TJ, Bless DM, Netsell R. A new technique for measuring velopharyngeal orifice area during sustained vowel production: an application of aerodynamic forced oscillation principles. J Speech Hear Res 1976; 19:601.

Hixon TJ, Saxman JH, McQueen HD. A respirometric technique for evaluating velopharyngeal competence during speech. Folia Phoniatr 1967; 19:203.

Horii Y. An accelerometric measure as a physical correlate of perceived hypernasality in speech. J Speech Hear Res 1983; 26:476.

Ibuki K, Karnell MP, Morris HL. Reliability of the nasopharyngeal fiberscope (NPF) for assessing velopharyngeal function. Cleft Palate J 1983; 20:97.

Iglesias A, Kuehn DP, Morris HL. Simultaneous assessment of pharyngeal wall and velar displacement for selected speech sounds. J Speech Hear Res 1980; 23:429.

Isberg A, Julin P, Kraepelien T, Henrikson CO. Absorbed doses and energy imparted from radiographic examination of velopharyngeal function during speech. Cleft Palate J 1989; 26:105.

Isshiki N, Honjow I, Morimoto M. Effects of velopharyngeal incompetence upon speech. Cleft Palate J 1968; 5:297.

Jones DL, Moon JB. Response characteristics of the velopharyngeal photodetector to known orifice cross-sectional areas. Annual convention. American Cleft Palate Association. San Francisco, 1989.

Karling I, Lohmander A, de Serpa-Leitao K, Galyas K, Larson O. Noram: calibration and operational advice for measuring nasality in cleft palate patients. Scand J Plast Reconstr Surg 1985; 19:261.

Karnell MP, Ibuki K, Morris HL, Van Demark DR. Reliability of the nasopharyngeal fiberscope (NPF) for assessing velopharyngeal function: Analysis by judgment. Cleft Palate J 1983; 20:199.

Karnell MP, Seaver EJ, Dalston RM. A comparison of photodetector and endoscopic evaluations of velopharyngeal functions. J Speech Hear Res 1988a; 31:503.

Karnell MP, Linville RN, Edwards BA. Variations in velar position over time: a nasal videoendoscopic study. J Speech Hear Res 1988b; 31:417.

Keller E. Ultrasound measurements of tongue dorsum movements in articulatory speech impairments. In: Ryalls JH, ed. Phonetic approaches to speech production in aphasia and related disorders. Boston: College-Hill, 1987.

Kelsey CA, Minifie FD, Hixon TJ. Applications of ultrasound in speech research. J Speech Hear Res 1969; 12:564.

Kent RD, Liss JM, Philips BJ. Acoustic analysis of velopharyngeal dysfunction in speech. In: Bzoch KR, ed. Communicative disorders related to cleft lip and palate. 3rd ed. Boston: College-Hill, 1989.

Kimes KR, Siegel MI, Mooney MP, Todhunter J. Relative contributions of the nasal septum and airways to total nasal capsule volume in normal and cleft lip and palate fetal specimens. Cleft Palate J 1988; 25:282.

Kuehn DP, Dalston RM. Cleft palate and studies related to velopharyngeal function. In: Winitz H, ed. Human communication and its disorders, a review 1988. Norwood, New Jersey: Ablex, 1988.

Kuehn DP, Dolan KD. A tomographic technique of assessing lateral pharyngeal wall displacement. Cleft Palate J 1975; 12:200.

Kuehn DP, Folkins JW, Cutting CB. Relationships between muscle activity and velar position. Cleft Palate J 1982; 19:25.

Kuehn DP, Folkins JW, Linville RN. An electromyographic study of the musculus uvulae. Cleft Palate J 1988; 15:348.

Kunzel HJ. Rontgenvideographische evaluierung eines photoelektrischen verfahrens zur registrierung der velumhole beim sprechen. Folia Phoniatr 1979; 31:153.

Landa LS, Shapiro G, Silverman SI, Storch CB. Radiation dosimetry for cleft palate patients. Cleft Palate J 1967; 4:308.

Larson PL, Hamlet SL. Coarticulation effects on the nasalization of vowels using nasal/voice amplitude ratio instrumentation. Cleft Palate J 1987; 24:286.

Lewis MB, Pashayan HM. The effects of pharyngeal flap surgery on lateral pharyngeal wall motion: A videoradiographic evaluation. Cleft Palate J 1980; 17:301.

Lowe AA, Gionhaku N, Takeuchi K, Fleetham JA. Threedimensional CT reconstructions of tongue and airway in adult subjects with obstructive sleep apnea. Am J Orthod Dentofac Orthop 1986; 90:364.

Lubker JF. An electromyographic-cinefluorographic investigation of velar function during normal speech production. Cleft Palate J 1968; 5:1.

Lubker JF. Velopharyngeal orifice area: a replication of analogue experimentation. J Speech Hear Res 1969; 12:218.

Massengill RM Jr, Quinn G, Barry WF Jr, Pickrell K. The development of rotational cinefluorography and its application to speech research. J Speech Hear Res 1966; 9:259.

McWilliams-Neely BJ, Bradley DP. A rating scale for evaluation of videotape recorded x-ray studies. Cleft Palate J 1964; 1:88.

McWilliams BJ, Bradley DP. Ratings of velopharyngeal closure during blowing and speech. Cleft Palate J 1965; 2:46.

McWilliams BJ, Girdany B. The use of Televex in cleft palate research. Cleft Palate J 1964; 1:398.

McWilliams BJ, Glaser ER, Philips BJ, Lawrence C, Lavorato AS, Beery QC, Skolnick ML. A comparative study of four methods of evaluating velopharyngeal adequacy. Plast Reconstr Surg 1981; 68:1.

Michi K, Suzuki N, Yamashita Y, Imai S. Visual training and correction of articulation disorders by use of dynamic palatography. J Speech Hear Dis 1986; 51:226.

Minifie FD, Hixon TJ, Kelsey CA, Woodhouse RJ. Lateral pharyngeal wall movement during speech production. J Speech Hear Res 1970; 13:584.

Moll KL. Cinefluorographic techniques in speech research. J Speech Hear Res 1960; 3:227.

Moll KL. "Objective" measures of nasality. Cleft Palate J 1964; 1:371.

Moon JB, Lagu RK. Development of a second-generation phototransducer for the assessment of velopharyngeal inadequacy. Cleft Palate J 1987; 24:240.

Moon JB, Smith WL. Application of cine computed tomography to the assessment of velopharyngeal form and function. Cleft Palate J 1987; 24:226.

Moon JB, Weinberg B. Two simplified methods for estimating velopharyngeal area. Cleft Palate J 1985; 22:1.

Müller EM, Brown WS Jr. Variations in the supraglottal air pressure waveform and their articulatory interpretation. Speech Lang Adv Basic Res Pract 1980; 4:317.

Oesch IL, Looser C, Bettex MC. Influence of early closure of soft palatal clefts on the pharyngeal skeleton: observation by CT scan. Cleft Palate J 1987; 24:291.

Ohkiba T, Hanada K. Adaptive functional changes in the swallowing pattern of the tongue following expansion of the maxillary dental arch in subjects with and without cleft palate. Cleft Palate J 1989; 26:21–30.

Parush A, Ostry DJ. Superior lateral pharyngeal wall movements in speech. J Acoust Soc Am 1986; 80:749.

PERCI. Microtronics Corp. PO Box 399 Carrboro, North Carolina 27510.

Pigott RW. Assessment of velopharyngeal function. In: Edwards M, Watson ACH, eds. Advances in the management of cleft palate. London: Churchill Livingstone, 1980.

Philips BJ, Kent RD. Acoustic-phonetic descriptions of speech production in speakers with cleft palate and other velopharyngeal disorders. Speech Lang Adv Basic Res Pract 1984; 11:113.

Reich AR, Redenbaugh MR. Relation between nasal/voice accelerometric values and interval estimates of hypernasality. Cleft Palate J 1985; 22:237.

Riski JE. Nasal airway interference: considerations for evaluation. Internat J Orofac Myol 1988; 14:11.

Riski JE, Warren DW. Study session. American Cleft Palate Association Convention, Williamsburg, 1988.

Sandham A, Solow B. Nasal respiratory resistance in cleft lip and palate. Cleft Palate J 1987; 24:278.

Scheier M. Die Bedeutung des Röntgenverfahrens fur die physiologie der sprache und der Stimme. Archiv Laryngol Rhinol 1909; 22:175.

Schwartz MF. Developing a direct, objective measure of velopharyngeal inadequacy. Clin Plast Surg 1975; 2:305.

Selley WG, Zananiri MC, Ellis RE, Flack FC. The effect of tongue position on division of airflow in the presence of velopharyngeal defects. Br J Plast Surg 1987; 40:377.

Shawker TH, Sonies BC, Stone M. Sonography of speech and swallowing. In: Sanders RC, Hill M, eds. Ultrasound annual. New York: Raven Press, 1984:237.

Shelton RL, Trier WC. Issues involved in the evaluation of velopharyngeal closure. Cleft Palate J 1976; 13:127.

Shelton RL, Beaumont K, Trier WC, Furr ML. Videoendoscopic feedback in training velopharyngeal closure. Cleft Palate J 1978; :6.

Shprintzen RJ. An invited commentary on the preceding article by Ibuki, Karnell and Morris. Cleft Palate J 1983; 20:105.

Shprintzen RJ. Evaluating velopharyngeal incompetence. J Childhood Commun Dis 1986; 10:51.

Shprintzen RJ. Nasopharyngoscopy. In: Bzoch KR, ed. Communicative disorders related to cleft lip and palate. 3rd ed. Boston: College-Hill, 1989.

Skolnick ML. Videofluoroscopic examination of the velopharyngeal portal during phonation in lateral and base projections—a new technique for studying the mechanics of closure. Cleft Palate J 1970; 7:803.

Skolnick ML. Velopharyngeal function in cleft palate. Clin Plast Surg 1975; 2:285.

Skolnick ML. Videofluoroscopic evaluation of the speech mechanism. Study Session at the Annual Meeting of the American Cleft Palate Association, Denver, 1982.

Skolnick ML. Commentary. Cleft Palate J 1989; 26:91.

Skolnick ML, Zagzebski JA, Watkin KL. Two-dimensional ultrasonic demonstration of lateral pharyngeal wall movement in real time—a preliminary report. Cleft

Palate J 1975; 12:299.

Smith BE, Weinberg B. Prediction of velopharyngeal orifice area: a re-examination of model experimentation. Cleft Palate J 1980; 17:277.

Smith BE, Weinberg B. Prediction of modeled velopharyngeal orifice areas during steady flow conditions and during aerodynamic simulation of voiceless stop consonants. Cleft Palate J 1982; 19:172.

Smith BE, Maddox CM, Kostinski AB. Modeled velopharyngeal orifice area; prediction during simulated stop consonant production in the presence of increased nasal airway resistance. Cleft Palate J 1985; 22:149.

Stevens KN, Kalikow DN, Willemain TR. A miniature accelerometer for detecting glottal wave forms and nasalization. J Speech Hear Res 1975; 18:594.

Strauss RP, Davis JU. Prenatal detection and fetal surgery of clefts and craniofacial abnormalities in humans: social and ethical issues. Annual meeting of the American Cleft Palate-Craniofacial Association. San Francisco, 1989.

Stringer DA, Witzel MA. Waters projection for evaluation of lateral pharyngeal wall movement in speech disorders. AJR 1985; 145:409.

Stringer DA, Witzel MA. Velopharyngeal insufficiency on videofluoroscopy; comparison of projections. AJR 1986; 146:15.

Stringer DA, Witzel MA. Comparison of multi-view videofluoroscopy and nasopharyngoscopy in the assessment of velopharyngeal insufficiency. Cleft Palate J 1989; 26:88.

Stuffins GM. The use of appliances in the treatment of speech problems in cleft palate. In Stengelhofen J, ed. Cleft palate the nature and remediation of communication problems. Edinburgh: Churchill Livingstone, 1989.

Subtelny JD, Pruzansky S, Subtelny J. The application of roentgenography in the study of speech. In: Kaiser L, ed. Manual of phonetics. Amsterdam: North Holland, 1957.

Subtelny JD, Worth JH, Sakuda M. Intraoral pressure and rate of flow during speech. J Speech Hear Res 1966; 9:498.

Taub S. The Taub oral panendoscope: a new technique. Cleft Palate J 1966; 3:328.

Van Demark DR, Kuehn DP, Tharp RF. Prediction of velopharyngeal competency. Cleft Palate J 1975; 12:5.

Warren DW. Aerodynamic assessment of velopharyngeal performance. In: Bzoch KR, ed. Communicative disorders related to cleft lip and palate. 3rd ed. Boston: College-Hill, 1989.

Warren DW. A quantitative technique for assessing nasal airway impairment. Am J Orthod 1984; 86:306–314.

Warren DW. Instrumentation. ASHA Reports No. 9, 1973:26.

Warren DW. PERCI: A method for rating palatal efficiency. Cleft Palate J 1979; 16:279.

Warren DW, Dalston RM, Trier WC, Holder MB. A pressure-flow technique for quantifying temporal patterns of palatopharyngeal closure. Cleft Palate J 1985; 22:11.

Warren DW, DuBois AB. A pressure-flow technique for measuring velopharyngeal orifice area during continuous speech. Cleft Palate J 1964; 1:52.

Weiss C, Blackley F. Feasibility of using computerized tomography in diagnosing nasopharyngeal closure. J Commun Dis 1981; 14:43.

Wilson FB. II. The importance of laryngeal visualization in voice management. In: Gerber SE, Mencher GT, eds. International perspectives in communication disorders. Washington: Gallaudet Press, 1988.

Wilson FB, Kudryk WH, Sych JA. The development of flexible fiberoptic video nasendoscopy (FFVN) clinical-teaching-research applications. ASHA 1986.

Yanagisawa E, Godley F, Muta H. Selection of video cameras for stroboscopic videolaryngoscopy. Ann Otol Rhinol Laryngol 1987; 96; 578.

Zimmerman G, Dalston RM, Brown C, Folkins JW, Linville RN, Seaver EJ. Comparison of cineradiographic and photodetection techniques for assessing velopharyngeal function during speech. J Speech Hear Res 1987; 30:564.

Zwitman DH, Gyepes MT, Sample F. The submentovertical projection in the radiographic analysis of velopharyngeal dynamics. J Speech Hear Dis 1973; 38:473.

12 | THE NATURE OF THE VELOPHARYNGEAL MECHANISM

A basic problem for individuals who have palatal clefts is defective velopharyngeal valving, that is, the oral and nasal cavities are not appropriately separated during speech, blowing, sucking, and swallowing. Unrepaired clefts are invariably associated with defective valving; even after surgical correction, some individuals continue to be unable to close the velopharyngeal valve during speech and, sometimes during vegetative activities as well. Thus it is important to understand the structure and function of the valve as a foundation for learning about the speech problems that accompany clefts. This chapter reviews the anatomy of the velopharyngeal valving mechanism and discusses normal valving and abnormal valving and its consequences. Useful relevant material is found also in Bateman and Mason (1984), Kahane and Folkins (1984), Zemlin (1988), and Cassell et al. (in press).

ANATOMY OF THE VELOPHARYNGEAL VALVING MECHANISM

The palate consists of hard and soft portions. The skeleton that comprises the hard palate includes the premaxilla, the paired palatine processes of the maxilla, and the paired palate bones (Fig. 12.1). The pterygoid bones, each with its lateral and medial plates and hamulus, are important to the palate in that they serve as anchors or supports for some of the velopharyngeal muscles. Foramina through the hard palate allow for the passage of nerves and blood vessels. The hard palate is covered with mucosa. The soft portion of the palate is composed primarily of muscles and is usually called the velum or soft palate.

Muscles of the Soft Palate and Pharynx

The muscles discussed in this section are all paired, one on each side of the head. However, our expression will be in the singular. The anatomical information presented here is not detailed. Rather, it is intended to summarize and review information needed for consideration of velopharyngeal function during speech. In this chapter, muscles are listed, briefly described, diagrammed, and categorized relative to function. Consideration is then given to innervation.

Tensor Veli Palatini

This muscle (Fig. 12.2) originates on the scaphoid fossa of the sphenoid bone of the cranium, attaches to the cartilaginous portion of the eustachian tube and to the medial pterygoid plate. A tendinous segment travels downward around the hamulus of the pterygoid bone and inserts into the palatine aponeurosis where it joins the tensor from the opposite side. Tensor fibers also insert into the hard palate. The palatine aponeurosis is fibrous connective tissue that extends from the hard palate to the free border of the soft palate. The aponeurosis serves as a firm plate to which muscles attach and against which they pull. The tensor opens the eustachian tube. It does not appear to contribute to velopharyngeal closure or to be involved in speech.

Levator Veli Palatini

This muscle (Fig. 12.2) originates on the petrous portion of the temporal bone at the base of the skull and descends in a frontomedial

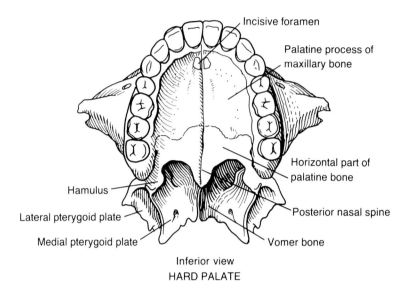

Inferior view
HARD PALATE

Figure 12.1 Inferior view of hard palate. Note that structures anterior to the incisive foramen make up the primary palate, while those posterior form the secondary palate. (From Dickson DR, Maue W. Human vocal anatomy. Springfield, IL: CC Thomas, 1970.)

direction, passing laterally to the torus tubarius, which is a mound of mucous membrane at the orifice of the eustachian tube. The levator inserts into the upper surface of the palatal aponeurosis in the middle third of the soft palate lateral to midline. The muscles from each side blend together. Levator fibers extend to the anterior third of the soft palate and posteriorly almost to the uvula. The paired levator muscles form a muscular sling that serves to raise the velum upward and backward to contact the posterior wall of the pharynx. There is controversy regarding the possible contribution of these muscles to medial movement of the lateral pharyngeal wall. The contributions of the levators and of the uvular muscles to the velar eminence or knuckle are evident in sagittal x-ray views of the normal palate during some activities.

Keller et al. (1984) reported neurological data from the palatal muscles in the dog in an attempt to better understand the relationship between the tensor and the levator. Additional data of this kind are needed to better understand velopharyngeal activity in speech and vegetative functions.

Musculus Uvulae

There is general agreement that the uvulus muscle gives needed bulk to the velum (Dickson,

1975; Azzam and Kuehn, 1977; Croft et al. 1978; Langdon and Klueber, 1978; Maue-Dickson and Dickson, 1980). Kuehn et al. (1988) report supporting data also, including EMG data that indicates the role of the muscle in normals is to provide velar extension during speech. Azzam and Kuehn (1977) concluded from a study of adult cadavers that two segments are separated by a septum. The musculus uvulae originates primarily from the palatal aponeurosis or raphe in the region of the second quadrant of the velum and extends posteriorly to the mucous membrane of the uvula. Some fibers originate from the hard palate. The musculus uvulae is located near the dorsal surface of the velum. This muscle is thought to contribute to the shape of the dorsal surface of the velum during function.

Palatopharyngeus

The two palatopharyngeus muscles (Fig. 12.2) form the posterior pillars of the fauces. Each arises from the pharyngeal wall and the side of the soft palate. Fibers reach the midline of the soft palate between the levator and tensor muscles. It is difficult at dissection to differentiate between the fibers of the palatopharyngeus and other muscles including the superior constrictor. Its functions include adduction of the posterior pillars, constriction of the pharyngeal isthmus, narrowing of the velopharyngeal orifice, raising of the larynx, and lowering of the pharynx. These muscles may contribute to the formation of Passavant's ridge.

Palatoglossus

This muscle (Fig. 12.2) extends from the oral surface of the soft palate to the side of the tongue. The two palatoglossus muscles form the anterior pillars of the fauces. They serve to pull the tongue

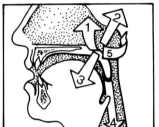

1. Tensor palatini
2. Levator palatini
3. Palatoglossus
4. Palatopharyngeus.
5. Superior pharyngeal constrictor

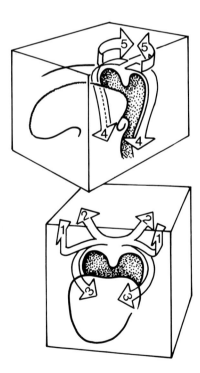

Figure 12.2   Schematic representation of the function of the muscles of the soft palate. The arrows indicate the approximate direction of their action and influence on the soft palate. (From Fritzell B. The velopharyngeal muscles in speech. Acta Oto-laryngol Suppl., 1969; 250.)

upward and backward, to constrict the pillars, and probably to lower the velum.

Superior Constrictor

This muscle (Figs. 12.3, 12.4) arises from the velum, medial pterygoid plate and hamulus, pterygomandibular raphe, mylohyoid line and adjacent alveolar processes of the mandible, and from the sides of the tongue. It inserts into the median pharyngeal raphe. Dickson and Maue-Dickson (1980) indicated that the superior fibers of the superior constrictor enter the velum with fibers of the levator veli palatini. Many of the origins of the superior constrictor are flexible, and the anatomy of the muscle is variable from person to person (Bosma, 1953).

The superior constrictor may contribute to medial movement of the lateral walls and anterior movement of the posterior pharyngeal wall. Controversy regarding its contribution to medial movement of the lateral walls is discussed later. The superior constrictor may also contribute to movement of the velum, tongue, hyoid bone, and larynx, and it may contribute to Passavant's ridge. The three constrictor muscles contribute to the formation of the pharyngeal tube.

Middle Constrictor

This fan-shaped muscle (Fig. 12.3, 12.4) extends from the median pharyngeal raphe to insert into the hyoid bone and stylohyoid ligament. This muscle overlaps the lower portion of the superior constrictor muscle and, in turn, is overlapped by the inferior constrictor muscle. It is thought to constrict the pharynx during deglutition and to move the hyoid bone posteriorly.

Inferior Constrictor

This muscle (Figs. 12.3, 12.4) consists of thyropharyngeal and cricopharyngeal portions. It extends from the median pharyngeal raphe to the thyroid and cricoid cartilages of the larynx. The inferior constrictor contributes to constriction of the pharynx in deglutition and to movement of the larynx upward and backward. Its most inferior fibers form the cricopharyngeus, which closes the esophagus and is thought to be important in esophageal speech.

Stylopharyngeus

This muscle (Figs. 12.3, 12.4) extends from the styloid process downward between the super-

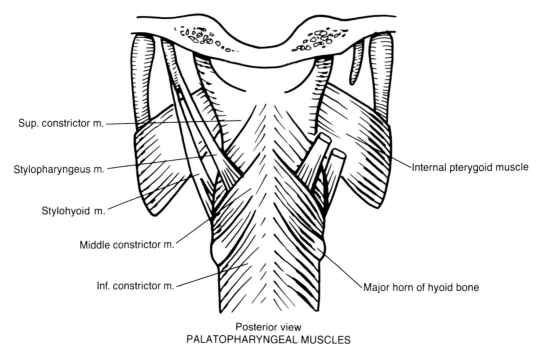

Figure 12.3   Palatopharyngeal muscles, posterior view. (From Dickson DR, Maue W. Human vocal anatomy. Springfield, IL: CC Thomas, 1970.)

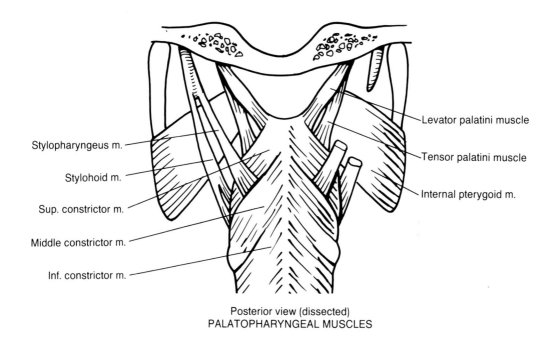

Figure 12.4   Palatopharyngeal muscles, posterior view (dissected). (From Dickson DR, Maue W. Human vocal anatomy. Springfield, IL: CC Thomas, 1970.)

ior and middle constrictor muscles into the lateral pharyngeal wall. It attaches to the thryoid cartilage of the larynx, and is thought to raise and widen the pharynx.

Salpingopharyngeus

This highly variable muscle is not always identified at dissection and may not even be present in some people. It arises from the torus tubaris at the opening of the eustachian tube and descends to join the palatopharyngeal fibers in the lateral pharyngeal wall. It may contribute to motion of the lateral pharyngeal wall, and its location is compatible with influence on the eustachian tube.

Muscles Used to Move the Lateral Pharyngeal Walls and to Form the Velar Eminence

There is controversy relative to the contribution of the levator veli palatini and the superior constrictor muscles to velopharyngeal closure. Understanding of the role of the musculus uvulae in velopharyngeal function has recently been increased. Selected literature pertinent to these issues is considered here.

Some authors attribute anterior movement of the posterior pharyngeal wall and medial movement of the lateral walls at the level of velopharyngeal closure to the superior constrictor. Shprintzen et al. (1975b) interpreted videofluoroscopic images to indicate that shelves form on the lateral walls during speech, that those shelves reflect the greatest range of motion of the lateral walls, and that they occur below the level of the most inferior fibers of the levator veli palatini muscles. They interpreted the literature to indicate that the most superior fibers of the superior constrictor are located where they could contribute to the shelf-like projections of the lateral walls. Iglesias et al. (1980) described simultaneous assessment of pharyngeal wall and velar displacement in normals by lateral radiography and frontal tomography. Low correlations were found between velar and pharyngeal displacement. They concluded that the superior constrictor muscle is an important contributor to velopharyngeal activity in normal speakers. Bell-Berti (1980) disagreed with that interpretation because the superior constrictor is positioned below the level where the velopharyngeal closure usually occurs. Her

1976 electromyographic data indicated that the superior constrictor contributed little to velopharyngeal closure. Dickson and Maue-Dickson (1980) discredited the superior constrictor as a mover of the lateral walls on the basis that its attachments do not lend the muscle to that function.

An alternative explanation of pharyngeal wall contribution to velopharyngeal closure was presented by Dickson (1972; 1975) and by Dickson and Maue-Dickson (1972). As summarized by Dickson and Maue-Dickson (1980), ". . . the inferior tip of the torus tubarius" is near the level of the hard palate and the levator "crosses lateral to it." Thus, the levator is positioned to influence the lateral walls of the pharynx by its action on the torus tubarius, whereas the superior constrictor is too low to contribute to velopharyngeal closure. They note that this is the most parsimonious explanation of lateral wall contribution to velopharyngeal closure. Movements of the torus tubarius have been described by Bosma (1953), and Lavorato and Lindholm (1976).

Kuehn et al. (1982) conducted EMG studies of five normal subjects and found that the level of levator activity was not directly related to velar position. They reported also that, in most instances, levator activity was related to activity in the palatoglossus and the palatopharyngeus. They also found activity in the superior constrictor, but on a more inconsistent basis.

Some additional data about the dynamic aspects of velopharyngeal closure are reported by Niimi et al. (1982).

We conclude that the relative contributions of the superior constrictor and the levator veli palatini muscles to movement of the lateral pharyngeal walls are not established at this time. The most commonly held view, however, is that the superior constrictors are influential.

As we have seen, elevation of the velum is attributed to the levator veli palatini muscles. The knuckled appearance of the velum in sagittal radiographs has been called the levator eminence because it was thought to reflect the activity of the levator fibers, which insert into the region of the velum that is part of the eminence. Recent information, however, suggests that the musculus uvulae may contribute to the velar eminence.

Simpson and Austin (1972) noted that contraction of the uvular muscle might account for an observed increase in the thickness of the soft palate during sustained /s/. Recently, evidence has been published that suggests that contraction of the musculus uvulae during speech contributes to the knuckled appearance of the velum. Dissection and histological studies led Azzam and Kuehn (1977) to conclude that contraction of the musculus uvulae may contribute bulk to the dorsal surface of the velum. Langdon and Klueber (1978) concluded from their anatomical studies in 15-month fetuses that the "combined vectors of the musculi levator veli palatini and palatopharyngeus" are such that they may serve as antagonists to the musculus uvulae. Interaction among these muscles may be responsible for the knuckled eminence of the elevated velum, and the eminence should probably be called the velar eminence.

On the other hand, Shprintzen et al. (1975b) wrote that the levator is positioned to contribute to the formation of the velar eminence: "The levator arises superior to the palate from where it courses in an anteroinferior direction to enter the velum through the lateral walls of the pharynx." The levator fibers enter the velum at the most inferior level of that muscle; they contribute to the sling which, when contracted, pulls the velum in a posterosuperior direction. The levator eminence represents the bottom of the sling. Since the mechanism of the eminence is not clear, we subscribe to the view that "velar eminence" is the preferred term.

Bosma (1986) presents drawings from meticulous, layer by layer dissections of the infant head—skeleton, nose, orbit, mouth, larynx, pharynx, and ear and auditory appartus. Information about the fetus as well as the term infant is presented, and the accompanying text provides information about morphological development. An extensive literature is reviewed and integrated. This book is particularly pertinent in an era when workers concerned with cleft palate patients give increasing recognition to the importance of the first 2 years of life to speech development. That development is influenced by the maturation of form and function of the speech mechanism, which continues for years beyond birth. It seems reasonable to expect some children to improve velopharyngeal function in association with maturation of the mechanism. Selected differences between infant and adult form, as described by Bosma, may be highlighted.

The levator muscles are nearly horizontal in their orientation, reflecting the spatial relation of the tympanic cavity and the palate in the fetus and infant. The cranial attachment of the levator muscle is slightly posterior to the insertion of the muscle into the palate. Accordingly, this muscle, designated as "levator" from its action in the adult, is principally a tensor and posteriorward mover of the pharyngeal (soft or muscular) palate in the fetus and infant; elevation of the pharyngeal palate is slight (p. 391).

In a footnote on the same page, he rejects the notion that the levator is activated by the facial nerves for speech and by the vagus nerves for swallow. "The motor innervation and the peripheral motor effector apparatus of the oral and pharyngeal area are pluripotential, apropos of performances."

Relative to motor performance of the pharyngeal palate, he wrote:

The mass of the infant's pharyngeal palate is greater in proportion to the adjacent pharynx. The palate also has a lesser range of motions; it is not elevated by its muscular action superior to the level of the oral palate (p. 292).

He described movement of the pharyngeal palate relative to pharyngeal wall and tongue:

In general, as the pharyngeal palate of the fetus and infant participates in valving of the palatopharyngeal and faucial isthmuses, the degree of its displacements are relatively less than in the child or adult. Reciprocally, the degree of displacement of associated structures, the constrictor wall and the tongue, increase. In the performances of infant swallowing and of the phonated, expiratory phase of crying, the constrictor wall is displaced extensively as it converges about the palate to close the palatopharyngeal isthmus; this greater displacement is seen particularly in the posterior wall. . .

VELOPHARYNGEAL MOTOR INNERVATION

Fritzell (1969) wrote that all palatal and upper pharyngeal muscles except the tensor and uvular muscles are innervated by the pharyngeal plexus, which is composed of branches from the glossopharyngeus and vagus cranial nerves and from the sympathetic trunk. The tensor is innervated by the mandibular branch of the trigeminal cranial nerve and the musculus uvulae by the lesser palatine nerves of the facial nerve. Nishio et al. (1976a and 1976b) studied motor innervation of the velopharyngeal mechanism in Rhesus monkeys by means of electrical stimulation and electromyographic EMG recording of responses. Palatopharyngeus responses to the stimuli were also observed by means of a nasal fiberscope. Dickson and Maue-Dickson (1980) interpreted the Nishio et al. findings as evidence that the uvular, levator, and superior constrictor muscles are innervated by both the facial nerve and the pharyngeal plexus. They suggested that facial nerve stimulation resulted in closure patterns similar to those associated with speech in the human, whereas stimulation of the vagus or glossopharyngeus resulted in swallow-like patterns.

The exact mechanism whereby velopharyngeal closure is achieved remains unknown. However, a great deal is known about velopharyngeal physiology. We turn next to that information.

VELOPHARYNGEAL FUNCTION

Knowledge about the structure and function of both normal and pathological velopharyngeal valving mechanisms is required if the speech pathologist is to understand and evaluate abnormal mechanisms and relate them to speech production. We are interested here in both the speech and the nonspeech function of the velopharyngeal mechanism, the contribution of the velum and pharyngeal walls to function, and in velopharyngeal closure requirements for normal speech.

Theories of Velar Function

Speech scientists have considered velar function in theoretical terms. Moll and Shriner (1967) hypothesized that the velum may function in only two modes, on and off. Postures intermediate between the elevated and rest positions are explained by timing variables and constraints inherent in the structures. Their hypothesis, which is more complex than presented here, has generated much research and discussion. However, later research combining cinefluorography and electromyography has not supported the hypothesis. Lubker's data (1968) supported Moll's earlier observation (1962) of systematic variation in velar motion and position with change in vowel height.

However, his data and those of Fritzell (1969) indicated that electrical activity in palatal muscles varies with velar height. He found the EMG signal to correlate from 0.69 to 0.83 with indices of velar motion for vowels. Lubker also found that velar height and other indices of velar motion do not differ between vowels sustained for 0.20 seconds and those sustained from 0.89 to 1.13 seconds. Lubker rejected the hypothesis that the velum functions in a binary fashion.

Seaver and Kuehn (1980) used electromyography to measure action potentials simultaneously in the levator, palatoglossus, and palatopharyngeus muscles. The speech performance studied was also filmed with sagittal cinefluorography. This study of normal function was directed to variation in velar height when the velopharyngeal port is closed in nonnasal utterances. The authors wrote:

Changes in velar positioning during the production of non-nasal speech are a result of the interaction of a number of variables operating simultaneously. Any attempt to relate only one of these variables to the activity of the velum may represent an oversimplification of this complex mechanical system.

Thus, their results are not compatible with the parsimonious on-off or binary hypothesis. Seaver and Kuehn suggested that variables in addition to those they studied should be considered. They mentioned tissue mass and elasticity as having potential importance. They described variability in movement patterns within and between subjects. Among their findings was the observation that velar height is greater for high vowels than for low vowels.

Lubker (1975) stressed the importance of considering the coordinated function of the several velopharyngeal muscles in velopharyngeal function during speech. He asserted that the velopharyngeal mechanism must be programmed centrally to coarticulate with other articulators. The velopharyngeal mechanism does not simply close for oral speech and then fall open when turned off for nasal consonants or silence. Rather, it elevates to different degrees, depending upon such variables as vowel height, voicing, and proximity to nasal consonants. Lubker wrote:

Velopharyngeal closure appears to be a complex and highly coordinated act. The muscles responsi-

ble function more or less forcefully to achieve more or less tight velopharyngeal closure. The tightness of the closure achieved is not a random variable, but is dictated by the speaker's needs, i.e., the production of a phoneme that is perceptually acceptable, and by certain physical constraints such as timing. Likewise, the variability of muscle effort is not random, but is also dependent partly upon the speaker's needs and partly upon what the velopharyngeal system has been required to do for the preceding phonemes. The clear implication is that of precise programming required in the central nervous system.

Lubker presented electromyographic data in support of his theory of velopharyngeal function.

More recently, attention has been given to the viewpoint that an individual may achieve a speech motor goal in different ways. Folkins (1985) discussed concepts of flexibility and plasticity relative to achievement of perceptually acceptable speech. Flexibility permits the talker to take alternate routes to perceptually acceptable speech. The individual may be able to adapt to a constraint within his or her motor control system. Plasticity comes into play when the individual must alter the motor control system to achieve a desired response. Research is also being directed to the hypothesis that speech motor control is directed to aerodynamic phenomena rather than acoustic goals (Warren, 1986).

The Velum

X-ray studies indicate that, in normal individuals, displacement of the velum upward and backward contributes to closure of the velopharyngeal port. Bzoch et al. (1959) studied 44 normal young adults during production of /p/, /b/, /f/, /w/, and /m/ and reported that the velum is highest at its middle segment and that its third quadrant meets the posterior wall of the pharynx in sealing the velopharyngeal port. They reported that, usually, the midpoint of contact between the velum and the posterior pharyngeal wall was 3 to 4 mm below the palatal plane. The highest point of contact was approximately at the palatal plane, and the highest point of the velar eminence was 4 to 5 mm above the palatal plane. Mazaheri et al. (1964) found velopharyngeal contact to be below the palatal plane in eight of ten normal subjects.

Velopharyngeal closure, as observed in the sagittal view from lateral radiographs, is completed before onset of phonation and is maintained until the person produces either a nasal consonant or a vowel adjacent to a nasal consonant or stops talking (Fig. 12.5). Even though velopharyngeal closure is maintained throughout the oral portions of an utterance, the velum moves upward and downward in coarticulation with other articulators (Moll, 1960). This motion appears to be neurally programmed so that closure is firmer for those sounds that require greater intraoral air pressure (Lubker, 1975).

Variation in velar displacement in different speech contexts has been of special interest to speech pathologists. Dickson and Maue-Dickson (1980) credited Bzoch with first reporting a relationship between velar and vowel heights. Warren and Hofmann (1961) found from cineradiographic research that the velum did not maintain firm contact with the posterior wall during the production of isolated sounds.

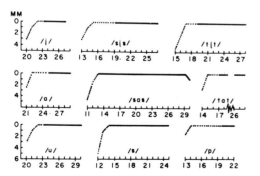
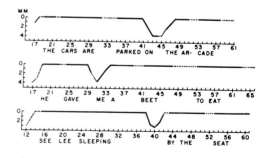

Figure 12.5 Curves illustrate palatopharyngeal gap in millimeters for each cine frame. Nonphonation frames are indicated by dotted lines. Frame numbers are indicated along the abscissa. Palatopharyngeal closure is complete except during utterance of nasal consonants. The subject is a normal speaker. (From Shelton RL, Brooks AR, Youngstrom KA. Articulation and patterns of palatopharyngeal closure. J Speech Hear Dis 1964; 29:395.)

Moll (1962) studied velar height, extent of contact between velum and posterior pharyngeal wall, and gap between velum and posterior pharyngeal wall for four vowels produced by ten normal adults. Data were obtained from cinefluorographic films exposed at 24 frames per second. The vowels /i/, /ae/, /u/, and /ae/, were studied in isolation and in CVC syllables produced in the carrier phrase, "Say—again." Each syllable was initiated or arrested with /p/. Fricatives, plosives, affricates, the liquid /l/, and the nasal /n/ appeared in either the releasing or arresting of each syllable.

Closure was not always achieved for vowels. Openings were observed on 30% of the isolated vowels, 13 to 15% of the vowels in oral consonant contexts, and 89% of the vowels in /n/ context. Velar height, which may be measured regardless of velopharyngeal closure, was greatest for vowels in non-nasal contexts. Mean velar heights were lowest in nasal contexts (8.4 mm) and ranged from 11.6 mm for the contexts free from consonants to 12.3 mm for /d_3/. Velar heights for the high vowels /i/ and /u/ averaged 12.4 mm each compared with 10.5 for /ae/, and 10.6 mm for /a/. Differences between high and low vowels were statistically significant, whereas differences among the high vowels were not. Data for extent of velopharyngeal contact were similar in pattern to those for velar height. Only the isolated vowel data were analyzed because the consonant context data were skewed.

Distance between the velum and the posterior wall was studied only for vowels in nasal contexts because most of the measures in other contexts were zero; that is, the velopharyngeal port was closed. Mean gaps were 2.45 mm for /i/, 2.03 mm for /u/, 4.6 for /ae/, and 4.0 for /a/. High vowels were not significantly different from one another; neither were the low vowels. However, the high vowels differed from the low vowels.

These data indicate that the function of the velum varies systematically with context. Moll noted that variability in velar height with the tongue height that determines vowel position may reflect the influence of the palatoglossus muscle which connects the two structures, or it may influence commands to the muscles that elevate the velum. Different vowels may require different degrees of velopharyngeal closure if hypernasality is to be avoided.

In another cineradiographic study, Moll and Shriner (1967) reported that the velum is elevated above its resting position for nasal consonants. They also reported that velar height varies with rate of syllable production in syllables composed of nasal consonants and vowels. The distance the velum moves between nasal consonant and vowel decreases as the rate of syllable production increases. Velar swing also decreases with increase in rate of production of strings of /t/ syllables. The velopharyngeal port opens between syllables produced at one and two syllables per second, whereas it remains closed when syllables are produced at a rate of four per second.

In a study using cinefluorography at 150 frames per second, Moll and Daniloff (1971) reported that some contact between the velum and the posterior pharyngeal wall was observed in normal young adult speakers during all oral consonants in NC*, NCC, NCCC, and NCN contexts. The last context sandwiches the oral consonant between two nasal consonants. Two of their subjects did not close on /w/ or /l/ when they occurred in NVC contexts. In most NVC sequences, movement of the velum toward closure began during the nasal consonant, during movement toward the vowel, or during vowel production. Other coarticulatory patterns were described by these authors. For example, in CN and CCN sequences, the velum moved toward opening just before or as the tongue tip moved toward the alveolar contact for /n/. They noted that in CVVN sequences, velar opening, which they associated with the nasal consonant, occurred as many as two vowels before the nasal even though a word boundary occurred within the sequence.

Kuehn (1976) studied the velopharyngeal function of two normal individuals uttering VCNV and VNCV syllables in the phrase "Say—again." The camera was operated at 100 frames per second. He noted that the speech sample was such that especially rapid velocities were probably obtained. His findings included the following information about context: (1) Subjects tended to drop the velum and show a large velopharyngeal opening on the /l/ in /alna/. (2) One subject dropped the velum on /s/ in /asna/. (3) The velum remained higher for nasal consonants in high-vowel than in low-vowel contexts. (4) One subject moved the tongue tip before the palate for some /s/ sounds in *say*, whereas the other subject always began velar movement "well in advance of tongue tip movement for those /s/ sounds." Kuehn also provided information about the speed of articulatory acts: (1) Velar movement was decreased during more rapid speech. (2) The velum generally moved more slowly than the tongue. (3) The farther a structure had to move, the faster it tended to move. (4) Speakers with large structures tended to move their articulators

---

*N = nasal consonant
 C = consonant
 V = vowel

---

farther and faster than individuals with smaller structures. Kuehn reported that measures of velocity, time, and distance varied considerably from speaker to speaker and from context too context. The pattern of velar movement was similar for each subject for contexts that were similar in place of articulation. The displacement of the velum to contact the pharyngeal walls is a major component of normal velopharyngeal closure.

Künzel (1979) used the velograph to study velar height in normal German speakers. He found velar heights to be greater for oral consonants than for vowels. He also reported greater height for plosives than for liquids. He found velar height to be greater in voiceless than in voiced plosives and in orally- than in nasally-released plosives. For example, in /lapn/ the release is oral, while in /lapm/ it is nasal. In the latter word, the position for /p/ is assumed but is not released. Rather, the syllable is released with the /m/. He described anticipatory and carryover coarticulation of velar movement, and he postulated that two types of coarticulation occur—passive and active. The difference in velar height for nasally and orally released stops was thought to reflect active neuromotor programming, whereas the modification of velar height during a vowel in anticipation of a consonant was seen by Künzel as passive. Elsewhere, Künzel (1977) had reported that maximum velar height is achieved earlier in nasally than in orally released plosives. In his 1979 paper, he cited publications which indicated that even in French, where opposition between nasal and oral vowels is phonemic, slight velopharyngeal openings during vowels do not impair communication. He considered airtight velopharyngeal closure to be essential to production of normal consonants.

Iglesias et al. (1980) obtained lateral still radiographs and frontal tomograms simultaneously as normal speakers sustained /z/, /n/, /i/, /u/, /a/, and /æ/. Velar displacement was measured in millimeters for the young adult subjects.

Displacement was significantly greater for /z/ and the high vowels than for the low vowels and for /n/, and it was greater for the low vowels than for /n/. Differences between front and back vowels were not statistically significant.

In summary, during speech the velum moves upward and backward contacting the posterior wall of the pharynx a bit below the palatal plane. This motion usually begins prior to the onset of an utterance. Closure is maintained until a nasal consonant is reached or the utterance is ended. However, the velum moves up and down in keeping with context (coarticulating with the tongue or achieving greater closure in keeping with aeromechanical requirements) even though closure is maintained. The elevated velum during speech, as viewed in a sagittal radiograph, is characterized by an eminence of knuckled appearance. The extent of velar displacement decreases with increased speech rate. The velum is higher in high than in low vowels and higher in consonants requiring intraoral air pressure than in vowels. There is variability among subjects in velar function.

Velar Stretch

Graber et al. (1959) observed that the length of the velum is greater during function than at rest. This "velar stretch" was studied by Mourino and Weinberg (1975). They compared cephalometric studies of 8- and 10-year-old children with reports in the literature concerning persons of other ages. Ninety percent of their subjects showed velar stretch during /u/, and 80 percent during /s/. All subjects closed the velopharyngeal port during /s/ but not during /u/. The 10-year-old children showed greater stretch than did the 8-year-olds. Adults studied by Simpson and Austin (1972) showed greater stretch than did the children studied by Mourino and Weinberg. The adults averaged a 20% increase in length during /s/ compared with rest, whereas the children showed a 10 to 13% increase. Mourino and Weinberg noted that in their subjects ". . . the length of the anterior portion of the soft palate measured during speech was not significantly different from anterior resting length." Simpson and Austin observed a significant increase in the functional length of the anterior portion of the soft palate in their group of normal adult speakers.

Further information about the relationship between age and velar stretch was provided by Simpson and Colton (1980), who studied adolescent subjects cephalometrically. Some of the subjects were at the peak of adenoid growth, whereas others showed the adenoid involution characteristic of young adults. They found that 11 subjects showed more stretch than the younger subjects of Mourino and Weinberg and less than the adults of Simpson and Austin. The stretch measures did not correlate significantly with need ratio, which was defined as pharyngeal depth divided by velar length at rest.

Simpson and Chin (1981) studied velar stretch during /a/, /u/, /ɛ/ and blowing in 20 normal speakers between 18 and 30 years of age. Stretch was measured from the nasal surface of the velum, as visualized in cephalometric radiographs, and from the velar midline. Stretch was greater for /u/ and blowing than for the other two vowels. No difference was observed between male and female subjects. In this study, the correlation between stretch and need ratio was 0.79 or greater. Some, but not all, stretch measures correlated significantly with velar height measures. The correlations ranged from 0.40 to 0.52. The authors concluded that velar stretch is a function of the act performed. They interpreted the context data to indicate that stretch results in order to prevent excess nasality.

These data indicate that the palate is stretched during function, that stretch is age-related, and that the stretch may not be equally distributed throughout the velum. Resting velar length does not compare with pharyngeal depth with respect to velopharyngeal closure because the velum is longer in function than at rest. Apparently, velar stretch occurs in an orderly pattern relative to context. Perhaps it interacts (coarticulates) with variables including velar height, pharyngeal wall movement, and others that account for some of the variance in velopharyngeal closure.

Pharyngeal Wall Movement

A number of investigators have attempted to determine the contribution of the movement of the pharyngeal walls to velopharyngeal closure. Wolfe (1942), Harrington (1944), and Hagerty and Hill (1960) conducted lateral x-ray studies and reported that there appeared to be little anterior movement of the posterior pharyngeal wall during the sustained speech activities of normal individuals. Iglesias et al. (1980) used midsagittal radiographs to study normal young

adults during production of /z/, /u/, /i/, /æ/, /a/, and /n/. They found that forward movement of the posterior pharyngeal wall ranged from 0.0 to 4.0 mm. Across subjects, the mean displacement value for /z/ was 1.3 mm as measured at a level above the palatal plane. All other mean values were less than 1.0. Measures were made at four levels, one at the palatal plane, one parallel to but above that plane, and two parallel to but below that plane.

Several studies have indicated that there is considerable movement of the lateral pharyngeal walls toward midline during speech. These movements are somewhat difficult to observe radiographically because of the superimposition of structures in radiographs. Radiopaque media have been used in some of these studies. Astley (1958) obtained data by frontal motion radiographs of lateral pharyngeal walls marked with barium paste. He concluded that there was medial movement of the lateral walls at about the level of the palate. Mason et al. (1973), using similar techniques, reported high variability in the symmetry of wall movement.

Detailed x-ray data regarding medial movement of the lateral pharyngeal walls was reported by Iglesias et al. (1980). They obtained simultaneous lateral still radiographs and frontal tomograms in 25 young adults, 20 females and five males, during rest and phonation of sustained /z/, /n/, /i/, /u/, /æ/, and /a/. Tomography permitted better definition of pharyngeal walls than do conventional sagittal radiographs. Individuals who would require more than three roentgens to complete the study because of skull size or density were excluded; this criterion ruled out larger male volunteers.

Medial displacement of the lateral pharyngeal walls was measured at four levels: Level 1: plane above and parallel to the palatal plane passing through "the point at which the superior margin of the pharynx was observed to change slope;" Level 2: the palatal plane; Level 3: a plane that dissected the distance between the palatal plane and the fourth level; Level 4: a level parallel to the palatal plane and positioned to pass through the inferior tip of the maxillary incisors and the lower part of the second cervical vertebra. As shown in Figure 12.6, the width of the pharynx at rest from Level 1 downward becomes wider and then narrower. The means and standard deviations for rest width at each level for males and females are reported in Table 12.1. Displacement of the lateral walls at the four levels is displayed in

Figure 12.7. The lateral walls move substantially toward midline in non-nasal contexts in most subjects. Two subjects produced little lateral movement, whereas others were similar in "absolute magnitude of lateral pharyngeal wall displacement." Greatest displacement was at Levels 2 and 3, which are at and just below the palatal plane. Except at Level 4, displacement for /n/ was significantly less than that for the other speech sounds. The authors stated that the subjects were variable in medial movement of the lateral walls in that some showed maximal displacement at Level 2 and some at Level 3. Some subjects sometimes showed maximal displacement at Level 2 and sometimes at Level 3, but none showed the maximal movement at Levels 1 or 4. The authors described the lateral wall displacement as taking the form of "a rather broad inbulging bilaterally." The largest mean bilateral displacements across subjects were approximately 50 percent of the pharyngeal width at rest. Four of the subjects produced slight outward (lateral) displacements of the lateral pharyngeal walls at Level 4 during /i/, /u/, and /z/. The authors discussed the stylopharyngeus as a dilator or expander of the lower pharynx and noted that their findings regarding medial movement of the lateral walls were similar to those of Harrington (1944), Isshiki et al. (1969), and Lavorato (1975). None of these authors identified the shelf-like projections described by Shprintzen et al. (1975b).

Minifie et al. (1970) used ultrasound with single-element transducers to study movement of the lateral pharyngeal walls 1 cm below the angle of the mandible. They stated that the configuration of the pharynx at this level is a factor in image clarity and that this location does not require

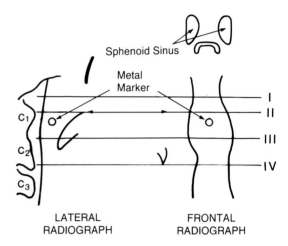

Figure 12.6 Illustration of the relationship between lateral-view and frontal-view radiographs. (From Iglesias A, Kuehn DP, Morris HL. Simultaneous assessment of pharyngeal wall and velar displacement for selected speech sounds. J Speech Hear Res 1980; 23:429.)

passage of the ultrasound beam through as much muscle and bone as would be involved if a higher placement were used. The amplitude of returning echoes decreases as the beam passes through more tissue. At this level, the lateral pharyngeal walls move outward or away from midline, especially during the production of some sounds.

Kelsey et al. (1969), also using ultrasound with the transducer location already described, found that in two of three subjects the walls moved laterally from rest during /ikiki/ utterances. Their subjects showed more medial movement of the lateral walls for the vowels than for the consonants studied. This same transducer location was used by Minifie et al. (1970) to study lateral pharyngeal motion in three normal adult males. Five vowels, including high and low vowels, were studied with six stop consonants in VCVCV utterances. They found that the lateral pharyngeal wall almost always moved outward during the consonants and inward during the vowels. There was little inward movement during high vowels, but substantial movement toward midline during low vowels. The authors advised that this movement pattern is not representative of levels other than the one studied. They interpreted their data to indicate that the amount of outward movement of the lateral pharyngeal walls on stop consonants is influenced by adjacent vowels.

The outward movement of the lateral pharyngeal walls observed in the ultrasound studies

TABLE 12.1   Means and Standard Deviations (in mm) of Pharyngeal Width at Rest for Males and Females

	Females		Males	
	Mean	SD	Mean	SD
Level 1	21.23	2.55	19.54	2.90
Level 2	25.46	2.71	22.60	4.44
Level 3	29.80	5.88	26.80	5.66
Level 4	25.00	6.72	25.07	5.64

From Iglesias A, Kuehn DP, Morris HL. Simultaneous assessment of pharyngeal wall and velar displacement for selected speech sounds. J Speech Hear Res 1980;23:429.

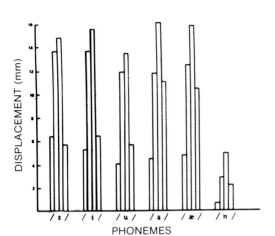

Figure 12.7 Bilateral (right plus left) lateral pharyngeal wall displacement for the utterances indicated. Values are means across subjects. Each group of bar graphs from left to right within groups represents displacement at Levels 1, 2, 3, and 4 respectively. (From Iglesias A, Kuehn DP, Morris HL. Simultaneous assessment of pharyngeal wall and velar displacement for selected speech sounds. J Speech Hear Res 1980; 23:438.)

differed from data obtained in the x-ray studies, which showed inward movement of the pharyngeal walls. Of course, the pharyngeal level at which the observations were made also differed. To resolve this difference, Zagzebski (1975) used ultrasound to compare lateral pharyngeal wall motion at the angle of the mandible and posterior to the mandible beneath the ear lobe or on the ramus of the mandible 1 cm below the ear canal. The second level was thought to correspond approximately to the level of velopharyngeal closure. This was confirmed for one subject through use of x-ray study. The subjects were three normal, English-speaking adults. The two levels were studied sequentially. The speech sample consisted of /pp/, /pip/, /mm/, and /mim/ in the phrase "Tape a ___ again."

Zagzebski (1975) found that transducer placement at the higher site gave results compatible with x-ray data, and placement at the lower site gave results compatible with previous ultrasound studies. Small discrepancies were explained in terms of variability in transducer placement and use of different speech samples. At the low transducer placement, low vowels involved mesial displacement of the pharyngeal wall, whereas, on the average, high vowels were produced with small outward displacement. Greater medial displacement of the pharyngeal walls occurred at the

higher than at the lower level studied. At the high level, the walls moved inward during high vowels in contrast to the small outward motion observed at the lower position. Contextual effects were also observed. At the level of velopharyngeal closure, less inward motion of the pharyngeal walls was observed on vowels in nasal contexts than when they occurred in non-nasal contexts. Zagzebski interpreted his data and the literature to indicate that both the superior constrictor and the levator muscles are involved in velopharyngeal closure.

Ryan and Hawkins (1976) placed an ultrasound transducer 5 to 10 mm above the angle of the mandible and behind the ramus. They noted that a lower transducer placement would miss movement in this area of velopharyngeal closure. They studied three normal adult males and two normal adult females. Subjects produced VCVCV strings composed of /a/ and /i/ combined with the consonants /p, t, s, m/ and /n/. The authors did not extract quantitative data from their ultrasound displays. Rather, their paper described problems that they experienced in using the equipment. They did, nonetheless, report descriptive information which indicates that the images they obtained portrayed movement patterns compatible with current understanding of velopharyngeal function. Medial movement was detected in non-nasal contexts, and data obtained from one subject indicated that pharyngeal wall displacement anticipated the onset of speech as reflected by an oscillographic voice trace. Ryan and Hawkins found no evidence of lateral wall motion outward from the rest position at the level of velopharyngeal closure during the production of non-nasal consonants.

Skolnick et al. (1975) reported information gathered with multitransducer ultrasound equipment which they designed and built. They evaluated three normal subjects, one of whom had undergone a frontal cinefluorographic study. "The transducer is vertically oriented to the lateral side of the neck with its upper edge just below the external auditory canal and over or just behind the superior portion of the mandibular ramus. The transducer covers the level from the nasal to the oral pharyngeal region." Results obtained with ultrasound were similar to those reported by Skolnick and associates in other papers based on frontal videofluoroscopy. During phonation, as illustrated in this paper, movement of the lateral wall toward midline occurs in the upper portion of the pharynx. During swallow, the entire length of the lateral wall moves toward midline. This report said nothing about motions of the lateral wall away from midline and beyond the resting position.

Hawkins and Swisher (1978) used a multielement transducer to study movement of the lateral pharyngeal walls in three adult subjects. VCVCV contexts were studied; nine consonants, four vowels, three diphthongs, and two sentences were used. Movements of three segments of the lateral pharyngeal wall were described; each segment was 3 cm in vertical height. Segment 1, the top segment, which encompassed the velopharyngeal port area, tended to move toward midline for 12 to 15 mm except when nasal consonants were involved, in which case there was little movement.

Segment 2 was similar to the first in direction and extent of movement except that, during vowels associated with nasals, the lateral wall moved laterally 3 to 5 mm in segment 2, as contrasted with a medial movement of the same distance in segment 1. Segment 3 sometimes moved in a direction opposite to segments 1 and 2. For segment 3, the authors reported a medial movement of 5 mm for /a/, a 5-mm lateral movement for /æ/, and lateral movement of 10 to 12 mm for /i/ and /u/. They reported that, except where diphthongs were involved, the lateral wall maintains its medial displacement at segment 1 until the utterance is completed. The authors also reported a wavelike motion during monosyllabic words wherein "greatest medial displacement began at the level of the velum" and then gradually moved down the lateral pharyngeal wall. Hawkins and Swisher (1978) interpreted their data as supporting the findings of Minifie et al. (1970) and Zagzebski (1975). Different movement patterns are observed at different levels of the pharynx.

Endoscopy has also been used to study movement of the lateral walls of the pharynx in normal individuals. Pigott (1969), using a rigid nasendoscope, observed little movement of the lateral or posterior pharyngeal walls during rapid speech. He reported that lateral gutters were sometimes seen. Gutters, termed the fossa of Rosenmüller, are characteristic of the lateral pharyngeal walls. Sometimes the gutters were blocked by mucus and sometimes they were open, leaving a gap 2 to 3 mm in diameter. Nasal emission was not present despite these openings. In some subjects, the gutters were blocked by movement toward the midline of the salpingopharyngeus muscles. Passavant's ridge was not seen in these 25 normal subjects between 11 and 45 years of age.

Using oral endoscopy, Zwitman et al. (1976) rated movements of the lateral pharyngeal walls of 34 normal individuals uttering "a pup pup." Four scale values were used. The percentage of subjects assigned to each of the values was as follows: 1. (little or no lateral wall movement), 17.6%; 2. (lateral walls fill lateral gutters) 56%; 3. (midline movement of the lateral walls past the sides of the velum), 17.6%; and 4. (lateral walls approximate), 8.8%. These observations were confirmed by cineradiography.

In summary, the lateral pharyngeal walls have long been known to move during speech. However, until recently, the importance of that movement to the accomplishment of velopharyngeal closure for speech was often overlooked. It is now well established that the walls do move toward midline in many normal individuals during speech. That movement is probably greatest at the level of velar elevation. Lateral wall movement is related to speech context, with greatest movement occurring in contexts in which velopharyngeal closure is especially important. The lateral walls, at a lower level, appear to move outward during speech.

Synchronization of Velar and Pharyngeal Wall Movements

There is considerable interest in determining whether the velum and the lateral pharyngeal walls move in synchrony. Bjork (1961) obtained transverse tomograms of 10 normally speaking adults at rest and as they sustained /m/, /n/ and /n/. The films obtained illustrated the velopharyngeal port, the velum, and the dorsum of the tongue. Bjork reported that closure of the velopharyngeal port involved medial displacement of the lateral pharyngeal walls as well as movement of the velum. He illustrated the contour of the velopharyngeal port in transverse display during different acts and presented a scatter plot showing a very strong linear relationship between the area of the transverse displays of the velopharyngeal port as measured in square millimeters and the sagittal axis of the velopharyngeal port. These data suggested that a linear measurement of the velopharyngeal gap in sagittal display provided a good index to the area of the velopharyngeal opening. However, as is evident below, this did not prove to be true for everyone.

Zwitman et al. (1973) studied velopharyngeal motion by motion x-ray filming of the subject in what they termed a submentovertical projection. This is similar to the baseview described in Chapter 11. They wrote that the posterior portion of the lateral pharyngeal walls moves medially to fill the lateral gutters. The illustrations in this paper give a different perspective relative to the lateral walls than is obtained with baseview. The angle at which these films are taken may influence the information obtained. The matter of which portion of the lateral pharyngeal walls moves medially seems to deserve more attention.

Shprintzen et al. (1974, 1975a, 1975b) illustrated a shelf-like configuration of the lateral pharyngeal walls in speech, whistling, and blowing, which they termed pneumatic activities. Their analysis of their x-ray data indicated that shelves, which occurred at the point of the greatest range of motion in the lateral walls, were located below the velar eminence. The authors wrote that, in pneumatic activities, "it appears that closure consists of elevation and posterior movement of the velum plus the medial movement of the LAPW (lateral aspects of the pharyngeal wall) around the lateral edges of the velum." They stated that closure seems to occur between the posterior third of the velum and the pharyngeal walls, not at the level of the velar eminence (Fig. 12.8). Shelf-like configurations were also illustrated by Mason et al. (1973), but their x-ray tracings of subjects sustaining vowels show less symmetry in the two lateral pharyngeal walls than do the tracings of Shprintzen et al. The appearance of a shelf-like configuration is controversial in that some investigators using x-ray techniques have not reported it. Iglesias et al. (1980) speculated that the radiopaque material used by Shprintzen to outline the lateral walls may have resulted in the artificial appearance of shelves. Another possible explanation is that the investigators studied different planes.

Zwitman et al. (1974) used an oral endoscope to describe velopharyngeal closure in 34 persons between 6 and 40 years of age. They had normal voice quality, and no oral pathology was mentioned. Four patterns of velopharyngeal closure were described.

1. Lateral walls move medially and fuse as the velum touches the approximated section of the lateral walls.
2. Lateral walls almost approximate, with the velum contacting the lateral walls and partly occluding the space between them. A small medial opening is observed in some cases.

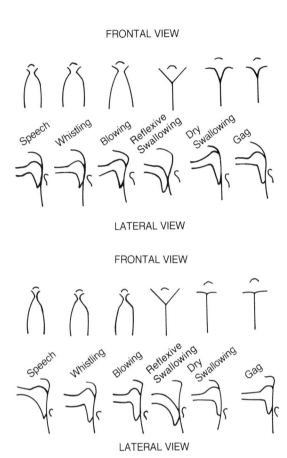

Figure 12.8 Tracings of frontal and lateral views during speech, whistling, blowing, reflexive swallowing, dry swallowing, and gagging. (From Shprintzen RJ, Lencione RM, McCall GN, Skolnick ML. A three-dimensional cinefluoroscopic analysis of velopharyngeal closure during speech and nonspeech activities in normals. Cleft Palate J 1974; 11:412.)

3. Lateral walls move medially, filling the lateral pharyngeal gutters and fusing with the raised velum as it contacts the posterior walls.
4. Lateral walls move slightly or not at all. Velum touches posterior wall at midline and lateral openings are observed during phonation.

Four of the subjects, one in each closure category, were studied by motion x-ray, which confirmed the patterns obtained with the endoscope.

Skolnick (1975) summarized descriptive research directed to motions of the pharyngeal walls in speech and other acts. These studies ultilized videofluoroscopic records in midsagittal, frontal, and base views. Skolnick described three patterns of velopharyngeal motion in normal persons who achieve closure: (1) simultaneous displacement of velum and lateral pharyngeal walls with roughly equal contributions from each or perhaps with a "somewhat greater velar than pharyngeal motion;" (2) a circular motion (with or without Passavant's ridge), characterized by relatively great medial motion of the lateral walls and a "shortened velum or reduced velar movement;" (3) a sagittal pattern wherein the lateral walls move markedly toward midline and the palate touches those lateral walls rather than the posterior wall. Skolnick acknowledged within subject variability in the contribution of velum and lateral walls to closure. Figure 12.9 shows the patterns he observed for both normal and pathological speakers.

Witzel and Posnick (1989) viewed patterns and location of velopharyngeal valving problems of 246 patients by nasopharyngoscopy. They reported that in these patients, a coronal pattern of closure was most often seen (60%), followed by a circular pattern (23%). Circular pattern with Passavant's ridge and sagittal pattern were seen infrequently (5% and 4%, respectively). The majority (66%) of velopharyngeal gaps detected were central.

The data reviewed here seem to establish that the lateral pharyngeal walls and the velum work synchronously to achieve velopharyngeal closure for speech, but that normal individuals differ in the relative contribution of velum and pharyngeal walls to closure. The study by Zwitman et al. (1974) suggests that medial motion of the more posterior portion of the lateral pharyngeal walls is especially important. Pigott (1969) also mentioned the lateral gutters of the pharynx. The presence of these gutters would seem to make medial movement of the lateral walls especially important. We trust that, in time, the interaction of the velum and the lateral walls during speech will be more precisely described.

Opening the Velopharyngeal Port

Little consideration has been given to the possible clinical significance of the mechanism whereby the velopharyngeal port is opened. However, the current interest in nasal airway obstruction associated with some pharyngeal flaps raises the possibility that attention to the structure and function of the opening mechanism could contribute to a patient's well-being. Bell-Berti (1980) observed that there are two possible mechanisms

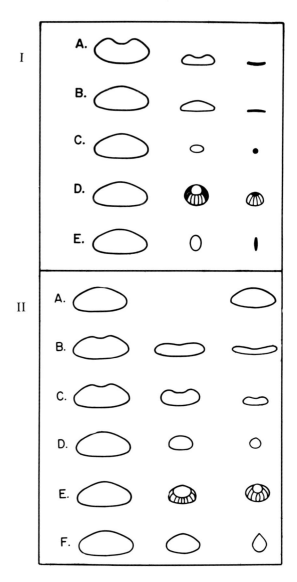

Figure 12.9 Schematic representation of sphincteric patterns of velopharyngeal competence, base view. Left column: contour of portal at rest; middle column: partial closure; right column: full closure. I. A, Normal subject. Note convex projection of uvula portion of velum into velopharyngeal portion at rest. B, Repaired cleft palate subject. Note absence of uvula muscle bulge at rest. Pattern of closure is coronal, similar to subject in A. C, Circular closure pattern, repaired cleft palate. D, Circular closure pattern with Passavant's ridge, repaired cleft palate. Ridge is represented by stippled and lined area in middle and extreme right columns. E, Sagittal closure pattern, repaired cleft palate. II. A, Essentially no velar or pharyngeal wall movement. B, Postadenoidectomy with good velar and almost no pharyngeal wall movement. C, Average coronal narrowing pattern. D, Circular narrowing pattern. E, Circular narrowing pattern with Passavant's ridge (lined areas). F, Sagittal narrowing pattern. (From Skolnick ML. Velopharyngeal function in cleft palate. Clin Plast Surg 1975; 2:285.)

of velopharyngeal port opening. The first is simple relaxation of the muscles involved in closure. Alternatively, contraction of muscles antagonistic to closure may be involved. The most likely muscles are the palatopharyngeus and the palatoglossus. Bell-Berti cited evidence that the palatopharyngeus muscles show more electromyographic activity during open than closed vowels. She thought the muscles might narrow the faucial isthmus for open vowels. The palatoglossus muscles appear to elevate the tongue dorsum and, during production of low vowels, to narrow the faucial isthmus. Bell-Berti concluded that velopharyngeal opening involves the natural tendency of tissue to return to its resting posture. In the velopharyngeal mechanism this occurs upon cessation of activity by the muscles that closed the valve. In some persons, contraction of the palatoglossus muscles may assist in this process.

Data presented and reviewed by Fritzell (1979) and Lubker (1975) are compatible with Bell-Berti's interpretation. They reported that levator electromyographic activity decreases or ceases prior to velopharyngeal port opening, and nasal sounds are sometimes preceded by activity in the palatoglossus muscle. Lubker noted that the palatoglossus has several functions, including elevating and stabilizing the tongue as well as depressing the velum. Fritzell wrote that this muscle is especially important to establishment of a velar-lingual seal, which is employed in breathing through the nose when the mouth is open. The function of the palatoglossus at a particular moment depends on the activity of other muscles. Lubker wrote that this muscle coarticulates with other muscles and that the coarticulation is centrally programmed. He described the levator as contributing to velopharyngeal opening by cessation of activity. Working in conjunction with the levator, the palatoglossus provides a "pull" on the velum. This coordination varies, depending on the phonetic context being articulated.

PATTERNS OF VELOPHARYNGEAL CLOSURE

In this section, we review reports concerning function of the velopharyngeal valve by persons with cleft palate or other velopharyngeal disorders. The literature does not lend itself to the structure-by-structure organization that we employed in considering normal function. Here the literature deals primarily with observations of closure of the valve.

Patterns of velopharngeal closure in patients with cleft palate have been charted from midsagittal cinefluorographic films using frame-by-frame measurements of the distance between the velum and the posterior pharyngeal wall (Bjork, 1961). Some patients with cleft palate present normal closure patterns in that they achieve closure prior to utterance onset and maintain it until a nasal consonant is produced or the utterance is finished. Some may usually or sometimes achieve closure but show velopharyngeal gaps whcre normal individuals would be closed (Shelton et al. 1964). Others may never achieve closure even though velopharyngeal motions are produced; still others may not move.

Skolnick (1975) identified three patterns of velopharyngeal closure from multiview x-ray studies of patients with cleft palate: (1) simultaneous movement of the velum and lateral walls, (2) a circular motion with relatively greater motion of the lateral walls than of the velum, and (3) a pattern in which lateral walls move toward midline, but the velum moves little. He wrote that similar movement patterns were evident in individuals who failed to achieve velopharyngeal closure. Skolnick described two additional patterns as well: (4) no movement of the velum or pharyngeal walls, and (5) motion of the velum in the absence of medial movement of the lateral pharyngeal walls. Figure 12-9B shows pathological patterns.

Shprintzen et al. (1977) described velar and lateral pharyngeal wall motions in five patients who failed to achieve velopharyngeal closure. Three of the five had cleft palates. The subjects ranged in age from 4 through 33 years. Each subject was taped by videofluoroscopy in the sagittal, frontal, and base views. Some of these patients moved the velum, but not the pharyngeal walls; others moved the lateral pharyngeal walls, but not the velum. The authors reiterated that medial movements of the lateral pharyngeal walls are essential to velopharyngeal closure.

Patients have been observed on cinefluorography to move away from velopharyngeal closure during the production of /s/ in words or sentences (Shelton et al. 1964; Brandt and Morris, 1965). Hagerty et al. (1968) hypothesized that poor velar movement prior to secondary surgical procedures may reflect functional surrender.

Other patterns have been reported wherein patients close on some non-nasal speech sounds, but not on others. Some patients often produce stops and /f/ correctly while emitting other pressure consonants nasally (Peterson, 1975). Van Demark et al. (1979) inferred that such a pattern is incompatible with velopharyngeal incompetence or even with marginal incompetence.

Some patients with cleft palate may use the velopharyngeal valving mechanism satisfactorily except when under stress. For some children, nasal emission limited to sounds from a phoneme or two may be a learned phonological pattern. Some patients resolve these patterns in short order with articulation training.

A number of investigators have looked at lateral wall motion using the endoscope. Zwitman et al. (1976) rated velar and lateral pharyngeal motions during "a papa pup" as observed through an oral telescope (endoscope) and cineradiography. They used a 4-point rating scale to evaluate both sets of data. Subjects were 31 individuals between 3 and 20 years of age with different degrees of velopharyngeal insufficiency. Twenty-three of the patients had had a cleft palate repair. Ninety percent of the velar ratings obtained with the two instruments agreed, as did 88% of the lateral wall ratings. Ratings of lateral pharyngeal wall motions were reported for 20 patients with cleft palate whose velar motions were categorized as 1, 2, 3, or 4, on a 4-point scale, which ranged from little or no wall movement through touch closure. More of the subjects with cleft palate fell into category 1 and fewer into categories 3 and 4 than did normal individuals also studied by these investigators. They reported that over one-third of their patients with cleft palate who had inadequate velar movement did not produce medial lateral pharyngeal wall motion.

Matsuya et al. (1979) studied 68 Japanese subjects with cleft aged 11 to 40 years for achievement of velopharyngeal closure during speech and nonspeech acts. A nasal fiberscope was used to observe the velopharyngeal mechanism. Their findings suggested a task hierarchy in which subjects are most likely to close during swallowing, then blowing, then on consonants, and finally on vowels.

Shprintzen et al. (1980) used nasopharyngoscopy in conjunction with still and super-8 motion picture photography to describe velopharyngeal motions in patients with facioauriculovertebral malformation complex (hemifacial microsomia).

They reported that 12 of 22 patients had velopharyngeal incompetence. Six of the subjects had cleft palates; the velopharyngeal openings were off midline in all but one subject. The authors reported that the pharyngeal walls move less well on the affected side than on the unaffected side and that, in three subjects, the unaffected side was ". . . seen to move past midline toward the affected side." The palate moved asymmetrically toward the unaffected side during speech. The authors inferred that the lateral gaps observed probably reflected hypoplasia of both the velar and pharyngeal muscle groups that contribute to veloparyngeal closure.

Osberg and Witzel (1981) used nasendoscopy to study velar and pharyngeal wall motion in patients with cleft who had had primary palatal surgery. One group consisted of six patients with ratings of 3 to 6 on a 6-point hypernasality scale; the other group consisted 13 persons whose ratings were 1 or 2. The subjects free from hypernasality moved toward closure with velar elevation; there was little lateral wall motion. The hypernasal subjects, on the other hand, approximated closure through medial movement of the lateral walls. One patient was able to shift from hypernasal to nonhypernasal voice; in doing so, he shifted from lateral wall to velar movement, and the shape of the opening changed from "a circular midline defect to a transverse slit-like gap." The authors offered an interpretation that slit-like openings associated with velar motion allow less air flow than circular openings with similar cross-sectional areas. The latter openings are associated with medial movement of the lateral pharyngeal walls. No reliability information about the endoscopic data are provided. Minifie et al. (1974) stated that particle velocity is most efficiently converted into sound pressure in circular orifices. Elliptical orifices are less efficient noise generators when the cross-sectional areas are the same. Warren (personal communication) questioned the work of Osberg and Witzel (1981) because nasal air flow was not measured, and the turbulent elements of speech air flow were not taken into account. Osberg and Witzel made explicit an hypothesis that has been speculated about informally from time to time. However, available data do not warrant their inference that the shape of the velopharyngeal orifice influences speech characteristics.

OTHER VELOPHARYNGEAL MOVEMENT PHENOMENA

Additional velopharyngeal movement phenomena have been described that are relevant to both normal and pathological function. These will be considered next. The first topic is Passavant's ridge.

Passavant's Ridge

A movement of pharyngeal tissue into the pharynx during speech was first reported by Passavant in the 1800s. He described the formation of a pad or ridge on the posterior wall of a patient with an unrepaired cleft palate. Glaser (1980) defined Passavant's ridge as:

. . . a localized anterior projection of the posterior pharyngeal wall as opposed to the generalized posterior pharyngeal wall motion seen within a broad inferior-superior range with little, if any, localized movement [Fig. 12.10]. The ridge is not a permanent projection, but instead is a "functional structure" which appears during certain velopharyngeal valving activities such as speech.

We will review reports descriptive of the structure and function of Passavant's ridge. Descriptions of the structure deal with such matters as the form of the ridge, its location, the function during which it occurs, and its consistency or frequency of occurrence with repetitions of an act. Function issues include: (1) How is the ridge formed physiologically? (2) What variables are related to it? (3) What variables influence it? (4) What functions does it serve? and (5) How is it acquired?

A distinctive form of pharyngeal wall movement, Passavant's ridge, is usually discussed in association with cleft palate rather than with normal subjects. Nonetheless, Passavant's ridge has been reported in many normal subjects. In radiographic research, Calnan (1957) reported Passavant's ridge in 20 percent of a group of 20 normal, adult subjects. Fletcher (1957) identified the ridge during phonation by three of ten normal children. Some of his subjects also produced the ridge when swallowing. Passavant's ridge in one normal subject was photographed through an oral endoscope (Shelton et al. 1975). The ridge was said to vary during voluntary velopharyngeal closure from slight to marked displacement and to occur in the absence of other forward movements of the posterior wall. The ridge was evident on the posterior wall and extended toward the lateral wall, disappearing behind the posterior pillar of the fauces. Passavant's inference that the ridge is a normal part of velopharyngeal closure for speech proved incorrect in that many normal persons, as well as many persons with cleft palate, do not produce the ridge.

Much of the research involving Passavant's ridge in pathological speakers has employed cine- or videofluorography. Before summarizing findings from several studies, we will consider the methodology employed in two studies that bear on several of the issues under consideration. Carpenter (1966) and Carpenter and Morris (1968) studied Passavant's ridge by cinefluorography in six subjects who had surgically repaired palatal clefts. The subjects ranged in age from 8 to 18 years. The pad was studied during utterance of /s/, /z/, /u/, and /æ/ under the following conditions: normal effort, rapid rate, half rapid rate, blowing, and swallowing. The pad was studied at various intervals before, during, and after 5 minutes of connected speech that included reading or repetition of three sentences constructed around plosive, fricative, or nasal consonants. This study was motivated in part by Calnan's report that Passavant's ridge is inconsistent and subject to fatigue and hence unsuitable for service as a mechanism compensatory for velopharyngeal insufficiency.

The second study to be considered for methodology was performed by Glaser (1980). This study was a descriptive analysis of multiview, videofluorographic tapes. The tapes were recorded in two settings for clinical purposes. Consequently, a standard set of performances was not recorded for each subject, and magnification was not controlled. The subjects were 29 persons, 4 through 30 years of age. Each subject presented Passavant's ridge. Twenty-two had surgically repaired cleft palates, one a repaired submucous cleft palate, one had velopharyngeal incompetence with no overt cleft, two post-tonsillectomy-adenoidectomy velopharyngeal incompetence, one had spastic dysphonia, and two were normal volunteers. No subject presented an unrepaired cleft, a pharyngeal flap, mental retardation, or hearing loss. Measurements were made from photographs of videofluorographic frames.

Shape

Passavant's ridge has been described as taking different configurations: shelf-like, semicircular, elliptical, and triangular. Glaser (1980) reported that in 81.8% of her subjects the ridge was usually perpendicular to the velum. In the remaining subjects the ridge was directed upward or downward. She reported that, among persons who have Passavant's ridge, a common pattern is for the ridge to take a crescent shape continuing along the lateral pharyngeal walls. In patients presenting this pattern, as viewed through baseview videofluorography, the velopharyngeal closure configuration is circular. Zwitman (1982a) differentiated between Passavant's ridge and the lateral pharyngeal wall. He said the two are demarcated by a hairline fissure visible through oral endoscopy.

Location

The location of the ridge is variable across subjects. Glaser (1980) recommended that the ridge be described relative to the velum (Fig. 12.10) rather than to the atlas because that reference is more pertinent to velopharyngeal closure. The location of the velum relative to the atlas is not constant across subjects, and within subjects it varies with age. For 69% of Glaser's subjects the ridge was commonly positioned opposite the vertical portion of the velum, and for 15 percent the ridge was positioned opposite the velar eminence. Glaser et al. (1979) reported that in 43 patients who produced the ridge, it occurred opposite the velar eminence in 4.7%, opposite the vertical portion of the velum in 58.1%, opposite the uvula in 25.6%, and below the uvula in 11.6%. In 72% of her 29 subjects, the ridge usually occurred at the "primary site of narrowing or closure," and 48% used the same constriction pattern for all speech tasks. She also identified instances in which the ridge is not in the primary region of velopharyngeal constriction.

Carpenter (1966) and Carpenter and Morris (1968) found the ridge to occur at the same level in nasal and non-nasal consonants, but to project further during the non-nasals. In some persons the ridge was located where it did not contribute to closure. In the Glaser et al, report (1979) the presence of a high-placed ridge was more frequently associated with hypernasality than was a low-placed ridge. Both Weiss (1972) and Glaser et

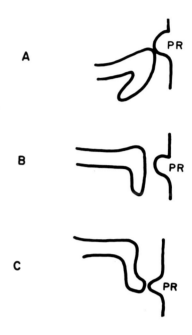

Figure 12.10 Passavant's ridge as a primary source of velopharyngeal narrowing or closure. Pattern A: velar eminence to Passavant's ridge; Pattern B: vertical portion of velum to Passavant's ridge; Pattern C: uvula to Passavant's ridge. (From Glaser ER, Skolnick ML, McWilliams BJ, Shprintzen RJ. The dynamics of Passavant's ridge in subjects with and without velopharyngeal insufficiency—a multiview videofluoroscopic study. Cleft Palate J 1979; 16:24.)

al. (1979) wrote that a low-positioned ridge that does not participate in closure may nonetheless partially deflect sound waves from the velopharyngeal port.

Functions in Which It Occurs

Descriptions of Passavant's ridge usually involve speech and swallow. The ridge is sometimes observed in other acts that involve velopharyngeal closure, for example, whistling and blowing. Descriptions of those acts will not be reviewed. Relative to swallow, we will simply acknowledge that the ridge has been observed and described. Carpenter (1966) did not observe the ridge during swallow in any of her subjects who presented it during speech, and the ridge was larger during swallow than during speech in those subjects who produced the ridge in both activities. In Glaser's research (1980) the superior boundary of Passavant's ridge during speech was higher than the corresponding boundary of the bulge observed during swallow. Posterior pharyngeal wall movement was lower in the pharynx during deglutition than during speech, and the bulge observed during swallow was less discrete than the ridge seen during speech. There may be a difference of opinion about whether the ridge in speech and the ridge in swallow are similar phenomena.

Consistency

The extent to which Passavant's ridge occurs in different speech acts and in repetitions of an act within an individual has been studied. Shelton et al. (1964) reported that their three subjects who produced Passavant's ridges did so during each phonation studied. Carpenter (1966) and Carpenter and Morris (1968) reported that the velum and pad assumed a phonation position that was maintained throughout an utterance except for phrasing interruptions. Movement was greater during consonants than vowels. The pad was not influenced by the task variations introduced by Carpenter and Morris during the production of isolated speech sounds. Indeed, patterns of performance were similar for all subjects under the various task conditions studied. Carpenter and Morris wrote:

... although the basic composition of the mechanism differed somewhat for each subject studied, pad activity was found to be consistent both within and between individuals. Admittedly, the internal consistency was greater, but if pad activity is considered as compensatory behavior, consistency within individuals, as compared to between, might be considered the more important factor.

Nonetheless, Passavant's ridge is not present throughout speech in all individuals in whom it appears. However, its presence seems related to speech context (Glaser, 1980).

The Physiological Formation of Passavant's Ridge

The physiological mechanism whereby Passavant's ridge is produced is uncertain. According to one viewpoint, muscle contraction pulling up on the pharynx results in a passive folding of tissue which constitutes the ridge. Glaser preferred an explanation that postulates a more active, muscular ridge. It should be noted that the concept of passive tissue does not explain the perpendicular orientation of the ridge to the velum that she observed in her study. She noted that different individuals may form the ridge by different means. She observed that no postmortem anatomical studies have been performed on persons known to have produced the ridge.

Calnan (1957) provided an excellent discussion about the phenomenon and a theoretical framework by which the mechanism could be considered part of velopharyngeal activity. He asserted that the ridge could not be part of the normal velopharyngeal mechanism because it is inconsistent in appearance; it frequently is too low in the velopharynx to assist in velopharyngeal competence; its activity is too "slow;" and it is prone to fatigue. In general, he maintained that use of Passavant's pad during speech was "uneconomical." Further, he concluded that only rarely does the pad function adequately for compensation purposes. Some of these issues will be discussed in the following paragraphs.

Variables Related to Passavant's Ridge

Investigators have been particularly interested in the relationship between measures of the ridge and measures of velopharyngeal structure and function. Shelton et al. (1964) reported that their three subjects who produced Passavant's ridge each presented a different pattern of velopharyngeal function as observed through use of lateral cinefluorography. One showed normal closure wherein closure was completed before the initiation of phonation and was maintained until phonation was terminated or a nasal consonant occurred. A second subject usually closed during the course of phonation, but breaks occurred that were not associated with nasal consonants or end of phonation. The third subject sometimes closed during the course of an utterance, but was usually open. Massengill et al. (1969) found no relationship between size of velopharyngeal port and presence of a Passavant's ridge in subjects with cleft palate. Nor was the occurrence of a ridge associated with cleft type or surgical procedure.

In Glaser's study, the depth of the ridge was related to the minimal velopharyngeal gap and to the gap between the ridge and the velum. These two measures may have been the same in some subjects. Velar elevation was related to area depth of Passavant's ridge. Among her 32 subjects with adequate baseview videofluoroscopic studies, 78.1% presented a circular pattern of velopharyngeal narrowing or closing, 15.6% had a coronal pattern, 3.1% oval patterns, and 3.1% had sagittal patterns. Passavant's ridge contributed to the coronal pattern. Glaser noted that we do not know whether the occurrence of Passavant's ridge is greater in older than in younger subjects.

A particularly important issue is the degree to which Passavant's ridge formation occurs in synchrony with movement of the velum and lateral pharyngeal walls toward closure. Carpenter (1966) reported that in connected speech the velum and ridge moved synchronously, but that motion of the ridge appeared to lag behind that of the velum in time. Synchrony of velum and ridge movement was reported by Glaser (1979) but was not observed by Calnan (1957).

Several authors have discussed the apparent influence of surgery or training on Passavant's ridge. Nylen (1961) described velopharyngeal function in patients with cleft palate before and after surgery. The ridge was observed preoperatively in 11 of 27 patients and after surgery in only six patients. He drew no causal interpretation of the relationship between surgery and the occurrence of Passavant's ridge. Zwitman (1982b), in an oral endoscopic study of patients before and after pharyngeal flap surgery, reported that ridge motion was reduced in all patients after the surgery. He wrote that the lateral segments of the ridge can contract even after the central portion of the ridge has been excised in pharyngeal flap surgery.

Weiss (1972) reported that Passavant's ridge was present in 2 of 16 patients who improved their velopharyngeal function through obturator reduction. Those patients may have presented the ridge prior to treatment. No radiographic studies were done prior to training. Glaser (1980) reported that ridge and no-ridge groups were not different to a statistically significant degree in terms of the number of persons with a history of speech therapy.

Acquisition of Passavant's Ridge

The means whereby the ridge is acquired are unknown. No one has described the development of Passavant's ridge in longitudinal observations in experimental studies directed to improvement of velopharyngeal function. Carpenter and Morris (1968) discussed occurrence of the ridge as learned behavior resulting from the occurrence of feedback or reinforcement. Alternatively, the ridge may be developed through unconscious problem-solving. If the ridge is compensatory, the question arises as to why some individuals do not develop the compensation. Also, a compensation hypothesis does not explain the occurrence of Passavant's ridge in normal individuals.

Function of Passavant's Ridge

It appears that Passavant's ridge does contribute to velopharyngeal closure in some of the patients who demonstrate the ridge. In their sagittal cinefluorographic study, Shelton et al. (1964) reported that the ridge contributed to closure in two of the three subjects showing a ridge. Ridges also contributed to closure or to reduction in velopharyngeal area in some subjects studied by Carpenter and Morris (1968). These investigators indicated that, in persons with repaired clefts, the pad functions as an addition to the closure mechanism and does not disturb the closure process. Earlier we reported that 72% of the subjects studied by Glaser (1980) produced their ridges at the site of velopharyngeal narrowing or closure. For 24%, the ridge was located at a secondary constriction site. In the final 4%, the ridge was located below the level of the velum.

We conclude from the literature reviewed that Passavant's ridge contributes to velopharyngeal closure in some patients who otherwise would not achieve closure. In that sense, the mechanism is compensatory for some persons. This ridge develops spontaneously in some, but certainly not all, individuals with velopharyngeal insufficiency. The important consideration, as Glaser concluded, is that there is high intra- and intersubject variability in the occurrence and configuration of Passavant's ridge and that each patient must be viewed on an individual basis.

Firmness of Velopharyngeal Closure During Speech

Another variable in velopharyngeal closure that has not received much study is the firmness of closure when closure is achieved. Nusbaum et al. (1935) studied the firmness of velopharyngeal closure during the production of English vowels by use of a device that allowed them to direct air pressure into the nose and a U-tube water manometer simultaneously. They reported that, for men, the pressures associated with the release of the velopharyngeal port in response to air pressure introduced during a vowel averaged 23 cm H_2O for /u/ and, for women, 16 cm H_2O. Unpublished exploratory research utilized placement of a pressure-sensing tube through the nose and velopharyngeal port as a means of studying firmness of closure.

Goto (1977) found that, in normal persons and in cleft palate persons with closure, tightness of velopharyngeal closure decreased from that observed in hard blowing to that associated with swallow when followed by pressure consonants and then by vowels. The strength of velopharyngeal closure was correlated with levator EMG activity. It was inferred from the data that, in normal individuals, firmness of velopharyngeal closure is produced by the levator.

The observation that small velopharyngeal openings are sometimes compatible with speech that is within normal limits suggests that firmness of velopharyngeal closure is not a clinically important variable. Alternatively, firmness of closure may be a factor in borderline valving mechanisms. Various authors have described nasal noises and snorts in addition to audible nasal emission (Bzoch, 1965; Trost, 1981). Some speakers may release air nasally after impounding some air orally for stops or fricatives. The resulting fricative or affricative noise would be different from audible nasal emission. If this does indeed happen, it may reflect a lack of firmness of closure.

Timing of Velopharyngeal Phenomena

The timing of velopharyngeal closure during speech production appears to bear upon the adequacy of the resulting speech signal. In normal function, the velum elevates, and closure is accomplished just before the initiation of an utterance that begins with a non-nasal sound, and in some persons, motion of the velum and formation of Passavant's ridge are synchronized. Kuehn and Moll (1976) reviewed the literature and presented data about timing patterns of the velum in normal subjects. They found a direct relationship between articulatory velocity and displacement.

Several investigators have raised the question of whether some aspects of velopharyngeal dysfunction reflect problems in timing of the

movements involved. For example, the velopharyngeal structures may be of sufficient size and position to achieve velopharyngeal closure, and they may be capable of normal range of motion. However, they may not be capable of normal rate of synchrony of movement, and hypernasality and other speech deficits may result (Netsell, 1969; Warren, 1967; Fritzell, 1969).

Warren and Mackler (1968) observed that the duration of oral port constriction for voiceless consonants is increased in subjects with cleft who have good closure compared to those with poor closure. Normal speakers used shorter durations for voiceless consonants than did either of the two groups with cleft palates. Duration was determined from measurements of intraoral pressure. Oral port constriction was greatest for voiceless fricative consonants. The authors hypothesized that speakers with cleft palate who had good closure extend the duration of oral port constriction to provide more acoustic cues and thus increase intelligibility. The speakers with poor closure do not use this compensatory phenomenon, presumably because it would be accompanied by an increase in nasal escape of air.

Rolnick and Hoops (1971) studied plosive phoneme duration spectrographically in 20 subjects with and without obturators. Duration was increased upon removal of the prosthesis. The increase in duration was seen as an attempt at compensation for poor velopharyngeal closure. Rolnick and Hoops did not compare their results with those of Warren and Mackler. Differences can be accounted for in terms of subject characteristics or the measurement procedures used. Warren and Mackler presented questions for investigation concerning increase in phone duration as a compensation for palatopharyngeal closure deficits.

Any theory that is sufficient to explain velopharyngeal function must account for timing phenomena. Central programming of the coordinated movements involved in velopharyngeal closure will be a topic of future research as will the extent to which timing problems can be modified, at least in part, by behavioral management.

Zimmerman et al. (1984) observed an association between hypernasality and the tardiness of velopharyngeal closure relative to voice onset and achievement of maximum vocal tract constriction. They inferred that lowering of the mandible and tongue may constrain movement of the velum.

Warren et al. (1985) studied temporal relationships between oral air pressure and nasal air flow in the word *hamper* as produced by groups of persons differing in velopharyngeal competency. Within a subgroup presenting borderline velopharyngeal adequacy, the occurrence of hypernasality was associated with overlap between nasal flow associated with /m/ and the pressure peak associated with /p/.

GENDER DIFFERENCES IN VELOPHARYNGEAL FUNCTION

McKerns and Bzoch (1970) measured the angle formed by the posterior nasal spine, the superior point of contact between the elevated palate and the posterior wall of the pharynx, and the inferior point of the uvula for normal men and women who ranged in age between 19 and 32 years. The measures were made from sagittal cinefluorographic film frames. They found the angle to be acute in males and more nearly a right angle in females. They also found the height of velar elevation to be greater in men than in women but extent of contact between the velum and posterior pharyngeal wall to be less in men. The inferior point of this contact was usually above the palatal plane in the men but not in the women.

Other investigators have also examined male-female differences. Kuehn (1976) studied the sagittal cinefluorographs of one normal male and one normal female and reported that the male's palatal displacement followed a steeper path than did the female's. Kuehn interpreted these data as agreeing with those of McKerns and Bzoch (1970) and Simpson and Austin (1972). Seaver and Kuehn (1980) compared their three normal young women and three normal young men relative to velopharyngeal function observed cinefluorographically at 100 film frames per second and by electromyography. A goal of this study was to identify variables that would predict velar height. The women changed velar height more than the men did. Tongue height appeared to be related to velar height in males. They wrote, "For the female subjects, palatoglossus was found to be the most consistent inferiorly positioned variable in the predictions of velar height change. In both sexes, the palatoglossus muscle was the least accurate predictor." Iglesias et al. (1980) studied normal speakers on simultaneous lateral still radiographs and frontal tomograms and found no difference between male and female young adults in angle of velar movement. They noted that their criteria for

subject selection differed from those used by McKerns and Bzoch (1970).

Thompson and Hixon (1979) compared normal male and female subjects from three to 37.5 years of age on nasal air flow during speech. They found that 70% of the persons who produced nasal flow at the midpoint of the initial vowel in /ini/ were female. They speculated that this finding reflected a biomechanical difference between the two sexes. However, as an alternative explanation, they postulated that females may be more tolerant of nasalization.

In summary, men and women appear to differ somewhat in velopharyngeal physiology. Even if this is so, to date, the difference has not been shown to require consideration in the management of pathological speakers.

Age and Velopharyngeal Function

Growth and maturation of structures constituting the vocal tract result in change in velopharyngeal function with increase in age. Key structural changes include downward and forward growth of the facial skeleton. As this occurs, the posterior border of the hard palate also moves downward and forward, and consequently the nasopharynx enlarges in anteroposterior and vertical dimensions (Fletcher, 1966). The velum is displaced along with the hard palate. In the infant, the velum tends to parallel the roof of the pharynx, whereas in the adult it is more nearly parallel with the posterior wall of the pharynx. With maturation, movement of the velum changes from a superior-inferior direction to a more anteroposterior direction. The velum increases in thickness and in length, but the rates of growth of those two dimensions are different (Fletcher, 1966). Another maturational variable that influences velopharyngeal function is growth of the adenoid until the individual is 9 to 15 years of age. The period of growth is followed by a period of adenoidal involution that continues until in most persons the adenoid is vestigial.

Maturation of the speech mechanism involves change in coordination or skill as well as change in size and relationships of structures. Thompson and Hixon (1979) reported that there was a trend for more older than younger subjects to show nasal flow at the midpoint of the initial vowel in /ini/. They interpreted this as reflecting increased motor skill allowing enhancement of anticipatory coarticulation. Their data indicated that even their youngest subjects closed the velopharyngeal port during non-nasal speech sounds.

AERODYNAMICS OF VELOPHARYNGEAL FUNCTION

In 1950, Black published important data about intraoral air pressure during speech production that greatly influenced subsequent research in cleft palate. Although later investigations showed that Black's data overestimated the magnitude of air pressures involved in sound production (Hardy, 1965), his findings led cleft palate researchers to the discovery that velopharyngeal physiology and the aerodynamics of speech were importantly related. Investigators discovered that misarticulation associated with cleft palate tended to involve sounds that Black showed to be associated with high intraoral air pressure in normals.

The aerodynamics of speech production and associated speech physiology have been the topics of a large number of investigations. Among the early studies were those of Arkebauer et al. (1967), Subtelny et al. (1966), Isshiki et al. (1968), Warren (1964), Warren and Ryon (1967), and Warren et al. (1969). The findings of these investigators point to important interrelationships among oral air pressure, oral and nasal air flow rate, subglottic air pressure, function of the velopharyngeal mechanism, and other structural and physiological characteristics of the vocal tract. Aeromechanical research has provided a means for estimating the area of velopharyngeal openings as well as for studying closure requirements for speech. The sections that follow pertain to the relationship between velopharyngeal opening and (1) oropharyngeal air pressure, (2) area and duration of oral port opening, and (3) nasal pathway resistance to air flow. Airway turbulence and nasal air flow are also considered.

Velopharyngeal Port Area and Oral Air Pressure for Speech

As the velopharyngeal port opens beyond 20 mm^2, air pressure in the mouth falls off rapidly (Warren and Dubois, 1964). Respiratory air flow also influences oral air pressure during speech. Figure 12.11 shows differential oral-nasal air pressure for different velopharyngeal areas. Pressures are shown at volume rates of respiratory air

flow of 0.426 and 0.240 L/sec. At a given velopharyngeal orifice area, differential air pressures are higher at the high air flow rate. However, in each case, the differential air pressure falls rapidly with increase in size of the velopharyngeal orifice. Warren and Ryon (1967), from research using a vocal tract analog producing simulated plosives, reported oropharyngeal pressures at different velopharyngeal orifice areas when respiratory air flows of 0.88 and 0.240 L/sec were employed. At orifices of 20 mm^2 and larger, very little air pressure was developed at the lower rate of respiratory flow. However, a pressure of 4 cm H_2O was developed at 0.240 L/sec when the velopharyngeal orifice was 20 mm^2.

Investigators have reported oral air pressures in the ranges of 3 to 8 cm H_2O for stop plosives and 3 to 7 for fricatives (Arkebauer et al., 1967). Moderately higher values were reported by Subtelny et al. (1966). The data provided by Warren and his colleagues indicate that oral air pressure peaks of this magnitude can be developed with velopharyngeal ports as large as 20 mm^2 if sufficient respiratory flow is employed and the mouth is closed. However, turbulence across the velopharyngeal orifice and nasal airway would probably cause noise at those flow rates. Clearly velopharyngeal ports greater in estimated area than 20 mm^2 are insufficient for impounding oral

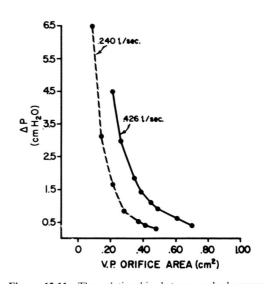

Figure 12.11 The relationship between velopharyngeal orifice area and oral-nasal differential air pressure at air flow rates of 0.240 and 0.426 L/sec. (From Warren DW, Devereux JL. An analog study of cleft palate speech. Cleft Palate J 1966; 3:103.)

air pressure for articulation, whereas lesser areas may permit build-up of the needed air pressures. This is not to say that lesser areas are satisfactory for normal speech. Warren and Ryon (1967) viewed the impact of the velopharyngeal mechanism on oral air pressure as dichotomous in the sense that increasing the velopharyngeal area beyond 20 mm² while holding other variables constant has little influence on oral air pressure.

Research by Isshiki et al. (1968) provided support for Warren's contention that velopharyngeal ports greater than 20 mm² will not permit unimpaired speech. These authors sought to identify the degree of velopharyngeal closure essential to speech by introducing velopharyngeal openings into normal speakers. The authors inserted tubes 4.5 cm in length through the velopharyngeal port and studied oral air pressure, nasal air flow, articulation, and nasality. The tubes were 0, 5, 7, 9, and 12 mm in internal diameter; the cross-sectioned area of the 5-mm tube was 19.6 mm². The critical degree of closure was to be defined in terms of observed alteration of speech as larger openings were introduced.

Peak oral air pressures of 9 and 8 cm H₂O were recorded with the 5- and 7-mm tubes. These oral air pressures are ample for articulation. However, the pressures measured with the 5-mm tube in use were accompanied by nasal air flows of between 200 and 300 cc/sec. The pressures seem high considering the amount of flow measured; however, information about rate of respiratory air flow was not reported. Nasal flow was observed with open tubes of each size, and larger flows were observed with progressively larger tubes. Misarticulation and hypernasality were associated with the 5-mm tube, and they became worse from tube to tube.

Isshiki et al. concluded that a port created by insertion of an open tube with a 5-mm diameter was sufficient to interfere with speech; consequently, a larger opening would not be acceptable. Since speech was somewhat hypernasal and articulation was affected in subjects wearing the 5-mm tube, it also seems unreasonable to accept 5-mm diameter openings (19.6 mm² area) as satisfactory for speech production. Openings between zero and 5 mm in diameter were not studied. It is possible that the pressure-sensing tube was partially collapsed by the velopharyngeal muscles. However, this seems unlikely considering the large nasal flows observed. Nasal leaks around the outside of the catheter were possible. The authors stated that the tubes were sufficiently long (4.5

cm) to prevent tissue from occluding either end of the tube.

Subtelny et al. (1966) found intraoral air pressure to be greater for children than for adult females and greater for adult females than for adult males. Brown and McGlone (1969), however, found no relationship between size of vocal tract and intraoral air pressure for speech activities. Vocal tract size was estimated for cephalometric radiographs and dental study models.

Intraoral air pressure is greater at higher than at lower speech intensities (Arkebauer et al., 1967; Brown and McGlone, 1969). Arkebauer wrote:

Impounding relatively high peak intraoral air pressures may not be the crucial problem of the speaker with a cleft. Rather, maintaining kinetic aerodynamic energy within the oral cavity over the time necessary to produce a continuant consonant may be the more significant problem.

Oral Port Opening, Intraoral Air Pressure, and Articulation

The opening of the oral port also influences oral air pressure during speech. Warren and Devereux (1966) demonstrated with the vocal

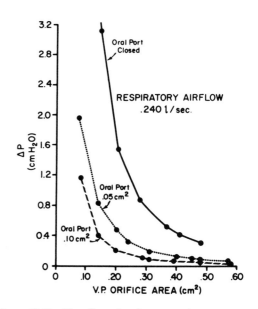

Figure 12.12 The effect of oral port opening on pressure-area relationships. Opening the oral port slightly for simulated fricatives significantly decreases orifice pressure unless air flow rate is increased. The difference in pressure is greatest when velopharyngeal orifice size is small. (From Warren DW, Devereux JL. An analog study of cleft palate speech. Cleft Palate J 1966; 3:103.)

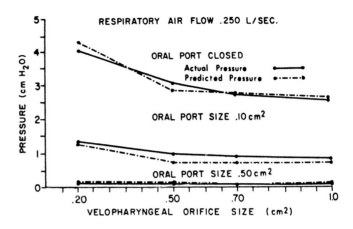

Figure 12.13 The relationship between velopharyngeal orifice area and oral air pressure under three oral port conditions: closed, 10 mm² opening, and 50 mm² opening. All data were obtained at a respiratory air flow of 0.250 L/sec. (From Warren DW, Ryon WE. Oral port constriction, nasal resistance, and respiratory aspects of cleft palate speech: an analog study. Cleft Palate J 1967; 4:38.)

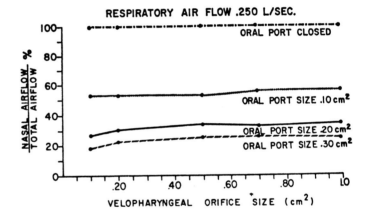

Figure 12.14 The percentage of total air flow that travels through the nose decreases with size of oral port opening essentially regardless of size of velopharyngeal opening. All data were gathered at a respiratory air flow of 0.250 L/sec. (From Warren DW, Ryon WE. Oral port constriction, nasal resistance, and respiratory aspects of cleft palate speech: an analog study. Cleft Palate J 1967; 4:38.)

tract analog that, at a respiratory air flow of 0.240 L/sec, oral-nasal differential air pressure declined as the oral port was opened to 5 mm² and then to 10 mm². Figure 12.12 shows interaction between oral port orifice and velopharyngeal orifice area in influencing oral-nasal differential air pressure as studied at a respiratory air flow rate of 0.240 L/sec. These studies suggest that a velopharyngeal opening of 20 mm² or less would have greater impact on fricatives than stops because there is an oral opening for fricatives and none for stops.

Similar data were reported by Warren and Ryon (1967). As reported in Figure 12.13, the amount of oral air pressure (as contrasted with oral-nasal differential air pressure in Fig. 12.12) available at a respiratory air flow of 0.250 L/sec was essentially zero at an oral port opening area of

50 mm² regardless of the size of the velopharyngeal orifice. When the oral port area of opening was 10 mm² and the velopharyngeal opening was 20 mm², about 1.4 cm H_2O was built up in the mouth. When the oral port was closed, however, about 4 cm H_2O pressure built up in the mouth, even though the velopharyngeal port was open to an area of 20 mm².

Warren and Ryon also reported evidence which indicated that, with increase in oral port opening, the percentage of total flow that passes through the nose decreases. For a given oral port size, the percentage of air passing through the nose was constant at velopharyngeal areas from 10 through 100 mm² (Fig. 12.14).

Speaking with clenched teeth and hence a nearly closed mouth may facilitate impoundment of oral air pressure but at the cost of increased nasal air flow. Articulatory gestures may be impaired also.

Nasal Pathway Resistance

High nasal pathway resistance, that is, resistance to air flow in the passages above the velopharyngeal port, may facilitate build-up of oral air pressure in individuals with velopharyngeal openings during speech. When the velopharyngeal port is closed, nasal pathway resistance has no effect on oral air pressure (Warren and Ryon, 1967). However, as the velopharyngeal port is opened, velopharyngeal resistance is decreased (Fig. 12.15). As the velopharyngeal port opens and velopharyngeal resistance decreases, nasal pathway resistance accounts for a greater segment of oral air pressure.

Warren and Ryon (1967) wrote that, for velopharyngeal areas in the range of 20 to 40 mm², "nasal resistance can account for as much as 30 to 90 percent of the oral pressure amplitude." They

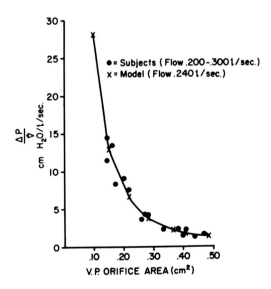

Figure 12.15 The relationship between velopharyngeal sphincter resistance (ordinate) to nasal airflow and orifice size (abscissa). The data presented for both subjects and the model indicate that sphincter resistance impedes nasal airflow significantly when orifice size is below approximately 0.2 cm². (From Warren DW, Devereux JL. An analog study of cleft palate speech. Cleft Palate J 1966; 3:103.)

varied nasal pathway resistance by placing inserts in the vocal tract analog. Their data indicated that oral pressures tend to increase at given velopharyngeal orifices and oral port orifices as nasal resistance increases from 2.5 to 5.2 to 9.8 cm H_2O/L/sec. For example, at a velopharyngeal opening of 20 mm² and an oral opening of 5 mm², oral pressures of 0.81, 1.29, and 1.30 cm H_2O were obtained under the three nasal pathway resistances (Table 12.2)

These values were obtained at a respiratory air flow of 0.2 L/sec. Resistance must be measured at a specified flow rate because whether the air flow is laminar and the relationship linear or the air flow turbulent and the relationship quadratic is determined by the flow rate (Warren et al. 1969).

Warren and Ryon (1967) reported that high nasal pathway resistance may explain why some persons with wide palatal clefts have fairly intelligible speech. Warren et al. (1969) compared normal and cleft palate individuals for nasal airway resistance and for the prevalence of such obstructions to nasal airflow as deviation of the nasal septum, vomerine spurs, thickening of the nasal mucosa, injection of the turbinates, nasal pathway atresia, or a combination of these. The subjects with cleft palate had surgically repaired clefts but no pharyngeal flaps. Nasal pathway obstruction was seen more frequently in persons with unilateral or bilateral complete clefts than in persons with cleft palate only.

Warren et al. (1974) reported data that indicated that surgical closure increases nasal airway resistance, that pharyngeal flaps increase it further, and that obturators also increase nasal airway resistance. Other research conducted in Warren's laboratory indicates that mouth breathing which may lead to malocclusion, is observed in a majority of persons with nasal airway resistance above 4.5 cm H_2O/L/sec.

More recently, Hairfield and Warren (1989) indicate that 60% of their adults with clefts had impaired nasal airway by their computation, whereas the same findings was obtained for only 3% of their adult normals.

The main clinical application of these findings is that an individual with obstructed nasal passages may be able to impound the oral air pressure needed for articulation even though there is marginally normal velopharyngeal competence.

**TABLE 12.2   Effects of Nasal Resistance on Oral Pressure Amplitude.
Three Nasal Resistances Were Used, all at a Flowrate of 0.2 L/sec.**

Size of Openings (cm²)		Pressure Readings (cm H₂O)		
Velopharyngeal Orifice	Oral Port	Nasal Component	Velopharyngeal Orifice Component	Oral Pressure
Nasal Resistance 1: 2.5 cm H₂O/L/sec				
0.05	0.0	0.56	8.42	8.98
0.05	0.05	0.23	2.80	3.03
0.20	0.0	0.51	0.74	1.25
0.20	0.05	0.36	0.45	0.81
0.40	0.0	0.48	0.31	0.79
0.40	0.05	0.37	0.19	0.56
Nasal Resistance 2: 5.2 cm H₂O/L/sec				
0.05	0.0	1.01	9.1	10.11
0.05	0.05	0.49	3.25	3.74
0.20	0.0	1.06	0.73	1.79
0.20	0.05	0.75	0.54	1.29
0.40	0.0	1.10	0.26	1.36
0.40	0.05	0.82	0.16	0.98
Nasal Resistance 3: 9.8 cm H₂O/L/sec				
0.05	0.0	1.95	8.55	10.50
0.05	0.05	0.61	3.04	3.65
0.20	0.0	2.19	0.68	2.87
0.20	0.05	0.93	0.37	1.30
0.40	0.0	2.13	0.27	2.40
0.40	0.05	0.94	0.12	1.06

Nasal Air Flow

Warren's research has stressed relationships among speech mechanism structure and aerodynamic measures with emphasis on oral air pressure as the dependent variable. However, he has also observed nasal air flow as a variable dependent upon areas of the velopharyngeal port and the oral port of the speech mechanism analog. Figure 12.16 shows decrease in nasal air flow with increase in oral port areas at three different velopharyngeal orifices. The change in size of the velopharyngeal port area had little influence on nasal air flow. The sizes were 10 mm², 50 mm², and 100 mm². These observations were made at a respiratory air flow of 0.250 L/sec. With the oral port closed, all the flow was nasal.

Nasal air flow data published by Thompson and Hixon (1979) indicated that 111 of 112 normal persons 3 through 28 years of age always presented zero nasal air flow and hence velopharyngeal closure during the oral consonants /s/, /z/, /t/, and /d/ as observed in strings of /Ci/ syllables and in /iCi/ syllables uttered in the carrier phrase "Say again." This was also true of sustained utterances of /i/, /s/, and /z/. Flow occurred during all nasal consonants and during vowels preceding nasal consonants suggesting the effects of assimilation. The authors suggested use of their /n/ data for normative purposes when possible velopharyngeal airway obstruction is being evaluated.

Respiratory Volume

Warren et al. (1969) measured respiratory volume and rate of respiratory air flow in normal persons and in patients with obturated cleft palate. Some of the latter achieved velopharyngeal ports of less than 20 mm² with their appliances in place. Respiratory volume increased from the normal speakers to the cleft palate speakers with presumably adequate closure to the cleft

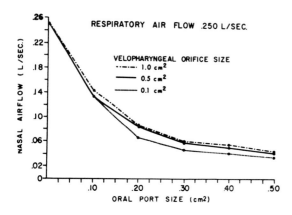

Figure 12.16 Relationship between oral port area and nasal airflow at three velopharyngeal orifice areas. Opening the oral port decreased nasal airflow at each velopharyngeal area studied. (From Warren DW, Ryon WE. Oral port constriction, nasal resistance, and respiratory aspects of cleft palate speech. Cleft Palate J 1967; 4:38.)

palate speakers with their appliances removed. The authors inferred that persons with palatal incompetence and intelligible pressure consonants use greater respiratory effort during speech; their volumes were nearly double those of normal subjects. The volumes recorded are influenced by air flow rate and amount of time used in the production of an utterance. Apparently, subjects with inadequate velopharyngeal mechanisms attempt to raise intraoral pressure for consonant production by increasing the rate of air flow.

Warren (1979) suggested that velopharyngeal openings greater than 20 mm² during speech permit so much nasal escape of air that oral air pressure sufficient for stops, fricatives, and affricatives cannot be impounded behind the velopharyngeal port. However, his research showed that speakers with velopharyngeal openings greater than zero but less than 20 mm² will sometimes but not always produce oral pressure sufficient for obstruents. The smaller the opening, the more likely it is that sufficient air pressure will be produced (Warren and Devereux, 1966).

An individual with a large velopharyngeal opening may be able to impound oral air pressure for speech if he or she has a nasal pathway obstruction. An individual may also compensate for a small velopharyngeal opening by increasing the rate of air flow during speech or by speaking with the mouth as nearly closed as possible. Unfortunately compensatory behaviors that serve to increase intraoral air pressure and hence to

facilitate articulation also serve to increase nasal emission of air. Audible nasal emission and other nasal noises result. If the velopharyngeal port almost closes, the speaker may gain greater intelligibility by using precise oral articulation rather than by trying to talk with the mouth closed or increasing the rate of air flow in an attempt to increase oral air pressure. Thus, attempting to compensate for small velopharyngeal openings may result in the trade of one set of speech problems for another.

BORDERLINE OR MARGINAL VELOPHARYNGEAL COMPETENCE

Failure of velopharyngeal function during speech is probably not a dichotomous phenomenon. Huber (1957) wrote that a speech mechanism may be satisfactory for "one or two syllable words in short sentences" but fail the speaker as linguistic development becomes more advanced. She noted that with language maturation the speech mechanism must accommodate demands for increased speech rate and complexity of coordination. Morris and Smith (1962) and McWilliams (1966) advanced the notion that some pathologic speakers show velopharyngeal function that is barely adequate or that is adequate inconsistently. Koepp-Baker (1971) noted that a person may achieve sufficient approximation of velopharyngeal closure to achieve "weak or transient oral occlusives" in careful speech but that with increased speech rate those sounds are omitted or replaced with glottal or pharyngeal sounds. Touch closure (McWilliams and Bradley, 1964; Van Demark et al. 1975) is a form of borderline competence. In many investigations that have employed the concept of borderline incompetence, that deficit is considered to be sufficiently modest that need for physical management is uncertain. Powers (1986) suggested that patients with marginal velopharyngeal closure show performance that is inconsistent or inconclusive.

Warren (1979) used the PERCI to estimate velopharyngeal orifice area. Eight patients with clefts and orifice areas of 10 to 20 mm² were classified as having borderline incompetence. He described the speech of this group as being marked by audible nasal emission, especially on fricatives when partial nasal airway obstruction was present. Hypernasality was present especially when the speakers reduced the oral airway by talking with small mouth openings. Presumably, under the condition of small mouth opening, an increased amount of acoustic energy travels into the nasal cavity. Warren also indicated that only rarely do individuals with velopharyngeal openings of less than 5 mm^2 have hypernasality and audible nasal emission. He recommended speech therapy for individuals with hypernasality and audible nasal escape when orifice areas are less than 10 mm^2. If therapy fails, he advocated surgery.

Subtelny (1968) described the speech of an adult male patient who wore an obturator to compensate for loss of velar tissue and part of the hard palate. The tissue had been removed because of cancer. All other speech structures were said to be normal. The obturator was constructed so that circular apertures of 2, 4, 6, 8, 10, and 12 mm diameter could be inserted into it, one at a time. The patient was studied for intelligibility under each aperture condition, with the pharyngeal section or speech bulb removed, and with the entire appliance removed. Fricative intelligibility fell from a loss of about 1% with a 2–mm diameter orifice to a loss of about 5% with a 4–mm orifice. Loss increased slightly with a 6–mm orifice and then declined with 8–, 10–, and 12–mm orifices. Regarding overall intelligibility, little loss was associated with change from no aperture to an aperture 4 mm in diameter. Intelligibility losses of about 10 and 26% were associated with the 12–mm aperture and the removal of the pharyngeal section. Bell-Berti (1980) noted that production of voice during obstruents requires expansion of the pharynx to achieve the needed difference in air pressure below and above the glottis. Some speakers may open the velopharyngeal port slightly to achieve the necessary pressure differential. This issue was discussed by Lubker (1975).

McWilliams et al. (1981) classified 48 subjects into nine groups based on speech characteristics and then estimated whether their velopharyngeal valving studies would show mechanisms that were competent, borderline, or incompetent. This study is discussed in greater detail in Chapter 23. It indicated that borderline capacities are associated with mild speech problems.

Morris (1972, 1984) suggested that individuals with borderline velopharyngeal competence may actually have different patterns of valving function. He described two different subgroups within the classification. One group, the "almost-but-not-quite (ABNQ)," represents relatively consistent function with a very small velopharyngeal opening always present. Presumably, the central feature of this subgroup is inadequate palatal length, unusual pharyngeal depth or width, or anterior displacement of the levators in the presence of neuromotor integrity.

The second group was labeled "sometimes-but-not-always (SBNA)." Their outstanding characteristic is inconsistency. They may sometimes achieve closure, but fail to do so at other times. Rate and phonetic context may partially account for this variability. Morris suggested that these subjects may give oral responses on single words, but have nasalized connected speech. They may give oral responses on speech tasks containing no nasal consonants, but show moderate or severe nasalization when required to include one or more nasal consonants. We add that others may be highly variable on repetitions of the same task. Presumably, the underlying factor is not a structural deficit but rather a disorder of timing whose etiology may be biomechanical or neurogenic or both. This subgroup is important clinically because diagnostic tests could indicate valving adequacy, yet significant speech problems, often unresponsive to therapy, could be present.

Morris did not offer evidence to support his hypothesized models, and not much information is available by which the validity of the models can be evaluated. The only relevant study to date is that of Hardin et al. (1986) in which they attempted to determine the extent to which the ABNQ subgroup can be identified from lateral still radiographs. They studied clinical findings of 50 patients who showed touch closure on the radiograph. Their findings did not support the ABNQ model, but rather indicated more variability in their subjects' behavior than the model predicts. They concluded that their choice of selection criterion (touch closure on still radiographs) may be too restrictive or unreliable, or that the model is too simplistic, or both. Further study of both subgroups is needed.

The concept of borderline velopharyngeal incompetence requires further development. Research is needed to enhance our understanding of patients with velopharyngeal openings between zero and 10 or even 20 mm^2 during the production of some or all pressure consonants. Investigators must control for dental malocclusions, fistulas, nasal passage features that may contribute to nasal noises, and other variables likely to influence the speech of the subjects. Clinical observations indicate that very small velopharyngeal openings may be associated with audible nasal emission and nasal noises. It is also possible that the availability of airtight velopharyngeal closure may be more important during speech development than it is for the maintenance of well-developed speech (Shelton et al., 1964; Isshiki et al., 1968). We occasionally hear preschool children who have articulation delay who produce nasal noises during some pressure consonants. Since these children appear to be physically normal, the question arises whether the precision of velopharyngeal closure increases with development during early childhood. However, nasal air flow data reported by Thompson and Hixon (1979) indicate that children as young as 3 years of age have airtight velopharyngeal closure during speech.

VELOPHARYNGEAL VALVING AND TONGUE POSTURE

Tongue function has been implicated in different ways in the disordered speech of some speakers with clefts (Morris, 1968). In early writings, some researchers felt that tongue innervation might be defective (Berry, 1949; Matthews and Byrne, 1953). Later, Fletcher (1978) hypothesized that misarticulation in those patients with poor diadochokinesis might be related to neurophysiological control of the articulators, especially the tongue. Fletcher found that lingual diadochokinesis accounted for more variance in articulation test scores than any other of several variables he studied.

There have also been suggestions that some patients who do not achieve velopharyngeal closure during speech use the tongue to support the velum or to fill space between the velum and posterior pharyngeal wall (Buck and Harrington, 1949). McWilliams (1966) wrote that the tongue sometimes serves as an obturator, a usage that limits its articulatory capacity.

McDonald and Koepp-Baker (1951) hypothesized that "at least some of the cleft-palate patient's nasality results from his persistent habit of elevating the mandible and dorsum of the tongue during speech." Later findings by Dickson (1969) contradicted this hypothesis. He found his most hypernasal subjects tended to carry the tongue low in the mouth and forward.

Tongue posture has been related to velopharyngeal competence by many authors. Shohara (1942) used palatography to identify changes in tongue posture of a patient with cleft palate subsequent to obturation. Prior to obturation there was no evidence of prepalatal, front alveolar, or dental contacts in articulation. Rather, sounds requiring those contacts were replaced by nonstandard sounds involving lateral, midpalatal, and back palatal contacts. After obturation, more anterior lingual contact was established.

Buck (1952, 1953) used still lateral radiographs taken during phonation of vowels to compare 20 normal persons and 20 with repaired clefts. Some of the data reported tongue height measured proportional to indices to subject size. Few statistically significant differences were found between the subject groups in tongue height or tongue retraction, and Buck concluded that previous concern about tongue carriage in patients with cleft palate may have been too great.

Subsequent research has indicated that some subjects with cleft palate elevate and retract the tongue relative to the lingual articulations observed in normal speakers. This apparently can be an unconscious attempt to obturate the velopharyngeal port. Powers (1962), in a cinefluorographic investigation, found that subjects with cleft palate who articulated poorly "tended to carry their tongues further back in the oral cavity than did subjects with good articulation." No difference was found relative to tongue height. Powers concluded that the occurrence of compensatory tongue postures is most likely to be observed in patients with deficient velopharyngeal function. Comparison of group means or measures of tongue posture in heterogeneous groups is likely to miss the compensatory tongue postures used by some patients. Perhaps this explains the negative results in Buck's 1953 study.

Brooks et al. (1965) found that cleft subjects who used tongue-pharyngeal wall contacts were inferior in articulation and velopharyngeal closure to those who did not have the posterior tongue posture.

In another cinefluorographic study, Brooks et al (1966) found that 13 of 28 subjects with velopharyngeal insufficiency contacted the soft palate with the tongue at some time during the speech sample studied. No normal subject did so. Two subjects were reported to show almost continuous tongue-velum contact during production of the sentences filmed. Subjects who showed linguavelar contacts did not differ to a statistically significant degree in sagittal velopharyngeal gap from subjects who did not show such contacts.

Wada et al. (1970) devised a means of studying relationships between velar and tongue movements and positions relative to the onset of isolated vowels and /kV/ syllables. The results suggested that poor closure may disrupt timing relationships between tongue and palate. Context is important to these relationships. The authors commented that "the tongue perhaps assumed positions to compensate for the velar disturbance or to assist the velar activity."

Lawrence and Philips (1975) used video-fluorography to study tongue contacts in 69 subjects with cleft palate, each of whom fell into one of three velopharyngeal categories: adequate, borderline, or inadequate. Forty-three of the 69 subjects showed deviant lingual contacts as defined by contrast between subject performance and textbook description of place of articulation for the sounds under study. Seventy-five deviant contacts were in a posterior direction, but 25 were in an anterior direction. Type of cleft was not related to the distribution of lingual contacts, nor was presence or absence of nasal emission. However, subjects showing linguavelar contacts were inferior to other subjects in velopharyngeal closure and articulation and were more likely to have hypernasality. Subjects who produced linguavelar contacts tended to have undergone their last velopharyngeal surgery later than subjects who did not produce those contacts. Linguavelar contacts were observed more frequently on /s/ than on any other of the consonants studied.

We conclude from all of these findings that some cleft palate speakers demonstrate patterns of tongue position and movement that are different from normal and that these patterns are most likely to be found in patients who have or have had velopharyngeal incompetence. Although it is difficult to prove, we also conclude that these patterns are compensatory for velopharyngeal incompetence. It follows then that early treatment for children with cleft palate should focus on the goal of providing velopharyngeal competence as early as possible and on teaching appropriate articulation patterns.

NONSPEECH ACTIVITIES

Speech pathologists are interested in descriptions of velopharyngeal function during non-speech activities such as swallowing, blowing, sucking, and puffing of the cheeks for their contributions to the understanding of oral physiology and because of the possibility that nonspeech function may be used clinically to enhance speech function.

Moll (1965) studied nonspeech oral activities in 10 adults by means of midsagittal cinefluorography utilizing a 24-frame-per-second camera speed. His subjects were filmed uttering six consonant-vowel-consonant syllables with the carrier phrase, "Say — again." Sucking and blowing were performed on an oral manometer with and without bleed. These activities were performed at the maximum pressure the individual could produce and at half that pressure. Barium was sucked through a straw with immediate swallow and with delayed swallow, and each subject was gagged. Dependent variables included velar height above a line extending from the anterior nasal spine (ANS) and the pterygomaxillary fissure (PTM) (Fig. 12.17) and superimposed tracings of the velum and the posterior wall during speech and nonspeech acts. Moll's data showed that sucking liquid, sucking on a manometer without a bleed opening, and puffing the cheeks tend to involve contact between the tongue and the velum and not velopharyngeal closure. In other words, the oral cavity is closed posteriorly by tongue-palate contact. Negative pressure for sucking or positive pressure for inflating the cheeks is accomplished by motions of the lips, cheeks, or a combination of these. It would be an error to generalize about

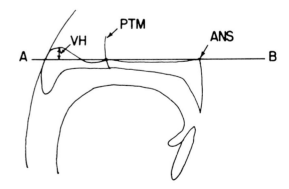

Figure 12.17 Line drawing showing the measure of velar height. (From Moll K. A cinefluoroscopic study of velopharyngeal function in normals during various activities. Cleft Palate J 1965; 2:112.)

velopharyngeal function for speech from observation of cheek puffing or sucking without benefit of a bleed. Velopharyngeal closure was achieved during speech, swallowing, and blowing with and without bleed at maximum and half maximum pressures. "Comparison of blowing and speech indicated that velar elevation is approximately 2 or 3 mm greater, on the average, for all of the blowing tasks." Moll noted that greater air pressure in the oral cavity associated with blowing might displace the velum upward or that the muscle(s) elevating the velum might be activated more vigorously during blowing.

Moll concluded that two patterns were evident in his findings: (1) contact between the velum and the posterior wall and (2) contact between "the tongue and the inferior surface of the hard and soft palates." Individuals with poor velopharyngeal closure may use the tongue to displace the velum toward the posterior pharyngeal wall. He also noted that swallowing, blowing, and gagging involve greater motion of the posterior pharyngeal wall than is observed in speech. Moll concluded that use of nonspeech tasks for the exercise of the velopharyngeal mechanism is a questionable practice. However, it is clear that more information is needed.

Shprintzen et al. (1974) utilized midsagittal and frontal videofluoroscopic recording to describe reflexive swallows in young normal adults relative to velar elevation and displacement of the lateral pharyngeal walls toward midline in the region of the soft palate during speech, whistling, blowing, reflexive swallowing, dry swallowing, and gagging. Their findings indicated that repeated swallows are highly similar within subjects and that different individuals also show similar motions during swallowing. The lateral walls touched less often during reflexive swallowing than for the other two acts (Fig. 12.8). Velar elevation was also less extensive during reflexive swallowing than during the other two acts.

The lateral pharyngeal walls do not usually make contact with each other during speech, whistling, and blowing, which, of course, require that the laryngopharynx and oropharynx be open for the passage of air and sound (see Fig. 12.8). Shprintzen et al. concluded that the velopharyngeal apparatus uses one mechanism for closure during speech, whistling, and blowing and another for swallowing and gagging. They termed these mechanisms pneumatic and nonpneumatic, and they hypothesized that a cleft palate person who

achieved closure during the nonspeech pneumatic activities of whistling or blowing, but not during speech, may be able to learn to achieve closure during speech.

CLOSURE ASSOCIATED WITH PHARYNGEAL FLAPS

Pigott (1969) used a nasoendoscope to study velopharyngeal function in 21 cleft patients 8 years of age or older. Satisfactory data could not

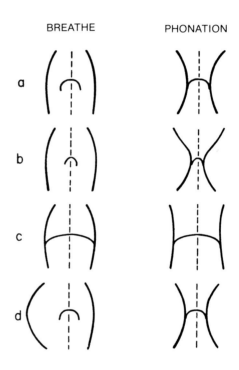

Figure 12.18 Line drawings of the lateral pharyngeal walls and pharyngeal flaps taken from frontal view radiographs of patients during breathing and phonation. Patients obtained velopharyngeal closure despite different relationships between lateral pharyngeal walls and flap. (a) Average width flap symmetrically placed between lateral pharyngeal walls. Both lateral walls touch flap during phonation. (b) Narrow pharyngeal flap. Velopharyngeal closure obtained with increased medial movement of lateral pharyngeal walls. (c) Excessively wide flap completely occluding velopharyngeal portal during respiration. Little lateral pharyngeal wall movement occurs with phonation. (d) Average width flap asymmetrically situated in velopharyngeal portal; right pharyngeal wall more lateral at rest than left one. During phonation, right lateral pharyngeal wall showed increased movement resulting in bilateral closure of the portals lateral to the flap. (From Skolnick ML, McCall GN. Velopharyngeal competence and incompetence following pharyngeal flap surgery; videofluoroscopic study in multiple projections. Cleft Palate J 1972; 9:1.)

be obtained from five other patients. The report described and illustrated closure of ports lateral to the pharyngeal flap, midline closure of the velopharyngeal port with lateral gutters remaining open, and closure of the velum and pharyngeal walls around an obturator. One patient who closed in midline while leaving the lateral gutters open showed nasal escape. Other patients achieved closure except for midline gaps.

Skolnick and McCall (1972), using multiview fluoroscopy, studied velopharyngeal valving in 33 patients who had had pharyngeal flaps. They, too, found movement of the lateral pharyngeal walls to be crucial in the achievement of closure. They concluded from the evaluation of the 22 incompetent patients in the series that the width of the flap, its vertical level, and its position in relation to the lateral pharyngeal walls on a horizontal plane are all relevant to the success or failure of the flap. We would add that the extent of movement in the soft palate is also a factor, since the palatoflap structure is often not static, but moves by action of the levators and that movement must also be in concert with lateral wall motion. Figure 12.18 shows line drawings of four different patterns of movement that they observed.

Schulz et al. (1973) utilized the Taub panendoscope to observe and describe patterns of closure lateral to a pharyngeal flap. They devised a scheme to classify and report openings and closure on each side of the flap. Ideally, the patient is open on each side at rest and closed on each side during speech. However, some individuals may always be open on both sides, some may always be closed; and some may be asymmetrical. These authors reported no reliability information about their procedure. In a large sample of cleft palate patients with pharyngeal flaps, all possible combinations will probably be observed. However, it is clear that the velopharyngeal mechanism must achieve closure but also permit nasal breathing if the pharyngeal flap is to be successful and that the motion of the lateral pharyngeal walls is intimately associated with closure of the lateral ports at the level of the flap. Thus, if the lateral walls do not move, if they move poorly, if the flap is not positioned ideally to interact with movement in the lateral walls, or if the flap is too narrow, the speech result will be less than ideal.

Reports have been made also by Zwitman (1982a, 1982b) about variation in velopharyngeal physiology and pharyngeal flap surgery.

SUMMARY

This discussion indicates both that considerable information about the velopharyngeal mechanism is available and that more is yet needed. For example, there is still controversy about the anatomy and physiology of the mechanism, even when normal. Indications are that there is wide variability in this regard in individuals with clefts, a fact that experienced cleft palate surgeons are all too familiar with. It is not yet clear to what extent this variability is important in velopharyngeal patterns and speech production, either before or after surgery. Questions about neuromotor influences seem particularly important, especially in patients who seem to show disorders in velopharyngeal function that appear to be primarily of timing.

By some standards, more information is available about velopharyngeal function than about velopharyngeal structure. Again, variability of function is highly evident in both the normal person and the person with a velopharyngeal disorder. Indeed, even with available information, we still have some difficulty identifying the demarcation between normal and abnormal velopharyngeal function. That is a special problem to the clinician. An especially confounding factor in considering velopharyngeal function is the potential impact of learning; that is how we can be certain in our evaluation of velopharyngeal function that we assess physiologic potential. This important question is a focus of the chapter on evaluation of velopharyngeal function.

REFERENCES

Arkebauer HJ, Hixon TJ, Hardy JC. Peak intraoral air pressures during speech. J Speech Hear Res 1967;10:196.

Astley R. The movements of the lateral walls of the nasopharynx: a cine-radiographic study. J Laryngol Otol 1958;72:325.

Azzam NA, Kuehn DP. The morphology of musculus uvulae. Cleft Palate J 1977;14:78.

Bateman HE, Mason RM. Applied anatomy and physiology of the speech and hearing mechanism. Springfield: CC Thomas, 1984.

Bell-Berti F. An electromyographic study of velopharyngeal function in speech. J Speech Hear Res 1976;19:225.

Bell-Berti F. Velopharyngeal function: a spatial-temporal model. In: Lass NJ, ed. Speech and language: advances in basic research and practice. Vol 4. New York: Academic Press, 1980:291.

Berry MF. Lingual anomalies associated with palatal clefts. J Speech Hear Dis 1949;14:359.

Bjork L. Velopharyngeal function in connected speech: studies using tomography and cineradiography synchronized with speech spectrography. Acta Radiol 1961; Suppl 202:1.

Black JW. The pressure component in the production of consonants. J Speech Hear Dis 1950;15:207.

Bosma JF. Correlated study of anatomy and motor activity of upper pharynx by cadaver dissection and by cinematic study of patients after maxillo-facial surgery. Ann Otol Rhinol Laryngol 1953;62:51.

Bosma JF. Anatomy of the infant head. Baltimore: Johns Hopkins University Press, 1986.

Brandt SD, Morris HL. The linearity of the relationship between articulation errors and velopharyngeal incompetence. Cleft Palate J 1965;2:176.

Brooks AR, Shelton RL, Youngstrom KA. Compensatory tongue-palate-posterior pharyngeal wall relationships in cleft palate. J Speech Hear Dis 1965;30:166.

Brooks AR, Shelton RL, Youngstrom KA. Tongue-palate contact in persons with palate defects. J Speech Hear Dis 1966;31:14.

Brown WS Jr, McGlone RE. Relation of intraoral air pressure to oral cavity size. Folia Phoniatr 1969;21:321.

Buck MW. An x-ray study of cleft palate oral and pharyngeal structures and their function during vowel phonation. Cleft Palate Bull 1952;2:5.

Buck MW. Facial skeletal measurements and tongue carriage in subjects with repaired cleft palate. J Speech Hear Dis 1953;18:121.

Buck MW, Harrington R. Organized speech therapy for cleft palate rehabilitation. J Speech Hear Dis 1949;14:43.

Bzoch KR. Articulatory proficiency and error patterns of preschool cleft palate and normal children. Cleft Palate J 1965;2:340.

Bzoch KR, Graber TM, Aoba T. A study of normal velopharyngeal valving for speech. Cleft Palate Bull 1959;9:3.

Calnan J. Modern views on Passavant's ridge. Br J Plast Surg 1957;10:89.

Carpenter MA. A preliminary study of Passavant's pad within the velopharyngeal mechanism. Unpublished Master's thesis. University of Iowa, 1966.

Carpenter MA, Morris HL. A preliminary study of Passavant's pad. Cleft Palate J 1968;5:61.

Cassell MD, Moon JB, Elkadi H. Anatomy and physiology of the velopharynx. In: Bardach J, Morris HL, eds. Multidisciplinary management of cleft lip and palate. Philadelphia: WB Saunders, in press.

Croft CB, Shprintzen RJ, Daniller A, Lewin ML. The occult submucous cleft palate and the musculus uvulae. Cleft Palate J 1978;15:150.

Dickson DR. A radiographic study of nasality. Cleft Palate J 1969;6:160.

Dickson DR. Anatomy of the normal velopharyngeal mechanism. Clin Plast Surg 1975;2:235.

Dickson DR, Maue-Dickson W. Velopharyngeal anatomy. J Speech Hear Res 1972;15:372.

Dickson DR, Maue-Dickson W. Velopharyngeal structure and function: A model for biomechanical analysis. In: Lass NJ, ed. Speech and language: advances in basic research and practice. Vol 3. New York: Academic Press, 1980:168.

Fletcher SG. A cinefluorographic study of posterior wall of the pharynx during speech and degluitition. Master's thesis. University of Utah, 1957.

Fletcher SG. Cleft palate: a broader view. J Speech Hear Dis 1966;31:3.

Fletcher SG. Diagnosing speech disorders from cleft palate. New York: Grune and Stratton, 1978.

Folkins JW. Issues in speech motor control and their relation to the speech of individuals with cleft palate. Cleft Palate J 1985; 22:106.

Fritzell B. The velopharyngeal muscles in speech. Acta Otolaryngol 1969; Suppl 250.

Fritzell B. Electromyography in the study of the velopharyngeal function—a review. Folia Phoniatr 1979;31:93.

Glaser ER. A multiview videofluoroscopic study of Passavant's ridge in patients with and without velopharyngeal insufficiency. Unpublished Doctoral dissertation. University of Pittsburgh, 1980.

Glaser ER, Skolnick ML, McWilliams BJ, Shprintzen RJ. The dynamics of Passavant's ridge in subjects with and without velopharyngeal insufficiency—a multi-view videofluoroscopic study. Cleft Palate J 1979;16:24.

Goto T. Tightness in velopharyngeal closure and its regulatory mechanism. J Osaka Univ Dent Sch 1977; 22:87. Cleft Palate J 1978;15:188 (abstract).

Graber TM, Bzoch KR, Aoba T. A functional study of the palatal and pharyngeal structures. Angl Orthodont 1959;29:30.

Hagerty RF, Hess DA, Mylin WK. Velar motility, velopharyngeal closure, and speech proficiency in cartilage pharyngoplasty: The effect of age at surgery. Cleft Palate J 1968;5:317.

Hagerty RF, Hill MJ. Pharyngeal wall and palatal movement in postoperative cleft palate and normal palates. J Speech Hear Res 1960;3:59.

Hairfield WM, Warren DW. Dimensions of the cleft nasal airway in adults: A comparison with subjects without cleft. Cleft Palate J 1989;26:9.

Hardin MA, Morris HL, Van Demark DR. A study of cleft palate speakers with marginal velopharyngeal competence. J Commun Dis 1986;19:461.

Hardy JC. Air flow and air pressure studies. Proceedings of the Conference: Communicative Problems in Cleft palate. ASHA Reports No. 1, 1965:141.

Harrington R. A study of the mechanism of velopharyngeal closure. J Speech Hear Dis 1944;9:325.

Hawkins CF, Swisher WE. Evaluation of a real-time ultrasound scanner in assessing lateral pharyngeal wall motion during speech. Cleft Palate J 1978;15:161.

Huber MW. A clinical approach to cleft palate speech therapy. West Speech 1957;21:30.

Iglesias A, Kuehn DP, Morris HL. Simultaneous assessment of pharyngeal wall and velar displacement for selected speech sounds. J Speech Hear Res 1980;23:429.

Isshiki N, Honjow I, Morimoto M. Effects of velopharyngeal incompetence upon speech. Cleft Palate J 1968;5:297.

Isshiki N, Honjow I, Morimoto M. Cineradiographic analysis of movement of the lateral pharyngeal wall. Plast Reconstr Surg 1969;44:357.

Kahane JC, Folkins JF. Atlas of speech and hearing anatomy. Columbus: Charles E. Merrill, 1984.

Keller JT, Saunders MC, Van Loveren H, Shipley MT. Neuroanatomical considerations of palatal muscles: tensor and levator veli palatini. Cleft Palate J 1984; 21:70.

Kelsey CA, Crummy AB, Schulman EY. Comparison of ultrasonic and radiographic determination of lateral pharyngeal wall displacement. Phys Med Biol 1969;14:332.

Koepp-Baker H. Orofacial clefts: their forms and effects. In: Travis LE, ed. Handbook of speech pathology and audiology. 2nd ed. New York: Appleton-Century-Crofts, 1971.

Kuehn DP. A cineradiographic investigation of velar movement variables of two normals. Cleft Palate J 1976;13:88.

Kuehn DP, Folkins JW, Cutting CB. Relationships between muscle activity and velar position. Cleft Palate J 1982;19:25.

Kuehn DP, Folkins JW, Linville RN. An electromyographic study of the musculus uvulae. Cleft Palate J 1988;25:348.

Kuehn DP, Moll KL. A cineradiographic study of VC and CV articulatory velocities. J Phonet 1976;4:303.

Künzel HJ. Videofluoroscopic evaluation of a photo-electric device for the registration of velar elevation in speech. (German) Folia Phoniatr 1979;31:153.

Künzel HJ. Some observations of velar movement in plosives. Phonetica 1977;36:384.

Langdon HL. Klueber K. The longitudinal fibromuscular component of the soft palate in the fifteen-week human fetus: Musculus uvulae and palatine raphe. Cleft Palate J 1978;15:337.

Lavorato AS. Normal lateral pharyngeal wall motion during velopharyngeal functioning: a cinefluorographic study. Doctoral dissertation. University of Pittsburgh, 1975.

Lavorato AS, Lindholm CE. Fiberoptic visualization of the motion of the eustachian tube cartilage. Am Acad Ophthalmol Otol, Las Vegas, 1976.

Lawrence CW, Philips BJ. A telefluoroscopic study of lingual contacts made by persons with palatal defects. Cleft Palate J 1975; 12:85.

Lubker JF. An electromyographic-cinefluorographic investigation of velar function during normal speech production. Cleft Palate J 1968;5:1.

Lubker JF. Normal velopharyngeal function in speech. Clin Plast Surg 1975;2:249.

Mason RM, Young EC, Stallworth W. The predictive value of lateral pharyngeal wall movement in speech diagnostics. J Speech Hear Assoc, Detroit, 1973.

Massengill R, Walker T, Pickrell KL. Characteristics of patients with a Passavant's pad. Plast Reconstr Surg 1969;44:268.

Matsuya T, Yamaoka M, Miyasaki T. A fiberscopic study of velopharyngeal closure in patients with operated cleft palates. Plast Reconstr Surg 1979;63:497.

Matthews J, Byrne MC. An experimental study of tongue flexibility in children with cleft palates. J Speech Hear Dis 1953;18:43.

Maue-Dickson W, Dickson DR. Anatomy and physiology related to cleft palate: Current research and clinical implications. Plast Reconstr Surg 1980;65:83.

Mazaheri M, Millard RT, Erickson DM. Cineradiographic comparison of normal to noncleft subjects with velopharyngeal inadequacy. Cleft Palate J 1964;1:199.

McDonald ET, Koepp-Baker H. Cleft palate speech: an integration of research and clinical observation. J Speech Hear Dis 1951;16:9.

McKerns D, Bzoch KR. Variations in velopharyngeal valving: the factor of sex. Cleft Palate J 1970;7:652.

McWilliams BJ. Speech and language problems in children with cleft palate. J Am Med Wom Assoc 1966;21:1005.

McWilliams BJ, Bradley DP. A rating scale for evaluation of video tape recorded x-ray studies. Cleft Palate J 1964;1:88.

McWilliams BJ, Glaser ER, Philips BJ, Lawrence C, Lavorato AS, Berry QC, Skolnick ML. A comparative study of four methods of evaluating velopharyngeal adequacy. Plast Reconstr Surg 1981;68:1.

Minifie FD, Hixon TJ, Kelsey CA, Woodhouse RJ. Lateral pharyngeal wall movement during speech production. J Speech Hear Res 1970;13:584.

Minifie FD, Abbs JH, Tarlow A, Kwaterski M. EMG activity within the pharynx during speech production. J Speech Hear Res 1974;17:497.

Moll KL. Cinefluorographic techniques in speech research. J Speech Hear Res 1960;3:227.

Moll KL. Velopharyngeal closure on vowels. J Speech Hear Res 1962;5:30.

Moll KL. A cinefluorographic study of velopharyngeal function in normals during various activities. Cleft Palate J 1965;2:112.

Moll KL, Daniloff RG. Investigation of the timing of velar movements during speech. J Acoust Soc Am 1971; 50:678.

Moll KL, Shriner TH. Preliminary investigation of a new concept of velar activity during speech. Cleft Palate J 1967;4:58.

Morris HL. Etiological bases for speech problems. In: Spriesterbach DC, Sherman D, eds. Cleft palate and communication. New York: Academic Press, 1968:119.

Morris HL. Cleft Palate. In: Weston AJ, ed. Communicative Disorders: An appraisal. Springfield: CC Thomas, 1972:128.

Morris HL. Types of velopharyngeal incompetence. In: Winitz H, ed. Treating articulation disorders: for clinicians by clinicians. Baltimore: University Park Press, 1984:211.

Morris HL, Smith JK. A multiple approach for evaluating velopharyngeal competency. J Speech Hear Dis 1962; 27:218.

Mourino AP, Weinberg B. A cephalometric study of velar stretch in 8 and 10 year old children. Cleft Palate J 1975;12:417.

Netsell R. Evaluation of velopharyngeal function in dysarthria. J Speech Hear Dis 1969;34:113.

Niimi S, Bell-Berti F, Harris KS. Dynamic aspects of velopharyngeal closure. Folia Phoniatr 1982;34:246.

Nishio J, Matsuya T, Ibuki K, Miyazaki T. Roles of the facial, glossopharyngeal and vagus nerves in velopharyngeal movement. Cleft Palate J 1976a;13:201.

Nishio J, Matsuya T, Machida J, Miyazaki T. The motor nerve supply of the velopharyngeal muscles. Cleft Palate J 1976b;13:20.

Nusbaum EA, Foley L, Wells C. Experimental studies of the firmness of velar-pharyngeal occlusion during the production of English vowels. Speech Monographs 1935;2:71.

Nylen BO. Cleft palate speech: a surgical study including observations on velopharyngeal closure during connected speech, using synchronized cineradiography and sound spectrography. Acta Radiol 1961;Suppl 203:1.

Osberg PE, Witzel MA. The physiologic basis for hypernasality during connected speech in cleft palate patients: A nasendoscopic study. Plast Reconstr Surg 1981;67:1.

Peterson SJ. Nasal emission as a component of the misarticulation of sibilants and affricates. J Speech Hear Dis 1975;40:106.

Pigott RW. The nasendoscopic appearance of the normal

palatopharyngeal valve. Plast Reconstr Surg 1969; 43:19.

Powers GR. Cinefluorographic investigation of articulatory movements of selected individuals with cleft palates. J Speech Hear Res 1962;5:59.

Powers GR. Cleft palate. Austin: Pro-Ed, 1986.

Rolnick MI, Hoops HR. Plosive phoneme duration as a function of palato-pharyngeal adequacy. Cleft Palate J 1971;8:65.

Ryan WJ, Hawkins CF. Ultrasonic measurement of lateral pharyngeal wall movement at the velopharyngeal port. Cleft Palate J 1976;13:156.

Schulz R, Heller JC, Gens GW, Lewin M. Pharyngeal flap surgery and voice quality factors related to success, and failure. Cleft Palate J 1973;10:165.

Seaver EJ, Kuehn DP. A cineradiographic and electromyographic investigation of velar positioning in non-nasal speech. Cleft Palate J 1980;17:216.

Shelton RL, Brooks AR, Youngstrom KA. Articulation and patterns of palatopharyngeal closure. J Speech Hear Dis 1964;29:390.

Shelton RL, Paesani A, McClelland KD, Bradfield SS. Panendoscopic feedback in the study of voluntary velopharyngeal movements. J Speech Hear Dis 1975; 40:232.

Shohara HH. Speech rehabilitation in a case of post-operated cleft palate and malocclusion. J Speech Hear Dis 1942;7:381.

Shprintzen RJ, Lencione RM, McCall GN, Skolnick ML. A three dimensional cinefluoroscopic analysis of velopharyngeal closure during speech and nonspeech activities in normals. Cleft Palate J 1974;11:412.

Shprintzen RJ, McCall GN, Skolnick ML. A new therapeutic technique for the treatment of velopharyngeal incompetence. J Speech Hear Dis 1975a;40:69.

Shprintzen RJ, McCall GN, Skolnick ML, Lencione RM. Selective movement of the lateral aspects of the pharyngeal walls during velopharyngeal closure for speech, blowing, and whistling in normals. Cleft Palate J 1975b;12:51.

Shprintzen RJ, Rakoff SJ, Skolnick ML, Lavorato AS. Incongruous movements of the velum and lateral pharyngeal walls. Cleft Palate J 1977;14:148.

Shprintzen RJ, Croft CB, Berkman MD, Rakoff SJ. Velopharyngeal insufficiency in the facio-auriculo-vertebral malformation complex. Cleft Palate J 1980;17:132.

Simpson RK, Austin AA. A cephalometric investigation of velar stretch. Cleft Palate J 1972;9:341.

Simpson RK, Colton J. A cephalometric study of velar stretch in adolescent subjects. Cleft Palate J 1980;17:40.

Simpson RK, Chin L. Velar stretch as a function of task. Cleft Palate J 1981;18:1.

Skolnick ML, McCall GN. Velopharyngeal competence and incompetence following pharyngeal flap surgery: a video-fluoroscopic study in multiple projections. Cleft Palate J 1972;9:1.

Skolnick ML. Velopharyngeal function in cleft palate. Clin Plast Surg 1975;2:285.

Skolnick ML, Zagzebski JA, Watkin KL. Two-dimensional ultrasonic demonstration of lateral pharyngeal wall movement in real time—a preliminary report. Cleft Palate J 1975;12:299.

Subtelny J. Evaluation of palatopharyngeal valving: Clinical and research procedures. In: Lencione RM, ed. Cleft palate habilitation: proceedings of the fifth annual symposium on cleft palate habilitation. Syracuse: Syracuse University Press, 1968:105.

Subtelny JD, Worth JH, Sakuda M. Intraoral pressure and rate of flow during speech. J Speech Hear Res 1966;9:498.

Thompson AE, Hixon TJ. Nasal air flow during normal speech production. Cleft Palate J 1979;16:412.

Trost JE. Articulatory additions to the classical description of the speech of persons with cleft palate. Cleft Palate J 1981;18:193.

Van Demark DR, Kuehn DP, Tharp RA. Prediction of velopharyngeal competency. Cleft Palate J 1975;12:5.

Van Demark DR, Morris HL, VandeHaar C. Patterns of articulation abilities in speakers with cleft palate. Cleft Palate J 1979;16:230.

Wada T, Yasumoto M, Ikeoka N, Fujiki Y, Yoshinaga R. An approach for the cinefluorographic study of the articulatory movements. Cleft Palate J 1970;7:506.

Warren DW. Compensatory speech behaviors in cleft palate: a regulation/control phenomenon. Cleft Palate J 1986; 23:251.

Warren DW. Velopharyngeal orifice size and upper pharyngeal pressure-flow patterns in normal speech. Plast Reconstr Surg 1964;33:148.

Warren DW. PERCI: a method for rating palatal efficiency. Cleft Palate J 1979;16:279.

Warren DW, Dalston RM, Trier WC, Holder MB. A pressure-flow technique for quantifying temporal patterns of palatopharyngeal closure. Cleft Palate J 1985; 22:1

Warren DW, Devereux JL. An analog study of cleft palate speech. Cleft Palate J 1966;3:103.

Warren DW, Duany LF, Fischer ND. Nasal pathway resistance in normal and cleft lip and palate subjects. Cleft Palate J 1969;6:134.

Warren DW, DuBois AB. A pressure-flow technique for measuring velopharyngeal orifice area during continuous speech. Cleft Palate J 1964;1:52.

Warren DW, Hofmann FA. A cineradiographic study of velopharyngeal closure. Plast Reconstr Surg 1961;28:656.

Warren DW, Mackler SB. Duration of oral port constriction in normal and cleft palate speech. J Speech Hear Res 1968;11:391.

Warren DW, Ryon WE. Oral port constriction, nasal resistance, and respiratory aspects of cleft palate speech: an analog study. Cleft Palate J 1967;4:38.

Warren DW, Trier WC, Bevin AG. Effect of restorative procedures on the nasopharyngeal airway in cleft palate. Cleft Palate J 1974;11:367.

Weiss CE. The significance of Passavant's pad in post-obturator patients. Folia Phoniatr 1972;24:51.

Witzel MA, Posnick JC. Patterns and location of velopharyngeal valving problems: A typical finding on video nasopharyngoscopy. Cleft Palate J 1989;26:63.

Wolfe WG. X-ray study of certain structures and movements involved in nasopharyngeal closure. Unpublished Masters thesis. University of Iowa, 1942.

Zagzebski JA. Ultrasonic measurement of lateral pharyngeal wall motion at two levels in the vocal tract. J Speech Hear Res 1975;18:308.

Zemlin WR. Speech and hearing science: anatomy and physiology. 3rd ed. Englewood Cliffs; NJ: Prentice-Hall, 1988.

Zimmerman GN, Karnell MP, Rettaliata P. Articulatory

coordination and the clinical profile of two cleft palate speakers. J Phonetics 1985;12:297.

Zwitman DH. Oral endoscopic comparison of velopharyngeal closure before and after pharyngeal flap surgery. Cleft Palate J 1982b;19:40.

Zwitman DH, Gyepes MT, Sample F. The submentovertical projection in the radiographic analysis of velopharyngeal dynamics. J Speech Hear Dis 1973;38:473.

Zwitman DH, Gyepes MT, Ward PH. Assessment of velar and lateral wall movement by oral telescope and radiographic examination in patients with velopharyngeal inadequacy and in normal subjects. J Speech Hear Dis 1976;41:381.

Zwitman DH, Sonderman JC, Ward PH. Variations in velopharyngeal closure assessed by endoscopy. J Speech Hear Dis 1974;39:366.

13 | LANGUAGE DISORDERS

Clifford (1979) pointed out that scant attention has been paid to language in children with cleft palates. He recommended that future research "take advantage of the sophisticated methodologies and theories of language development and acquisition, going beyond the rudimentary aspects (description of language behavior) so frequently emphasized in cleft palate literature." Intelligence, cognition, mother-child interaction, sensory integration, and environment, among other variables, require definition as they operate singly and together to influence language acquisition. As will be seen in the discussion which follows, attempts have been made to control for some of these variables and to explore others. However, since the study of language development generally is still in a relatively crude state, it is not surprising that the numerous interacting variables have been difficult to examine and understand even in children who do not have the complications of clefting. Shames and Rubin (1979) suggested that "the shortcomings of research on language in cleft palate children . . . are directly traceable to the shortcomings of language research in general." They go on to say:

A cleft palate population is homogeneous only with respect to specific structural abnormalities. This population appears to be remarkably heterogeneous with respect to indirect correlates to cleft palate, such as parental attitudes, child-rearing practices, medical and hospitalization histories, and speech and language stimulation and reinforcement.

In addition, we would add that children with clefts are heterogeneous in the nature of the original deformity, the outcome of treatment, presence and type of other congenital abnormalities, the degree to which hearing loss is controlled,

intelligence, social experience both at and away from home, genetic characteristics, and family constellation. In truth, children with clefts are far more dissimilar than they are similar; and the same factors that combine to make language possible in all children are operative for children with clefts. Thus, if the experience of having a cleft is not in some way detrimental to language development, these children should not be substantially different from their noncleft peers. Therefore, the early research, which attempted to find out if there were differences, was a reasonable stage in the evolution of language research in children with clefts. Unfortunately, too little effort has been made to move further to understand the variations observed within the context of other aspects of development (McWilliams, 1973).

The studies discussed in the sections that follow cannot be viewed as conclusive, but they represent the present state of the art.

DIFFERENCES BETWEEEN VERBAL AND PERFORMANCE IQS

The discussion about intelligence in Chapter 8 indicates that, in the past, a number of studies have rather consistently found that performance IQ as measured by one of the Wechsler forms was higher than verbal IQ (Goodstein, 1961; Lamb et al., 1973; Ruess, 1965; Ruess and Lis, 1973; Wirls, 1971). These findings led to the conclusion that the differences provided some evidence of language deficits in children with clefts. Clifford (1979) stated that these studies are frequently used to bolster the position that poor speech has resulted in poor verbal performance.

McWilliams (1970) suggested that we refer to "intellectual depression" until we better understand the origins of reduced scores on intelligence tests and that it was premature to conclude that such reductions were either permanent or irreversible. Indeed, (McWilliams and Musgrave, 1972), found no verbal-performance differences even when speech was defective. McWilliams and Matthews (1979) also reported no such discrepancies in a study designed to determine the extent to which mental development is related to other factors such as cleft type and the presence or absence of other congenital abnormalities. Leeper et al. (1980), in an extensive study of 103 adults, found no significant differences between verbal and performance IQs. The fact that differences between verbal and performance IQ, once assumed to be almost invariable in children with clefts, are now being found less frequently argues strongly for the position that language deficits may not be of a "primary" nature in children who are not otherwise impaired. Rather, they reflect problems emerging from a complex of factors that are not necessarily innate to children with clefts. As care improves and more relevant variables are brought under control, fewer marked symptoms of disruption in verbal performance manifest themselves. However, these early findings triggered our concern about language development and communication skills in children with clefts.

STUDIES OF ORAL LANGUAGE BEHAVIOR

The first studies of the development of communicative skills in older children with clefts stressed articulation proficiency and vocabulary size. Later, limited attention was paid to other aspects of language usage.

One of the early studies of language was that of Spriestersbach et al. (1958). They evaluated 40 children with clefts between the ages of 3.5 and 8.5 years and compared them with published norms for mean length of response (Templin, 1957), for structural complexity (McCarthy, 1930), and for vocabulary as measured by the Ammons Full Range Picture Vocabulary Test. The authors concluded that the children with clefts had a shorter mean length of response than the normative group but that their structural complexity did not differ. The children were also somewhat reduced in vocabulary usage but not in vocabulary recognition. Thus there was no evidence of overall language retardation, but deviations in expressive behavior were found.

Later, Morris (1962) expanded the study to include 107 children between the ages of 2 and 15.5 years. The methods of analysis were similar to the earlier study with the addition of correlations with a number of variables such as age, intelligence, speech competence, socioeconomic status, social maturity, and type of cleft.

Children up to age 8 were statistically less adequate than the normative samples on the Ammons Picture Vocabulary Test, mean sentence length, complexity of structure, variety of words used, and articulation skills. In this second study, vocabulary recognition was also reduced. These same trends held for children over the age of 8, but differences were not always statistically significant. The fact that articulation skills were correlated with language abilities only until the age of 7 suggests that errors after that age may have been related to physical characteristics. Spontaneity of expression, unlike the other characteristics, decreased with increasing chronological age. Although the children improved in usable communicative skills, they grew increasingly unable to respond verbally without inhibition.

Important though these findings were, no single measure correlated with other measures well enough to be used as an indicator of language functioning. This is not surprising. Shames and Rubin (1979) pointed out that Morris's results supported their view that language involves a number of interacting yet not completely interdependent developmental processes. One wonders what the outcome of the Morris study might have been had the factor of hearing been better controlled. Although, as we shall see, there is danger in overemphasizing the influence of ear disease, neither can we afford to ignore it.

Nation (1970a) used the Peabody Picture Vocabulary Test to assess both comprehension and usage in 25 children with clefts, 25 of their siblings, and 25 normal controls, all ranging in age from 34 to 63 months. As would be expected, comprehension was greater than usage in all groups. The normals in this study performed better than the siblings and the siblings better than the subjects with clefts. Nation concluded that "cleftness" affects vocabulary development.

In a companion study, Nation (1970b) examined the relationship between vocabulary as measured by the Peabody and other variables that might affect vocabulary development. Hearing loss and length of period of hospitalization were both significantly related to vocabulary measures, whereas socioeconomic status and the age at surgery were not.

These two studies included only preschool children, and subjects could have hearing losses as great as 30 dB in their better ears. Just how severe the losses were is not known. In addition, the reliability of the Peabody Picture Vocabulary Test has been shown to be highly questionable for use with children with clefts (McWilliams, 1974; Watson and Severson, 1976).

Shames et al. (1966) and Shames and Rubin (1971, 1979) tested 75 children with clefts and 75 noncleft children between the ages of 1.5 and 5.5 years. They used a standardized interview composed of 135 stimulus episodes based on Skinner's 1957 model of verbal behavior (echoic, mand, tact, intraverbal, autoclitic). The stimuli elicited socially usual responses including greeting, asking and answering questions, making assertions or denials, asking for help, responding to unusual behavior on the part of the examiner, providing reasons or qualifications, identifying emotions, offering response chains, and imitating stimuli presented by the examiner.

The children with clefts were 1.0 to 1.5 years behind noncleft children in responding as expected until about the age of 3 years, 9 months, when the group with clefts began to resemble their noncleft peers. By 4 years, 3 months, the groups were similar. By 5 years, 3 months, both groups responded to the items with 90% accuracy.

This study provided useful information about the order in which these various behaviors emerged in both groups. The earliest response was the *echoic* followed by the *tact* or naming. Asking for something, the *mand,* appeared next, followed by the *intraverbal* or chains of responses and idioms, and lastly, by the *autoclitic,* which Skinner defined as "verbal responses about verbal responses."

This study showed that children with clefts master Skinner's forms of verbal behavior at a slower pace than do their peers but that they overcome these lags and are similar to others by age 4 years, 3 months. In spite of this, the children with clefts maintained a higher grammatical error rate at all age levels, a result consistent with other studies indicative of slight language differences.

In a similar study, Warr-Leeper et al. (1988) evaluated 27 children by means of the Test of Pragmatic Skills (Shulman, 1985). In this study, the preschool children with clefts were not different from their peers but the cleft children of school age were less competent.

Exactly why these differences occurred is not clear, but they are at odds with the results of Shames and Rubin (1971, 1979). The difference in sample size is one possible explanation. Another is that differences that have washed out in the later preschool years may again be apparent at school age. Shames and Rubin did not continue their study into those years. It is also possible that the children under investigation were not comparable in terms of other relevant variables.

Smith and McWilliams (1968a,b) administered the Illinois Test of Psycholinguistic Abilities (ITPA) to 136 children with clefts ranging in age from 3 years to 8 years, 11 months of age. In comparison to ITPA normative data, the children demonstrated general psycholinguistic depression with particular weaknesses in vocal expression, gestural output, and visual memory.

In a longitudinal study of the efficacy of two different surgical procedures, Musgrave et al. (1975) unexpectedly learned that the children showed significant gains over time on a number of variables including scores on the ITPA. In a period of 2 years, the children moved from mean scores on the ITPA of 87 and 93 to 105 and 108, well within normal limits when compared with ITPA norms. Thus, when the same children are followed over a period of time, their ITPA psycholinguistic quotients appear to change significantly for the better. This apparent "catching up" was also suggested by Zimmerman and Canfield (1968), but they offered no data in support of their hypothesis.

The ITPA is not a language test in that it does not test linguistic performance *per se.* Rather, it tests behaviors that are thought to be relevant to linguistic development and certainly to learning and cognition. In fact, the ITPA is useful in identifying children with a variety of learning disabilities. For this reason, among others, investigators have sought more direct means of assessing language in children generally, as well as in children with clefts.

Faircloth and Faircloth (1971), in a study of children with clefts, concluded that "the child who strives for articulophonetic accuracy" reduces sentence length, word length, and sentence "complexity," while the child who "relies on language structure for intelligibility" uses a wider variety of linguistic constructions. These conclusions were based on a sample of 10 subjects with clefts from differing backgrounds, so the study, while of interest, is not conclusive. In fact, logic leads to the hypothesis that bad articulation in association with shorter, less involved sentences would increase intelligibility, whereas subjects able to articulate accurately would not be so constrained.

Pannbacker (1975) shed some light on the Faircloth study when she compared 20 adults with repaired clefts with 20 normal adults on a number of different language measures. The subjects with clefts were inferior to the normals on mean length of sentence, number of words in the longest response, mean length of the five longest responses, number of different words used, and the intelligibility of speech. However, for the subjects with clefts, there were significant correlations between intelligibility and mean length of response, number of words in the longest response, mean number of words in the five longest responses, the number of different words used, and scores on the vocabulary subtest of the Wechsler Adult Intelligence Scale. These findings for adults are in contrast to those of Faircloth and Faircloth (1971) for children and appear to have somewhat greater face validity.

Bland (1974) contributed to the resolution of this issue when she compared preschool subjects who had clefts and intelligible speech with a group of noncleft preschoolers on the Northwest Syntax Screening Tests, a verbal imitation test, and Developmental Sentence Scoring. She found no differences between the two groups. This study, together with that of Pannbacker (1971), casts doubt upon the conclusions of Faircloth and Faircloth and indicates the need for more definitive investigations in this area.

In a small but valuable study, Horn (1972) undertook a transformational analysis of the language output of three children with palatal clefts between 4 and 6 years of age and three normal children of similar age. She described the output of the children with clefts as immature. The rules that the children used were "clearly indicative of rules applied in the early stages of language acquisition." The differences were still present at age 5 but were less marked. The three normal children in the study had more advanced linguistic behavior; they demonstrated this through a decreased use of restricted forms and a greater proportion of grammatically correct transformations.

Horn also administered the ITPA to the six children. As in most other studies using this

instrument, the children with clefts were generally inferior to the noncleft children on the nine subtests but were least adequate in encoding. Like other writers, Horn speculated about the role of hearing problems, poor mother-child relationships, inhibition, parental overprotection, and inferior speech modeling. No conclusions could be drawn about causation since none of the variables had been investigated or controlled for. However, the relative improvement over time was again noted.

Brennan and Cullinan (1974) compared 14 children with clefts and 14 noncleft children at a mean age of 8 years, 10 months, and 8 years, 11 months, respectively on tasks involving object identification and naming. Once again, the children with clefts performed less well than did their controls. This study is of special interest because the cleft children, who were older than those of some earlier investigations, appeared to remain at somewhat of a disadvantage.

Whitcomb et al. (1976) explored the language functioning of 8 children with clefts and 8 normal children between 5 and 6 years of age. The children with clefts, although they had normal hearing and intelligence, were less competent on both the Developmental Sentence Scoring and the Length-Complexity Index (Shriner and Sherman, 1967). Discrepancies between these two small groups were obvious on both instruments but were more marked on the Length-Complexity Index. Again, these preschool children did less well than did their noncleft peers. The study stressed verbal output, and, regardless of what else has changed, it is probable that many children with clefts suffer from a reduction in the amount and complexity of their verbal productions.

STUDIES RELATING LANGUAGE BEHAVIOR TO HEARING

The consistency with which otitis media occurs in infants with palatal clefts and the strong evidence of fluctuating hearing losses, particularly in the early years, have led researchers to speculate about a possible relationship between otitis media and variations in language and speech development. Indeed, similar speculations about otitis media in children who do not have clefts are liberally represented in the literature.

Early landmark studies (Holm and Kunze, 1969; Clark, 1976; Zinkus et al., 1978), for the most part, supported a relationship between early ear disease and later developmental differences. However, the studies were often faulted on methodological grounds, and disagreement was the rule (Paradise, 1980, 1981; Ventry, 1980; Bluestone et al., 1983).

An extensive review of this topic can be found in a monograph on otitis media and child development (Hanson and Ulvestad, 1979), in which there are papers by Horowitz (1979) and Menyuk (1979). Horowitz reviewed the bases for the assessment of intelligence, commenting on the difficulties that can be encountered in attempting to relate a condition such as otitis media to the development of skills assessed by an intelligence test. Menyuk (1979) considered design factors in the assessment of language development in children with otitis media. She critically reviewed the existing literature, stressed the complexity of the issues, and identified various factors in normal language development, all of which are operative for children with clefts.

In a later paper (1980), Menyuk concluded that otitis media probably does have repercusions, but perhaps only for some children. She suggested that the age when the child experiences otitis media, the frequency and duration of the episodes, the extent of the accompanying hearing loss, the child's environment including socio-economic status, physical care, linguistic and psychological stimulation, and the basic cognitive competence of the child may all interact with the otitis media to create problems in some children but not in others. Using her criteria, children with clefts appear to be at increased risk.

Horowitz (1980) extended the argument with the suggestion that hearing loss that fluctuates in severity further complicates the understanding of this complex issue and may, in reality, increase the risk for children with clefts. She wrote:

. . . The infant with recurrent otitis media and periodic hearing loss experiences an inconsistent environment in terms of the clarity of auditory input. . . If consistent and repeated auditory input is important to language and cognitive development, then the child with recurrent otitis media is likely to be missing important experiences. The cumulative effects of recurrent otitis media could be critical depending upon the time during development when there is a high incidence and upon caretaker skills.

RECENT STUDIES OF NONCLEFT CHILDREN

Studies Relating Language Behavior to Hearing

Recent studies of otitis media and various aspects of development have not resolved the issues that were apparent earlier. Silva et al. (1982) compared 47 5-year-old children with bilateral otitis media with 355 otologically-normal children. Significant differences favoring the children free of otitis media were found on measurements of articulation, verbal comprehension, motor development, and intelligence. There was, however, no difference between groups on verbal expression. The differences found, while significant, were very small, and their practical significance must be questioned.

The group with otitis media also demonstrated increased dependency, shorter attention spans, weaker goal orientation, greater restlessness and destructiveness, and were more often disobedient and not liked by other children. The magnitude of these differences is unclear.

Silva et al. (1986) continued to follow the children described in the 1982 report through ages 7, 9, and 11. When mean IQs over the span of the study were combined, there was no significant difference between groups. However, differences in both receptive and expressive language and articulation were significant as were reading scores, all favoring the group free of otitis media. Behavior problems as reported by parents did not differ, but teachers reported significantly more problems in the group with otitis media.

It is important to note that hearing thresholds were significantly different in the two groups, although real differences averaged approximately 11 dB at age 5, 8 at age 7, and 6 at 9 and 11, differences that would not appear to have major clinical significance unless there was marked fluctuation, as there might have been. Again, this study points to differences that may be more impressive in their statistical than in their practical implications; but the data do support the evidence of some relationships even though they may be subtle.

Teele et al. (1984), in a well designed prospective study, followed children from birth and tested 205 at age 3. Children who had had prolonged middle-ear effusion had significantly lower scores on the Peabody Picture Vocabulary Test and on auditory comprehension and verbal ability quotients, subtests of the Zimmerman Pre-school Language Scale, when compared to those who had spent little time with middle-ear disease. These differences were especially marked in children from higher but not from lower socioeconomic levels.

Teele et al. found no differences between groups on measures of articulation, intelligibility of connected discourse, number of grammatical transformations, or mean length of utterance.

The authors concluded that time spent with middle-ear effusion in the first year of life was far more relevant to outcome at age 3 than at other time periods, even though it is common clinical practice to place tubes after the first year. Once again, the evidence of subtle differences in children with middle-ear disease emerges, but there is also information here to support the conclusion that many aspects of language and communicative development seem not to be affected. Confusion remains.

The problem is compounded by Roberts et al. (1988) who examined the relationship between otitis media during the first 3 years of life and subsequent speech development in 55 socioeconomically disadvantaged children attending a research day-care program. They found no significant relationship between otitis media in early childhood and the number of common phonological processes or consonant errors in the preschool years. However, the number of days of otitis media before age 3 was associated with the number of phonological processes used between the ages of $4^1/2$ and 8 years, suggesting that phonological processes tend to drop out more slowly for children with histories of otitis media. The authors suggest that these relationships are modest but warrant the monitoring of children with such histories. These authors also found no relationship between early otitis media and verbal or academic functioning at $3^1/2$ to 6 years of age (Roberts et al., 1986).

Wallace et al. (1988) compared 15 babies with normal otoscopic findings at least 80% of the time during the first year of life with 12 infants who had bilateral positive findings more than 30% of the time during the same period. They found no significant differences at 1 year of age between the two groups on the Bayley Scales of Infant Development or on the receptive scale of the Sequenced Inventory of Communication Development. However, the group with more episodes of otitis media was significantly lower than their peers on the expressive scale of the same test. The authors conclude that language intervention may be appropriate for infants who are prone to ear disease during the first year of life.

We conclude from these studies of noncleft children that middle-ear disease probably does have subtle developmental ramifications and that, even though some of the statistically significant differences are not likely to have profound implications in later functioning, an issue that still remains to be explored, the best course is to control the ear disease whenever possible. Programs of language intervention may be advisable in extreme cases but not in the absence of otological intervention.

Studies of the Interaction Between Ear Disease and Language Development in Children with Clefts

Given the evidence just reviewed for children who do not have clefts, it would be surprising if children with clefts and an almost universal occurrence of middle-ear disease did not provide data of similar magnitude and similar confusion, and that sums up the current state of our knowledge about this issue.

Galkowski et al. (1970) studied 95 cleft children aged 7 to 14 years, divided into two groups on the basis of hearing. Eighty-two percent of those without major losses were "delayed" in vocabulary, syntax, and vocabulary development, while 90% of those with "marked losses" showed such delays. These percentages are high, and it is suspected that the subjects had other significant problems, particularly in view of the fact that children between 7 and 14 have, for the most part, relatively stable hearing levels. The results of this study, conducted in Poland, are difficult to interpret because the methodologies are not specified.

Axton (1972) evaluated 26 selected children from the Smith and McWilliams study (1968a, b) between 4 years and 5 years, 11 months, of age. These subjects, who had not had active ear care from birth, were compared to 31 others of similar age who had had intensive ear care. On the ITPA, the mean for the group having aggressive ear care was significantly higher than for the other group.

The most significant differences were in manual expression and auditory sequential memory. Verbal expression was also better but remained somewhat below ITPA norms.

The children who had not had ear care were also audiologically inferior to those who had been treated from birth. However, since active, ongoing ear care depended on the regularity with which parents kept appointments, parental interest may have been a confounding factor. While this was a small study, it points to a tentative relationship between ear disease and performance on the ITPA.

Bless et al. (1972) reported the results of two studies designed to investigate the language and related skills of children with clefts. They indicated that children with hearing losses showed language deficits. Later, Saxman and Bless (1973) examined 60 cleft and noncleft children, all with normal hearing at the time of the study, between the ages of 3 and 8 years, and matched for age, sex, and socioeconomic level. The authors wisely used a variety of language tests. They found no significant differences between groups on any of the tests. One may speculate, however, that the children, particularly if they had histories of repeated and poorly controlled middle-ear disease, might have shown earlier language deficits as did the cleft children with hearing losses studied in their 1972 investigation. Without more compelling evidence of the hearing status of the subjects over time, these conclusions remain tentative.

Hubbard et al. (1985) evaluated 24 closely matched children between 5 and 11 years of age. Management of their palatal clefts had been equivalent, but ear care had differed. One group had had aggressive ear care on an ongoing basis and initial myringotomies at 3 months, while the other had not been consistently followed and had had myringotomies at a mean age of 30.8 months or, as in two cases, not at all. The children who had had active ear care from birth had significantly better hearing and consonant articulation than did their matched controls. However, the groups did not differ on verbal, performance, or full-scale IQs as determined by the Wechsler Intelligence Scale for Children, Revised, on social maturity measured by the Vineland Social Maturity Scale, on self esteem indicated by the Coopersmith Self-Esteem Inventory, or on behaviors reported in response to the Child Behavior Checklist. This study did not support the hypothesis that cognitive, language, and psychosocial development are adversely affected by otitis media.

A modest relationship between otitis media and subsequent language development in children both with and without clefts is suggested by the research conducted to date. However, as Menyuk (1980) suggested, otitis media may place some children at greater risk for language deficits than it does others.

Bishop and Edmundson (1986) found the same interactions that others have reported but were reluctant to draw the same conclusions. Instead, they speculated that otitis media alone may not be a crucial determinant of language disorder but that it may interact with other risk factors so that it becomes important if the child is already vulnerable because of a hazardous perinatal history. They pointed out that most language research has explored one etiological factor at a time and that we need to design studies specifically to look for interactions among variables. From their own data, they were particularly impressed with family histories of language disorders in first-degree relatives and suggested that it might be fruitful to look for a genetic component in some of these problems.

We concur with the view of Bishop and Edmundson and must conclude that the evidence of a one-to-one relationship between otitis media and language deficits does not exist for children with or without clefts. Rather, it is probable that many language disorders are associated with multiple causal factors including genetics, parent-child interactions, variations in neural integrity, intelligence, social competence, social responses to various handicaps, life experience in and out of clinics, and otitis media, among many other things.

This interpretation of the literature, on the other hand, in no way denies the importance of providing adequate ear care to children in general and, specifically, to children with clefts, who are at high risk for ear disease, hearing loss, and the complications that occur when otitis media is not treated. It is clinically desirable to minimize possible negative factors, wherever they occur, in order to maximize the child's developmental potential.

THE EVIDENCE FOR LANGUAGE-BASED LEARNING DISABILITIES

Richman and Eliason (1986) summarized the literature suggesting the probability of language-based learning disabilities in children with clefts. Of special interest is Richman's work (1980). He assessed 57 children who had a lower verbal than performance IQs. He found that one group of children demonstrated only an expressive deficit, whereas another group had a more generalized deficit that involved both receptive and expressive abilities and disturbances in associative reasoning. These problems occurred most often in males with cleft palate only.

A later study by this group (Richman and Eliason, 1984) confirmed the greater language deficit in 24 children with cleft palate only than in 24 with clefts of both the lip and palate. Criteria for participation in the study included at least average full-scale IQ on the WISC, reading at least one year below grade level on the Wide Range Achievement Test, grade placement between third and sixth, absence of other contributing conditions, and hearing loss no greater than 30 dB in the poorer ear. Since the data were not analyzed with reference to hearing loss, questions must be raised about the possible role of hearing losses of that magnitude in this study. It will be remembered that Silva et al. (1986) found an increase in reading deficits in noncleft children with otitis media.

Children with clefts of the lip and palate were significantly higher on memory for words and sentences and language-association tasks such as auditory association, word fluency, and picture association. There were no differences in visual-perceptual, visual-motor, or graphomotor skills as had been suggested in earlier studies (Smith and McWilliams, 1968a, b).

Richman and Eliason also investigated the nature of reading problems in these 48 children. There were no differences between groups on word recognition, but children with cleft palate only were below the group with cleft lip and palate in reading comprehension and made significantly more nonphonetic errors, whereas the group with both lip and palatal clefts made more phonetic errors.

The authors concluded that children with clefts of the lip and palate and reading disabilities appear to have only peripheral speech problems related primarily to phonetic reading errors. They also demonstrate good reading comprehension skills, are within normal range on neuropsychological tasks, and have no signs of symbolic language deficiencies. Children with cleft palate only, when they have reading disabilities, demonstrate significantly more sight-word errors and reduced reading comprehension, suggesting the possibility of a basic language deficiency.

Richman et al. (1988) strengthened their

position in a study of 172 cleft children in elementary school. They learned that reading problems occurred in 48.6% of children with clefts of the lip and palate and in 53.3% of those with cleft palate only between the ages of 6 and 7 years. Between 8 and 9, the percentages decreased to 22.7% and 37.5% respectively. Between 10 and 13, the 8.6% for children with clefts of the lip and palate matched the rate for the general population, while those with palatal clefts only showed a rate of 33.3%. Thus, both groups showed a decrease in reading disabilities with increase in age, but the palate-only group retained a significant number of impaired readers.

There is less evidence about writing abilities in children with clefts than there is about reading. Ebert et al. (1974) found no differences between the writing skills of 23 children with clefts who had a mean age of 7 years, 7 months, and 23 matched controls with a mean age of 7 years, 9 months. All subjects had hearing within normal limits at the time they were tested, and they were matched for intelligence and socioeconomic level. The Myklebust Picture Story Language Test was administered. The authors suggested that, since written language skills are logically related to linguistic competence, subjects with clefts appear "to have access to words and structures which they may not call upon for purposes of verbal communication." We are very far from knowing why, and the findings of Kommers and Sullivan (1979), which showed a decline in writing skills with an increase in chronological age, lead to new concerns.

It is possible that the children in the study by Ebert et al. were too young for differences in writing skills to manifest themselves in the way they might in older children. This issue requires further exploration as does performance in other academic areas including mathematics, which clinical experience suggests may also be at increased risk.

Richman et al. (1988) make a strong case for the inclusion of psychological-educational assessments as part of team management and for studies addressing the best approach to those problems, which appear to reflect central language disabilities. We concur.

CURRENT STATE OF THE ART AND FUTURE RESEARCH NEEDS

It is clear that many different studies over the

past 30 years have found evidence of mild language deficits in children with clefts, especially if they have clefts of the palate only. However, these studies have not been in agreement about the nature or extent of these differences, nor have we yet successfully specified the origins of the language problems when they are found to be present. By the same token, we have written too little about cleft children who do not have language deficits, and we have not explored how the variables in their lives differ from those in the lives of children who function less than ideally in language skills. It is clear that the time has come to stop describing what we know to be present to one degree or another and to begin searching for explanations of a multifactorial nature, including social-emotional dimensions and hearing loss that may interact in unique ways to cause problems in some but not all children with clefts.

Of particular interest would be studies designed to explore language usage or sociocommunicative skills (Chapman and Hardin, in press). Chapman and Hardin discuss this aspect of language behavior in terms of ability to use language for communication. However, it is important to remember that inability to develop communicative skills and unwillingness to become involved in certain interpersonal interactions can easily be confused clinically and often are. Thus, we would like to see studies of communicative behaviors and the way in which they may vary under differing sets of stimuli. Nonetheless, Chapman and Hardin are wise to suggest the use of the model proposed by Fey (1986) as a means of exploring communicative behavior in children with clefts.

In this model, conversational assertiveness, described as the ability or willingness to take a conversational turn when there has been no direct solicitation from the conversational partner, and conversational responsiveness, or the child's response when invited to take a turn, are both examined.

This system describes children as active conversationalists when they both initiate and respond to the efforts of others, as passive conversationalists when they respond but do not initiate, as inactive communicators when they rarely initiate and are also underresponsive, and as verbal noncommunicators when they initiate but are underresponsive to others. Chapman and Hardin

suggest that their clinical experience indicates that children with clefts can most often be described as passive or inactive communicators. While we know cleft children with and without speech and language problems who fit each of the four categories, we agree that the model is a fascinating one and one that lends itself to research purposes. Of special interest would be relating these conversational styles to various indicators of language and speech deficits and to the many other variables that may help to establish conversational modes. Information from such a study might help to delineate the most reasonable approaches to treatment as well as to clarify the origins of some of the variations we continue to find even though we understand them poorly.

It is clear that the final evidence of the relationship of otitis media to language deficits is still not in. Of special concern is the failure in many past studies to specify the degree of hearing impairment. There is likely to be a vast difference between two children who both have otitis media but one of whom has a hearing loss of 15 dB and the other a loss of 45 dB. Another problem is the fact that middle-ear disease fluctuates and that investigations that take evidence of hearing impairment or of middle-ear fluid only on the day testing is done may not be recognizing differences in children with chronic ear disease as opposed to those with acute problems. Future studies should control many such variables as well as consider the interaction among variables.

Much more research is needed with respect to the learning disabilities which may be prevalent in certain but not all children with clefts. It is relevant here to define differences between children who have innate neuropsychological deficits as opposed to those who, for reasons of poor self esteem or social penalty, are unable to perform academically as well as their native abilities dictate. The interaction among these factors is difficult to explore, but it is a challenge that we must try to meet.

As clinicians, we should be aware of the possibility of language disabilities in children with clefts, understand the necessity for careful evaluation, and be prepared to intervene when it is appropriate to do so. We should also be aware that language intervention is not invariably required and recognize those children who are better served if we do not intervene.

REFERENCES

Axton S. Hearing loss, otological care, and language retardation in cleft palate children. Masters thesis, University of Pittsburgh, 1972.

Bishop DVM, Edmundson A. Is otitis media a major cause of specific developmental language disorders? Br J Disord Commun 1986; 21:321.

Bland J. A language comparison of intelligible preschool children with cleft palate and noncleft palate preschool children. Masters thesis, University of North Carolina, 1974.

Bless D, Saxman J, Evanowski S. Influence of hearing loss on vocabulary comprehension in children with palatal cleft. Unpublished study, 1972.

Bluestone CD, Klein JO, Paradise JL, et al. Workshop on effects of otitis media on the child. Pediatrics 1983; 71:639.

Brennan D, Cullinan W. Object identification and naming in cleft palate children. Cleft Palate J 1974; 11:188.

Chapman KL, Hardin MA. Considerations about language in children with cleft lip and palate. In press.

Clark M. Hearing: a link to IQ? Newsweek 1976; June 14:46.

Clifford E. Psychological aspects of cleft lip and palate. In: Bzoch KR, ed. Communicative disorders related to cleft lip and palate. Boston: Little, Brown, 1979:37.

Ebert PR, McWilliams BJ, Woolf G. A comparison of the written language ability of cleft palate and normal children. Cleft Palate J 1974; 11:17.

Faircloth S, Faircloth M. Delayed language and linguistic variations. In: Grabb W, Rosenstein S, Bzoch K, eds. Cleft lip and palate. Boston: Little, Brown, 1971:805.

Fey ME. Language intervention in young children. San Diego: College-Hill Press, 1986.

Galkowski T, Gassowski P, Grossman J. Influence of hearing disorders on development of speech in children with cleft lip and palate. Folia Phoniatr 1970; 22:72.

Goodstein LD. Intellectual impairment in children with cleft palate. J Speech Hear Res 1961; 4:287.

Hanson DG, Ulvestad RF. Otitis media and child development. Ann Otol Rhinol Laryngol 1979; Suppl 60:88.

Holm V, Kunze L. Effect of chronic otitis media on language and speech development. Pediatrics 1969; 43:833.

Horn L. Language development of the cleft palate child. J S Afr Speech Hear Assoc 1972; 19:17.

Horowitz FD, Leake H. Design factors in the assessment of intelligence. Ann Otol Rhinol Laryngol 1979; 88 (Suppl 60):

Horowitz FD. Effects of otitis media on cognitive development. Ann Otol Rhinol Laryngol 1980; 89 (Suppl 68):264.

Hubbard TW, Paradise JL, McWilliams BJ, Elster BA, Taylor FH. Consequences of unremitting middle-ear disease in early life. N Engl J Med 1985; 312: 1529.

Kommers M, Sullivan M. Written language skills of children with cleft palate. Cleft Palate J 1979; 16:81.

Lamb M, Wilson F, Leeper H. The intellectual function of cleft palate children compared on the basis of cleft type and sex. Cleft Palate J 1973; 10:367.

Leeper HA, Pannbacker M, Roginski J. Oral language characteristics of adult cleft palate speakers compared on the basis of cleft type and sex. J Commun Dis 1980; 13:133.

McCarthy D. Language development of the preschool child. Minneapolis, MN: University of Minnesota Press, 1930.

McWilliams BJ. Psychosocial development and modification. ASHA Reports No. 5, 1970:165.

McWilliams BJ. Language problems. ASHA Reports No. 9, 1973:41.

McWilliams BJ. Clinical use of the Peabody Picture Vocabulary Test with cleft palate pre-schoolers. Cleft Palate J 1974; 11:439.

McWilliams BJ, Matthews HP. A comparison of intelligence and social maturity in children with unilateral complete clefts and those with isolated cleft palate. Cleft Palate J 1979; 16:363.

McWilliams BJ, Musgrave R. Psychological implications of articulation disorders in cleft palate children. Cleft Palate J 1972; 9:94.

Menyuk P. Design factors in the assessment of language development in children with otitis media. Ann Otol Rhinol Laryngol 1979; 88 (Suppl 60):78.

Menyuk P. Effect of persistent otitis media on language development. Ann Otol Rhinol Laryngol 1980; 89 (Suppl 68):257.

Morris HL. Communication skills of children with cleft lip and palate. J Speech Hear Res 1962; 5:79.

Musgrave R, McWilliams BJ, Matthews H. A review of the results of two different surgical approaches for the repair of clefts of the soft palate only. Cleft Palate J 1975; 12:281.

Nation J. Vocabulary comprehension and usage of preschool cleft palate and normal children. Cleft Palate J 1970a; 7:639.

Nation J. Determinants of vocabulary development of preschool cleft palate children. Cleft Palate J 1970b; 7:645.

Pannbacker M. Language skills of cleft palate children: a review. Br J Disord Commun 1971: 6:37.

Pannbacker M. Oral language skills of adult cleft palate speakers. Cleft Palate J 1975; 12:95.

Paradise JL. Otitis media in infants and children. Pediatrics 1980; 65:917.

Paradise JL. Otitis media during early life: How hazardous to development? A critical review of the evidence. Pediatrics 1981; 68:869.

Richman LC. Cognitive patterns and learning disabilities in cleft palate children with verbal deficits. J Speech Hear Res 1980; 23:447.

Richman LC, Eliason M. Type of reading disability related to cleft type and neuropsychological patterns. Cleft Palate J 1984; 21:1.

Richman LC, Eliason MJ. Development in children with cleft lip and/or palate: intellectual, cognitive, personality, and parental factors. In: McWilliams BJ, ed. Seminars in speech and language. Current methods of assessing and treating children with cleft palates. New York: Thieme, 1986.

Richman LC, Eliason MJ, Lindgren SD. Reading disability in children with clefts. Cleft Palate J 1988; 25:21.

Roberts JE, Burchinal MR, Koch MA, Footo MM, Henderson FW. Otitis media in early childhood and its relationship to later phonological development. J Speech Hear Dis 1988; 53:424.

Roberts JE, Sanyal MA, Burchinal MR, Collier AM, Ramey CT, Henderson FW. Otitis media in early childhood and its relationship to later verbal and academic performance. Pediatrics 1986; 78:423.

Ruess AL. A comparative study of cleft palate children and their siblings. J Clin Psychol 1965; 21:354.

Ruess AL, Lis EF. A multidimensional study of handicapped children. Final Report to Maternal and Child Health Services. Health Services and Mental Health Services Administration, Department of Health, Education and Welfare, Grant No. MC-R- 170007-04-0, 1973.

Saxman J, Bless D. Patterns of language development in cleft palate children aged three to eight years. Presented at 31st Annual Meeting of the American Cleft Palate Association, Oklahoma City, 1973.

Shames G, Rubin H. Psycholinguistic measures of language and speech. In: Bzoch K, ed. Communicative disorders related to cleft lip and palate. Boston: Little, Brown, 1971:201.

Shames G, Rubin H. Psycholinguistic measures of language and speech. In: Bzoch K, ed. Communicative disorders related to cleft lip and palate. 2nd ed. Boston: Little, Brown, 1979:202.

Shames G, Rubin H, Kramer JC. The development of verbal behavior in cleft palate and non-cleft palate children. Presented at the Annual Meeting of the American Cleft Palate Association, Mexico City, 1966.

Shriner T, Sherman D. An equation for assessing language development. J Speech Hear Res 1967; 10:41.

Shulman BB. Test of pragmatic skills. Tuscon, Arizona, 1985.

Silva PA, Chalmers D, Stewart I. Some audiological, psychological, educational and behavioral characteristics of children with bilateral otitis media with effusion: a longitudinal study. J Learn Dis 1986; 19:165.

Silva PA, Kirkland C, Simpson A, Stewart IA, Williams SM. Some developmental and behavioral problems associated with bilateral otitis media with effusion. J Learn Dis 1982; 15:417.

Skinner BF. Verbal Behavior. New York: Appleton-Century-Crofts, 1957.

Smith RM, McWilliams BJ. Psycholinguistic abilities of children with clefts. Cleft Palate J 1968a; 5:238.

Smith RM, McWilliams BJ. Psycholinguistic considerations of the management of children with cleft palate. J Speech Hear Dis 1968b; 33:27.

Spriestersbach DC, Darley FL, Morris HL. Language skills in children with cleft palate. J Speech Hear Res 1958; 1:279.

Teele DW, Klein JO, Rosner BA, The Greater Boston Otitis Media Study Group. Otitis media with effusion during the first three years of life and development of speech and language. Pediatrics 1984; 74:282.

Templin M. Certain language skills in children: their development and interrelationships. Institute of Child Welfare Management, Ser 26. Minneapolis: University of Minneapolis Press, 1957.

Ventry IM. Effects of conductive hearing loss: Fact or fiction. J Speech Hear Dis 1980; 45:143.

Wallace IF, Gravel JS, McCarton CM, Ruben RJ. Otitis media and language development at 1 year of age. J Speech Hear Dis 1988; 53:145.

Warr-Leeper G, Crone L, Carruthers A, Leeper H. A comparison of the performance of preschool children with cleft lip and/or palate on the test of pragmatic skills. Presented at the Annual Meeting of the American Cleft Palate-Craniofacial Association, Williamsburg, Virginia, 1988.

Watson C, Severson R. The Peabody Picture Vocabulary Test as a measure of intelligence in children with palatal problems. Cleft Palate J 1976; 13:357.

Whitcomb L, Ochsner G, Wayte R. A comparison of expressive language skills of cleft palate and non-cleft palate children: a preliminary investigation. J Okla Speech Hear Assoc 1976; 3:25.

Wirls CJ. Psychosocial aspects of cleft lip and palate. In: Grabb WC, Rosenstein SW, Bzoch K, eds. Cleft lip and palate: Boston: Little, Brown, 1971:119.

Zimmerman J, Canfield. Language and speech development. In: Stark R, ed. Cleft palate. a multidiscipline approach. New York: Harper and Row, 1968:220.

Zinkus PW, Gottlieb M, Schapiro M. Developmental and psychoeducational sequelae of chronic otitis media. Am J Dis Child 1978; 132:1100.

14 | DISORDERS OF PHONATION AND RESONANCE

This chapter deals with two major aspects of voice—phonation and resonance. Both are likely to be impaired when there is velopharyngeal incompetence caused by cleft palate or any other condition that leads to the coupling of the oral and nasal cavities during speech. Resonance disorders are, however, often the major focus of concern.

VOICE PRODUCTION

As a prelude to the consideration of phonation and resonance in people with velopharyngeal incompetence, the student should recall that the acoustic characteristics of voice are generated in the larynx. Pulses of respiratory air are released into the supraglottic portion of the vocal tract as the vocal cords vibrate. The fundamental frequency of voice is dependent upon the length of the cords interacting with mass and tension. These pulses excite supraglottic air, and the sound wave travels omnidirectionally at a much greater speed than that of the aeromechanical wave that initiated it. Minifie (1973) likened these phenomena to the wave appearing in the water when a swimmer dives into a pool. This wave is accompanied by an acoustic wave, which can be heard before the wave reaches the listener. Both waves are established by the same force, but the waves differ in speed and direction.

In speech, the voice signal is transmitted through the vocal tract, which includes the pharyngeal, oral, and nasal cavities. These tissues are covered by mucosa and are shaped by their skeletal frameworks. They are influenced by any condition that alters their impedance, which is defined as the amount of energy that is accepted or rejected per unit of time. Impedance is deter-

mined by the interaction of three major factors in the resonating system: mass, stiffness or compliance, and resistance or viscosity. The structure and configuration of the tract will determine the spectrum (frequency emphasis) of the resulting tone. Acoustic features resulting from resonation in the supraglottic cavities are called "formant frequencies." Vowels are complex tones, that is, they are composed of the fundamental frequency enriched by overtones that are harmonics of the fundamental tone.

During the production of normal non-nasal speech, the velopharyngeal port is closed, or nearly so, and impedance is high for the transmission of the sound wave into the passages superior to the portal. When the portal is open, as it normally is for nasal consonants and the vowels adjacent to them, impedance is reduced, and the unimpeded sound wave moves freely into the nasal passages, provided the nasal passages themselves do not present increased resistance resulting from some degree of blockage. When velopharyngeal incompetence is present, impedance at the velopharyngeal port is always reduced; the sound wave is deflected into the nasal passages when it is inappropriate, and hypernasality is the result. Thus, it is clear that the velopharyngeal valve, for the production of normal speech, must be capable of opening and closing with the demands of speech.

In both normal and incompetent speakers, the sound wave that passes through the velopharyngeal port is further modified by pathway variations that alter mass, stiffness, or resistance. For example, resonance is altered when the normal person has an infection of the upper respiratory tract. The degree of change is dependent on the severity of tissue involvement. In addition to their ability to move into all parts of the resonating system, sound waves are also capable of traveling through tissue. For this reason, normal resonance is marked by some head resonance arising from the nasopharyngeal and nasal passages.

Voice production is a highly integrated, automatic behavior that requires the finely tuned interaction of the respiratory system, the laryngeal structures, and the supraglottic vocal tube with both its oral and nasal branches. A problem in one part of the system is likely to be reflected elsewhere.

TERMINOLOGY

Individuals with velopharyngeal incompetence have traditionally been described in the literature as having hypernasal voice quality. It should be remembered that hypernasality is not a problem associated with phonation but is the result of alterations that occur when the oral and nasal cavities are coupled when they should be separated by action of the velopharyngeal valve. Hypernasality is not, in this sense, a voice problem if that implies phonation. Zemlin (1968) recognized the controversy over this issue and suggested that the phrase "vocal quality disorders" be reserved for problems having to do with abnormal patterns of vocal fold behavior and that "voice disorders" be used to designate hypernasality. We find this terminology somewhat confusing. Thus, in this book, "phonation disorders" refers to a problem that occurs at the level of the larynx, a disorder of phonation. Hypernasality and other disturbances that occur supraglottally will be referred to as "resonance disorders." Phonation and resonance together comprise voice quality.

PHONATION

Prevalence of Phonation Disorders in Noncleft Speakers

Phonation disorders are found in both children and adults. However, the subjective nature of assessment, the semantics of describing phonation that listeners agree is aberrant in some way, and the difficulty of following up with examinations of the larynx and of the speech signal pose problems of interpretation. Senturia and Wilson (1968), in a study of 32,500 children, determined that 6% had phonation disorders. Wilson (1971) estimated an occurrence of 6% in elementary and junior-highschool children, but he thought that only 1% were in need of therapy.

The phonation disorder described as hoarseness has also been explored by several investigators. Baynes (1966) studied 1012 elementary school children and found that 7.1% were hoarse, whereas Yairi et al. (1974) placed the percentage at 13, with only between 2.4 and 3.4% of clinical importance. Silverman and Zimmer (1975) reported chronic hoarseness in 38 of 162 children (23%) from kindergarten through eighth grade. Nine of the 38 were laryngoscoped, and seven of these (78%) had vocal-cord nodules. This was higher than the 57% reported by Shearer (1972). It is obvious that the criteria used to define "chronic hoarseness" is not sufficiently well standardized to interpret the differences in outcome of these studies.

Few studies of phonation disorders in adults appear in the literature. Laguaite (1972) assessed 428 patients between 18 and 82 years of age. She reported that 7.2% of the males and 5% of the females had voice disorders worthy of laryngeal examination. Brindle and Morris (1979), in a study of 112 adults aged 17 to 80, found that 2.7% had phonation patterns that were "clearly abnormal." They interpreted their data to mean that such disorders are more prevalent in children than in adults and pointed out that maturation alone may resolve problems in a number of cases.

The criteria for establishing that a phonation disorder is present are of major concern in determining the frequency of these problems in both children and adults. The lack of adequate laryngeal data further complicates our ability to view variations from an objective perspective. However, most investigators, directly or indirectly, agree that the most frequently encountered problems are those associated with vocal hyperfunction (Aronson, 1980; Boone and McFarlane, 1988).

Prevalence of Phonation Disorders in Speakers with Clefts

McDonald and Baker (1951), Westlake (1953), and Hess (1959) all recognized faulty phonation as an important attribute of the speech of people with palatal clefts. McDonald and

Baker pointed out that laryngoscopic examinations often reveal "hyperemia" and "hyperplasia" of the vocal folds in adult patients.

The occurrence of phonatory disorders in individuals with clefts is not well understood because it may vary from one sample to another depending on such variables as velopharyngeal competence and the criteria for determining the presence of a phonatory deviation. It is clear, however, that phonation disorders are more common than in normals. Brooks and Shelton (1963) reported an occurrence of 10% of 76 children while Takagi et al. (1965), in a retrospective study, found only 0.6% in 1061 cleft patients over a wide age range. Marks et al. (1971) identified laryngeal dysfunction in 34% of 102 subjects over 6 and under 20 years of age. More males than females were thought to have phonatory deviations.

Deering (1984) investigated the prevalence of dysphonia in 38 subjects with clefts and found that 50% had aberrant phonation. Of these, 23.7% were described as hoarse, 13.2% as harsh, and 10.5% as breathy. D'Antonia et al. (1988) examined 85 patients to determine the prevalence of perceived phonatory symptoms and/or laryngeal abnormalities. Forty-one percent of the subjects had evidences of laryngeal or phonatory abnormalities.

Although data differ from study to study as do methodologies, the evidence overwhelmingly supports the conclusion that phonation deficits are considerably more common in subjects with clefts than in those without clefts.

The Nature of Phonation Disorders Associated with Velopharyngeal Incompetence

Hoarseness

In 1969, McWilliams et al. provided information about 43 children with cleft palates and hoarseness. Thirty-two of the 43 children with chronic hoarseness were successfully laryngoscoped, and 84% had positive vocal-cord findings. The most usual pathological condition was bilateral vocal-cord nodules, which occurred in 23 or 71.9% of the children. Other pathological conditions included posterior glottal chink, bilateral vocal cord hypertrophy, slight anterior edema, and improper approximation of the vocal cords. The child with edema was laryngoscoped a second time 4 months later and, at that time, had bilateral nodules.

One case of particular interest was that of a boy who wore a prosthetic appliance that permitted air leakage. In order to evaluate his velopharyngeal valving capabilities more completely and at the request of the referring clinic, we undertook a trial period of speech therapy. During the course of the therapy, his voice became increasingly hoarse. Laryngoscopy revealed large bilateral nodules. This observation led us to speculate that attempts to compensate for inadequate velopharyngeal valving—as was demanded by speech therapy—might be related to the onset of the vocal-cord nodules.

A relationship between faulty valving, hoarseness, and speech therapy was reinforced when it was discovered that 16 of the 22 children with vocal-cord nodules had had speech therapy prior to the diagnosis of laryngeal pathology. For this reason, the velopharyngeal valving capabilities of all 32 chronically hoarse children were evaluated by lateral videofluoroscopy. Seven of the 32 children with known vocal-cord pathology had velopharyngeal-valving capacities that were considered at that time to be adequate for speech, although they achieved only touch velopharyngeal closure, which we have since recognized as a borderline valve. None had the partial or total blending of structures seen in unequivocally competent mechanisms. At that time, base-view videofluoroscopy was not available, so it is not known what deficiencies might have been revealed if the orifice had been viewed *en face*. However, touch closure is often associated with small midline openings for patients whose lateral views show closure but whose speech is not consistent with a competent mechanism.

Nineteen children fell clearly into the borderline-valving classification. Seven had touch closure combined with inconsistency in achieving closure, and one had touch closure with improper timing. Eleven had wider openings in the hyperextended position, and six failed to achieve closure under any circumstances, although the openings were very narrow.

It is of interest to note that the laryngologist did not hear hoarseness in eight children (in addition to the 32 studied). Seven of these were laryngoscoped, and all had normal vocal cords. The hoarseness previously heard appeared to have been acute rather than chronic as in the other subjects.

Children with cleft palates associated with chronic hoarseness are likely to have vocal-cord pathology, particularly bilateral vocal-cord nodules, and this combination leads to a suspicion of velopharyngeal-valving deficits. Children with clefts and hoarseness or have any other evidence of velopharyngeal-valving deficiencies should probably *not* be subjected to the stresses of speech therapy for hypernasality because of the chance that they will compensate laryngeally. Vocal-cord nodules appear to be a danger signal and to provide evidence of a need for further evaluation of the valving mechanism and consideration of secondary management.

Since this was not a study of prevalence, no claim is made that children with clefts have vocal-cord nodules any more or less frequently than children who do not have clefts. Nodules are not infrequent in childhood and occur also in adults. Fitzhugh et al. (1958) reported that 134 of 300 cases (44%) with benign vocal-cord lesions had nodules. Such nodules usually reflect vocal misuse of a hyperfunctional nature. In children, the condition has been popularly called the "screaming-child syndrome." It is our contention, however, that hyperfunction of the vocal apparatus can spring from a variety of causes and that the attempt to compensate for velopharyngeal incompetence is one possible precipitating factor. Many children so affected are virtually unable to increase vocal intensity and regularly demonstrate the elevated larynx and neck tension typical of the hyperfunctional speaker.

In a second investigation by McWilliams et al. (1973), 27 of the subjects who had participated in the previous study were recalled for reevaluation at an average of 4.7 years following their initial assessment. At follow-up, 70% had retained their vocal-cord abnormalities. The eight subjects who demonstrated normal cords at the time of the second study continued to have hoarseness. Subjects who no longer showed vocal-cord pathology but retained hoarseness had an average age of 15 years, 8 months, as opposed to an average of 12 years, 1 month, for those children who retained the vocal-cord abnormalities. This difference was statistically significant and indicated that age probably played a role in the remission of the nodules. Surgical removal of the nodules was usually ineffective unless attention was also given to the faulty velopharyngeal-valving mechanism. When the valve was altered, as it was in seven children, the phonation problem was usually eliminated. No patient failed to show improvement when the valve was made more competent. Vocal-cord pathology also showed improvement following attention to the valve. Nodules either disappeared or were reduced in size.

Since children with velopharyngeal-valving problems retain their vocal-cord nodules longer than do noncleft children, whose transitional age has been placed at 11 years (Senturia and Wilson, 1968), the hypothesis of a relationship between velopharyngeal incompetence, the development of hoarseness, and vocal-cord abnormalities appears to be valid.

Greenberg (1982) surveyed 200 speech-language pathologists, of whom 70 responded, about the number of children in their programs with hoarseness. Hoarseness was reported in 5% of 121 hearing-impaired children, 3.3% of 3,244 articulatory cases, 3.7% of 191 stutterers, and 15.8% of 38 subjects with cleft palates. It is of interest that the speech-language pathologists referred 42% of children with articulation disorders and 43% of the stutterers for unspecified medical evaluations but referred none of the children with clefts. This failure to recognize the possible meaning of hoarseness in a child with a cleft may result in ill-advised or fruitless therapy.

The deviations discussed here have been variously labelled hoarseness, breathiness, aspirate quality, huskiness, or hoarseness with aperiodic aphonia. In some extreme cases, what approaches a glottal fry is also heard. Individuals with the most serious disturbances will have occasional breaks in voice accompanied by aphonia and then a return to hoarseness. These periodic breaks and aphonia appear to be associated, usually, with larger bilateral vocal-cord nodules and with relatively greater degrees of velopharyngeal-valving deficits.

Nodules are of special concern because they are indicators of vocal hyperfunction, but also because Scherer et al. (1982), noting that a growth on the vocal fold may change the shape, mass, viscosity, and stiffness of the fold so that the two vocal folds are biomechanically unequal, examined the pressure-flow relationships in rigid models of the laryngeal airway with different simulated growths on the vocal folds. They found that nonobstructive growths on the vocal folds may not be associated with greater respiratory effort, which may be necessary if the growths are obstructive. However, growths anywhere in the larynx may result in altered flow patterns in the glottis sufficient to create asymmetric glottal-wall pressures. Thus, the driving forces on the folds may be changed, augmenting motion asymmetries caused by the tissue asymmetries and resulting in loss of vocal control. In addition, they suggest, laryngeal growths may alter the mechanicoreceptor system and neurological control of the larynx. Although this was a pilot study, it serves to demonstrate the complex issues that are involved when growths on the vocal cords occur. Scherer et al. point to the need for more complete studies in this area, and we suggest that they are also required in systems incorporating velopharyngeal incompetence.

Soft-Voice Syndrome

Because of loss of pressure through the velopharyngeal port, some cleft patients have difficulty creating voice of sufficient loudness for conversational purposes. Reduced loudness may be a compensatory strategy for some, whereas others seem unable to achieve increased intensity under any circumstances. Patients with this characteristic may have little nasal escape, even though their valving mechanisms are deficient. Those who succeed in increasing loudness must use subglottic pressures higher than normal, leading to elevated nasal emission and perceptions of hypernasality.

Bzoch (1979) alluded to this problem in his discussion of "dysphonia characterized by aspirate voice." He found this "weak and aspirate" voice in 323 of 1000 cleft patients and speculated that these voices were developed to compensate for velopharyngeal incompetence in order to improve intelligibility.

There are few data to support the association between reduced loudness and velopharyngeal-valving deficits, nor are we sure how often it occurs. However, it is a feature of phonation heard clinically and should be recognized as a possible indicator of a deficient valving mechanism.

Monotone

Often accompanying the soft-voice syndrome is the monotonous voice with little pitch variation. Patients with this problem cannot demonstrate pitch variation of more than three or four tones and do not do so even when they attempt to sing. Once again, this problem is identified on the basis of clinical experience only. It should be systematically studied relative to its physiological and psychological origins, and its occurrence in various populations of subjects with velopharyngeal-valving problems should be determined.

Strangled Voice

This problem is not one of the more common phonation disorders found in patients with valving problems, but it is encountered often enough to warrant mention here. Strangled voice appears to be associated with an attempt to be non-nasal in the presence of velopharyngeal incompetence of sufficient magnitude to lead inevitably to hypernasality. Phonation is associated with extreme tension in the abdominal, diaphragmatic, thoracic, laryngeal, and supraglottal muscles. It is almost as if the person were trying to retain breath and talk at the same time. The tension is so great that it can be observed by videofluoroscopy in the form of taut, hyperextended structures that maintain their positions over protracted time periods. The introduction of relaxation into the system results in an increase in hypernasality. One patient, a teenage boy, developed this compensatory method of producing voice in response to speech therapy undertaken to eliminate hypernasality. His mother, incidentally, considered the therapy a success and indicated that he "used to have nasality." Signs of this extreme effort and hyperfunction should be carefully monitored, even though it is an issue about which we still have very few data.

Sometimes confused with strangled voice is the rare phenomenon of speaking on inhalation, a symptom that should bring the valving mechanism into question.

Studies of Phonation in Speakers With Clefts

Vibrating Patterns of Vocal Cords

Zemlin (1968) reviewed the early literature on nasality, a disorder of resonance, and noted that there was considerable speculation about the possibility that hypernasality might have its origins in the larynx. He cited Curry (1910) as believing that one of the causes of nasality could be increased laryngeal tension. Other writers have suggested that nasality might be, at least in part, the result of some aberration in the vibratory pattern of the vocal folds. Fletcher (1947) noted the opening phase of the vocal cords to be different when hypernasality is present (Fig. 14.1) and the pattern of movement to be asymmetrical with greater movement in the right than in the left fold.

Hamlet (1973), using ultrasound, investigated the characteristics of vocal-fold vibrations in 11 normal subjects, both children and adults. The task of the subjects was to attempt to match the loudness and pitch of nasal and non-nasal vowels. Hamlet's goal was to measure the open quotient of the vocal vibratory cycle and peak-to-peak amplitude of the sound waves. She found that, at equal levels of sound intensity, the open quotient of nasalized vowels was comparable to the open quotient for vowels that were not nasalized but that were produced during loud phonation. In the subjects for whom the degree of mouth opening was controlled, the difference between the two modes of speaking was increased. She interpreted her data to mean that glottal tightness was revealed in a reduced open quotient. This "strong muscular adductory force" might contribute to vocal abuse, which would in turn lead to hoarseness, harshness, and vocal nodules secondary to hypernasality. There might also have been a respiratory component interacting with the laryngeal.

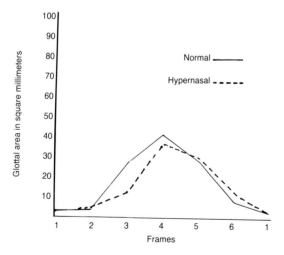

Figure 14.1 Schematic of the modes of vocal fold vibration during normal and hypernasal voice production. (From Fletcher WW. A high-speed motion picture study of vocal fold action in certain voice qualities. Master's thesis. University of Washington, 1947.)

Zajac et al. (1987) used electroglottography to examine voice production in 12 children with clefts. There were significant positive correlations between both cycle-to-cycle amplitude variations (shimmer) and cycle-to-cycle period variations (jitter) and nasality. Correlations between jitter and phonation ratings and shimmer and nasality were positive but not significant. This study points to a relationship between laryngeal behaviors as assessed by perturbation measures and hypernasality.

In a later paper, Zajac (1988) explored jitter and shimmer in normal male subjects using normal resonance, exaggerated nasal resonance, normal intensity, and increased intensity. Results indicated that increased intensity contributed to an increase in jitter, while nasalization contributed to an increase in shimmer.

These studies add to the mounting evidence suggesting alterations in laryngeal behavior in the presence of velopharyngeal-valving deficits.

Respiration

Bzoch (1964) discussed the hoarseness and breathiness associated with pharyngeal flaps and speculated that this aspirate phonation might occur as a response to hypernasal distortions and might represent an effort to mask hypernasality. Bzoch's hypothesis was supported in part by Curtis (1968), who wrote that a hypernasal speaker would have to expend more than the usual effort to attain a given intensity. If such effort were not made, speech would not be loud enough to be easily heard.

House and Stevens (1956) and Fant (1960) demonstrated a 5 to 10 dB drop in vowel amplitude in the presence of significant degrees of oronasal coupling. Curtis (1968) suggested that losses of this magnitude can probably be compensated for only by appreciable increases in both subglottic pressure and vocal effort. This conclusion is supported by Warren et al. (1969) who reported that subjects with clefts use twice the air volume during speech production without their appliances as they do when the appliances are in place.

Additional evidence of altered respiratory demands was supplied by Tronszynska (1972) who found that, on the average, people with palatal clefts demonstrate more breath units during speech than do normals. They noted that the difference in rates between the two groups becomes increasingly exaggerated with speech therapy. This finding lends support to the apparent increase in phonatory compensations as a function of speech therapy designed to move speech closer to normal in spite of valving deficits.

Bernthal and Beukelman (1977) studied the behavior of normal speakers when velopharyngeal openings were experimentally introduced. They concluded that "as velopharyngeal orifice area increases, the effective damping of the vocal tract is increased and the amplitude of the acoustical energy radiated from the speech mechanism is reduced." This results in an increase in vocal effort and in the potential for laryngeal abuse in individuals with velopharyngeal-valving deficits if they are to maintain loudness.

Leder and Lerman (1985) used acoustical methods to examine laryngeal function in normal and cleft speakers with and without evidences of hypernasality. Hypernasal speakers with clefts demonstrated voicing characteristics on voiceless consonants, and this was interpreted as symptomatic of vocal abuse. We are in agreement with Peterson-Falzone (1988), who suggested that this explanation ignores the more fundamental probability that the aerodynamics of the vocal tract in the presence of velopharyngeal-valving deficits play a major role. Increase in subglottic pressures and changes in laryngeal vibratory patterns both may be implicated.

D'Antonio et al. (1988) evaluated laryngeal and phonation characteristics in 85 patients with evidences of deficient velopharyngeal valving from 3 to 52 years of age. They assessed subglottic pressures aerodynamically and compared them against normative data for 70 children reported by Lotz and Netsell (1986). Seventy-one percent of the patients with known vocal-cord nodules, 58% of those with other laryngeal and phonatory findings, and 25% of those with phonatory symptoms but no pathology showed elevations in subglottic pressures. The authors point out that Lotz et al. (1984) found excessive subglottic pressures for 17 children with vocal nodules and that those authors speculated that increased respiratory effort could be a causal factor in the formation of nodules for some patients.

Although this conclusion appears to be justified on the basis of present information about subglottic pressures in subjects with clefts, it does not take into account evidence from data based on the simulation of growths on a model of the larynx (Scherer et al., 1982). These authors indicate that an increase in subglottic pressure may be unnecessary if the growth does not directly obstruct the glottis. On the other hand, they point out that the growth may alter the driving forces of the folds, creating or augmenting motion asymmetries. Thus, the singer or speaker may experience loss of vocal control as the result of asymmetrical intraglottal pressures even when there are no extra respiratory demands. This work has relevance to speakers with clefts and suggests the need for more precise studies that take into account location, size, and nature of vocal pathologies.

Studies reporting slower speaking rates for subjects with clefts (Lass and Noll, 1970; Tarlow and Saxman, 1970; Forner, 1983) may be partially explained by the respiratory adjustments required when velopharyngeal valving is faulty. Forner, in fact, working from a motor-control perspective, found that subjects with hypernasality and decreased intelligibility demonstrated significantly longer voice-onset times than subjects who had fewer evidences of defective valving.

McWilliams (1985) suggested that the velopharyngeal valve must be viewed as part of an integrated vocal system and that we must determine the extent to which structural and functional attributes of the whole system work in concert with velopharyngeal valving to create speech variations. Respiration is certainly a major component in that interactional system.

Warren (1986) hypothesized that speech aerodynamics conform to patterns characteristic of a regulating system and that the compensatory behaviors found in people with clefts are manifestations of regulation and control strategies. Warren suggests in this model that functionally and anatomically distinct parts of the speech system are constrained to act together to achieve the goal of maintaining appropriate pressures. In people with clefts, accommodations are required if pressure is to be regulated despite losses at the velopharyngeal portal. He points out that control of air-flow rate and movements of the articulators provide the resistance required to maintain pressures. In speakers with clefts, attempts to regulate pressures often result in highly defective speech patterns, which are perpetuated even after the mechanism has been modified.

This hypothesis is attractive and offers an explanation of the alterations found in respiration and phonation as they relate to all other aspects of speech production.

In a later study of 137 subjects with clefts

who had adequate closure and of 74 with closure deficits ranging from borderline through inadequate, Laine et al. (1988) demonstrated that, as inadequacy increased, airflow rate also increased, even though intraoral pressure decreased. The rates of increase were dramatic, with mean airflow rates of 26.8 for the adequate group, 101.0 for the adequate/borderline group, 167.5 for the borderline/inadequate speakers, and 397.2 for the inadequate speakers. The Spearman correlation coefficient between airflow rate and orifice area was 0.94. Nasal pressure increased in proportion to the decrease in intraoral pressure, and the combined nasal and oral pressures remained constant.

The authors considered the latter finding to be of major significance because it reflects an attempt to maintain an "appropriate magnitude of upper airway resistance in spite of lowered velar resistance." This study lends support to Warren's 1986 theory that compensatory strategies associated with velopharyngeal inadequacy follow regulation/control strategies.

Frequency

Curtis (1968) hypothesized that pitch ranges might be reduced by velopharyngeal incompetence. With the air loss in the vocal system, the greatest subglottic pressure possible with maximum effort would produce less output energy than would be the case if velopharyngeal closure were achieved. Since increases in both subglottic pressure and vocal effort are closely related to increases in intensity and to pitch elevation, it is logical to assume that the speaker with velopharyngeal incompetence might have a somewhat high voice with limitations in the lower part of the pitch range.

Dickson (1962) lent support to this theory when he reported measurements of fundamental frequencies for vowels produced by males who were either normal speakers, had functional nasality, or had cleft palates. His most nasal speakers tended to have higher fundamental frequencies than did those who were least nasal. Flint (1964), on the other hand, reported lower fundamental frequencies for females with clefts as compared to normals and no differences for male subjects. Tarlow and Saxman (1970) found no differences between normal children and those with clefts between the ages of 7 and 9 years.

Rampp and Counihan (1970) were in general agreement with Flint. Females with clefts had lower mean fundamentals for the vowels /i/ and /u/ than did their normal controls. Differences between normal and male subjects with cleft palates were small and directionally inconsistent. Thus, we still know too little about the effects of velopharyngeal incompetence on the frequency of the voice or whether any observed effects are direct or indirect. Variations in findings cannot be easily explained except to say that samples and methodologies have both varied in these studies. It is probable that frequency varies along with other characteristics, both physiological and perceptual.

We do not recommend either raising or lowering pitch as a therapeutic strategy for obscuring hypernasality. Sherman and Goodwin (1954) failed to find significant changes in the perception of hypernasality when pitch was raised or lowered, and changing pitch may be injurious to the larynx.

Summary

While the exact occurrence of phonatory disorders in speakers with clefts is not known, it is clear that they are more prevalent in this group than they are in the general population and that they are manifested in a variety of ways. These include hoarseness, reduction in loudness, monotony, and sometimes extreme systemic tension. Although much remains to be learned about voice production in these patients, data now available suggest alterations in vocal-cord vibratory patterns and differences in respiration. These variations are most marked when velopharyngeal incompetence is also present. The best probable explanation lies in the vocal-tract interactions necessary for the regulation of pressures.

RESONANCE

Resonance, an acoustical phenomenon, is a complex attribute of speech that is not completely understood. Simply, it may be defined as "the vibratory response of a body or air-filled cavity to a frequency imposed upon it" (Wood, 1971). Thus, resonance is a physical rather than a perceptual phenomenon, but there is no completely acceptable general term that can be used to identify the perceptual aspects of the speech signal as it varies under a variety of resonating conditions. For this reason, "resonance" is used here to describe the perceptual as well as the physical attributes of speech. The student should realize, however, that we would prefer to use a different word if we had one. A parallel to this may be drawn between the physical term *intensity* and its psychophysical counterpart *loudness*. *Intensity* refers to sound pressure levels that can be measured, while *loudness* is used to describe an auditory perception.

Some writers have suggested a way around this semantic dilemma by using the designation "oral-nasal balance" (McDonald and Baker, 1951) when referring to problems of resonance. That is a satisfactory solution so long as its meaning is clarified to permit definitions of nasal characteristics that are either increased or decreased.

The terms "hypernasality," "nasalization" and "nasalance" also appear in the literature with reference to disorders marked by an increase in nasal resonance, which is a major characteristic of speakers with velopharyngeal incompetence. The literature on this topic is voluminous. Less well documented are other types of resonance disorders that also occur. These issues are discussed in the sections that follow.

Defective Resonance

Speech that is not outstanding in any of its resonance characteristics depends upon the integrity of the vocal tract, including the supraglottal structures. Anything that upsets the ideal relationship between the oral and nasal cavities will be reflected in the speech pattern. For example, too much nasal resonance coupled with reduced oral resonance increases the perception of nasality, whereas an increase on the oral side may serve to decrease it.

For reasons already noted, speakers do not have speech patterns that are either normal or abnormal with respect to resonance. Rather, like all other attributes of speech, resonance characteristics form a continuum. Normal resonance is marked by some nasal resonance. One person may sound slightly more hypernasal than another in paired-comparison judgments, but both may be considered by the majority of listeners to be normal speakers. Given just a bit more nasality, one might well fall into a borderline classification, where some listeners would consider the speech to

be normal while others would think that it was disordered. As nasal quality increases, the speech moves further from the mean in the direction of a greater degree of deficiency. Those with hypernasality may be placed along a continuum from least to most defective, and so it is with all of the other disorders of resonance—as it is with other speech attributes as well.

Hypernasality

Hypernasality occurs when the oral and nasal cavities are coupled when they should not be. The result is that the sound wave is diverted into the nasal airways, and speech sounds as if it is coming through the nose. Early clinicians recognized that hypernasality was a logical sequela if the velopharyngeal port could not be closed. However, resonance and other speech problems associated with velopharyngeal incompetence cannot be summed up by saying that an individual is hypernasal. We must first understand the complexities and contradictions inherent in the question of resonance and its relationship to voice and articulation. Kantner made a profound statement in 1948: "The final decision as to whether an individual is 'nasal' is still, I believe, to be reached by someone's *subjective judgment*." This is still true regardless of how much additional information we bring to bear on the subject.

Resonance problems should not be confused with atypical air flow, although the two conditions usually occur together. When the velopharyngeal port cannot be closed, high-pressure consonants are likely to be accompanied by visible and, in more serious cases, audible nasal escape—unless, of course, the air stream is prevented from moving freely through the nasal passages by nasal obstruction. The nasal emission referred to throughout this book is evidence of velopharyngeal incompetence but is not synonymous with hypernasality.

Hypernasality is a phenomenon associated primarily with vowels, which are differentially affected by the shift from a primary laryngeal-pharyngeal-oral system to a laryngeal-pharyngeal-nasal-oral system, with the competing oral and nasal cavities both playing roles in the resonating aspects of speech and serving to alter the acoustic signal so that its spectrographic characteristics are changed and the auditory perception of the signal is recognized as "different."

Factors Responsible for Hypernasality

Curtis (1968) was accurate when he said:

All of the consequences of excessive nasalization...result from one cause, viz., inadequate velopharyngeal function.

The *primary* cause of hypernasality is the coupling of the oral and nasal cavities regardless of how the phenomenon may be displayed instrumentally. As Curtis pointed out, this fundamental truth "is not likely to be changed by any new discoveries concerning the acoustic process of speech generation." However, what that speech signal ultimately becomes will also depend in part upon conditions other than oral-nasal coupling (Dalston and Warren, 1986). Some related factors are respiratory effort and the degree of tension in the subglottal, glottal, and supraglottal structures, including the oral and the nasal pharynx. Superimposed on these elements will be the positioning of the tongue, which, riding high posteriorly (McDonald and Baker, 1951), may essentially block oral access of the sound stream and effectively reduce or almost eliminate the possibility of oral resonance, thus decreasing the relative oral-nasal balance. The extent to which this occurs in speakers with clefts remains unclear, however. In fact, Dickson (1969) reported that most hypernasal speakers use an anterior tongue carriage. This subject is covered in detail in Chapter 12.

Other behaviors will obviously also be involved. Constriction of the oral port by mandibular positioning, limited movement, increased tension, and lip function further serve to restrict or minimize the oral components of speech. Since cleft speakers have a tendency to restrict the size of the cavity (Falk and Kopp, 1968) by the strategies already described, their hypernasality springing from velopharyngeal incompetence may be increased. In addition, the size of the velopharyngeal portal during speech will, in relationship to respiratory effort and other tract features, dictate the air and energy loss into the nasal cavities.

As we have seen, the nasal cavities themselves have characteristics that also affect resonance. There is even evidence that, in normals, the nasal valve acts as a respiratory brake during expiration (Hairfield et al. 1987). Some speakers with velopharyngeal incompetence may also achieve some modification in the speech signal by this means.

Nasal cavities are complex in normals and are rendered more so in individuals with clefts. Warren et al. (1969a) found higher airway resistance in subjects with clefts even prior to surgery. Hairfield et al. (1988) reported that 68% of 85 children and adults with cleft lips and palates were oral, predominantly oral, or mixed oral-nasal breathers, whereas only 32% were nasal or predominantly nasal breathers. The authors attributed this obligatory mouth breathing to such things as a constricted maxilla, large tonsils, a posterior pharyngeal flap, or scarring of the pillars.

It is probable, however, that alterations in the nasal airways are present in fetal specimens as early as 8 to 21 weeks postmenstrual age. Siegel et al. (1987), using computer reconstruction, produced three-dimensional representations of the nasal capsule, nasal septal cartilage, and nasal airway in 20 normal human fetuses and 9 fetuses with clefts. Qualitative assessment revealed that nasal-capsule development in the specimens with clefts appeared to be asymmetrical. The septum was enlarged and distorted and was flanked laterally by reduced nasal airway passages. In those with unilateral clefts, the airway on the cleft side was often enlarged and irregularly shaped. However, they found no significant differences in growth rates or size of the nasal capsule between those with clefts and the normal specimens.

In a subsequent study (Kimes et al., 1988), these researchers, in an effort to explain their earlier findings, assessed the relative contributions of the nasal septum and nasal airway to capsule size. They found that the nasal septum in fetal specimens with clefts was enlarged by 45%. The septum was wider, not taller or longer. Mean airway volume, as might be expected, was smaller by 43%. Thus, it is clear that velopharyngeal valving and resonance characteristics are likely to be modified by increased nasal resistance.

Such factors as the thickness of the soft palate and the vertical depth of the contact between the velum and the pharyngeal walls may be factors in hypernasality even though the precise nature of these variations remains to be specified. We have seen individuals with hypernasality in the presence of what looked to be closure accomplished by a thin velum or with a limited contact between the velum and the pharyngeal walls. In Chapter 12, reference was made to borderline closure and to probable variations in the strength of the seal. The conditions discussed here may reflect these kinds of valving deficits.

Recognition of the influences of the entire vocal tract including oral-nasal coupling on the perception of hypernasality is not new. Schwartz (1979) suggested that:

... listening to a nasalized vowel involves listening not only to the features produced by the nasal-coupling condition but also to normal variations of quality which are unrelated to nasal coupling.

In short, the degree to which hypernasality is perceived by a listener will depend on the characteristics of the entire vocal tract and not only on the size of the functional opening in the velopharyngeal valve (Curtis, 1968).

Occurrence

In considering the speech of individuals with palatal clefts, it is important to remember that many do not have hypernasality because they do not have defective velopharyngeal valving. The achievement of adequate closure is the goal of all surgical management of the soft palate, and valving integrity is accomplished in many centers for many children. The speech pathologist should not start with the false assumption that people with repaired palatal clefts are hypernasal. Many are free of hypernasality entirely; some have only mild hypernasality; a few are moderately affected; and fewer still have severe hypernasality. Our clinical expectation should be that speech following palatal repair will be normal or nearly so. If that is not the outcome, explanations should be sought.

Influence of Oral-Nasal Coupling on the Perception of Vowels

Understanding the influence of the entire vocal tract as it interacts with velopharyngeal valving helps us see that hypernasality as a vowel phenomenon does not mean that all vowels will be similarly affected. Some vowels will be more vulnerable to oral-nasal coupling than will others (Curtis, 1968), and they will be affected in a variety of ways by context.

When a patient says /a/, he has a relaxed mandible, a lowered tongue, and an increased oral-pharyngeal space, all likely to be combined with lesser levels of tension throughout the system than is true for certain other vowels such as /i/, a

high front vowel involving an increase in tongue tension and reduction in the size of the pharyngeal and oral spaces. The integrity of /i/ cannot be well maintained in the presence of even small degrees of velopharyngeal incompetence, while /a/ may be relatively unaffected by greater degrees of incompetence. The vowel /u/ is also sensitive to coupling of the oral and nasal cavities. Thus, /i/ and /u/ are likely to be more seriously impaired by velopharyngeal incompetence than are most other vowels, although, usually, none escapes completely.

Hess (1959), Spriestersbach and Powers (1959), Carney and Sherman (1971) all found that high vowels were perceived as more nasal than low vowels. Van Hattum (1958) did not support that finding but did state that vowels produced by constriction in the anterior part of the tongue, e.g., /i/, were perceived as more nasal than back vowels.

Moll (1968) pointed out that the aforementioned conclusions for speakers with clefts—and, presumably, with velopharyngeal incompetence from any other cause—do not coincide with those for both nasal and non-nasal subjects who do not have clefts. Several studies have shown that those subjects were less nasal on high than on low vowels (Lintz and Sherman, 1961). On the other hand, as in speakers with clefts, front vowels were perceived as more nasal than back vowels. These studies point to the differential effects of hypernasality on vowels, especially for some speakers, and may offer new insights into valving integrity. Thus, vowels should be carefully evaluated in combination with assessment of the velopharyngeal valve.

Although hypernasality affects the perceptual characteristics of vowels, vowels tend to retain enough of their features to be recognizable at least in the context of speech (Moll, 1968). Waterson and Emanuel (1981), however, reported that, when an adult female with an obturated palatal cleft produced vowels in isolation with varying sizes of openings in the speech bulb, vowel intelligibility was interfered with, although not in a linear manner. Fortunately, the isolated vowel is not usually a major factor in connected discourse. While vowels are altered when they are nasalized, they are less negatively affected by oral-nasal coupling than are the pressure consonants, especially /s/, followed by other fricatives, affricates, and plosives (McWilliams, 1958). Chapter 15 goes into greater detail on this issue. Suffice it to say here that these consonant deficiencies are related to velopharyngeal incompetence but are not equated with hypernasality. Velopharyngeal competence is required for accurate consonant production (Shelton et al., 1968), and relatively small openings may be associated with reduced intraoral pressure, especially on /s/. As incompetence increases, plosives may be affected (Subtelny and Subtelny, 1959).

Influence of Other Speech Dimensions on Perception of Hypernasality

The close harmony between velopharyngeal incompetence and the extent to which consonant articulation is adversely affected leads to one of the profound clinical dilemmas with which we are faced. When we hear seriously disordered articulation, we tend to perceive increased hypernasality (McWilliams, 1954). Bzoch (1979) went so far as to suggest:

The general impression of hypernasality in the speech of a patient is related to mode of phonation, to precision of articulation of the consonant sounds, to age and to sex, to general fundamental frequency of voice, to the speech sample studied, to rate of articulation of speech, to the subject's level of fatigue or anxiety, and also to velopharyngeal insufficiency. Only if the term hypernasality is defined and strictly limited to the detectable distortion of syllabic elements in speech due to the effects of atypical coupling of the nasal resonating cavities produced under conditions of clear phonation and normal articulation can hypernasality be reliably identified or logically discussed in clinical or speech science research (p. 180).

We tend to agree in general with this statement but point out that various equal-appearing-intervals scales have been used reliably (McWilliams, 1954) to rate hypernasality. The question remains, however, as to the extent to which hypernasality was actually evaluated. This issue is addressed in Chapter 17. Schwartz (1968, 1979), because of the confusion in identifying the various components, even questioned the validity of the term hypernasality. However, since the human ear does seem to detect elements that are eventually perceived as hypernasality and since, in its pathological state, these appear to be associated with velopharyngeal incompetence, it is doubtful that the terminology will be dropped from the clinical lexicon. We must, however, be aware of factors other than

resonance that may influence our perceptions of hypernasality.

The consonant context in which a given vowel is placed may influence perceived hypernasality, especially in cases in which valving is marginal or borderline rather than grossly incompetent. Crosby (1952) found that judges could not effectively select cleft from noncleft speakers when the vowels were embedded only in nasal consonants. The subjects with clefts did not sound unlike normal subjects when they produced vowels adjacent to nasals for which the oral and nasal cavities are normally coupled. Larson and Hamlet (1987) report similar results.

On the other hand, Lintz and Sherman (1961) wrote that vowels adjacent to plosives in the speech of both nasal and non-nasal speakers without clefts were perceived as less nasal than were the same vowels adjacent to fricatives, especially sibilants. In the same study, however, vowels adjacent to *voiced* consonants were perceived as more nasal than those adjacent to voiceless consonants. Although it is not clear whether these findings hold for cleft speakers with or without velopharyngeal incompetence, consonant context does play a role in the extent to which nasality is perceived by a listener. Moll (1968) concluded that it would be difficult to repeat the Lintz and Sherman study on normal articulating speakers with clefts because misarticulation influences the perception of hypernasality.

The relationship of perceived nasality to vocal pitch has also been considered as noted in the section on phonation. Some writers have felt that changing pitch might reduce the perception of hypernasality. However, as early as 1934, Kelly did not confirm a relationship between the perception of nasality and pitch. Hess (1959) also failed to find a strong relationship between habitual pitch and the degree of perceived nasality. In spite of that, he reported that there was a reduction in the perception of nasality when pitch was raised 1.4 times the habitual level and then rated on a 7-point scale. The difference was statistically significant but was less than half a scale value, which, in practical terms, is very little real improvement.

Sherman and Goodwin (1954) studied individuals with "functional" hypernasality. Thus, there was probably no consonant disintegration. The subjects each read a passage at his or her habitual pitch level and then at lower and higher levels. There was a slight improvement for males at lower pitches on forward play of the tapes but not on backward play. There were no other significant differences. The authors were unimpressed with the importance of these results but speculated that there might be a reversal for speakers with clefts, since one of their patients had shown improvement at a higher pitch. However, this is a dubious possibility since quite a few slightly hypernasal boys have been observed clinically to sound more nearly normal following puberty, when the voice is lowered.

The best conclusion that can be drawn from these studies is that too little is yet known to permit a working clinical hypothesis about pitch and its relationship to the perception of nasality. We suspect that future studies of pitch in speakers with velopharyngeal incompetence should be related to information about perceived hypernasality and the integrity of the velopharyngeal valve. No research to date has specified these variables.

The relationship of perceived nasality to intensity of voice must also be considered. One aspect of voice in speakers with velopharyngeal incompetence is low volume and difficulty in making the voice louder as was noted earlier. Curtis (1968) and House and Stevens (1956) showed that nasal quality is characterized by a decrease in the intensity of vowels because of an increase in the absorption of acoustic energy. Hess (1959) reported that listeners rated hypernasality as less severe for vowels produced at 85 dB than for the same vowels produced at 75 dB. However, as Moll (1968) pointed out, the interpretation that "nasality changes because intensity changes" may not be valid since Hess had all vowels produced at the same intensities, a condition that does not occur in normal connected discourse, and since many subjects had difficulty producing high vowels at 85 dB.

There is theoretical justification for this finding in the work of Stathopoulos (1986), who found that both children and adults produce comparable intraoral air pressures when speaking at the same intensity levels. As we have seen, clinically, many speakers with velopharyngeal incompetence seem unable to increase loudness. Those who are able often do so at the cost of increasing both nasal escape and the impression of hypernasality. The increased air flow resulting from the increased respiratory effort is lost through the ineffective velopharyngeal portal instead of altering intraoral pressures. On the other hand, speakers who substitute breathiness for loudness may sound less hypernasal when asked to increase loudness.

As with other elements that may or may not contribute to the extent to which hypernasality is perceived, the speech pathologist is reminded to experiment carefully to determine whether alterations in loudness seem to make a difference but to exercise restraint in adopting the technique for therapeutic purposes. The voice mechanism is highly vulnerable to stress, and patients with clefts are unusually susceptible when velopharyngeal incompetence is present.

The relationship of perceived nasality to rate was investigated by Jones and Folkins (1985), who studied the effects of rate on the perception of disordered speech including hypernasality in six children with clefts between 7 and 10 years of age and found, in support of the earlier work of D'Antonio (1982), that the perception of disordered speech did not increase as a function of increased rate. It would be of interest to repeat this study using subjects representative of a continuum of valving capabilities since it is possible that the outcome might be different or that some speakers might experience difficulty when attempting to increase rate. This latter problem is observed clinically, but it is not known whether it is related to structure and function, to personality, or to both. Certainly, as mentioned earlier, some speakers with clefts adopt a slower than usual speaking rate.

The relationship between perceived nasality and palatal movement during speech production was explored by Karnell et al. (1985), who used lateral cinefluorography to study a variety of structural movements in four adult female subjects with repaired palatal clefts, two with hypernasal speech and two without. All four subjects showed touch closure in the midsagittal plane. It is possible, of course, that the subjects were not comparable in their velopharyngeal-valving capacities since lateral views examine closure in only one plane.

The subjects produced target syllables embedded in a carrier phrase and designed to produce a range of nasalization. The two subjects judged to be most nasal showed velar movements similar to those found in normal speakers, that is, the velum was lowered near the time of prevocalic constriction release. Neither of the two subjects judged to be least nasal lowered the velum during the production of the target syllables.

The authors speculated that some speakers with clefts may minimize perceptible nasality by avoiding normal palatal movements. This is an issue worthy of further study, but it clearly suggests that speakers may adopt a variety of strategies to minimize the negative effects of oral-nasal coupling.

Hypernasality is a resonance phenomenon that arises primarily from the coupling of the nasal and oral cavities for speech requiring separation. However, other attributes of the speech signal such as context, pitch, intensity, and certain physical characteristics of the system may be influential in minimizing or maximizing the perception of hypernasality.

Instrumental Correlates of Perceived Hypernasality

Hypernasality is psychologically real to listeners, who agree remarkably well in rating that characteristic in speech samples (Starr et al., 1984). If we are to account for as much variance as possible in global impressions of disordered speech, we must measure hypernasality as well as articulation, phonatory characteristics, rate, and rhythm and their physiological and acoustical correlates. Understanding and treating hypernasality depend upon the ability of the clinician to quantify it or describe it reliably and validly.

Since hypernasality is a perceptual phenomenon, any instrumental measurement must be validated against perceptual ratings. This is necessary in order to ascertain that the instrumental measurement is responsive to the same phenomenon that is perceived by listeners. Unfortunately, obtaining reliable perceptual data relative to hypernasality is dependent, as is shown in Chapter 17, on deriving mean ratings from specially trained panels of listeners. Although these mean ratings often achieve adequate reliability, ratings assigned by individual speech pathologists working under clinical conditions are often not reliable. Instrumental measurements that correlate highly with the average ratings of a group of listeners may be used to confirm or negate the opinions of a speech pathologist working alone.

Four instruments, information from which has been correlated with or related to perceived hypernasality, are considered here.

Spectrography has been applied extensively by a number of researchers (Curtis, 1942; Hattori et al., 1958; Fant, 1960; and Dickson, 1962) in studies designed to specify the acoustic characteristics of hypernasality. There is general agreement that the intensity of the first format of the spectrograph is often weakened when hypernasality is present (House and Stevens, 1956; Dickson, 1962; Schwartz, 1979). Fant (1960) concluded that this reduction in the intensity of the first formant is the most consistent spectral finding when speech is perceived by the listener to be excessively nasal; Schwartz (1979) concurred with this interpretation of the literature. This reduction, which varies from one vowel to another, is shown in Figure 14.2 for the vowel /i/.

A second characteristic, although one that is more variable than the reduction of the intensity of the first formant, is the presence of antiresonances. Antiresonances are sharp drops in the intensity of a portion of the spectrum. Figure 14.2 shows antiresonance during the production of /i/ at about 2100 Hz, where the second formant has been eliminated. Extra resonances may also be seen on the spectrograph. Note that feature between formants one and two for the vowel /i/ in Figure 14.2. A fourth feature often seen is a shift in frequency of the vowel formants. Figure 14.2 shows these slight frequency shifts for each of the formants in the vowel /i/.

Peters (1963) asked 100 listeners to judge the vowel /æ/ produced by 32 normal adult males. When the judgments were compared to the acoustical analysis of the speech productions, it was found that differences in perception were related to frequency locations and the intensities of the

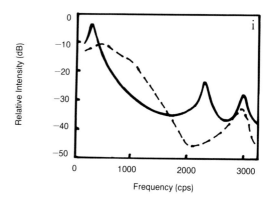

Figure 14.2 Overall spectra of a normal (solid line) and a nasalized (dashed line) production of /i/. (From Schwartz MF. Acoustic measures of nasalization and nasality. In: Bzoch KR, ed. Communicative disorders related to cleft lip and palate. 2nd ed. Boston: Little, Brown, 1979:263.)

first three formants—two variables influenced by coupling of the oral and nasal cavities. In short, when so-called normal speakers were thought to have some nasal elements in their speech patterns, these showed up on spectrograms in ways that were much like the tracings of people with pathological hypernasality, indicating that velopharyngeal closure and nasality are not binary qualities, i.e., either present or absent. Rather, each is distributed along a continuum.

Philips and Kent (1984) indicated that the spectrograms of nasalized vowels show low-frequency nasal formants below F1, a weakening and slight increase in frequency of F2, a reduction of overall energy, a reduction of F2 amplitude, and an increase in formant band widths. Thus, nasalized vowels are characterized by low-frequency energy and reduced intensity. The authors express the view that nasalization makes it more difficult to differentiate among vowels acoustically.

Spectrographic analyses of nasal and non-nasal vowels have shown considerable variability from subject to subject and from one vowel to another so that it is difficult to describe unequivocally the features of nasality. Dickson (1962) examined /i/ and /u/ in the words "beet" and "boot" as produced by 20 normal speakers, 20 speakers with "functional" nasality, and 20 speakers with cleft palates and hypernasality. Narrow-band spectrograms and narrow-band sections of each vowel were measured to determine formant peak frequency, intensity of the first formant, formant band width at half power, fundamental frequency, frequency location of any harmonic energy between regular vowel formants, and the frequency and intensity of the individual harmonics of the vowels. *None* of these measurements consistently differentiated the least nasal from the most nasal subjects. All of the measurements derived occurred in some of the least nasal, some of the moderately nasal, and some of the most nasal speakers. Variability in the acoustic characteristics of nasality was the rule. Three factors, however, were felt to be inconsistently related to hypernasality: loss of power, increased damping, and the addition of resonances and antiresonances. Dickson suggested that the inconsistencies were probably related to the differences in the physical properties of the subjects' resonating systems, a concept we should remember when considering any aspect of hypernasality.

We have come full circle to discover that both perceptual and instrumental studies of nasality point to an interplay among many physical and physiological characteristics that alter the speech signal in a variety of ways. However, the fundamental source of hypernasality remains the coupling of the oral and nasal passages. Recognizing this, Bjork and Nylen (1961) took lateral cineradiographs simultaneously with tape recordings that were analyzed spectrographically. Although these authors had a sizeable sample of cleft and noncleft children and adults, they did not attempt to determine anything about group characteristics. Instead, they presented discussions about "representative cases."

It is of interest to note that a 6-year-old girl with velopharyngeal incompetence and "open nasality" showed "very poor" detail in the "upper frequency range" of the spectrograph. Following a pharyngeal flap, the valve appeared to be normal as did her spectrogram. Although it is difficult to determine the exact features of the spectrogram that made it "normal," it is apparent that speech and velopharyngeal closure changed together and that those changes were reflected in the spectrogram. Thus, once again, the efficiency of the velopharyngeal sphincter is implicated in the etiology of hypernasality. When the valve is not capable of separating the nasal and oral cavities, the two will be coupled, and the resonating characteristics of the entire pharyngeal-nasal tract will be reflected in the resulting speech. Why should we be surprised to learn that there is variability in hypernasal vowels? There is variability in almost everything from one speaker to another. That is why it is so difficult to read a message from a voice print and why we can identify each other's voices as unique.

Oral-nasal sound-pressure levels (SPL) have been studied by several researchers seeking correlates of perceived hypernasality. This technique uses microphones to record oral and nasal sound pressure levels. To detect the nasal signal, a probe tube is attached to a condenser microphone, and this tube is placed in the most patent nostril. A second microphone is placed in front of the mouth. The signal from each microphone is amplified and then graphed by use of level recorders, which provide pen traces from which SPL may be determined. The difference between oral SPL and nasal SPL or the quotient obtained by dividing oral SPL into nasal SPL is correlated with the mean ratings of hypernasality provided by a panel of listeners.

Weiss (1954) employed probe microphones to

measure oral and nasal SPLs during speech. These data were then correlated with perceived nasality as rated by 14 listeners using a paired-comparison technique. Oral SPL minus nasal SPL correlated with perceived hypernasality at 0.94 and nasal SPL divided by oral SPL correlated with perceived hypernasality at 0.91. These substantial correlations suggested the clinical use of oral and nasal SPL measures as indices of perceived hypernasality.

Shelton et al. (1967) demonstrated that subjects with clefts produced high nasal SPLs when their obturators were removed. Shelton et al. (1969) showed that subjects differing in velopharyngeal competence also differed on SPL measures. The less adequate the valving mechanism, the greater the nasal SPL. Nonetheless, these measurements are ambiguous as indices to hypernasality and to velopharyngeal competence.

Tonar (the oral-nasal acoustic ratio) (Fletcher, 1970) brought advancements to the measurement or oral and nasal sound intensity as indices to hypernasality. This instrument is described in detail in Chapter 11.

Fletcher and his associates have conducted a number of studies indicating that Tonar is an adequate index to perceived hypernasality and is useful as a biofeedback apparatus. Fletcher and Bishop (1970) reported a rank-order correlation of 0.74 between ratings of hypernasality and Tonar measurements, which Fletcher (1978) termed *nasalance*. The subjects were 20 children with surgically repaired cleft palates. These authors also reported that the ratio between oral and nasal sound energy varies depending on the frequency band studied. The Tonar analyses associated with the correlation of 0.74 cited above involved ". . . spectrum analyzers at central frequencies of 1250 Hz and 1750 Hz and a 1.0 K Hz half band width."

In 1972, Fletcher reported that Tonar II, a second-generation instrument, was capable of tracking the resonant frequency of the individual nasal cavity. His original intent had been to use the same fixed frequency filtering arrangement with all patients. In 1976, Fletcher reported a correlation of 0.91 between nasalance scores and mean ratings obtained by the psychophysical method of magnitude estimation. This computation involved dividing the nasal signal by the sum of the nasal and oral signals. He had previously divided the oral into the nasal measurements. The subjects were 23 children with surgically repaired palatal

clefts. The listeners were college students who were enrolled in introductory speech courses. Fletcher concluded that the nasalance measure was an adequate index to perceived nasality.

Tonar is sometimes used as an index to velopharyngeal function, but empirical support for that application is lacking. Although Fletcher (1972) discussed hypernasality relative to the ability to close the velopharyngeal valve, in 1978, he reported that two measures of velopharyngeal valving accounted for only 30% of the variance in subjects' nasalance.

Warren et al. (1981) obtained Tonar II measures and listener judgments of hypernasality in normal adults and children and in patients who had clefts and adequate velopharyngeal closure, borderline competence, or velopharyngeal incompetence as measured by the pressure-flow technique. The results showed a clear tendency for orifice area and nasalance covary. However, the relationship was not as strong in the borderline group. Tongue position altered nasalance but only in younger subjects. Listener judgments of nasality also covaried with Tonar assessments, but intelligibility did not.

Dalston and Warren (1986) studied the interrelationships among Tonar II, pressure-flow, and listener judgments of hypernasality in 124 children and adults. They found correlations of 0.80 between pressure-flow and listener judgments; 0.76 between Tonar II and listener judgments; and 0.74 between Tonar II and pressure-flow. Both instruments sometimes failed, usually in borderline cases, to agree with speech ratings; and these disagreements were most often in the direction of identifying as adequate speakers with high ratings of hypernasality. Dalston and Warren suggested that basing treatment decisions on agreement between the two instruments reduces the error to a minimum.

The desirability of using two instruments supports the conclusion of McWilliams et al. (1981), who compared pressure-flow and videofluoroscopy with speech ratings and with each other. In this study, two manometric techniques were also assessed and were found to be worthless in identifying speakers with or without hypernasality.

It is clear that Tonar is an instrument that correlates highly but not perfectly with speech ratings and with other commonly used instruments. A third-generation instrument known as the nasometer is a much more sophisticated device connected to a microcomputer using software that permits instantaneous statistical calculations useful in documenting clinical impressions and for research purposes. As data are generated from this new instrument and compared to information from other instruments, more definitive statements can be made about its applicability. However, there is little doubt that it will prove to be at least as reliable as its predecessors. It is likely that it will be well accepted and used in specialty clinics.

The accelerometer has been available for many years (Hultzen, 1942). Recently, however, there has been a renewal of interest in the device as a means of detecting and displaying nasalization. Stevens et al. (1975), attached an accelerometer weighing only 1.8 grams and with a flat frequency response from 8 to 20,000 Hz to the nose where it responded to vibrations on the nasal surface. The signal was amplified, filtered, rectified, and smoothed. They were able to demonstrate a progressive increase in nasalization from the utterance "his father," through "his mother," and "my money."

Later, Stevens et al. (1976) presented data regarding the accelerometric assessment of nasalization in hearing-impaired and normally hearing children. They found that the nasal accelerometer is influenced by the intensity of speech and that this problem is not unequivocally resolved by relating nasalization to an index of energy detected by a voice microphone. This is so because speech amplitude varies with different speech sounds and decreases with nasalization. However, the authors did not consider this to be an important problem so long as the speaker was successful in maintaining nearly constant vocal effort. They reported a correlation of 0.78 between ratings of velopharyngeal closure and nasalization, a measurement that was computed by determining one-half of the sum of the nasalization values obtained from accelerometer readings taken during utterances loaded with nasal consonants and utterances containing no nasals.

Garber and Moller (1979) employed this technology with normal individuals and those with clefts or hypernasality following adenoidectomy. Although their main purpose was to determine whether filtering of auditory feedback to the patient altered hypernasality, they also correlated nasality ratings and measurements in three subjects with normal voices, three with mild hypernasality, and three with severe hypernasality. All had

satisfactory articulation. The correlation for the two measures was 0.77 under conditions that tended to assure a wide range of scores.

In one part of the study by Garber and Moller, hypernasality was reported for normal subjects as they read sentences and talked spontaneously with no filtering, with low-pass filtering with cut-off frequencies of 1000, 500, and 300 Hz, and with high-pass filtering with cut-off frequencies of 500, 1000 and 2000 Hz. A correction was made for variability associated with change in vocal intensity. For the normal subjects during spontaneous speech, nasalization was significantly lower with low-pass filtering at 300 Hz than for any other condition. During sentence reading, nasalization was lower under the 300-Hz-condition than under the 500- or 2000-Hz, high-pass conditions. For the subjects with clefts, during reading, nasalization was lower at the 300-Hz, low-pass condition than during any of the other filtering conditions. Small but statistically significant differences in nasalization under certain filtering conditions were interpreted to mean that nasalization is under feedback control. However, the authors pointed out that perceptual ratings were not used to study changes in nasalization under the different filtering conditions.

Horii (1980) summarized a number of problems associated with accelerometers. As noted by Mease (1961) and Leeper (1966), the vibrations that can be detected depend upon tissue characteristics of the speaker; skin-sensor contact characteristics such as the pressure, angle, and torque; and phonatory intensity. For these reasons, nasal vibrations, he suggested, were not comparable from one speaker to another or from utterance to utterance within the same speaker. In addition, it was not possible to determine a point separating normal from deviant speech.

In order to solve these problems, Horii proposed the use of an index based on the ratio of nasal amplitude to vocal amplitude derived from two accelerometers placed on the external surface of the nose and neck. He referred to the index as the Horii Oral-Nasal Coupling Index (HONC).

This theoretical paper was followed by a study (Horii and Lang, 1981) of 10 normal young women reading the zoo and rainbow passages. The zoo passage was read with normal voice and with simulated moderate and severe hypernasality, which was rated on a 5-point scale. Subjects were studied with the accelerometer on the surface of the nose, and voice amplitude was obtained from a neck accelerometer and from a regular microphone positioned approximately 12 centimeters in front of the lips.

The HONC values were computed by dividing the root-mean square amplitude of the nasal signal by the root-mean square amplitude of the voice signal and multiplying by K, the correction factor derived from the ratio between the root-mean square amplitudes of the nasal and voice signals acquired during the production of /m/.

The two systems for detecting the voice signal correlated with each other at 0.89, and the rank-order correlations between voice ratings and instrumental quotients was 0.81. The HONC technique appeared to be a reasonably reliable and safe technique for the instrumental assessment of hypernasality.

Redenbaugh and Reich (1985) simplified the HONC methodology with their Nasal Accelerometric Vibratory Index (NAVI) using accelerometers on the nose and anterior neck. Analog circuitry provides a normalized nasal-throat voltage ratio. A voltage range of 0 mV to 1000 mV permits the measurement of responses from no nasal coupling to maximum nasal coupling. They reported a correlation of 0.91 between NAVI values and hypernasality as determined by direct-magnitude estimation.

Reich and Redenbaugh (1985) applied their system to the study of 12 children with velopharyngeal incompetence ranging from mild to very severe as determined by 20 graduate students in speech and hearing sciences using a 5-point equal-appearing-intervals scale. One normal male and two normal females served as controls. Both forward- and backward-play were used with similar results.

The Spearman rank-order coefficient for each of the two conditions was 0.92. Correlations between NAVI values and speech ratings were moderate to strong and were significant at the 0.05 level of confidence. The correlation between NAVI values and ratings of hypernasality for an obstruent-loaded sentence was 0.90. Since HONC and NAVI values compare favorably, (Redenbaugh and Reich, 1985), the authors conclude that the NAVI system provides useful indirect information relative to nasal resonance. Reich and Redenbaugh paid close attention in this study to issues of reliability so that the impressiveness of their data is enhanced.

In summary, all of these instruments offer certain information about hypernasality but do not correlate perfectly with what is perceived. The spectrographic technique provides variable data that have greater research than clinical applicability. SPL is not recommended for clinical use at this time. Tonar II, the nasometer, and accelerometers yield data that correlate with perceived hypernasality sufficiently well to warrant clinical and research application within limits. Unfortunately, there is still no instrument to replace either the human ear or human judgment. Additional research is needed to establish the predictive validity of these instruments as they apply to patients with hypernasality and to establish their relationship to other techniques for assessing the velopharyngeal valve.

Reduced Nasal Resonance

Hyponasality and Denasality

Hyponasality, a reduction in nasal resonance, is heard when the nasal airway itself is partially blocked or the entrance to the nasal passages is partially occluded, as might occur if moderately large adenoids were present. If the nasal airways were completely occluded, speech would be denasal, meaning that nasal air flow associated with /m, n, and η/ would be eliminated and the sound wave altered; the nasal consonants would approach but not match /b, d, and g/.

When either hyponasality or denasality is heard, speech pathologists may be lulled into thinking that the velopharyngeal valve is intact. In reality, the valve may be faulty, but the increased nasal resistance minimizes its effects. The role of the velopharyngeal valve is obscured until the nasal airway is corrected, at which time the defective valve becomes apparent as the speech takes on the characteristics of velopharyngeal incompetence, i.e., visible or audible nasal escape, hypernasality, and reduced intraoral pressure.

Cul-de-Sac Resonance

Cul-de-sac resonance is really a variation of hypo- and denasality. It differs only in the place of obstruction and in the way the speech sounds. A cul-de-sac is defined as a blind pouch or a passage with only one outlet. The speech has a muffled characteristic, which you can hear in your own speech if you repeat the CV chain "mi, mi, mi" and then, continuing to produce the chain, pinch your nostrils tightly together. You will hear and feel the airstream necessary for the nasals as it enters the open airway, but you will trap it by the tight anterior constriction. The resonating cavity, normally an open tube, thus becomes a cul-de-sac with concomitant changes in its resonating properties.

Speech pathologists should be aware that people with complete clefts of the lip and palate are at high risk for intranasal conditions capable of changing the architecture of the airways and, thus, their acoustical properties. To the extent that these problems alter the nasal cavities, speech will be influenced. In addition, nasal emission may be minimized or eliminated.

Hyper-Hyponasality

McWilliams and Philips (1979) described resonance characterized by elements of both hypo- and hypernasality. This phenomenon was also reported by Millar (1980). Hyper-hyponasality occurs in patients with velopharyngeal incompetence in combination with increased nasal resistance that is not great enough to eliminate nasal resonance entirely but is too great to permit nasal consonants to maintain their integrity. Instrumental assessment of this problem is long overdue.

Summary

Resonance disorders occur frequently in patients with clefts. Although there are many normal speakers in this population, this outcome is not universal. Even among the most successful speakers, vestiges of resonance variations often remain. These include: hypernasality, which is the most commonly heard disorder and which springs from the coupling of the oral and nasal cavities; hyponasality, which is related to the increased nasal resistance typical of these speakers; cul-de-sac resonance, also caused by an increase in nasal resistance, but resistance that is anterior rather than posterior; and a combination of hyper- and hyponasality.

The perception of these resonance disorders is influenced by other dimensions of the speech signal such as articulation, context, and phonation. Frequency, intensity, and rate have also been implicated, but data are inconclusive.

Instrumental means for assessing hypernasality and other resonance disorders are gradually being perfected and are gaining in popularity. However, they have not yet replaced the human ear and must be validated against perceptual judgments. To date, no single instrument has proven to be ideal by itself.

REFERENCES

Aronson AE. Clinical voice disorders. New York: BC Decker, 1980.

Baynes RA. An incidence study of chronic hoarseness among children. J Speech Hear Dis 1966; 31: 172.

Bernthal JE, Beukelman DR. The effect of changes in velopharyngeal orifice area on vocal intensity. Cleft Palate J 1977; 14:1.

Bjork L, Nylen BO. Cineradiography with synchronized sound spectrum analysis. Plast Reconstr Surg 1961; 27:397.

Boone DR, McFarlane S. The voice and voice therapy. 4th ed. Englewood Cliffs, NJ; Prentice-Hall, 1988.

Brindle BR, Morris HL. Prevalence of voice quality deviations in the normal adult population. J Commun Dis 1979; 12:439.

Brooks A, Shelton R. Voice disorders other than nasality in cleft palate children. Cleft Palate Bull 1963; 13:63.

Bzoch K. The effects of a specific pharyngeal flap operation upon the speech of 40 cleft palate persons. J Speech Hear Dis 1964; 29:111.

Bzoch KR. Etiological factors related to cleft palate speech. In: Communicative disorders related to cleft lip and palate. 2nd ed. Boston: Little, Brown, 1979.

Bzoch KR. Measurements and assessment of categorical aspects of cleft palate speech. In: Communicative disorders related to cleft lip and palate. 2nd ed. Boston: Little, Brown, 1979.

Carney PJ, Sherman D. Severity of nasality in three selected speech tasks. J Speech Hear Res 1971; 14:396.

Crosby CA. Audience differentiation of recorded samples of cleft and non-cleft palate speech. Master's thesis. University of Wisconsin, 1952.

Curry SS. Mind and voice. Boston: Expression Company, 1910.

Curtis JF. An experimental study of the wave-composition of nasal voice quality. Ph.D. thesis. The University of Iowa, 1942.

Curtis JF. Acoustics of speech production and nasalization. In: Spriestersbach DC, Sherman D, eds. Cleft palate and communication. New York: Academic Press, 1968.

Dalston RM, Warren DW. Comparison of Tonar II, pressure flow, and listener judgments of hypernasality in the assessment of velopharyngeal function. Cleft Palate J 1986; 23:108.

D'Antonio LL. An investigation of speech timing in individuals with cleft palate. Ph.D. thesis. University of California at San Francisco, 1982.

D'Antonio LL, Muntz H, Providence M, Marsh J. Laryngeal/voice findings in patients with velopharyngeal dysfunction. Laryngoscope 1988; 98:432.

Deering KM. The occurrence of phonatory disorders among cleft palate speakers. Master's thesis. University of Akron, 1984.

Dickson DR. An acoustic study of nasality. J Speech Hear Res 1962; 5:103.

Dickson DR. A radiographic study of nasality. Cleft Palate J 1969; 6:160.

Falk ML, Kopp GA. Tongue position and hypernasality in cleft palate speech. Cleft Palate J 1968; 5:228.

Fant G. Acoustic theory of speech production. Hawthorne, NY; Mouton, 1960:139.

Fitzhugh GS, Smith DE, Chiong AJ. Pathology of 300 clinically benign lesions of the vocal cords. Laryngoscope 1958; LXVIII:855.

Fletcher SG. Theory and instrumentation for quantitative measurement of nasality. Cleft Palate J 1970; 7:601.

Fletcher SG. Contingencies for bioelectric modification of nasality. J Speech Hear Dis 1972; 37:329.

Fletcher SG. Nasalance vs listener judgments of nasality. Cleft Palate J 1976; 13:31.

Fletcher SG. Diagnosing speech disorders from cleft palate. New York: Grune and Stratton, 1978.

Fletcher SG, Bishop ME. Measurement of nasality with TONAR. Cleft Palate J 1970; 7:610.

Fletcher WW. A high-speed motion picture study of vocal fold action in certain voice qualities. Master's thesis. University of Washington, 1947.

Flint R. Fundamental vocal frequency and severity of nasality in cleft palate speakers. Master's thesis. University of Oklahoma, 1964.

Forner L. Speech segment durations produced by five and six year old speakers with and without cleft palate. Cleft Palate J 1983; 20:185.

Garber SR, Moller KT. The effects of feedback filtering on nasalization in normal and hypernasal speakers. J Speech Hear Res 1979; 22:321.

Greenberg R. The incidence of hoarseness among children enrolled in speech therapy. J PA Speech Lang Hear Assoc 1982; XV:20.

Hairfield W, Warren DW, Hinton V, Seaton D. Inspiratory and expiratory effects of nasal breathing. Cleft Palate J 1987; 24:183.

Hairfield W, Warren DW, Seaton D. Prevalence of mouth breathing in cleft lip and palate. Cleft Palate J 1988; 25:135.

Hamlet SL. Vocal compensation: an ultrasonic study of vocal fold vibration in normal and nasal vowels. Cleft Palate J 1973; 10:267.

Hattori S, Yamamoto K, Fujimura O. Nasalization of vowels in relation to nasals. J Acoust Soc Am 1958; 30:267.

Hess DA. Pitch, intensity and cleft palate voice quality. J Speech Hear Res 1959; 2:113.

Horii Y. An accelerometric approach to nasality measurement: a preliminary report. Cleft Palate J 1980; 17:254.

Horii Y, Lang JE. Distributional analyses of an index of nasal coupling (HONC) in simulated hypernasal speech. Cleft Palate J 1981; 18:279.

House AS, Stevens KN. Analog studies of the nasalization of vowels. J Speech Hear Dis 1956; 21:218.

Hultzen LS. Apparatus for demonstrating nasality. J Speech Hear Dis 1942;7:5.

Jones DL, Folkins JW. Effect of speaking rate on judgments of disordered speech in children with cleft palate. Cleft Palate J 1985; 22:246.

Kantner CE. Diagnosis and prognosis in cleft palate speech. J Speech Dis 1948; 13:211.

Karnell MP, Folkins JW, Morris HL. Relationships between the perception of nasalization and speech movements in speakers with cleft palate. J Speech Hear Res 1985; 28:63.

Kelly JP. Studies in nasality. Arch Speech 1934; 1:26.

Kimes K, Siegel M, Mooney M, Todhunter J. Relative contributions of the nasal septum and airways to total nasal capsule volume in normal and cleft lip and palate fetal specimens. Cleft Palate J 1988; 25:282.

Laguaite JK. Adult voice screening. J Speech Hear Dis 1972; 37:147.

Laine T, Warren DW, Dalston RM, Hairfield WM, Morr KE. Intraoral pressure, nasal pressure and airflow rate in cleft palate speech. J Speech Hear Res 1988; 31:432.

Larson P, Hamlet S. Coarticulation effects on the nasalization of vowels using nasal/voice amplitude ratio instrumentation. Cleft Palate J 1987; 24:286.

Lass N, Noll J. A comparative study of rate characteristics in cleft palate and noncleft palate speakers. Cleft Palate J 1970; 7:275.

Leder SB, Lerman JW. Some acoustic evidence for vocal abuse in adult speakers with repaired cleft palate. Laryngoscope 1985; 95:837.

Leeper HA. The relations between the vibrations of the nasal bones and severity of simulated nasality; a methodological investigation. Unpublished Master's thesis. Purdue University, 1966.

Lintz LB, Sherman D. Phonetic elements and perception of nasality. J Speech Hear Res 1961; 4:381.

Lotz W, Netsell R. Developmental patterns of laryngeal aerodynamics. Presentation, Midwinter meeting of the Association for Research in Otolaryngology, Clearwater, FL, 1986.

Lotz W, Netsell R, D'Antonio L, et al. Aerodynamic evidence of vocal abuse in children with vocal nodules. Presentation, ASHA, San Francisco, 1984.

Marks C, Barker K, Tardy M. Prevalence of perceived acoustic deviations related to laryngeal function among subjects with palatal anomalies. Cleft Palate J 1971; 8:201.

McDonald E, Baker HK. Cleft palate speech; an integration of research and clinical observation. J Speech Hear Dis 1951; 16:9.

McWilliams BJ. Some factors in the intelligibility of cleft palate speech. J Speech Hear Dis 1954; 19:524.

McWilliams BJ. Unresolved issues in velopharyngeal valving. Cleft Palate J 1985; 22:29.

McWilliams BJ, Bluestone CD, Musgrave RH. Diagnostic implications of vocal cord nodules in children with cleft palate. Laryngoscope 1969; 79:2072.

McWilliams BJ, Glaser ER, Philips BJ, Lawrence C, Lavorato AS, Berry QC, Skolnick ML. A comparative study of four methods of evaluating velopharyngeal adequacy. Plast Reconstr Surg 1981; 68:1.

McWilliams BJ, Lavorato AS, Bluestone CD. Vocal cord abnormalities in children with velopharyngeal valving problems. Laryngoscope 1973; 83:1745.

McWilliams BJ, Philips BJ. Audio seminars in speech pathology: Velopharyngeal incompetence. Philadelphia: WB Saunders, 1979.

Mease RP. The relationship between vibrations of the nasal bones and ratings of nasality in cleft palate speakers.

Unpublished Master's thesis. Pennsylvania State University, 1961.

Millar R. Cleft palate and communication disorders. Ear Nose Throat J 1980; 59:54.

Minifie FD. Speech acoustics. In: Minifie FD, Hixon TJ, Williams F, eds. Normal aspects of speech, hearing, and language. Englewood Cliffs, NJ: Prentice Hall, 1973.

Moll KL. Speech characteristics of individuals with cleft lip and palate. In: Spriestersbach DC, Sherman D, eds. Cleft palate and communication. New York: Academic Press, 1968;61.

Peters RM. Dimension of quality for the vowel /ae/. J Speech Hear Res 1963; 6:239.

Peterson-Falzone S. Speech disorders related to craniofacial structural defects: Part 2. In: Lass N, McReynolds L, Northern J, Yoder D, eds. Handbook of Speech-Language Pathology and Audiology. Toronto: BC Decker, 1988; 493.

Philips BJ, Kent R. Acoustic-phonetic descriptions of speech production in speakers with cleft palate and other velopharyngeal disorders. In: Lass N, ed. Speech and language: advances in basic research. New York: Academic Press, 1984.

Rampp DL, Counihan DT. Vocal pitch intensity relationships in cleft palate speakers. Cleft Palate J 1970; 3:846.

Redenbaugh MA, Reich AR. Correspondence between an accelerometric nasal/voice amplitude ratio and listeners' direct magnitude estimations of hypernasality. J Speech Hear Res 1985; 28:273.

Reich AR, Redenbaugh MA. Relation between nasal/voice accelerometric values and interval estimates of hypernasality. Cleft Palate J 1985; 22:237.

Scherer RC, Titze IR, Linville R, Hueffner D, Shaw K. The effects of vocal cord growths on pressure-flow relationships in the larynx. In: Titze I, ed. The Proceedings of the Voice Foundation 1982. Presentation at the 11th Symposium: Care of the Professional Voice. New York City: The Voice Foundation, 1982.

Schwartz MF. The acoustics of normal and nasal vowel production. Cleft Palate J 1968; 5:125.

Schwartz MF. Acoustic measures of nasalization and nasality. In: Bzoch KR, ed. Communicative disorders related to cleft lip and palate. 2nd ed. Boston: Little, Brown, 1979:263.

Senturia BH, Wilson FB. Otorhinolaryngologic findings in children with voice deviations. Preliminary report. Ann Otol Rhinol Laryngol 1968; 77:1027.

Shearer WH. Diagnosis and treatment of voice disorders in school children. J Speech Hear Dis 1972; 37:215.

Shelton RL Jr, Hahn E, Morris HL. Diagnosis and therapy. In: Spriestersbach DC, Sherman D, eds. Cleft palate and communication. New York: Academic, 1968.

Shelton RL, Knox AW, Arndt WB Jr, Elbert M. The relationship between nasality score values and oral and nasal sound pressure level. J Speech Hear Res 1967; 10:549.

Shelton RL, Arndt WB Jr, Knox AW, Elbert M, Chisum L, Youngstrom KA. The relationship between nasal sound pressure level and palatopharyngeal closure. J Speech Hear Res 1969; 12:193.

Sherman D, Goodwin F. Pitch level and nasality. J Speech Hear Dis 1954; 19:423.

Siegel M, Mooney M, Kimes K, Todhunter J. Analysis of the size variability of the human normal and cleft palate fetal nasal capsule by means of 3-dimensional computer reconstruction of histologic preparations. Cleft Palate J 1987; 24:190.

Silverman EM, Zimmer CH. Incidence of chronic hoarseness among school-age children. J Speech Hear Dis 1975; 40:211.

Spriestersbach DC, Powers GR. Nasality in isolated vowels and connected speech of children with cleft palates. J Speech Hear Res 1959; 2:40.

Starr CD, Moller KT, Dawson W, Graham J, Skaar S. Speech ratings by speech clinicians, parents and children. Cleft Palate J 1984; 21:286.

Stathopoulos ET. Relationship between intraoral air pressure and vocal intensity in children and adults. J Speech Hear Res 1986; 29:71.

Stevens KN, Kalikow DN, Willemain TR. A miniature accelerometer for detecting glottal waveforms and nasalization. J Speech Hear Res 1975; 18:594.

Stevens KN, Nickerson RS, Boothroyd A, Rollins AM. Assessment of nasalization in the speech of deaf children. J Speech Hear Res 1976; 19:393.

Subtelny J, Subtelny JD. Intelligibility and associated physiological factors of cleft palate speakers. J Speech Hear Res 1959; 2:353.

Takagi Y, McGlone R, Millard R. A survey of the speech disorders of individuals with clefts. Cleft Palate J 1965; 2:28.

Tarlow A, Saxman JA. Comparative study of the speaking fundamental frequency characteristics in children with cleft palate. Cleft Palate J 1970; 7:696.

Tronczynska J. Electrorhinopneumography as an objective method of assessment of velopharyngeal insufficiency in cleft palate patients. Folia Phoniatr 1972, 24:371.

Van Hattum RJ. Articulation and nasality in cleft palate speakers. J Speech Hear Res 1958; 1:383.

Warren DW. Compensatory speech behaviors in cleft palate: a regulation/control phenomenon. Cleft Palate J 1986; 23:251.

Warren DW, Dalston R, Trier WC, Sakata R, Holder MB. Effects of palatopharyngeal incompetency on oral-nasal resonance and listener judgment. Paper presented at the 4th International Congress on Cleft Palate and Related Craniofacial Anomalies, Acapulco, 1981.

Warren DW, Duany LF, Fischer ND. Nasal pathway resistance in normal and cleft lip and palate subjects. Cleft Palate J 1969; 6:134.

Warren D, Wood M, Bradley D. Respiratory volume in normal and cleft palate speech. Cleft Palate J 1969; 6:449.

Waterson T, Emanuel F. Observed effects of velopharyngeal orifice size on vowel identification and vowel nasality. Cleft Palate J 1981; 18(4):271.

Weiss AL. Oral and nasal sound pressure levels as related to judged severity of nasality. Unpublished Doctoral dissertation. Purdue University, 1954.

Westlake H. Understanding the cleft palate child. Quart J Speech 1953; 38:165.

Wilson FB. The voice disordered child. Lang Speech Hear Serv Schools 1971.

Wood KS. Terminology and nomenclature. In: Travis LE, ed.

Handbook of speech pathology and audiology. New York: Appleton-Century-Crofts, 1971:19.

Yairi E. Incidence of hoarseness in school children over a one-year period. J Commun Dis 1971; 7:321.

Zajac D. Effects of nasalization/intensity on voice perturbations. Presented at ASHA, Boston, 1988.

Zajac D, Linville R, McWilliams BJ. An electroglottographic analysis of velopharyngeal incompetent speakers. Presented at ASHA, New Orleans, 1987.

Zemlin WR. Speech and hearing science. Englewood Cliffs, NJ: Prentice Hall, 1968.

15 | ARTICULATION, PHONOLOGY, AND INTELLIGIBILITY

Psychological experimentation often fails, not through failure in the experimental method itself, but because theory that is supposed to mediate the events under consideration is not sufficiently detailed to make any single experiment easily interpreted.*

Misarticulation is an important speech disorder in many patients with cleft palate. A primary purpose of this chapter is to review the empirical literature concerning how persons with cleft palate articulate and misarticulate as they employ the speech sound system in communication. Most of the empirical literature about the speech of patients with cleft palate has been written from a phonetic perspective. This trend continues even given the recent interest among speech-language pathologists in phonology. Phonetic analyses utilize observer perception to learn about how individuals produce sounds in speech, and perception is supplemented by instrumental study of speech production and acoustics. Much is known about movements of the vocal folds, velum and pharyngeal walls, tongue, mandible, and lips in voice and articulation. These movements, which are precisely coordinated with one another and with air flow from the lungs, produce a continuous alteration of the shape of the vocal tract. The resulting constrictions permit the impounding and releasing of air pressures and flows essential to the production of obstruent consonants and the resonances needed for sonorants. Movements associated with sounds perceived to

* Deese J. *Psychology as Science and Art.* New York: Harcourt, Brace, Jovanovich, 1972.

occur sequentially actually co-occur or coarticulate and assimilate or take on characteristics of one another. Some coarticulation is physiologically determined and some reflects conventions of the speaker's language (Daniloff et al., 1980; Kent, 1988).

If articulation involves complex patterns of movement of several structures, then in disordered articulation, movements depart from the patterns that are accepted in the speaker's community. The articulators either do not pass through sites required for acceptable articulation or they are not accompanied by whatever voicing, resonance, and intraoral air pressure that are needed. Nasal airflow may be present where it should not be. A phonetic-articulatory emphasis in study of the speech associated with palatal clefts is necessary because of the influence of velopharyngeal closure failures, fistulas, malocclusions, nasal pathway obstruction, hearing loss, faulty oral somatesthesia, and other variables associated with clefts.

Phonetic studies do not, however, show how the talker uses phonemic contrasts in the expression of meaning nor the orderliness of the sound pattern as viewed from a linguistic perspective. Speech development and production are influenced by linguistic constraints (Elbert, 1984; Bernthal and Bankson, 1988) which should be taken into account to understand well the patient with cleft palate. As Locke (1983) noted, multiple influences—including those of a linguistic nature—determine the sound system of children with clefts. For example, speech may be nasalized because of velopharyngeal incompetence but other articulatory characteristics such as final consonant deletion may occur because the individual has not yet developed needed knowledge of the sound system of the language. This could reflect experience, neural underpinnings of phonology, or a combination. Furthermore, a child's phonological structure could influence his or her velopharyngeal movement pattern, and limitations of velopharyngeal structure and function may influence what children store about the sound system.

Some authors have adopted phonological terminology for use in discussion of those speech patterns specifically associated with cleft palate (see for example Trost-Cardamone, 1986). However, others have argued, and we agree, that phonetic and phonological components of a child's sound pattern should be considered separately (Hawkins, 1985; Stengelhofen, 1989; Albery, 1989). Hewlett (1985, p. 160) differentiated between phonetic disorders that involve faulty expression of adequate phonological knowledge and phonological disorders that involve misrepresentation of words in the speaker's mind. Grunwell (1985, p. 169) stated that "...phonetics and phonology coexist semiautonomously but interact independently." In summary, several British authors see phonetics and phonology as equal and distinct but interacting. Those authors have used that organization effectively in the study of cleft palate speech, and that organization is appropriate to this chapter. Both phonetic and phonological perspectives should be considered in studying the speech of patients with cleft palate.

Study of abstract phonological constructs has led to clinically useful insights and to clinical phonology which is concerned with sound patterns and the expression of meaning by individuals with communication disorders. In clinical phonology, ideas drawn from psychology, linguistics, and other fields are interwoven with information from speech-language pathology, and the product is revised and polished. Eclecticism has long been a hallmark of speech pathology. Borrowing from linguistics is justified if only because phonological concepts have contributed to identification and understanding of disordered sound patterns of children and to increased use of phonemic contrasts in therapy.

Nonetheless, in applying phonological constructs to cleft palate speech, there is a danger of getting lost in multiple phonological viewpoints, abstractions, and assertions contradictory to data (Lubker, 1984; Folkins and Bleile, in preparation). Milroy (1985) stated that the generative phonolo-gist is concerned with mental organization of language not with its physical or psychological correlates, and he suggested that it is unlikely that mentalistic claims of a generative linguistic nature can be tested empirically. Some generative theorists are interested in the power of their constructs to explain language but not in the psychological reality of the phenomena they study. Hewlett (1985) indicated that generative analysis is directed to the data—speech produced by a speaker— and not to the speaker. This suggests that attempts to apply phonological theory in the study of disordered speech might result in a mismatch. Foster et al. (1985) (see also Harris and Cottam, 1985) indicated that phonological theory, including the segment thereof concerned with distinctive features, pertains to mentalistic or psychological constructs and not to the physiology of speech. They suggest that speech-language pathologists who have used phonological theory have misinterpreted it in physiological-phonetic terms. In amalgamating information from phonology into speech pathology we have altered borrowed ideas. Rather than apologizing for that alteration, we look for reapproachment of linguistic and motor control theory within a neurobiological framework. Some linguists and motor performance-learning specialists use similar abstractions or schemas in their theory building. Cognitive scientists appear to be moving toward a unified theory that will account for learning, perception, motor control, language, and other variables (Waldrop, 1988). We hope that new theory brings clarity to the current complexity (Szent-Gyorgyi, 1964).

Within clinical phonology, a physical inability to produce certain speech sounds is assumed when a talker does not produce those sounds, even when provided with models for imitation and with information about how they are produced. This is an articulatory or phonetic problem. Phonological disability involves a loss of phonemic contrast. For example, two or more phonemes may be merged into one (Hawkins, 1985). Phonological misarticulation involves a failure to use some sounds appropriately and consistently even though they are produced correctly under some conditions.

Shriberg and Kwiatkowski (1988) wrote that deletion and substitution of sounds that are sometimes produced correctly have been taken as the hallmark of phonological error. The misarticulations are not considered to be phonetic in nature because the child has demonstrated the ability to produce the sounds correctly. However, this distinction may not apply to misarticulating individuals with cleft palate. Some patients continue to misarticulate even though successful treatment of the cleft has been provided and they produce sounds correctly during stimulability testing. The continued use of misarticulations established prior to habilitation of the speech mechanism may reflect some combination of sensorimotor and linguistic variables. Hewlett (1985) wrote that, in cleft palate speech, substitutions and omissions of an apparent phonological origin "may not be the result of phonological problems but the responses of an unimpaired phonology in seeking to circumvent problems of production. This, then, would be a case of an articulatory disorder which is (partially) manifested in substitutions of a phonological origin" (p. 164).

The clinical phonologist seeks to inventory the sounds the child can articulate, their distribution in syllables of different shapes, and the sounds that are used in a contrastive (phonemic) fashion in language expression (Elbert and Gierut, 1986). Similarly, those of us serving children with cleft palate are interested in the phonetic skills of those patients and with their use of the sound system in the expression of meaning. Clinical phonological conceptualization has emphasized study of the earliest development of the sound system, and this has influenced study of the sound systems of young children with clefts (O'Gara and Logemann, 1988). The emphasis on development invites a search for maturation and learning variables that are likely to influence articulation development—topics considered later in this chapter. We acknowledge the improbability of establishing the exact cause of sound system disorder in any individual; etiology sometimes refers to the grouping of individuals who share characteristics (Hubbell, 1981).

Many speech pathologists have adopted the practice of describing sound patterns in terms of phonological *processes* and *rules* (see Chapter 18). Shriberg and Kwiatkowski (1980) used *rule* in reference to regularities observed in language and natural *process* to explain or account for sound changes. (See also Kent, 1988.) Phonological processes may explain or at least describe the correspondence between a child's immature or misarticulated speech and that of normal adults in the child's community.

Dinnsen (1984) used *rule* and *process* synonymously as theoretical abstractions useful in explaining the correspondence between a talker's abstract knowledge of the sound system (underlying representation) and the speech produced. He indicated that the concept of process is not needed unless the correspondence between two phonological levels is of interest. That interest in turn leads to study of whether children with phonological disorders have adult-like knowledge of the sound system or knowledge perhaps idiosyncratic to the individual.

Establishing rules of correspondence between children's surface speech and their underlying knowledge of the sound system proves to be difficult. Elbert (1984) stated that a child has knowledge of a given sound if it appears somewhere in the individual's speech as in morphophonemic alternation (/dɔ/ for *dog*; /dɔgi/ for *doggy*) or during stimulability testing. However, Smith (1981) wrote that determination of the abstract knowledge or representation that theoretically underlies a child's productive sound system "is virtually impossible." He questioned the value of most rules written to transform an underlying representation into a surface representation. Grunwell (1985) characterized existing assessment procedures as primarily descriptive rather than explanatory. Smith (1981) wrote that description of phonological behavior whether in reference to rules and processes or other terms does not explain it, and he suggested that explanation be sought at the phonetic level before one turns to the phonological level. "It is much easier to create a label, assign it to the psychological or cognitive realm, and call it an "explanation" than to delve further into acoustic, aerodynamic, and/or physiological factors that may more accurately and realistically account for phonological data" (p. 11). He acknowledged that explanation will not always be found at the phonetic level. It seems to us that the speech clinician's search for phonological processes in children's speech is a search for patterns of sound usage shared by two or more sounds.

Statements that phonological concepts are useful in the description, evaluation, and treatment of patients with cleft palate (Stoel-Gammon and Dunn, 1985) remain largely assertions. Clinical phonology is new and developing. Its time on stage has not been sufficient for resolution or even clear identification of conceptual differences among ideas expressed through similar terminology but based on different theoretical foundations (Milroy, 1985; Connell, 1988; Fey, 1988). For many children the phonological disorder is part of a larger language problem (Stoel-Gammon and Dunn, 1985 p. 126; Shriberg and Kwiatkowski, 1988). If, in fact, the segment of the cleft palate population with extensive language disability is small, that observation argues against a major phonological emphasis in the study of cleft palate speech.

Certainly, the application of theory in treatment of disordered speech requires empirical tests, and the speech pathologist is necessarily concerned with the speaker as well as with his or her speech. Speech pathology includes a search for subject variables that correlate with speech phenomena and for interactions among subject, speech, and treatment variables. To be important, the relationships must make sense intellectually and facilitate the making of correct predictions (clinical decisions) and the development of effective treatments. Within this field, there is an abiding interest in rules of correspondence between abstract, theoretical constructs used to explain speech and the observations from which those constructs are inferred (Shontz, 1965). That interest is essential to attempts to develop valid measures that will support inferences about patients. The test of hypotheses and theory in speech pathology is an empirical one. Does the theory or model contribute to thinking in such a fashion that a more effective or efficient therapy results?

In summary, the disordered speech presented by some persons with clefts has been investigated and understood primarily in physiological-phonetic terms. Orderly patterns have been identified among articulation, velopharyngeal structure and function, aeromechanics, and other variables. This information has proved valuable in the conceptualization of multidisciplinary treatments for patients with clefts. Phonological-linguistic variables may also be involved in a patient's disordered sound pattern, and they may interact with physiological influences. Consequently, the speech-language pathologist serving patients with clefts should be alert to the phonological side of sound system disorders.

In this chapter, attention will be given to phonology as it bears on the patient with cleft palate. We will strive to use the terms *articulation* and *phonology* as they were employed by authors cited. Behavioral and cognitive factors are consi-

dered relative to their contribution to the sound system disorders that are presented by some speakers with cleft palate. Physiological influences on articulation and other speech behaviors are discussed in Chapter 12 and elsewhere. This chapter ends with a review of information about the intelligibility of speakers with cleft palate.

ARTICULATION DISORDERS ASSOCIATED WITH CLEFT PALATE

Articulation has been studied extensively in patients with cleft palate, and the information gained is reviewed in some detail. We attempt to characterize the articulation patterns of individuals with palatal clefts. Some articulation trends are strong, presumably trustworthy, and have face validity. Others, however, are weak and must be regarded with caution even though their recurrence suggests reliability of observation (Gilbert et al., 1977).

Identification of trends that occur from one study to another is sometimes difficult because different procedures have been used to study similar problems. For example, a variety of criteria has been used in the selection of subjects. In some studies, patients with different types of clefts were grouped together; in others, more homogeneous subject groups were used. Studies differ also in the quality of the techniques used to measure velopharyngeal valving. Some investigators studied only misarticulating subjects; others lumped together speakers with normal articulation and those with articulation errors. Studies have differed in the techniques used to measure articulation so that there are variations in the sounds and contexts studied. Different stimuli have been used to elicit responses and different criteria to score the responses. The studies have also differed on many other important variables, including research design. Thus, it is not always possible to equate one investigation with another. However, in spite of these understandable variations and limitations in methodology, patterns do emerge which should be understood and used clinically.

Occurrence of Disordered Articulation

The data cited here report counts of numbers of articulation errors. Later we will consider the articulation of different types of sounds and also the nature of articulation errors associated with cleft palate.

In general, individuals with cleft palate are at high risk for disordered articulation. As a group, they tend to articulate less well than normal persons. Bzoch (1965) reported that 5-year-old children with cleft palate articulated less well than 3-year-old normal children. Fletcher (1978) reported scores on the Iowa Pressure Articulation Test for 70 children with cleft palate aged 5 to 15 years for whom he judged velopharyngeal function to be normal or nearly so. The average score was similar to the test norm for age 3.5 years. Some subjects articulated with skill superior to that reflected by the group mean score, and many subjects with clefts have normal articulation (McWilliams, 1960). However, as Riski (1979) concluded, even following secondary surgical procedures, acceptable articulation and resonance are not established in all patients with cleft palate. McWilliams and Musgrave (1977) reported that articulation abilities in children with clefts usually lag behind those of physically normal children. Van Demark et al. (1979) studied subjects with cleft palate longitudinally. Between the ages of 3 and 8 years the subjects' articulation scores were below available norms. The subjects were studied through age 18 years, and many continued to misarticulate at 18. Normal individuals achieve mature articulation by age 8 or earlier as do some children with clefts.

Philips and Harrison (1969) conducted a cross-sectional study intended to describe speech maturation in 74 children with cleft palate and to compare their maturation with that of 127 normal children. They reported that the children with clefts made many more articulation errors than did normal children. They noted that the articulation scores of 94% of preschool children with cleft palate aged 3 years and older were inferior to the mean articulation scores of normal children of the same ages. They also noted that children with cleft palate from 60 to 71 months of age were inferior to normal children 36 to 74 months of age on all measures studied excepting percentage of errors on aspirants. The authors reported that the design of their study did not allow determination of the extent to which hearing loss, adequacy of velopharyngeal function, age at time of palatal repair, or other variables contributed to the articulation problems. Indeed, velopharyngeal function was not known except to the extent that it could be

inferred from speech production. No articulatory data were collected regarding nasal emission, nasal noises, glottal stops, pharyngeal fricatives, or other articulatory phenomena thought to be particularly likely to occur in individuals with velopharyngeal dysfunction.

Patterns of Misarticulation

The characteristics of speech associated with velopharyngeal insufficiency have been known for a long time. In an insightful article published in 1928, Berry referred to the "nasal character of all sounds," nasal emission, lack of intraoral air pressure, misarticulation of /s-z/, and especially severe hypernasality on the high vowels /i/ and /u/. She noted that the high vowel nasality is contrary to that reported in phonetics texts for normal speakers, but that high tongue posture probably directs the voice through any existent velopharyngeal opening and into the nasal passage. She also used pneumographic recordings to study movement of the abdomen and chest in cleft palate patients.

Bzoch (1979) tallied the speech characteristics in 1000 cleft palate patients he evaluated over a period of several years. Characteristics observed included laryngeal and pharyngeal substitution errors, consonant distortions from audible nasal emission, lisping, and other articulation distortions associated with hearing loss. Developmental misarticulation and delayed speech and language development were observed, and some patients had nasal and facial grimaces that interfered with communication.

Nasal Emission

Hypernasality and nasal emission are both speech characteristics associated with poor velopharyngeal structure and function. Hypernasality is discussed in Chapter 14. Nasal emission of air may be associated with reduced oral breath pressure for pressure consonants, and the combination of hypernasality and reduced oral breath pressure may mask place and manner of articulation faults (Wells, 1971). Data reported by Warren (1986) indicate that most patients maintain the ability to produce intraoral air pressure (3 cm H_2O) minimally sufficient for obstruent production. The literature differentiates among several degrees and types of nasal emission.

Inaudible Nasal Emission. Normally, most speakers produce connected discourse without evidence of nasal air escape except on the nasal /m/, /n/, and /ŋ/, where such air escape is appropriate. Speakers who do not achieve sufficient closure for production of the pressure sounds may demonstrate "visible" nasal escape from one or both nostrils for obstruents. This escape, though inaudible, may fog a cold mirror held at the nose, and thus, is sometimes referred to as "visible" nasal escape. The contexts in which this inappropriate nasal emission occurs should be carefully noted since this is one of the indicators of either a velopharyngeal valve that is not completely competent or of a symptomatic oronasal fistula.

Audible Nasal Emission. Audible nasal emission is the sound created when air being exhaled through the nasal passageways becomes turbulent and generates noise. You can create audible nasal emission by exhaling forcibly. This rush of air creates a noise that becomes a part of the speech signal generated and influences how it is perceived by listeners. It is a more serious problem than inaudible nasal escape along and may indicate the need for attention to velopharyngeal valving.

When marked intranasal resistance to air flow is present, the speech sound, which may be produced normally even though it has nasal air flow as a complicating factor, may be accompanied by extra turbulent noises, which we refer to as *nasal turbulence* (McWilliams, 1982). In these cases, clearing the nasal airway, sometimes simply by blowing the nose, may eliminate the noise, but it will not eliminate the airflow through the faulty valve, and the resulting emission may still be audible. It must be stressed that nasal turbulence is a severe form of audible nasal escape and that the noise generated is distracting to listeners. It points to a faulty velopharyngeal valve and to increased resistance in the nasal airway.

Nasal emission may also occur in an affricate-like or snort form. Morley (1970) wrote that the "nasopharyngeal snort" results from the passage of air through a sphincter which is closed but not tightly so. Thus, velopharyngeal closure may be sufficient for the impounding of intraoral air pressure for obstruents, but they may be released nasally rather than orally. This may reflect weak closure of the velopharyngeal port. Morley stated that these snorts often accompany /s/ sounds and other fricatives but can be associated with other sounds as well.

We have noticed that some patients direct air nasally with a tongue gesture. Closure of the nares during the nasal emission completely stops air flow. Peterson (1975) cited elevation of the tongue body or tongue dorsum in her description of nasal emission as a component of sibilant misarticulation. Riski (personal communication) described posterior nasal frication that results when the tongue occludes the oral cavity and the airstream is driven nasally. He indicated that this maneuver is involved in phoneme-specific nasal emission where a competent mechanism fails to close; however, we think it also occurs in some individuals with physiological velopharyngeal disability.

We should point out that the extent of the velopharyngeal opening associated with audible nasal emission may vary from less than 5 mm^2 (McWilliams and Philips, 1989) to completely open. McWilliams and Musgrave (1977) warned that other speech disorders, such as lateralized /s/ associated with dental anomalies, may easily be confused with audible nasal emission and attributed mistakenly to a faulty valve. This occurs because both types of errors are associated with an alteration in the direction of the airstream for speech but for different reasons. The speech pathologist should be alert to the need for careful study when nasal escape is audible.

Nasalized consonants have orderly patterns as studied spectrographically (Philips and Kent, 1984; Ericsson, 1987). Evidence of nasalization varies with the severity of velopharyngeal incompetence, but some distortion is obligatory. Leakage of air through the open velopharyngeal port may be associated with voicing during the stop gaps of voiceless stops. A stop gap is a moment of silence that precedes the release of a stop. Philips and Kent (1984, p. 140) stated that the resulting nasal murmer may make a stop resemble a nasal consonant. In cleft palate speech, the stop gap may be increased in duration, and the burst associated with release of plosive stops may be weak or missing. Also, the "antiresonances and increased damping associated with nasalization may obscure transitions into and out of the stop-gap segment" (Philips and Kent, 1984, p. 137) (Fig. 15.1). Nasal emission during stops and fricatives appears on the spectrogram as an interval of high frequency frication; it may be weak in intensity. Ericsson (1987) also described frication-

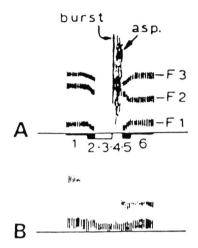

Figure 15.1 Stylized spectrograms to illustrate (A) acoustic features of a normal production of a voiceless stop, and (B) acoustic features of a strongly nasalized stop for which voicing does not cease. The acoustic segments in (A) represent: (1) a preconsonantal vowel, (2) formant transitions from the preconsonant vowel into the stop, (3) voiceless stop gap, (4) interval of noise containing both noise burst and aspiration (asp.), (5) formant transitions from stop into postconsonantal vowel, and (6) postconsonantal vowel. Most of the acoustic features represented in (A) disappear in the nasalized production in (B). (From Philips BJ, Kent RD. Acoustic-phonetic descriptions of speech production in speakers with cleft palate and other velopharyngeal disorders. Speech Lang Adv Basic Res Pract 1984; 11:113-168.)

alization of stops and partial devoicing of voiced stops.

Nasal emission will be a problem in the speech of persons with velopharyngeal incompetence unless the individual resorts to use of compensatory articulation, which is usually an unsatisfactory solution to the problem. Compensatory articulation is discussed later in the chapter.

Sounds Most Frequently Misarticulated

In two descriptive studies, McWilliams (1953) and Spriestersbach et al. (1956) described the articulation of heterogeneous groups of adults and children with palatal clefts. Consonants misarticulated more than 60% of the time by the children studied by Spriestersbach were /z/, /s/, /θ/, /ts/, / ʃ /, / dʒ /, /ð/, /s/, and / ʧ /. The consonants correctly articulated at least 80% of the time were /m/, /h/, /n/, /j/, and /ŋ/. Table 15.1 summarizes these data. In the McWilliams study, the most frequently misarticulated sounds were /s/ (63%), /z/ (61%), /d / (48%), and / ʧ / (44%). Only 11% of the /p/ sounds sampled and 9% of the /b/ sounds were misarticulated.

The /s/ is the speech sound most frequently and most consistently misarticulated by individuals with cleft palate (McWilliams, 1953, 1958). Byrne et al. (1961), also reported that their subjects correctly produced only 50% of the /s/ items studied. Using a different test, Fletcher (1978) reported that his subjects misarticulated 46, 43, and 49% of the /s/ sounds studied in the initial, final, and medial positions of words, respectively. His subjects most frequently misarticulated the blends str-(67%), st-(63%), sk-(63%), sp-(61%), and -ks (61%). The subjects of Van Demark et al. (1979) most frequently misarticulated fricatives and affricatives, and /s/ had an especially low percentage of correct productions across the ages studied.

Error Types

In the 1950s and 1960s research descriptive of cleft palate speech tended to categorize errors as substitutions, omissions, and distortions.

McWilliams (1953, 1958) found that, of 1814 misarticulated sounds produced by adult subjects with palatal clefts, 1436 were distortions, 335 were omissions, and 43 were substitutions. Similarly, in

TABLE 15.1   Rank Order of Consonants (Classified According to Place of Articulation) in Terms of Percentage of Correct Responses by a Group of 25 Subjects with Palatal Clefts

Labial		Labio-dental		Lingua-dental		Post-dental			Velar		Glottal	
1 (m)	96%											
						2.5	(n)	88%			2.5 (h)	88%
						4	(j)	86%				
									5 (η)	80%		
6 (w)	77%											
7 (b)	73%											
8 (p)	70%											
									9 (g)	64%		
		10 (f)	63%									
						11	(l)	60%				
		12 (v)	59%									
						13	(d)	58%				
						14	(r)	57%				
									15 (k)	53%		
16 (hw)	42%											
						17	(t)	39%				
						18	(ʃ)	38%				
				19.5 (ð)	37%	19.5	(dʒ)	37%				
						21	(ʒ)	30%				
						22	(tʃ)	29%				
				23.5 (θ)	23%	23.5	(s)	23%				
						25	(z)	21%				

From Spriestersbach DC, Darley FL, Raus V. Articulation of a group of children with cleft lips and palates. J Speech Hear Dis 1956; 21:436.

a study by McDermott (1962), most cleft palate speakers between 8 and 18 years of age produced distortions of /s/. He classified 70% of the /s/ sounds he studied as distortions, 23% as correctly articulated, 5% as omitted, and 1% as replaced by other sounds. Van Demark (1966) observed from his study of cleft palate children between 5 and 14 years of age that nasal distortions were frequently produced. Nasal distortions accounted for 25% of the articulation errors found, distortions 30%, omissions 29%, substitutions 13%, glottal substitutions 2%, and nasal substitutions 1%. Bzoch (1956) observed that nasal distortions persist with age, whereas other distortions tend to decrease in frequency of occurrence.

Clearly, distortion errors do not account for all misarticulated sounds produced by individuals with cleft palate. In their study of cleft palate children between 3 and 8 years of age, Spriestersbach et al. (1956) reported that omissions occurred most frequently followed by substitutions and distortions, in that order.

Type of error has been found to vary with whether single consonants or blends are being tested. Spriestersbach et al. (1961), in a study of children between the ages of 3 and 17 years found more omissions and distortions and fewer substitutions for blends than for single elements. Distortions occurred more frequently and substitutions less frequently for singleton fricatives and affricates than for singleton stop plosives. As Moll (1968) concluded, consonants in blends tend to be omitted when they are misarticulated, whereas the articulation errors on singleton fricatives and affricates are frequently distortions. When substitutions occur, the manner of production is often maintained as is the case when glottal stops replace standard stops. Only rarely are glottal stops substituted for fricatives, which do not share a similar manner of production.

If the misarticulation associated with cleft palate primarily reflects anatomical defects, the speaker would be expected to produce the best possible approximation of the target sound. This logic could account for sound distortions. As Locke (1980) pointed out, a distorted [s] is usually a form of /s/ and reveals "knowledge of which phoneme is appropriate." Use of distortions could reflect the individual's best effort to meet the phonological standard of his community. Substitution of a glottal stop for a perceptually similar sound such as /k/ or /g/ would be compatible with this reasoning as would omission or slighting of consonants to avoid nasal emission or because the air source is exhausted. Final consonant deletion, sometimes termed the open syllable, has been interpreted as evidence of a grammatical-cognitive problem (Panagos, 1974). However, this phenomenon could have multiple origins. For example, speakers with velopharyngeal insufficiency could delete final consonants as a means of avoiding nasal emission, because the available air pressure has been depleted, or because sounds lacking normal oral air pressure could be interpreted as omissions even though some energy marked the final consonant. Bernthal and Weiner (1976) demonstrated that acoustic energy is often present where articulation evaluators have reported speech sound omission.

Manner and Place of Articulation

Moll (1968) reported that velopharyngeal incompetence is more likely to interfere with some manner classifications than with others. He concluded that, within different manner-of-production categories, sounds involving lingual contacts tended to be more defective than those involving only the lips. When substitutions occur in cleft palate speech, the manner of production is often maintained as in the case when glottal stops replace standard stops. The tendency for nasal consonants to be correctly articulated, most fre-

TABLE 15.2   Number of Times each Phoneme was Tested, Consistency of Correct Articulation, and Consistency of Incorrect Articulation for the Total Group of 154 Subjects. Percentages of Consistently Correct Productions are also Given for the Different Manner-of-Production Categories

Phoneme	Frequency of Occurrence	% Consistently Correct	% Consistently in Error
Plosives (pl)			
t	23	67.9	1.3
d	12	66.6	3.2
p	4	81.3	4.5
b	4	84.2	1.3
k	9	63.9	8.4
g	4	67.3	13.6
category percentage		69.0	
Fricatives (fr)			
f	5	74.1	9.1
v	4	69.1	12.9
s	11	23.7	38.9
z	5	32.4	40.9
ʃ	1	44.6	56.5
ð	6	68.2	7.8
Θ	1	51.9	48.1
category percentage		47.7	
Nasals (na)			
m	9	98.8	—
n	20	97.1	—
η	2	75.6	12.3
category percentage		96.2	
Glides (gl)			
l	6	84.5	3.2
r	5	80.5	7.1
j	5	92.3	—
w	7	96.6	—
h	5	98.3	—
ʍ	1	95.4	4.5
category percentage		90.8	

From Van Demark DR. Consistency of articulation of subjects with cleft palate. Cleft Palate J 1969; 6:254.

TABLE 15.3 Percentages of Misarticulations by Cleft Palate and Normal Subjects, According to Type of Error and Age Level

Error Types for Single Consonant Elements	Cleft Palate			Normal		
	36–47 mos.	48–59 mos.	60–71 mos.	36–47 mos.	48–59 mos.	60–71 mos.
	N 27	N 16	N 21	N 25	N 51	N 51
Fricatives	0.98	0.83	0.73	0.49	0.35	0.28
Affricatives	0.92	0.84	0.70	0.42	0.21	0.12
Glides	0.71	0.46	0.39	0.30	0.18	0.13
Plosives	0.70	0.43	0.31	0.06	0.02	0.02
Aspirants	0.44	0.25	0.07	0.02	0.01	0.01
Nasals	0.38	0.30	0.24	0.05	0.01	0.03
Voiced	0.87	0.70	0.57	0.35	0.24	0.17
Unvoiced	0.86	0.68	0.56	0.29	0.17	0.15
Initial	0.69	0.48	0.39	0.25	0.17	0.13
Medial	0.78	0.63	0.48	0.26	0.16	0.13
Final	0.84	0.68	0.59	0.31	0.25	0.15
Indistinct production	0.17	0.16	0.16	0.04	0.04	0.04
Substitutions	0.27	0.22	0.22	0.18	0.11	0.08
Omissions	0.33	0.20	0.10	0.05	0.02	0.01

From Philips BJ, Harrison RJ. Articulation patterns of preschool cleft palate children. Cleft Palate J 1969; 6:245.

quently followed in order by glides, plosives, and fricatives, was cited earlier. Van Demark (1969) and Van Demark et al. (1979) reported the percentage of correct articulation for these four categories as observed in cleft palate subjects (Table 15.2). Philips and Harrison (1969) also reported the percentages of misarticulated sounds in each of several articulatory categories by cleft palate and normal subjects in three age groups (Table 15.3). These findings indicated that persons with clefts are especially likely to articulate fricatives and affricatives poorly.

Fletcher (1978) analyzed articulation data from 70 subjects with cleft palates by factor analysis revealing a sibilant-nonsibilant contrast. Fletcher sorted the sounds he studied into three categories: (1) sibilants —/s, z, ʃ, tʃ, and dʒ/, (2) nonsibilant fricatives—/Θ, ð, v, and f/, and (3) plosives—/p, b, t, d, k/ and /g/. He wrote that this classification resulted in more homogeneous groupings of sounds than the more traditional assignment of sounds to fricative and affricative categories. Fletcher reported mean error percentages of 47.4 for sibilants, 24.0 for nonsibilant fricatives, and 17.3 for plosives, findings consistent with those of McWilliams (1953, 1958) and Spriestersbach (1956).

Counihan (1956) rank-ordered sounds from least to most frequently misarticulated as follows: lip sounds, tongue-tip simple sounds, tongue-tip complex sounds, and back-of-tongue sounds. Moll (1968) pointed out that tongue-tip complex sounds include fricatives and affricates. Logemann (1983) stated that children with cleft palate who are between 24 months and 5 years tend to have articulatory placement errors but correct manner of articulation. They maintain manner by placing articulation posterior to fistulas or velopharyngeal opening. Older children present accurate articulatory placement but manner errors in the form of faulty release of stops, fricatives, and affricates.

Investigators have studied whether persons with cleft palate are more likely than normal individuals to misarticulate /r/ and /l/. These sounds are sometimes listed as liquids and sometimes as glides. The misarticulation of these sounds would be difficult to account for directly in terms of velopharyngeal incompetence, since they do not require high intraoral air pressure.

McWilliams (1958), in her study of cleft palate adults, found 13 of 48 subjects to misarticulate /r/, and they misarticulated from 5 to 47% of the number tested. No subject misarticulated all

/r/ sounds. Pitzner and Morris (1966) found that individuals with cleft palate who had poor velopharyngeal closure were more likely to misarticulate these sounds than were those with palatal clefts who had good velopharyngeal function. That conclusion is compatible with Van Demark's (1969) finding that children with low oral manometer quotients produced liquids correctly less frequently than did individuals with higher quotients. Philips and Harrison (1969) (Table 15.3) found a high percentage of glide errors in their preschool children with cleft palate. Indeed, percentages of errors on glides and plosives were similar in the three age groups they studied. Van Demark et al. (1979) reported that cleft palate speakers misarticulate /r/ and /l/ more often than do normal individuals. Van Demark and Van Demark (1967) compared the articulation of children with cleft palate who had good velopharyngeal function and children with functional articulation disorders. The latter group more frequently misarticulate glides and also used more sound substitutions.

Moll (1968) observed that consideration of manner of articulation contributes special insights regarding the speech of individuals with clefts and that study of place of articulation may be confounded by manner of articulation. However, defects associated with cleft palate may influence both manner and place of articulation. For example, nasal air leakage associated with velopharyngeal incompetence may particularly impair frication while also encouraging articulation placement posterior to a fistula or to an opening of the velopharyngeal valve. Thus, manner requirements that are difficult for the speaker with velopharyngeal incompetence to achieve may be associated with articulation errors that involve a shift in place of articulation.

Patterns of misarticulation as they relate to place and manner may also be interpreted in phonological terms. Phonemic substitutions within a manner category involve a shift in placement. These errors (and also distortions involving consonant release or placement shift insufficient for change in phoneme) may reflect adjustments to a faulty mechanism in the presence of a satisfactory phonological system. An observation of Platt et al. (1980) written in consideration of dysarthria may apply to cleft palate speech. They concluded that within-manner errors of place and voicing, as contrasted with between-manner errors, suggest the presence of competent

phonological knowledge but articulatory imprecision.

Study of both place and manner of articulation provides valuable information which helps us understand the articulation and phonology of persons with clefts.

Voicing

Individuals with clefts appear to misarticulate voiceless sounds more frequently than the voiced cognates (Spriestersbach et al., 1956; McWilliams, 1953, 1958). Sherman et al. (1959) found that glottal stops were used more frequently to replace voiceless than voiced consonants. However, the percentages of voiced and voiceless sounds misarticulated by the younger subjects in the study by Philips and Harrison (1969) were most equal (see Table 15.3). Spriestersbach et al. (1961) found that voiced stops and affricates were better articulated than were their voiceless counterparts but that the reverse was true for fricatives. Moll (1968) noted that the relative difficulty of voiced and voiceless consonants may change with age. He also noted that voicing and manner of production may interact to influence articulation. It is also possible that voicing masks placement errors that are evident to the ear when they occur in voiceless members of cognate pairs (Sherman et al., 1959; Kent, 1982).

Vowel Articulation

Moll (1968) noted that cleft palate speakers tend to articulate vowels adequately unless nasalization is considered to be an articulation error. Since nasalization is not phonemic in English, Moll would classify it separately from vowel misarticulation. However, Klinger (1956) reported that listeners identified only 53% of the vowels produced by persons with cleft palate, whereas 70% of the vowels produced by normal speakers were identified correctly. Cullinan and Counihan (1971) questioned studies which indicate that persons with clefts articulate vowels with few or no errors and noted that these studies may have been confounded by contextual cues to vowel identification. They studied the ability of listeners to identify the vowels /a, i,/ and /u/. Vowels produced by normal speakers were correctly identified 79% of the time, whereas for subjects with cleft, the vowels were recognized in only 53% of the utterances. The source of this loss of vowel intelligibility in speakers with clefts has not been established. However, Cullinan and Counihan noted that tongue height and mouth opening may be adjusted to compensate for velopharyngeal opening.

Hypernasality may degrade vowel intelligibility. Philips and Kent (1984) stated that nasalized vowels show low-frequency nasal formants below F1 (the first formant), a weakening and small increase in frequency of F2, a reduction of overall energy, a reduction of F2 amplitude, and increase in formant band widths. Thus nasalized vowels are characterized by low-frequency energy and reduced intensity. The authors indicated that nasalization makes it difficult to differentiate among vowels.

Van Demark et al. (1979) found that subjects with clefts misarticulate vowels more frequently than do subjects without clefts. Fletcher (1978) concluded that persons with cleft palates show "considerable variability" in tongue placement for vowels. His statement was based on cephalometric, radiographic study of tongue posture during the production of isolated /a/, and /i/. In spite of these findings, relatively few children with or without palatal clefts require articulation training for vowels. Severe vowel misarticulation may differ in etiology from other patterns of misarticulation.

Variability in Articulation

Information about variability in articulation is important in the study of articulation disorders. It is used to help define the severity of the disorder and to plan remediation. Consistent misarticulation, that is, the misarticulation of all sounds from one or more phonemes, is thought to be more severe than misarticulation patterns wherein errors are inconsistent. Stimulability testing is used to differentiate between patients who can and those who cannot produce correctly articulated sounds. Poor stimulability and consistent misarticulation may reflect a physiological inability to produce the sounds, whereas inconsistent articulation may reflect immature knowledge of the sound system. Inconsistent misarticulation is not likely to be random. Phonological analysis often shows the articulatory behavior to be orderly and context-dependent. While such a pattern could be

expressed in terms of rules and processes, its origin could very well be in the physiology of the oral mechanism.

The Influence of Context

The influence of context on articulation proficiency has been studied by a number of investigators. Most of the studies have been of normal speakers or of speakers with articulation disorders but with presumably normal oral structures, but some context information is also available about cleft palate speakers. For example, as has already been noted, cleft palate speakers are more likely to misarticulate sounds in blends (clusters) than as singletons. Spriestersbach et al. (1956) found this to be true for their heterogeneous 3 to 8 year old children with cleft palates or cleft lips and palates. A similar trend was found by Spriestersbach et al. (1961). Here, 71% of the singletons were correctly articulated as compared to 64% of the consonants in blends. Differences in percentages correct for the two conditions were statistically significant.

Morris et al. (1961) sorted subjects with clefts into good- and poor-closure groups on the basis of wet spirometer ratios and cephalometric x-rays taken during the production of /s/ or /u/. In this study, only subjects in the poor-closure groups differed in the correctness of consonants as singletons or as members of blends. Target sounds were studied in 11 singleton items, 11 two-element blends, and 11 three-element blends. For the good-closure group, the mean numbers of correct responses were 9.7, 9.2 and 9.0 for the three conditions, whereas, for the subjects with poor closure, the means were 6.0, 5.4, and 3.9 respectively.

Bzoch (1965) found that two-consonant blends better differentiated cleft palate and normal children than did fricatives or plosives. He noted that these results were compatible with those of Counihan (1956, 1960), Starr (1956), and McWilliams (1953, 1958).

McDermott (1962) found that subjects who produced /s/ correctly one or more times were more likely to be correct in words where /s/ appeared as a singleton (42% correct) than as a blend (30% correct). In addition, /s/ was more frequently articulated correctly in two-element than in three-element blends. These results were statistically significant. For /s/ in a variety of blends, the percentages correct ranged from a high of 40% to a low of 22%. McDermott sorted his clusters into three categories, /sC-/, /Cs-/, and /-sC/, and found no statistically significant differences in correctness of /s/ articulation among the three categories. The /s/ was more frequently articulated correctly in /sn-/ blends than in /-ns/ blends.

A reasonable conclusion from these findings is that cleft palate speakers are more likely to misarticulate a given speech sound when it occurs in a cluster than when it occurs as a singleton. It would be interesting to know to what extent these errors involve distortions as contrasted with cluster reduction. The latter is considered to be phonological in nature. Spriestersbach and Curtis (1951) reported that consonant blends somehow facilitate articulation proficiency. That facilitation is not evident in the data reviewed here concerning the speech of children with clefts.

Data about articulation in the initial, medial, and final positions in words are also available for cleft palate speakers. Counihan (1960) and Bzoch (1965) examined the articulation of consonant sounds in these positions. Bzoch's subjects were between 3 and 6 years of age, whereas Counihan's ranged from 13 through 23 years. Each author sampled various consonant sounds. Bzoch found a trend toward more frequent misarticulation of sounds in the medial position than in either of the other positions. Counihan found no relationship between misarticulation and word position.

Starr (1956) analyzed the articulation of cleft palate speakers between 6 and 11 years of age. He classified articulation errors as substitutions, omissions, indistinct productions, and indistinct productions resulting from nasal emission. Omissions occurred more frequently in the final than in the initial or medial positions, whereas the other errors occurred with equal frequency in all three positions. Byrne et al. (1961) reported the percentage of correct consonant singletons produced by children with cleft palate in the initial, medial, and final position of words. The percentage of correct responses by position varied from sound to sound, but differences were generally small.

McDermott (1962) reported that /s/ is articulated correctly more often in syllable releasing than arresting positions. He recommended that the clinician study the individual patient's speech pattern to identify contexts associated with relatively high proportions of correct and incorrect responses. Morris et al. (1961) concluded that the position of sound elements in articulation test words does not relate strongly to the distinction

between subjects with good and those with poor velopharyngeal closure. Nor did position in test word influence the discriminatory power of two- and three-element blends.

Additional context variables have also been studied. Bless et al. (1978) commented that individuals with velopharyngeal incompetence are most likely to misarticulate consonants that are adjacent to nasal sounds, whereas individuals with marginal velopharyngeal incompetence may nasalize oral consonants adjacent to nasals through assimilatory relationships.

The evidence cited indicates that misarticulating individuals with cleft palate like other misarticulating persons are inconsistent in their misarticulation in the sense that a given sound may sometimes be correctly produced and sometimes misarticulated. However, this "inconsistency" occurs in orderly patterns. The studies reviewed did little to classify subjects according to the severity of oral structural deformities or phonological development each of which would be involved in the overall sound pattern. Subjects with cleft palate who had oropharyngeal structures that function normally or nearly so may have articulation characteristics similar to those of children free from physical disability.

Consistency

Analysis of the consistency of misarticulation in cleft speakers has been based on procedures that define consistency as the percentage of speech sounds from a particular phoneme that an individual articulates correctly or incorrectly. Moll (1968) pointed out that only individuals who produce all responses correctly or incorrectly are consistent and that the individual who misarticulates a speech sound correctly 50% of the times it is uttered is maximally inconsistent. Consistency may also pertain to whether or not a speaker always makes the same sort of error on a particular sound, and a sound may be consistently or inconsistently articulated in repetitions of the same context. As McWilliams (1953, 1958) observed, the number of times a sound is tested will influence findings of consistency. The concepts of consistency and context are related.

Spriestersbach et al. (1956) found a heterogeneous group of children with cleft palate to be generally inconsistent in consonant production. Different sounds were misarticulated in different ways; indeed a given child would misarticulate a given sound in different ways. For the subjects as a group, 27% of the consonants were always articulated correctly and 20% were always misarticulated.

McWilliams (1953, 1958) found that adults with cleft palate were also inconsistent. She reported that, of 23 consonants tested, only nine were misarticulated by some subjects each time the phonemes were attempted. Since the sounds appeared in the test battery in the same frequency with which they occur in conversation, some of those sounds were sampled only once or twice each. She concluded that most of her subjects were able to produce all sounds correctly some of the time and that they were most nearly consistent in their misarticulation of sibilants.

McDermott (1962), in his study of /s/ articulation by cleft palate speakers, reported that 10 of 54 subjects articulated between 43 and 60% of their /s/ sounds correctly. Children with manometer ratios of 0.90 or higher were more consistent in /s/ articulation than were those with lower ratios.

Van Demark (1969) reported information about the percentage of sounds consistently correct across 154 subjects and the percentage of subjects who consistently misarticulated each of the sounds studied. His findings indicate that some sounds were misarticulated each time they were used by certain subjects. That is, some subjects consistently misarticulated certain sounds, especially fricatives. However, the subjects as a group articulated most sounds correctly most of the time. Fricatives had especially low percentages of correct productions across subjects. The trends cited above are not applicable to all individuals with clefts because some may differ in oropharyngeal physiology from the subjects studied.

Stimulability

Stimulability in speakers with cleft palates has been given little attention in research. McDermott (1962) reported that cleft speakers articulated /s/ correctly more frequently when it was imitated in response to an examiner than when it was produced spontaneously. This was true whether the production was an isolated sound or in a syllable or word.

Philips and Harrison (1969) compared articulation development in normal and cleft palate children. Imitative articulation of 24 consonants

in CV syllables was sampled by having the subject listen to a syllable three times and then produce it. Correct responses were scored one, questionable responses one-half, and incorrect responses zero. Responses were scored separately for "articulation placement and resultant acoustic signal." In a second imitative task, responses were obtained by asking each child to repeat pictured test words after an examiner three times. The best production of the target sound in each set was scored as correct, omitted, substituted, or indistinct. For each age subgroup and each measure, children with clefts were inferior to noncleft children, but the older children with clefts performed better than their younger counterparts. These data indicate that children with clefts are less stimulable for correct articulation than are normal children.

Speech Rate

Speech rate in speakers with cleft palate has received relatively little study. McDermott (1962) found that /s/ was articulated less accurately as rate of syllable production increased. He thought that slow rate afforded the subject greater opportunity to compensate for structural defects. Lass and Noll (1970) compared the speech rates of young adults with palatal clefts with those of normal individuals. A power-level recorder operated at 30 mm per second was used to measure rate as each subject read a passage several times as they engaged in 2 minutes of impromptu speaking. The subjects with cleft palate tended to speak more slowly than the normal individuals and to show greater variability on the measures studied.

Philips and Kent (1984, pp. 123 and 121) reviewed literature which shows that increase in speaking rate involves change in range of movement, duration of pauses, and duration of steady-state segments such as vowels and fricatives. Articulators differ in their speed of movement and in the movements they can produce. For example, in speech the tongue moves faster and participates in a greater variety of movements than does the velopharyngeal apparatus. Therefore, motor control involves the coordination of articulators moving at different rates. Observation of speech variation with change in rate is considered to offer a means for investigation of motor control for speech.

Forner (1983) stated that segment durations reflect ability to coordinate speech gestures and also "the interactions of the mechanism's components to meet segmental and suprasegmental requirements of meaningful speech" (p. 185). Therefore, she compared 5- and 6-year-old children with and without clefts for speech segment and stop gap durations and for voice onset time measured spectrographically. Subjects with clefts were variable in nasality and intelligibility. She stated that children the age of her subjects should evidence adult-like voice onset time distinctions for voiced and voiceless stop cognates. Inferential statistics are reported, but many of the descriptive data are not included. As compared with the normal children, the children with clefts prolonged segments in single word and nasal sentence contexts. Cleft subjects who were hypernasal and relatively unintelligible had longer voice onset times than did cleft subjects with less disordered speech. The cleft and noncleft groups did not differ significantly in overall CV segment duration. The author and also Linville (1984) discussed the findings in terms of theories that may explain speech motor control.

Jones and Folkins (1985) studied the influence of increased speaking rate on judgments of severity of disordered speech. Their subjects were between 7 and 10 years of age; six had cleft palate and two were normal. The speech sample consisted of three sentences that differed in phonetic complexity; one sentence was free from nasal and pressure consonants. The other two had both. Increased speaking rate was not associated with change in ratings of the severity of the speech disorder. The authors concluded that the flexibility and plasticity (Folkins, 1985) of the subjects' speech mechanisms were sufficient to permit the subjects to adapt to the demands of the increased speaking rate. We anticipate future research investigating rate, timing, and constraints to increase understanding of the control of speech and velopharyngeal function in patients with clefts.

Reduced speech rate is thought to result in interruptions of velopharyngeal closure. Colton and Cooker (1968) found nasality ratings to be higher in normal and hearing-impaired individuals when reading word by word than when reading at a normal rate. They thought the velopharyngeal seal might be broken at the slower rate. This inference was also drawn by Hutchinson et. al. (1978).

Articulation and Velopharyngeal Closure

This section is concerned with the relation-ship between velopharyngeal closure or function and articulation and the extent to which velopharyngeal valving inadequacies account for the misarticulation found in some cleft palate patients.

Other variables being equal, individuals who fail to achieve normal velopharyngeal closure articulate less well than persons who do achieve it. Also, those with larger openings generally articulate more poorly than individuals with smaller openings. These relationships are identifiable even with relatively crude tests for the assessment of velopharyngeal function. For example, subjects with cleft palates who have poor velopharyngeal closure, as indicated by still cephalometric radiographs and manometric tests, are inferior in articulation to cleft palate subjects with better performance on those measures (Powers, 1962). Van Demark (1966) reported a similar trend for cleft palate speakers classified into low, medium, and high velopharyngeal closure groups on the basis of manometer ratios.

Van Demark (1974) described velopharyngeal function and articulation in Danish and American children. Subjects in each group were sorted into competent, marginally competent, and incompetent groups. This classification was based partly on speech characteristics, but also on intraoral inspection, oral manometer ratios, and lateral radiographs taken during production of /s/ or /u/. Mean data for the Danish subjects showed that articulation test scores of competent subjects were better than those of either of the other two subgroups, and the marginal groups articulated better than the incompetent group. The American subjects who achieved closure or marginal performance articulated better than the incompetent group, but did not differ from one another to a statistically significant degree.

Measures of velopharyngeal function, such as cephalometric indices to the gap between the soft palate and the posterior pharyngeal wall during speech, tend to correlate only moderately with articulation. As an example, Spriestersbach and Powers (1959) correlated articulation data with cephalometric measurements of velopharyngeal gap and with spirometric and manometric data. The subjects were 103 boys and girls with palatal clefts with or without lip involvement ranging in age from 5 through 15 years. The correlations reported ranged from 0.40 to 0.53.

A correlation of 0.50 is a rough average of the correlations between velopharyngeal function and speech that have been reported in the literature (Morris, 1968). This level of correlation indicates that velopharyngeal function accounts for only 25% of the variance in articulation. Velopharyngeal valving as measured in three dimensions might account for more of the variance in articulation measures. Replication of research correlating velopharyngeal competence, articulation, intelligibility, and hypernasality would update our understanding of those relationships if the velopharyngeal measure captured the contributions of both the velum and the pharyngeal walls to velopharyngeal closure. However, it seems likely that variables in addition to velopharyngeal valving account for substantial amounts of the articulation variance in patients with clefts.

The linearity of the relationship between articulation and velopharyngeal closure has also been studied. Shelton et al. (1964) found a higher correlation between articulation scores and velopharyngeal function determined from sagittal cinefluoroscopy when the data were analyzed by use of the Eta procedure rather than the Pearson correlation. This suggests that the relationship is nonlinear. Brandt and Morris (1965) correlated articulation scores with velopharyngeal gaps taken from lateral head radiographs during production of /u/ and /s/. In this study, the correlations ranged from 0.50 to 0.60. Most of the analyses were not compatible with the hypothesis of a nonlinear relationship between articulation and velopharyngeal function. However, if Warren (1967) was correct in stating that increase in velopharyngeal port beyond 20 mm^2 is not linearly related to an increase in nasal air flow, then a nonlinear relationship between velopharyngeal function and articulation could be expected.

The research cited above has examined relationships between speech and velopharyngeal closure by analyzing only one pair of variables at a time. Multivariate research has also been carried out and is discussed next.

Research by Van Demark (1964, 1966) was directed to the identification of articulatory patterns in 154 children who had cleft palates with or without cleft lip, and were between 5 and 14 years of age, had not undergone adolescent voice change, and were free from hearing loss as measured by a screening procedure. Articulatory factors attributable to velopharyngeal dysfunction and those that reflected learning or maturational influences were differentiated.

In the 1964 report, Van Demark identified two clusters of variables within each of which variables correlated moderately or highly with one another. One cluster consisted of stop-plosive and fricative misarticulation and nasal distortions. Van Demark reasoned that these articulation errors were related to velopharyngeal dysfunction. A second cluster included glides, nasals, and semivowels. This cluster was interpreted to represent defects in maturation or learning.

A multiple correlation of 0.88 resulted when stop misarticulation from the velopharyngeal cluster and glide misarticulation from the maturational-learning cluster were correlated with an articulation defectiveness rating. These results indicated that a substantial percentage of the variance in articulation defectiveness is accounted for by velopharyngeal function and maturation-learning. It is of special interest that the factor related to valving made a contribution to the severity of the articulation problem three times greater than did the factor related to maturation and learning.

Van Demark (1966) reanalyzed his data using factor analysis rather than multiple correlations. Analyses were computed for the total group of subjects and for subgroups with low, medium, and high manometer quotients. The ages of these subjects were also entered into the analysis. Again he concluded that the severity of articulation defectiveness is related primarily to two factors, one representing velopharyngeal dysfunction and the other maturation. Factor analyses of individuals in the low, medium, and high manometer groups indicated that the high quotient group did not show a velopharyngeal factor, whereas both velopharyngeal function and maturation seemed to influence the articulation of members of the other two groups.

The data reinforced Van Demark's earlier conclusion that although velopharyngeal dysfunction together with defective maturation and learning are involved in the articulation problems of individuals with clefts, faulty valving emerges as a major source of their errors. Maturation and learning may also be influential in children who appear not to have valving deficits.

In another multivariate study, Fletcher (1978) collected articulation data and other measures including physiological indices to place of articulation. Statistical analysis was conducted to identify a relatively small group of nonarticulatory variables that accounted for as much articulation test variance as possible. Fletcher studied cleft children who ranged in age from 5 to 15 years. He administered the Iowa Pressure Articulation Test supplemented by seven items. Fletcher obtained 103 measures on each subject. In addition to articulation, he evaluated dentition, including malocclusion and fistulas, morphology and mobility of the tongue; syllable repetition time or diadochokinesis; and cephalometric variables. He then submitted the data to a multivariate statistical analysis to identify which 10 measures from the four categories just listed accounted for the most variance in articulation. A coefficient of determination indicated that polysyllable diadochokinesis, palate-pharyngeal contact, velopharyngeal gap, class of cleft, linguapharyngeal aperture, tongue retraction, tongue fronting, vertical interincisor aperture, horizontal interincisor aperture, and velar retraction, in that order, accounted for 79 percent of the variance in articulation.

In summary, the first of the two multivariate studies cited provided information suggesting that articulation errors have their origins both in velopharyngeal function and in learning. The second study suggested that physical and physiological variables in addition to velopharyngeal function also contribute to disordered articulation in cleft palate speakers. These correlational studies are causal in orientation. Theories implicitly or explicitly held by the authors undoubtedly influenced the choice of measures, and that influenced the findings. Each author used multivariate analysis of numerous measures, but the variables studied and the outcomes are quite different. These studies complement each other and help us understand the complicated interactions that must be taken into account in the clinical management of cleft palate speakers.

As we stated earlier, some speech distortion is obligatory in the presence of velopharyngeal incompetence. Certain articulation error types, for example distortion by audible nasal emission, indicate failure of velopharyngeal closure. Thus, consideration of error type helps the clinician to understand the origins of a given child's speech pattern. Nonetheless, two individuals may respond to similar disability in different ways— strategies are considered later in the chapter—and an individual may persist in errors associated with velopharyngeal incompetence even after surgery has provided a potentially competent mechanism.

Hardin et al. (1986) examined several speech and nonspeech measures for their ability to predict speech proficiency at age 14 years. Their subjects were cleft palate individuals with intelligence quotients no lower than 85 and without sensorineural hearing loss or multiple congenital anomalies. The predictor variables, which were measured between 4 and 13 years of age, included articulation test scores, information about manner of production and error type, ratings of articulation defectiveness and nasality, gender, type of primary palatoplasty, age at palatoplasty, and whether the patient had a pharyngeal flap. Multivariate statistical procedures were used in a search for a subset of predictor variables that accounted for large percentages of the predicted variable. The authors noted that speech proficiency across subjects at age 14 years was restricted in range—a condition that limits the study. Gender itself accounted for 40% of the variance in judged speech proficiency—the females showed better speech proficiency than did the males. The most efficient subsets of predictors measured at different age levels accounted for 50 to 75% of the variability in the predicted variable. However, except for gender, what constituted an efficient subset of predictors changed from age level to age level.

Articulation Errors Related to Type of Cleft

Spriestersbach et al. (1961) found better speech in patients with cleft lip and palate than in persons with cleft palate only. This is compatible with the facts that some patients with cleft palate alone present extensive horseshoe-shaped clefts with significant tissue deficiency and that persons with cleft palate alone are much more likely to present associated congenital deformities than are patients with cleft lip and palate (Ross and Johnston, 1972; McWilliams and Matthews, 1979).

On the other hand, patients with unilateral or bilateral complete clefts are subject to maxillary collapse, protrusion of the premaxilla, or both. These conditions present their own hazards to articulation. Studies cited by Moll (1968) and additional information collected by Morley (1970), McWilliams and Musgrave (1977), and Fletcher (1978) suggest that patients with clefts of the soft palate alone are likely to have less severe articulation problems than are other patients.

Morley (1970, pp. 126 to 127) reported that 42% of the children with bilateral complete clefts,

23% of those with unilateral complete clefts, and 18% of those with postalveolar clefts required speech therapy. Using Veau's classification system, Fletcher (1978) reported the following percentages of correct articulation responses: soft palate only—91%; soft and hard palate—72%; unilateral lip and palate—64%; and bilateral lip and palate—49%. As cleft severity increases from the soft palate only, to soft and hard palates, to unilateral complete clefts, to bilateral complete clefts, the severity of speech problems also increases.

We cannot predict with any accuracy the future speech of patients with cleft palate at the time of their birth. Many variables in addition to the severity of the cleft will influence future speech. If all other variables could be controlled, we would expect the severity of speech disorder to correlate positively with the severity of cleft. Function of the velopharyngeal mechanism after surgery is logically more important to speech than type of cleft and extent of malformation at birth. Even then, inspection of a patient's speech mechanism is no substitute for study of his or her speech.

Our clinical experience indicates that cleft lip alone is almost never responsible for articulation problems. When the cleft lip is associated with bilateral alveolar clefts, or with a very short, tight upper lip, the individual may be unable to close the lips over the anterior teeth for bilabial consonants. However, this problem is rare and appears to resolve spontaneously with lip growth and as dental and surgical treatment improve the position of the premaxilla. Children with deficient tissue in the middle of the upper lip may substitute labiodental sounds for bilabials. These labiodental productions may be indistinguishable to the ear from their bilabial counterparts, but they are readily apparent to the eye. Young children with lip deficiencies may omit bilabial consonants.

McWilliams (personal communication, 1983) reports one unusual case where a fistula communicated between the oral cavity and the upper lip via a narrow channel sealed only by mucosa. As /s/ was produced through the channel created by the fistula, air passed into the upper lip, and the mucosa bubbled forth like a small balloon. Again, this was visually as well as acoustically distracting.

Developmental Trends

Cross-sectional studies show improvement in articulation with increase in age. This trend is shown in Table 15.3. Van Demark (1969) reported the percentage of correctly articulated sounds in four categories based on manner of articulation. The results show that cleft speakers, evaluated in three age groups, improve with increase in age, especially for plosives and fricatives. They also show that the lowest percentage of correct responses was for fricatives. The relative positions among the manner categories remains constant in regard to number of articulation errors. Van Demark et al. (1979) reported longitudinal data which indicated that their subjects with cleft palate improved their articulation beyond age 10 years. The rate of improvement slowed after age 10, and about 80% of the items tested were produced correctly by age 16. At that age their subjects produced 98% of the plosives correctly, but that level of proficiency was not achieved for fricatives and affricates. Various services including speech training were available to the subjects in these studies although the effects of intervention were not explored.

Riski and DeLong (1984) analyzed longitudinal recordings of children's responses to the Templin-Darley articulation screening test. Children from the Lancaster Cleft Palate Clinic with different sorts of clefts were compared; those with and without pharyngeal flaps were studied separately. Children with cleft lip only were homogeneous in articulation and normal in articulation development. The children with clefts were heterogeneous. Some children developed articulation on normal schedule; those with more severe clefts articulated less well. Those with pharyngeal flaps were slower in articulation development than were those who did not require flaps. The authors noted that their subjects' performance was strikingly similar to that of Iowa subjects (Van Demark et al., 1979) at 3 and 4 years of age but that the Lancaster children articulated better than the Iowa children from ages 5 through 8. The Lancaster children had received palatal repair at earlier ages than the Iowa children. No gender difference was found.

Bzoch (1956) observed that nasal distortions persist with age whereas other distortions tend to decrease in frequency of occurrence. Philips and Harrison (1969) noted that indistinct productions, substitutions, and omissions occurred in roughly equal percentages among the articulation errors found in their study of children from 36 to 71 months of age. However, the percentage of omissions declined with age: 33% of the sounds of children 36 to 47 months of age were omitted, compared with 20 and 10% for children 48 to 59 and 60 to 71 months of age. Percentages of items replaced by other sounds or by distortions remained very similar throughout the age range studied. Milisen (1954) reported that apparently normal children with functional misarticulation also tend to shift from omissions and substitutions to distortions with increase in age.

In 1956, Counihan reported that his subjects over 16 years of age actually articulated less well than younger children with clefts. Perhaps that difference reflected improvement in care which benefited the younger subjects. Van Demark et al. (1979) compared data from 16-year-old patients with data McWilliams reported in 1958 for adults with a mean age of 24.6 years. The articulation tests used in the two studies were different, but the sounds were similarly rank ordered for number of correct responses. The subjects in the Van Demark study correctly produced several sounds at substantially higher percentages than did McWilliams' subjects. Van Demark et al. attributed the differences in percentage of correct responses to improvements in treatment. Similarly, Renfrew (1960) found substantially better speech in school-aged children with clefts observed from 1953 to 1960 than in children seen between 1946 to 1953.

Karnell and Van Demark (1986) reexamined the patients described by Van Demark et al. in 1979 and reported longitudinal articulation data. Subjects' performance on the Iowa Pressure Articulation Test (IPAT) was reported in terms of percentage of responses that were correct, oral distortions, nasal distortions, glottal stops, pharyngeal fricatives, omissions, and substitutions. Articulation defectiveness during conversational speech was rated on the basis of a seven-point, equal-appearing intervals scale. Ratings of articulation defectiveness improved throughout the study but with rate of improvement decreasing markedly after about 10 years of age. The data showed that on average the subjects did not achieve "...what speech pathologists may consider perfectly normal speech at age 16 years. However, such deficits probably are not so severe by this age as to require intervention" (p. 287). Errors in each of the articulation test categories studied occurred infrequently during observations made in the older years. Glottal stops and pharyngeal fricatives occurred infrequently at any time in the study. Nasal distortions also occurred infrequent-

ly, but their occurrence did increase slightly after age 10 in a subgroup, the members of which scored below 20% on the IPAT at age 4 years and did not have secondary surgery of the velopharyngeal mechanism before age 8. Members of this subgroup tended to become slightly worse at about 12 years of age.

We conclude from the findings cited above that cleft palate speakers improve with age and that there has been considerable improvement in treatment methods during the past 35 years. From the findings reviewed, it is difficult to tell the severity of articulatory problems remaining in older children with cleft palate. Recent research has been directed to the speech of children with clefts during the first 2 years of their lives. That work is reviewed next.

Development of a child's sound pattern is thought to involve interaction over time among a number of variables including those in both physiological and linguistic categories (Hubbell, 1981, p. 112). This hypothesis of interaction has been applied in support of very early operative treatment of cleft palate. Philips and Kent (1984) and Moller et al. (1987) suggested that the speech distortions associated with velopharyngeal incompetence including the unrepaired cleft have negative influence on the patient's developing sound system. Philips and Kent (1984) noted that prephonemic development of the sound system may be studied by phonetic methods, and they reported acoustical information about the cry of an infant with cleft palate and information about babbling in association with velopharyngeal incompetence.

Dorf and Curtin (1982) demonstrated through use of narrow phonetic transcription that children whose palatal clefts were repaired prior to 12 months of age were less likely to show compensatory articulations than were children operated later. Unfortunately, they reported their data in such a way that it is not possible to tell how great the magnitude of difference in use of compensatory articulation was between the two groups. Further study of individual subjects indicated that whether use of compensatory articulations developed depended on the extent of development prior to operation. For example, among children operated after 12 months of age, those with slower development of the sound system were less likely to develop compensatory articulation. Cohn and McWilliams (1983) reported a lower occurrence of gross errors for children operated at an average age of 18 months than Dorf and Curtin reported for children repaired below 12 months.

Ainoda et al. (1985) described articulation status and change in 87 Japanese children who had been operated for cleft palate or cleft lip and palate. Age at operation averaged 15.2 months with a range from 1 to 22 months; speech was reevaluated at about 4 years of age and for most of the children again between 4 and 9 years (average 6 years). The children received no speech therapy, but parents were encouraged to provide speech stimulation at home. Articulation proficiency was evaluated from observation of conversation, sentences, words, and consonant-vowel syllables. The subjects were divided into two groups. In one group the children's speech was developing normally, whereas in the other group speech development was abnormal. Ninety-eight percent of subjects in the first group and 90% of those in the second group were considered competent in velopharyngeal closure. Data reported show that glottal stops appeared between 6 and 18 months and palatalized articulation at about 2 years. Articulation tended to improve over time with greatest reduction in nasal articulation and then glottal stops. Palatalized articulation was least likely to disappear.

O'Gara and Logemann (1988) phonetically transcribed the vocalizations of babies with cleft palate at selected ages from 3 to 36 months. Diacritic symbols were used to signify posterior nasal fricatives, pedicle flap fricatives, and "freely expressed nasal air emission with no intraoral consonant constriction but nasal path of air emission..." Two subgroups were observed— greater tissue-operation at or before 12 months and lesser tissue-operation after 12 months. The transcriptions were analyzed to determine the percentage of occurrence of several phonetic responses such as place of consonant articulation, manner of consonant constriction, and how stops and fricatives were produced.

The greater tissue-early operation subgroup was superior to the lesser tissue-later operation group in development of the sound system, but both groups were slower than members of a group of normal subjects described by other authors. Various trends were described. The use of glottal place of articulation declined over time; use of other articulatory places tended to increase. Overall, the use of oral stops and fricatives increased during the study period. Labial articulatory

places were used more frequently than lingual places. "Both groups evidence a spurt in use of nasal fricatives at 30 to 31 months of age, possibly related to the increased language requirements for fricative differentiation" (p. 133). Narrow phonetic transcription provided information that contributes to the understanding of speech associated with cleft palate.

Grunwell and Russell (1988) indicated that studies of prespeech vocalization in children with clefts (Olson, 1965; Dorf and Curtin, 1982; O'Gara and Logemann, 1988, and Mousset and Trichet, 1985) showed continuity in speech characteristics from pre- to postoperative observations, a tendency for these children to use posterior articulatory placement, and a tendency for children repaired early to present better speech than children operated late. The children operated early were less likely to use compensatory articulation.

Grunwell and Russell (1987) studied prespeech vocalizations of three children with clefts. The authors were interested in differentiating between phonetic deviance and the function of the phonological system. The data are relevant to understanding of the development of the sound system and also to understanding the immediate impact of surgical repair of the palate on vocalization. The children were first recorded 2 to 6 days before operative repair of the palate which was done at from 11 months to 14 months of age. Four postoperative recordings were also made and analyzed. Recordings were made of 5 minutes of vocalization during play and 5 minutes of vocalization during interaction with a parent. The authors devised an instrumental means of identifying vocalizations and measuring their durations. They also performed phonetic analyses that provided place and manner information relative to speech-like vocalizations, and they reported percentage of occurrence of monosyllables, disyllables, and polysyllables, and the syllable shapes that were used most frequently and next most frequently during each recording.

The data showed a tendency for performance to decrease on each measure for the recording following operation and then for improvement to occur thereafter. Thus, the analysis procedure was sensitive to a transient change for the worse in vocalization following surgery. Performance during the final recordings tended to be better than that sampled during the initial recording. These findings are tentative in that only one preoperative recording was made and, for two measures, performance was poorer in sample five than in sample four. Also, the first postoperative recording was postponed for subject two. The data showed the early occurrence of glottal stops, frequent use of glides and velar approximates, and almost exclusive use of open syllables. The authors noted that the children used the "whole range of articulatory placements...(bilabial through glottal)...[and that] the whole range of articulatory stricture types" was also used. Use of frontal bilabial and apical/laminal contoids (consonant-like) was infrequent compared with the performance of normal children. It appears that the articulatory placements of children with clefts are more posterior than those of normal children by 1 year of age.

In a second paper concerning two of the three subjects in the study just cited, Grunwell and Russell (1988) attempted to determine if the children's phonetic patterns can be attributed to physical defects and related variables. They hypothesized that variables identified in postoperative recordings but also present in preoperative recordings of prespeech vocalization are logically physiological-phonetic rather than linguistic-phonological in origin. This could indicate that physiological variables influence phonological patterning and phonemic expression. The study was also intended to have a predictive component whereby problems could be identified in prespeech vocalization and therapy instituted early. Grunwell's (1985) phonological assessment procedures were used to study the children's phonetic inventories, contrastive use of speech sounds, phonotactic (syllable shape) patterns, use of phonological processes, and other variables. The data were interpreted to indicate that phonetic variables restrict phonological development. Differences between the two children supported earlier assertions that the children with clefts are heterogeneous in speech.

Estrem and Broen (1989) used phonetic transcription of speech samples to compare the word-initial sounds used by six normal children and six children with clefts. The children were studied as they progressed from the use of 6 to 10 words through the use of 50 words. Although the six children with clefts were variable in both velopharyngeal competence and patterns of sound usage, certain trends were observed. The children with clefts frequently targeted and used sonorants (nasals, vowels, and approximates /w, j, r, l, h./) and used obstruents (stops, fricatives, and affricates) infrequently. The normal children made more frequent use of obstruents. The children with clefts tended to favor [- coronal] consonants whereas the normal children made more use of [+ coronal] consonants; [- coronal] sounds are said to be made at the periphery of the vocal tract and include velars, glottals, and labials. Late in the comparison period, differences between the two groups were small and may have been a matter of chance. The authors concluded, "Deviant production patterns, characteristic of the speech of children with cleft palate appeared very early in the speech of some children." They inferred that the children with clefts used various strategies in choosing words that began with different speech sounds.

There appears to be growing acceptance of the assumption that what a child learns about speech prior to palate repair may negatively influence phonological development even after successful primary surgery. An alternative hypothesis is that children catch up in development of the sound system after operation at about 18 months of age. Speech development is thought to involve a shift from organization based on word-sized units to organization based on rule-governed sound-sized segments. Perhaps velopharyngeal incompetence present after that shift has an especially persistent influence on later development of the sound system. The shift is thought to occur when the child is between 12 and 18 months of age (Schwartz, 1984).

COMPENSATORY ARTICULATION PATTERNS AND STRATEGIES

Pharyngeal and palatal fricatives and some glottal stops are classed as articulatory substitutions compensatory for poor velopharyngeal structure or function (Morris, 1968). Bzoch (1979) applied the term *gross substitutions* to these articulatory behaviors. Moll (1968) noted that pharyngeal or palatal place of misarticulation is often inferred from what is heard and not directly observed by the clinician. Erroneous inferences may be drawn about just how the speaker is producing some sounds. Folkins (1985) wrote that *compensation* has different meanings and should be defined when used. He stated that in reference to cleft palate speech, *compensation* refers not to movements but to phonetic units perceived by a listener. "*Compensatory articulation* refers to substitutions by a speaker with cleft palate that are perceptually unacceptable..." (p. 113). In reference to velopharyngeal disability during speech production, Philips and Kent (1984, p. 162) defined *compensatory articulation* in reference to "...behaviors which are thought to be learned and habituated [automatized] for productions of speech sounds when, due to VPI, normal productions cannot be achieved." They differentiated between compensatory articulation and sound alterations forced by failure of velopharyngeal closure. For example, in the presence of velopharyngeal openings, /p/ will be nasalized or produced in a continuant fashion with a nasal murmer and partial voicing. These alterations are not compensatory but are obligatory because of the velopharyngeal opening. Philips and Kent (p. 128) noted that an individual might use nonphonetic markers to compensate for a missing articulatory skill associated with velopharyngeal disability. Prosodic variables may serve that purpose. Warren (1986) postulated that compensatory speech behaviors used by patients with clefts are manifestations of a physiological regulation-control mechanism that serves to maintain a normal aerodynamic environment even though the velopharyngeal mechanism is disabled.

This section reviews descriptions of compensatory articulations and also the authors' various inferences about strategies speakers adopt in order to cope with velopharyngeal incompetence.

The early appearance of glottal stops in the speech of children with cleft palate was cited above. Cohn and McWilliams (1983) gathered articulation data on 204 children with clefts. None of the 105 children with unilateral clefts had pharyngeal misarticulations, and only one (less than 1%) had glottal stops. Seven of 109 subjects (6%) with isolated palatal clefts had pharyngeal errors, and only five (4.5%) had glottal errors. There was only one nasal snort in the entire group of 204. These children had had surgical closure of their palates by 18 months of age, and none had ratings indicative of severe hypernasality.

Morley (1970) distinguished between pharyngeal and glottal fricatives. The former involved use of frication between the tongue dorsum and the pharyngeal wall, whereas the latter is "made with increased frication between overtense vocal cords." The glottal fricative "may be produced with slight tongue protrusion." In English, pharyngeal fricatives are rare other than in the speech of persons with cleft palate or related conditions.

Trost (1981) described three types of compensatory articulation which she recommended be added to the list of articulation patterns characteristic of individuals with cleft palate or other velopharyngeal valving faults. Her observations were based on auditory perception and the use of cephalometric radiographic studies. The first compensatory production she described was the substitution of a pharyngeal stop for /k/ and /g/. She noted that the location in the vocal tract of this stop, which is produced with tongue and pharyngeal wall, is influenced by the phonetic context in which it occurs. The second compensatory production described was mid-dorsum palatal stop, which is similar in vocal tract location to /j/. When used, it is substituted for /t/, /d/, /k/, or /g/. The distinction between the voiced and voiceless members of cognate pairs replaced by the mid-dorsum palatal stop is lost, thus making phonemic distinctiveness dependent upon nonsegmental cues. The third type of articulation described by Trost was a lingualveolar nasal fricative produced with an open or incompletely closed velopharyngeal port, accompanied by nasal emission, and distinctive because of audible frication. This is similar to the nasal snort discussed earlier, and it could be obligatory rather than compensatory. Trost and also Henningsson and Isberg (1986) noted that some speakers with clefts use two places of articulation simultaneously. For example, some individuals make tongue tip gestures for /t/ while producing glottal stops. Only glottal stops and pharyngeal fricatives were found by Trost to co-occur with normal articulatory placement. Phonetic symbols used in the transcription of sounds made in the back of the vocal tract are presented in Figure 15.2 (Pullum and Ladusaw, 1986). Distinctions among these sounds would be difficult to make without radiographic analysis.

Remarkable articulatory movements have been reported by several other authors. Kawano et al. (1985) described a 20-year-old Japanese cleft lip and palate patient who replaced /s/ and /ʃ/ with an unusual laryngeal fricative. Nasopharyngoscopic and videofluoroscopic recordings showed that the laryngeal fricative was produced with a constriction formed by the depressed epiglottis and the elevated arytenoid cartilages. The velopharyngeal port was open during production of these sounds but nearly closed during

Symbol	Definition
ħ	Voiceless pharyngeal central fricative.
ʕ	Voiced pharyngeal fricative.
ɦ	Voiced or murmured glottal fricative or approximate.
ɧ	Voiceless fricative articulated with simultaneous velar and palato-alveolar friction.
ɰ	Voiced velar median (central) approximate.
ç	Voiceless palatal central fricative. Articulated posterior to [ʃ] (palato-alveolar) and [ɕ] (alveolo-palatal) but not as far back as [×] (velar).
ɕ	Voiceless alveolo-palatal central laminal fricative. Articulated between [ç] (true palatal) and [ʃ] (palato-alveolar).

Figure 15.2 Phonetic symbols that may be useful for the transcription of unusual articulations employed by some individuals with cleft palate. (Source: Pullum GK, Ladusaw WA. Phonetic symbol guide. Chicago: University of Chicago Press, 1986.)

stops. This patient had not undergone palato-plasty until he was 8 years of age. The authors observed a similar phenomenon in four additional patients.

Fletcher (1985) described a patient with an unrepaired cleft of the soft palate and of approximately 28 mm of the hard palate. The cleft was 18 mm wide at the posterior border of the hard palate. This man's total phoneme intelligibility was 79%, and 91% of his /s/ sounds were intelligible. Electropalatography indicated that this speaker narrowed the constriction for sibilant fricatives. For example, "…/s/ in *seed* was spoken with a groove only 2 to 3 mm wide." Normal talkers used a groove 6 to 10 mm wide.

Shelton and McCauley (1986) described a woman who had an unrepaired cleft of the secondary palate and who wore a hinge-type speech prosthesis. The pharyngeal section of the prosthesis was raised by use of the tongue and the two segments of the cleft velum. The velar segments or halves maintained the elevation. The authors noted that the appliance may have been constructed to take advantage of existing movements, but they also indicated that learning probably influenced her performance. For example, bumping the section upward with her tongue and "catching" it with the velar halves would appear to involve an element of learning.

From frontal and lateral cineradiographic studies, Henningsson and Isberg (1986) determined that velopharyngeal closure is impaired—particularly movement of the lateral pharyngeal walls is reduced—during glottal stops and co-occurrence of glottal stops and other articulatory gestures. They concluded that velopharyngeal openings during these sounds may give a false impression of inability to close the velopharyngeal port. If closure is present during other speech sounds, velopharyngeal function during glottal stops should be observed for change during the course of articulation therapy directed to the correction of the glottal stops.

In a companion paper, Isberg and Henningsson (1987) reported that the width and size (area mm_2) of uncovered fistulas of the hard palate correlated significantly (r = 0.78 and 0.55; p <0.05) with movements of the lateral pharyngeal walls. They found that lateral wall movement increased when the fistula was covered and when place of articulation was anterior to the fistula.

Several of the papers just cited indicate that the velopharyngeal mechanism may be left open during compensatory articulation. An individual velopharyngeal closure pattern may reflect insufficient structure, failure to use available structure in a normal pattern, or a combination. This relates to the topic of velopharyngeal surrender which is discussed later in the chapter. Next we review descriptions of strategies adopted by speakers in response to velopharyngeal disability.

Morley (1970) described two speech patterns found in patients with cleft palates who had had palatal surgery after speech development. One pattern involved good place of articulation and intelligible speech in association with nasal emission and consonant weakness resulting from lack of intraoral breath pressure. The second pattern involved not only nasal escape, but also nasal snort, glottal stops, pharyngeal fricatives, nasal grimace, and other articulatory substitutions.

Hewlett (1985, p. 164) hypothesized that individuals with developmental speech sound disorders associated with anatomical deformities are characterized by phonological avoidance strategies, whereas persons with acquired deformities apply compensatory strategies. For example, he observed a 15-year-old boy with an acquired velopharyngeal incompetence. This boy compensated for nasal air leakage by increasing overall air flow. Presumably a younger child with a congenital defect is more likely to avoid nasal escape by deleting obstruents or replacing them with other sounds. The speech clinician attempts to identify the sound pattern of each patient.

Hutters and Brondsted (1987) reported the results of narrow phonetic transcription of the speech of five Danish children ranging in age from 4.2 to 5.2. The children presented palatal clefting ranging from cleft of the palate only to bilateral complete cleft. Speech samples obtained as each child played with a parent were videorecorded. The speech patterns identified were classified according to three "strategies" to be summarized below. The speech of the first child was characterized by use of glottal stops for stops and fricatives, and both progressive and regressive assimilation were noted. Child two also used glottal stops—mostly for stop consonants. The glottal stops were produced in combination with the correct supraglottal articulatory gesture. Stop articulation was described as variable. This subject used several variants of /s/ including a nasal fricative and /s/ accompanied by audible nasal emission, [s̃]. Child three often produced stops correctly, but he also replaced stops with voiced nasal consonants and with voiceless nasal fricatives. Fricatives were variably produced but often involved nasal frication. Voiced oral consonants tended to be nasalized, and progressive and regressive assimilation

were present. Velars were sometimes fronted and accompanied by assimilation of nasality. Child four tended to replace stops and fricatives with nasal consonants or [h]. Glottal stops were also observed. This child's speech was said to be "frequently interrupted by superficial snatching of breath." Child five misarticulated relatively few sounds. However, he replaced the velars (/k/ and /g/) with /h/ and partially devoiced [g̊], and he fronted [g̠]. The speech of these children was characterized by reduced accuracy and reduced number of phonemes.

The speech patterns of the children were classified in terms of three strategies for responding to velopharyngeal dysfunction—present or past. The first is a passive or do-nothing strategy. The velopharyngeal dysfunction is permitted its influence, that is, nasalization and nasal frication are allowed to occur. However, the pattern varies with phonetic category. Sonorants are nasalized, voiced stops are "realized as voiced nasal consonants" (p. 127), voiced fricatives are nasalized and produced with reduced air pressure, and unvoiced obstruents are produced with nasal frication. Aspirated stops may be heard as unvoiced nasal consonants with a degree of nasal frication. The authors stated that in Danish /b/, /d/, and /g/ are unvoiced and unaspirated. Two active strategies involve compensation or camouflage. Compensation involves substitution of sounds produced with constrictions posterior to the velopharyngeal valve, and camouflage involves weak articulation including breathy phonation.

Recent studies cited above illustrate the wealth of information that can be derived from narrow phonetic transcription of running speech. Confidence in such analysis is increased as it agrees with information derived from instrumental analysis. Hutters and Brondsted (1987) assert that comparison of patterns of cleft palate speech across speakers of different languages will provide information about which phonetic and phonological difficulties are unavoidable and which are language-dependent.

Explanation of compensatory or gross articulation errors and other articulatory and phonological patterns is a continuing and speculative enterprise. Of two children with similar velopharyngeal and dental mechanisms, one may produce gross substitutions and the other not. Velopharyngeal insufficiency is related to these substitutions, and phonological variables, motor control variables, perception, and learning are probably factors. Phonology and learning will be considered in the next sections.

Phonological Patterns

As stated earlier, there is currently much interest in understanding delayed and disordered sound patterns in phonological terms. For example, misarticulation is often inconsistent in that a sound from a given phoneme may be articulated correctly sometimes and misarticulated sometimes, but careful study of the patient's speech is likely to show an orderly pattern. Ingram (1976) stated that the speech of cleft palate patients is patterned and may be described in phonological terms. He concluded from the Philips and Harris (1969) data that processes characteristic of deviant speech tend to persist in cleft palate speakers.

Little use has been made of distinctive features and phonological processes in the study of patients with cleft palate speech. Singh et al. (1981) used seven distinctive features to analyze articulation data from 1077 children receiving speech services in schools. The data analyzed were articulation profiles obtained by speech-language pathologists using different articulation tests. Only substitutions and omissions were evaluated. The subject group included 18 children with cleft palate. Consideration of the percentage correct by feature showed that the group with cleft palates presented a profile different from that of other misarticulating subgroups. The children with clefts performed best on the labiality feature and poorest on the front-back feature.

Hodson et al. (1983) described the sound pattern on a 5-year-old boy with a repaired cleft of the soft and hard palate and highly unintelligible speech. Phonological analysis showed that the boy omitted singleton obstruents from both pre- and postvocalic positions, omitted and fronted velar consonants, reduced and deleted consonant clusters, deleted stridency by omitting strident consonants or replacing them with spots, and misarticulated liquids by omission, gliding, stopping, nasalizing, and vowelizing. Glottal substitutions were also used. Perhaps consideration of patterns such as these helps the clinician to understand the speech of patients with clefts.

Lynch et al. (1983) used confusion matrices to study the substitution patterns of two misarticulating children with repaired bilateral clefts of the lip and palate. The children were videorecorded interacting with their parents, and the children's speech was transcribed phonetically. Recordings were made when they were between 29 and 37 months of age and again when they were between 5 and 7 years of age. The articulation of word-initial consonants was analyzed in terms of place and manner of articulation, and phonological processes that characterized the speech of each child were identified informally. The authors concluded that the analyses helped them to differentiate between developmental articulation errors and those reflecting velopharyngeal insufficiency.

Powers et al. (1984) submitted 1-hour running speech samples of four children with repaired clefts to several speech analyses: phonetic inventory, phonological process, and idiosyncratic pattern. The children were between 3 years, 2 months and 3 years, 11 months of age. A key finding was that the children were similar in phonetic inventory but differed in use of phonological processes. For example, use of fricatives and affricates was restricted in all four children, but while one child used stopping only 8% of the times where it might have occurred another child used it 48%. This suggests that the children were similar in ability to produce sounds but differed in their linguistic use of their phonetic skills. The child thought to have the best language used the fewest processes. Backing, which is said to be an unusual process, was used by three of the four subjects and influenced most alveolar and palatal obstruents. Substitution of posterior for anterior place of articulation has been explained as a compensation for velopharyngeal and fistula leaks. However, three of the subjects in this study were free from audible nasal emission, and all four were thought to be free of "significant problems in velopharyngeal closure." The authors were conservative in interpreting the origin of the children's process usage but noted that an organizational-linguistic phenomenon may have influenced the children's speech. No attempt was made to measure phonological knowledge underlying the processes.

Foster et al. (1985), in a letter concerning problems in the clinical application of phonological theory, suggested that the studies by Singh et al. (1981), Hodson et al. (1983) and Lynch et al. (1983) were not compatible with the phonological theory on which their vocabulary and procedure were based because the authors offered no reason to think that the speech disorders of their patients with clefts were psychological or linguistic in nature. The study by Lynch et al. was more phonetic than linguistic, but the title carries the word *phonological*. That usage is in keeping with the move from *articulation disorder* to *phonological disorder*. Altogether, some of the studies cited here and the letter by Foster et al. suggest that clinical phonology and phonology are quite different fields of study.

Phonological theory and analysis have contributed little to the understanding or treatment of cleft palate speech to date. Nonetheless, cognitive-linguistic variables probably interact with orofacial variables including velopharyngeal function to influence the sound pattern of individual patients. Use of various phonological pattern analyses procedures may help the clinician to recognize and understand patterns that involve multiple phonemes in the speech of patients with clefts. Information gained from such analyses may supplement phonetic information, data about the speech mechanism, and other information from the speech evaluation to help the clinician classify patients and plan treatment that will correct disordered sound patterns in an efficient fashion.

Discussion

We have reviewed information about articulation disorders associated with cleft palate. Individuals with cleft palate are at risk for articulation disorders that persists beyond the period of articulatory-phonological development, and many of them show articulatory faults associated with velopharyngeal incompetence or other conditions that result from cleft palate. Nonetheless, not all children with cleft palate demonstrate all of these error types; indeed, many of them show normal articulation. A major inference to be drawn is that the population of persons with cleft palate is highly heterogeneous in articulation; the speech pathologist may expect patients with cleft palate to vary widely in their articulation proficiency. Those who misarticulate will differ in the error patterns they present.

ETIOLOGICAL INFLUENCES CONTRIBUTING TO MISARTICULATION

From the review above, it is evident that attempts to explain the origins of misarticulation by patients with cleft lip and palate must account for a variety of findings including delay in the development of articulation skills, nasalization of speech sounds that normally are oral, oral distortions usually of sibilants, gross substitutions such as glottal stops and pharyngeal fricatives, and misarticulation of liquids. Palatal clefts influence articulation and the sound system as soon as they start to develop, but children respond to clefts and related conditions in different ways.

It is known that velopharyngeal incompetence and other oropharyngeal pathology contribute to disordered articulation in patients with clefts. We think that unless velopharyngeal closure is achievable during running speech, some impairment of speech, including articulation, will occur (Morris, 1968). These views are based on theory, data, and clinical observation. Morris (1968) wrote that opinions about etiology are likely to be inferences based on known relationships and logical interpretation. Some causal inferences, for example, are based on knowledge of the physiology and acoustics of normal speech production. If normal speech is known to require a mechanism that can impound air pressure in the mouth, then what is likely to happen if that mechanism fails to hold air because of velopharyngeal defect or malfunction? Sound energy and air are likely to escape through the nose with resultant hypernasality, audible nasal emission, and reduction of the oral breath pressure needed for fricatives, affricates, and stops.

We are especially likely to accept a causal hypothesis if one phenomenon always follows another and does not occur in the absence of the other. Nasal emission of air during speech is always observable in patients with congenitally abnormal velopharyngeal mechanisms unless the pathology has been corrected or the nasal passages are closed. Other sorts of evidence provide support to a causal hypothesis regarding the influence of velopharyngeal incompetence on articulation. In experiments of nature such as the loss of velopharyngeal tissue to disease or accident, the acquired pathology damages speech in a predictable manner. Also, mechanical and acoustical models have served as analogs to the speech mechanisms in tests of hypotheses about the function of the velopharyngeal port. When surgical repair of a cleft palate or prosthodontic treatment alters articulation, that change suggests that the velopharyngeal mechanism has influenced articulation. Thus, treatments serve to test causal hypotheses.

We concluded earlier in this chapter and in Chapter 12 that defects in the peripheral mechanism interacting with a motor control system and with a cognitive-linguistic system influence the development and use of the sound system by children born with palatal clefts.

The multivariate work of Van Demark (1964, 1966) indicates that learning influences the speech of patients with cleft palate. Behavioral and cognitive learning concepts used in the explanation of the origins of misarticulation are considered next. Maturation and learning may seldom be solely responsible for articulation problems in patients with clefts, but neither is their influence ever absent. That speech mechanism variables cannot by themselves account for the misarticulation associated with cleft palate may be inferred from knowledge that articulations such as gross substitutions are not present in all persons with incompetence and that they are observed in some persons who at least some of the time achieve velopharyngeal closure during speech. Some patients persist in misarticulation after successful surgical and dental treatments of the velopharyngeal mechanism, whereas others do not.

Additional articulatory phenomena appear to reflect learning. For example cine- and videofluorographic films and tapes have shown speakers using part of the tongue for articulation while, at the same time, using another tongue part to support the velum or a loose obturator. The laryngeal fricative reported by Kawano et al. (1985) was described earlier. Same patients show palatal surrender (Hagerty et al., 1968) or what Morris (1968) termed *the discouraged* /s/ where the patient moves away from closure during /s/ sounds. Other patients show better velopharyngeal function during /s/ than on any other sound (Shelton et al., 1964). Some persons with clefts maintain closure in nasal contexts (Karnell et al., 1985: Shelton and McCauley, 1986), perhaps because the speaker is unable to open and close the velopharyngeal valve at a normal rate. Denasalization of a nasal consonant may be more acceptable than nasalization of nearby sounds. Nasal emission during a phoneme or two in the absence of evident velopharyngeal pathology invites a learning explanation. Even should a physiological component be identified in patients with this phoneme-specific nasal emission, the patient's response to the pathology would be an important contributor to the speech disorder. Nonetheless, it is difficult to establish just how these behaviors were acquired. Next we differentiate between maturation and learning as components of development.

Maturation and Learning

Articulation, like many other capabilities that people acquire, involves development. In this discussion, we use the word *development* to encompass both maturation and learning. The difference between the two has long been controversial in psychology. Maturation is associated with growth of the central nervous system in a satisfactory environment (Kagan et al., 1978). Learning, on the other hand, is dependent on experience. Galambos and Morgan (1960) wrote that maturation tends to have greater influence on early behavior and learning on later behavior but that the two overlap and interact. Neural connections established through maturation are thought to be more difficult to alter than those established through learning. Some now conceptualize development as a lifelong process.

Bosma (1985) described the ontogeny of postnatal performance of pharynx, larynx, and mouth including mechanisms of neurological maturation. Increase in discrimination and precision of motion accompanies brain development. Inhibition of response is achieved. Bosma stated that "...the developmental changes in the pharynx, larynx, and mouth reflect maturation in the representations of their performances in the developing brain and also their own growth and structural changes" (p. S15). Smith (1981, p. 151) suggested that biological maturation rather than linguistic learning influences much phonological development. Rather than learning the phonology of their language, children may experience expansion of the sound system through biological maturation. Speech production capability is increased through neurological, anatomical, and physiological development that continues into the second decade of life. Smith suggested that different investigators look at different parts of sound system development and that no real explanation of that development exists. Kent (1984) discussed speech development in terms of the coemergence of language and a movement system. He stressed the importance of "musculoskeletal and neural maturation" rather than conventional linguistic contrasts. However, he also cited active discovery or problem solving on the part of the developing child as he or she interacts with the physical and biosocial environments (p. R893). Like Kent, Elbert (1984) referred to interaction between the phonetic (physiological) and the cognitive aspects of speech. As she stated, it is unlikely that the child remains passive while physical changes take place and the phonological system emerges phoneme by phoneme.

Behavioral learning constructs such as antecedent and reinforcing stimuli, contiguity among stimuli and responses, and generalization (Mowrer, 1982; Elbert and Gierut, 1986) are powerful variables in some forms of treatment but do not seem to provide precise, prospective explanations for the misarticulation patterns described earlier. A person may appear to adopt or discover a response to a velopharyngeal valving disability that he or she finds rewarding, but that hardly constitutes an explanation. Cognitive concepts are also important to the understanding of phonological and articulatory development and disorder. No currently available explanation of sound system development or failure thereof is satisfactory. Newmeyer (1986, pp. 74-75) wrote that generativists use the concept of inborn or innate knowledge because the child learning language is not provided with stimuli that would permit the acquisition of the abstract knowledge. that underlies language usage. Rather than seeking to explain the origins of cleft palate speech in any final fashion, we would attempt to understand evaluation and treatment relative to their contribution to treatment effectiveness.

We presume that maturational and innate mechanisms are related. Miller (1965) stated that the child is predisposed to pay attention to language, to remember it, and to use it, and that the child learns language by using it and testing hypotheses about it. Langacker (1967) stated that linguistic experience doesn't shape language but rather activates inborn linguistic competence. To the extent that language is too abstract and develops too rapidly for explanation in stimulus-response-reinforcement learning terms, its acquisition involves an innate predisposition.

This is not to say that experience is unimportant to language acquisition. Bzoch (1979) wrote that children's predisposed progression through the stages of speech and language development is dependent upon experience with other people. Fey (1988) and Connell (1988) suggested that because of the abstractness of language, the clinician charged with helping a language-impaired child is hard pressed to know what to do. (The articulation side of language is more manageable.) Connell cited the so-far unsuccessful search for "triggers" that set "parameters that control language characteristics." Fey would not set out to teach the child language rules but rather would structure an environment that gives the child the opportunity to extend language skills through problem-solving experience.

Investigators attempting to explain the articulation problems of some cleft palate speakers seem, at least implicitly, to draw on such behavioral concepts as reinforcement. However, psychologists concerned with language have turned to cognitive concepts of learning. These appear to be more compatible with the nature of language and the speed of language development.

Behavioral and Cognitive Learning

Both behavioral and cognitive learning concepts may contribute to understanding of disturbed articulation patterns. Important variables in behavioral explanations of learning include reinforcement and generalization. A reinforcing stimulus is one that increases the frequency of occurrence of the responses that it follows; it is likely to occur close in time to the response. This definition has been criticized as being untestable, but reinforcing stimuli remain powerful tools in all forms of therapy for communicative disorders and in the etiology and maintenance of defective speech patterns.

Reinforcement has been used to explain some of the articulation errors produced by children with cleft palates. Parents, pleased with the appearance of compensatory articulation behavior in their children's speech, may knowingly or unknowingly reinforce it. Bzoch (1979) suggested that articulation learning might be negatively influenced by lack of reinforcement of early speech efforts, failure of parents to understand and respond to early speech efforts, deliberate discouragement of speech pending completion of surgery, acceptance of poor speech at least until physical treatment is completed, and anticipation of the child's needs which obviates the need for speech. Each of these variables functions in a reinforcement mode. Morris (1968) noted that communication failure may cause the child with cleft palate to speak less and hence to show less rapid or complete speech development.

Morris (1972) also hypothesized that some persons with velopharyngeal incompetence utilize glottal stops as a means of avoiding nasal distortions. This type of misarticulation may reflect speaker preference albeit at an unconscious level. The performance may reflect past reinforcement. To test this hypothesis, Paynter and Kinard (1979) asked normal children, cleft palate children with velopharyngeal incompetence but without compensatory articulation, and cleft palate children with both velopharyngeal incompetence and compensatory articulation to indicate preference for test words with nasal emission or with compensatory articulation. The normal children and cleft palate children without compensatory articulation preferred the test words with compensatory articulation, but the cleft palate children with compensatory articulation preferred the nasally emitted articulation.

This research was extended by Paynter (1987) and by Bradford and Culton (1987) using the stimulus tape employed by Paynter and Kinard. Normal children, children with clefts, and the parents of these children tended to favor compensatory articulation over audible nasal emission. The finding that children using audible nasal emission and their parents tend to prefer compensatory articulation argues against preference as a variable motivating use of a particular type of articulation error. Bradford and Culton suggested that the findings might be limited to the stimulus recording used. Paynter wrote that there was enough inconsistency of response in the parent groups to suggest that it is unlikely that use of compensatory articulation resulted from orderly reinforcement by parents.

Different meanings of *generalization* are used in the symposium summarized by Fey (1988). One participant in the symposium, Warren (1988), considered generalization as a part of a soft behaviorism wherein learning is considered in terms of behavioral learning strategies, present knowledge base, environmental variables, and cognitive processes. He appeared to be using both behavioral and cognitive concepts within experimentation that utilizes operational definition of variables and control of confounding variables. Another participant, Johnston (1988) noted the importance to learning research and hence to therapy of considering subject and language variables as well as training variables. She indicated that generalization reflects properties of the stimuli and also the learner's prior knowledge.

Generalization is involved in disordered articulation. In generalization learning, similar stimuli may elicit the same response, and related responses may be associated with a particular stimulus (Mowrer, 1982). Pitzner and Morris (1966), Van Demark et al. (1979) and others have speculated that the misarticulation of high-pressure consonants may generalize to other sounds. Such generalization may account for some articulation errors in cleft palate speakers and may, perhaps, be mediated by shared distinctive features. Placement compensations for velopharyngeal valving dysfunction may also generalize from one speech sound or sound class to others. The speech pathologist working with articulation expects generalization from newly learned behaviors to influence articulation responses not directly taught. Nonetheless, the clinician should be alert for unwanted generalization, which is also known to occur. Articulation generalization reflects perception, reinforcement, and other variables and is studied in its own right. It, in turn, is a part of transfer, a more comprehensive construct that pertains to the influence of past learning on current learning.

Although authors writing about cognitive language learning use expressions suggesting that the learner is making conscious decisions, it is highly probable that children use strategies in acquiring language without conscious intention (Snyder and McLean, 1976). This appears to be true of the normal acquisition of phonetic skills and phonological patterning. The child with velopharyngeal insufficiency may hit upon compensatory ways of producing difficult sounds. This may include learning to use the tongue to support the defective velum as the child unconsciously attempts to match the adult speech model. Reinforcement from others in the environment might at that point become a factor in the child's speech learning.

It is assumed that children learn language by testing hypotheses and evaluating feedback and that this process occurs instinctively and below the level of consciousness. Leonard (1985, p. 8) cited the viewpoint that the child is "...an active learner who creates knowledge from the environmental input, rather than...a more passive learner whose acquisition of phonology is simply a linear progression of unfolding abilities." The learning is generative in that it allows children to acquire rules which, in turn, allow the perception and production of language units not previously experienced. Kent (1985) discussed speech acquisition as a self-organizing process influenced by several kinds of variables: genetic, physical, psychosocial, and learning.

Winitz and Reeds (1975) integrated behavioral learning and cognitive-linguistic concepts in a way that accorded reinforcement an important role in language acquisition. They said that there is a relationship between parental approval and language growth in that parents simplify the speech they direct to their young children, and children are rewarded for processing language addressed to them.

Articulatory and phonological development do not depend upon carefully programmed sequences of antecedent and reinforcing stimuli. To conceptualize the child's speech and language development as something achieved through behavioral engineering with the child a passive participant is at best an incomplete viewpoint. At the same time, reinforcement and generalization are important topics for the speech pathologist concerned with therapy.

Very little has been written about the speech maturation variables of individuals with cleft palate. Ewanowski and Saxman (1980) cited evidence that children with clefts start speech sound development slowly and then accelerate this development with the passage of time. They stated that that pattern is the reverse of what is observed in physically normal children. An issue that recurs in the literature on speech and language disorders is whether the communication disorder of an individual is a matter of delayed development, deviant structure, or a combination. McDonald (1964) conceptualized the disordered articulation of physically normal individuals as arrested development; the misarticulation was not something the child had learned in error. A child with cleft palate may show arrested speech development; however, compensatory articulatory deviations are something acquired in response to impaired structure and function, and they are undesirable.

Physiological deficits contribute to departure from normal phonetic and phonological development, and psychological variables influence the resulting speech pattern. However, if the child has adult-like knowledge of the sound system, we expect his or her speech pattern to bear an orderly and predictable relationship to that of the language spoken in the patient's community. For example, dental deformities associated with a cleft of the alveolar ridge may prevent production of normal sibilants. The distorted sounds that replace normal sibilants should represent the closest approximation to the community pattern that the patient can learn with his existing speech mechanism. Treatment of the defect in the mechanism, however, may not be sufficient to correct the speech disorder. The patient must also learn new articulatory gestures and must incorporate those gestures into his phonological pattern.

Discussion

Many children with clefts have normal articulation, and some may have developmental articulation disorders similar to those seen in many physically normal children. We know of no reports of such children. The etiology of articulation disorders in most children with cleft palate who do misarticulate involves the cleft and its physical sequelae. Physical and psycholinguistic variables influence the child's response to the cleft, and many articulatory patterns are observed.

Identification of causal variables and their patterns of interaction is difficult. While it is clear that the anatomical and physiological differences which occur in persons with clefts are major contributors to disordered articulation, the clinician should identify the child's overall sound pattern and give attention to psycholinguistic variables that may have influenced that sound pattern and that are likely to be important in any speech therapy that is needed.

INTELLIGIBILITY

Intelligibility, or how well the speaker is understood by listeners, has often been measured in cleft palate speakers. Wells (1971) wrote that measurement of intelligibility was once the most commonly used procedure for assessing the effects of palatal surgery on speech.

Intelligibility is influenced by many variables including articulation, hypernasality, voice quality, phonemic content, stress, accent, intonation, rate, and duration patterns (Fletcher, 1978), not to mention syntax, semantics, and pragmatics (Hewlett, 1985). The relationship between language variables and intelligibility is reviewed in Chapter 13. Shriberg and Kwiatkowski (1982) noted that listener as well as speaker variables influence intelligibility as does the context of the speech sample and the quality of instrumentation when recordings are used to study intelligibility.

Misarticulation is perhaps the greatest contributor to intelligibility loss although it is possible to articulate quite poorly and still speak intelligibly.

Measurement of Intelligibility

Intelligibility is measured by use of psychophysical scaling or "write-down" procedures wherein the subject is recorded producing lists of syllables, words, or sentences. Often phonetically-balanced material devised for assessment of telephone equipment or hearing loss has been used. Recordings are played to listeners who write down what they hear. The number or percentage of correct responses is the intelligibility index.

Subtelny and Subtelny (1959) had seven speech pathologists write down what they heard on the recordings of 27 cleft palate individuals speaking 48 CV and VC syllables. In a later study (Subtelny et al., 1961), the 48 syllables and phonetically balanced words lists were used.

Prins and Bloomer (1965) had a panel of listeners evaluate the intelligibility of cleft palate speakers recorded reading a 50-item word list selected at random from the Fairbanks Rhyme Test. Three scores were derived: number of words misidentified, number of errors in different consonant sound classes, the type of error in each consonant class. This procedure was used in a second study by Prins and Bloomer (1968), who reported a rate-rerate correlation coefficient of 0.88 for number of errors. This was based on the reratings of 12 tapes by the raters, who were college sophomores untrained in phonetics. These raters were asked to write down both the entire word and only the initial consonant in the test word. For the second task, the score sheet provided the remainder of the word: (d)ot. Results obtained with and without word cues were similar. There was a slight tendency toward reduction in error scores when listeners evaluated a tape the second time. The authors noted that a requirement that observers guess when they were not certain probably contributed to disagreements among listeners.

Subtelny et al. (1972) noted that assessment of intelligibility by write-down techniques is so time-consuming that the technique is more appropriate to research than to clinical application. Therefore, they evolved rating scales for use by the clinician in rating articulation, intelligibility, nasal emission, and other characteristics of speech in cleft palate patients. They described their scales as reliable and recommended that they be applied to conversational speech samples. It should be noted, however, that the reliability of such scales cannot be specified from one listener group to another. The reliability of the listeners must be individually established regardless of the rating technique used. Subtelny et al. (1972) correlated the intelligibility ratings derived from the rating scales with intelligibility ratings obtained by the write-down technique, and a correlation of 0.70 resulted.

Other speech pathologists have also used rating procedures in the study and assessment of the speech of persons with cleft palate. Wells (1971) recommended the use of a seven-point scale to rate intelligibility in different situations including casual conversation and emotional expression. Ratings should be made as the listener both listens to and watches the speaker and then on the basis of listening alone. Ratings can be made by persons who are familiar with the patient's speech and by those who are not.

In addition to testing articulation and performing pattern analyses relative to the patient's speech, the speech pathologist often employs rating scales to describe speech and changes in speech. For example, the Templin-Darley Tests of Articulation include the following descriptive intelligibility scale: readily intelligible, intelligible as listener knows topic, words intelligible now and then, and completely unintelligible.

Shriberg and Kwiatkowski (1982) used tapes of running speech in the assessment of intelligibility. The speech was divided into utterance units, which were played to listeners one at a time. The listener wrote down each utterance verbatim and was then told what a speech clinician's understanding of the passage was. Each utterance was processed in this fashion through the end of the speech sample. Weiss et al. (1980) developed an intelligibility index based on the percentage of words that listeners consider to be intelligible in the patient's running speech. A recording is played to the diagnostician or to a panel of listeners who count the number of unintelligible words.

Intelligibility Characteristics Associated with Cleft Palate

In the Subtelny studies cited in the previous section, intelligibility correlated significantly with stop errors but not with fricative or glide errors. There was a tendency for intelligibility to decrease as velopharyngeal opening increased. The opening was measured through use of sagittal cephalometric radiographs, and the correlation coefficients between intelligibility and velopharyngeal gap were not strong: 0.57 for overall intelligibility, 0.51 for stop intelligibility, and 0.21 and 0.35 for fricatives and glides respectively. Subjects with velopharyngeal gaps between 0.5 and 3.0 mm, were similar in intelligibility to individuals who achieved velopharyngeal closure. Persons with gaps between 3.5 and 7.0 mm had much greater losses in intelligibility.

Prins and Bloomer (1965) reported that their subjects with cleft palate, submucous cleft palate, and idiopathic velopharyngeal incompetence were not homogeneous on intelligibility measures. Some children were more frequently misunderstood on words containing the vocalic consonants, whereas others were most unintelligible when stops, sibilants, and other fricatives were used. Later, Prins and Bloomer (1968) reported the following mean error percentages on a word-intelligibility measure for cleft palate subjects: plosives 10.4, nasals 5.0, fricatives 9.3, sibilants 4.4, affricates 6.4, and vocalics 16.1. The subjects with cleft palate had an overall error rate of 12% compared with 1.4% for normal speakers. A matrix showing error distribution indicated that listeners heard substitutions within as well as across manner-of-production categories and that the subjects with clefts were more frequently perceived to have substituted a nasal for a nonnasal than were the normals.

Philips and Harrison (1969) rated connected speech intelligibility of normal and cleft palate children between 24 and 71 months of age. Ratings were based on a five-point descriptive scale, with 1 indicating always intelligible. Each group improved with age, but, in all subgroups, cleft palate speakers received poorer ratings than the noncleft speakers. For the total groups, the means and standard deviations were 3.83 and 1.04 for the cleft palate subjects and 2.20 and 0.93 for the normal subjects.

Moore and Sommers (1975) studied intelligibility and hypernasality in VCV syllables constructed from 21 consonants and six vowels. Each syllable was rated for each variable on a seven-point equal-appearing interval scale. Sixteen subjects from 3.8 to 13.5 years of age had all undergone surgical repair of their clefts. The authors presented data that indicated a progressive decrease in intelligibility across the vowels from low to high. The total change was about one-half of one scale value. Vowel height was more important to vowel intelligibility than was front-to-back position. No statistically significant differences were found in any possible combination of plosives, glides, and fricatives. Significant differences in intelligibility among consonant pairs were reported. For example, /s/ differed in intelligibility from one other consonant, /h/. Intelligibility ratings of glides, stops, and fricatives tended to be correlated within specific vowel contexts. One hundred and thirty-eight of 153 correlations were statistically significant, and the significant correlations ranged from 0.52 to 0.97.

Fletcher (1978) obtained intelligibility data on 68 children who had undergone surgical repair of their clefts, but had had no secondary surgery such as pharyngeal flap. Their scores on the NU-6 lists ranged from 29 to 98% correct with a mean of 64.3% and a standard deviation of 24.8. The distribution of scores was skewed toward the higher end. All but 26% of Fletcher's subjects had intelligibility scores above 50% and presumably could carry on conversations. Fletcher assumed that the subjects with lower scores suffered impaired ability to communicate orally. He cited other data which indicate that, on the average, cleft palate persons achieve intelligibility percentages of about 70 and that, in the absence of effective remediation, intelligibility is likely to plateau at about the seventh year of life. He reported a correlation of 0.27 between age and intelligibility. This depends, however, upon the population studied.

Several authors have correlated ratings of intelligibility with other speech measures. McWilliams (1953, 1954) had 48 adult cleft subjects each record one of 12 lists of words, phrases, and short sentences containing the 23 major consonants in proportions comparable to their occurrence in conversational speech. These speech samples were played for three auditors whose reliability was predetermined. They wrote down exactly what they understood each speaker to say. The percentage of words misunderstood constituted the scores. These scores correlated with both number of articulation errors and nasality ratings at 0.72 ($p < .01$).

Phillips (1954) had both speech pathologists and lay persons rate the intelligibility and articulation of 14 female cleft palate speakers who ranged from 17 to 35 years of age. Intelligibility and articulation were rated from an auditory recording alone and from a recording combined with a facial photograph. The intelligibility ratings under the two stimulus conditions were highly correlated for both groups of observers—0.96 for speech pathologists and 0.99 for the lay group. The intelligibility ratings of both groups were highly correlated— 0.97 for the auditory-visual and 0.97 for the auditory stimuli. There were no statistically significant differences in mean ratings. Articulation and intelligibility ratings were also correlated. The rank order correlation coefficients for the four correlations computed were: experienced group—auditory 0.91, experienced group—visual-auditory 0.81, lay group—auditory 0.83, and lay group—visual-auditory 0.84.

A key finding of Moore and Sommers (1975) was that intelligibility and nasality relationships were context specific. A correlation of 0.56 was found between intelligibility and nasality ratings when measures were collapsed across vowels and consonants. However, when these two variables were correlated within each VCV syllable studied, only 62 of 324 correlations achieved statistical significance. The authors concluded that the hypernasality-intelligibility relationships are highly context dependent.

Subtelny et al. (1972) noted that a speaker can be rated as intelligible, but as having a severe articulation disorder. Fifty-five percent of their subjects were rated as normal or only mildly deviant in intelligibility, but only 21% were found to have normal or mildly deviant articulation. Only 4% of the subjects had speech that was rated as unintelligible, but 34% had severely defective articulation. Intelligibility ratings were skewed to the good end of the scale and articulation ratings to the poor end. The authors noted that nasalized speech and perceptible nasal emission do not necessarily result in loss of speech sound identity.

Subtelny et al. (1972) noted that although intelligibility, articulation, and nasality are correlated, the correlations reported in the literature vary greatly. They recommended that clinicians assess each one and not concern themselves with predicting one measurement from another. The overall rating of intelligibility, which is a global rating, has merit both in the clinic and for research purposes.

REFERENCES

Albery L. Approaches to the treatment of speech problems. In: Stengelhofen J, ed. Cleft palate: the nature and remediation of communication problems. Edinburgh: Churchill-Livingstone, 1989.

Ainoda N, Yamashita K, Tsukada S. Articulation at age 4 in children with early repair of cleft palate. Ann Plast Surg 1985; 15:415.

Bernthal JE, Bankson NW. Articulation and phonological disorders. 2nd ed. Englewood Cliffs, NJ: Prentice-Hall, 1988.

Bernthal JE, Weiner FF. A re-examination of the sound emission— preliminary considerations. J Child Comm Dis 1976; 1:132.

Berry MF. Correction of cleft-palate speech by phonetic instruction. Quart J Speech 1928; 14:523.

Bless DM, Ewanowski SJ, Paul R. A longitudinal analysis of aerodynamic patterns produced by speakers with cleft palates. Annual Convention, ASHA, San Francisco, 1978.

Bosma JF. Postnasal ontogeny of the pharynx, larynx, and mouth. Am Rev Respir Dis 1985; 31 (Suppl 10):

Bradford PW, Culton GL. Parents' perceptual preferences between compensatory articulation and nasal escape of air in children with cleft palate. Cleft Palate J 1987; 24:299.

Brandt SD, Morris HL. The linearity of the relationship between articulation errors and velopharyngeal incompetence. Cleft Palate J 1965; 2:176.

Byrne MC, Shelton RL, Diedrich WM. Articulatory skill, physical management and, classification of children with cleft palates. J Speech Hear Dis 1961; 26:326.

Bzoch KR. An investigation of the speech of pre-school cleft palate children. Doctoral dissertation. Northwestern University, 1956.

Bzoch KR. Articulatory proficiency and error patterns of preschool cleft palate and normal children. Cleft Palate J 1965; 2:340.

Bzoch KR. Measurement and assessment of categorical aspects of cleft palate speech. In: Bzoch KR, ed. Communicative disorders related to cleft lip and palate. Boston: Little, Brown, 1979.

Cohn ER, McWilliams BJ. Early cleft palate repair and speech outcome—letter to the editor. Plast Reconstr Surg 1983; 71:442.

Colton RH, Cooker HS. Perceived nasality in the speech of the deaf. J Speech Hear Res 1968; 11:553.

Connell PJ. Induction, generalization, and deduction: models for defining language generalization. Lang Speech Hear Serv Schools 1988; 19:282.

Counihan DT. A clinical study of the speech efficiency and structural adequacy of operated adolescent and adult cleft palate persons. Unpublished Doctoral dissertation. Northwestern University, 1956.

Counihan DT. Articulation skills of adolescents and adults with cleft palates. J Speech Hear Dis 1960; 25:181.

Cullinan WL, Counihan DT. Ratings of vowel representatives. Percept Mot Skill 1971; 32:395.

Daniloff RG, Schuckers RG, Feth LL. The physiology of

speech and hearing: an introduction. Englewood Cliffs: Prentice Hall, 1980.

Dinnsen DA. Methods and empirical issues in analyzing functional misarticulation. In: Elbert M, Dinnsen D, Weismer G, eds. Phonological theory and the misarticulating child. ASHA Monographs No. 22, 1984.

Dorf DS, Curtin JW. Early cleft palate repair and speech outcome. Plast Reconstr Surg 1982; 70:74.

Elbert M. The relationship between normal phonological acquisition and clinical intervention. Speech Lang Adv Basic Res Pract 1984; 10:111.

Elbert M, Gierut J. Handbook of clinical phonology: approaches to assessment and treatment. San Diego: College-Hill Press, 1986.

Ericsson G. Analysis and treatment of cleft palate speech: some acoustic-phonetic observations. Linkoping, Sweden: Linkoping University Medical Dissertations No. 254, 1987.

Estrem T, Broen PA. Early speech production of children with cleft palate. J Speech Hear Res 1989; 32:12.

Ewanowski SJ, Saxman JH. Orofacial disorders. In: Hixon TJ, Shriberg LD, Saxman JH, eds. Introduction to communication disorders. Englewood Cliffs, NJ: Prentice-Hall, 1980.

Fey ME. Generalization issues facing language interventionists: an introduction. Lang Speech Hear Serv Schools 1988; 19:272.

Fletcher SG. Diagnosing speech disorders from cleft palate. New York: Grune and Stratton, 1978.

Fletcher SG. Speech production and oral motor skill in an adult with an unrepaired palatal cleft. J Speech Hear Dis 1985; 50:254.

Folkins JW. Issues in speech motor control and their relation to the speech of individuals with cleft palate. Cleft Palate J 1985; 22:106.

Folkins JW, Bleile KM. Taxonomies: biological, phonological, and speech motor. In process.

Forner LL. Speech segment durations produced by five and six year old speakers with and without cleft palates. Cleft Palate J 1983; 20:185.

Foster D, Riley K, Parker F. Some problems in the clinical application of phonological theory. J Speech Hear Dis 1985; 50:294.

Galambos R, Morgan GT. The neural basis of learning. In: Field J, ed. Handbook of physiology Section 1: neurophysiology Vol. 3. Washington, DC: American Physiological Society, 1960.

Gilbert JP, McPeek B, Mosteller F. Statistics and ethics in surgery and anesthesia. Science 1977; 198:684.

Grunwell P. Comments on the terms "phonetics" and "phonology" as applied in the investigation of speech disorders. Br J Disord Commun 1985; 20:165.

Grunwell P, Russell J. Vocalisations before and after cleft palate surgery: a pilot study. Br J Disord Commun 1987; 22:1.

Grunwell P, Russell J. Phonological development in children with cleft lip and palate. Clin Linguist Phonet 1988; 2:75.

Hagerty R, Hess D, Mylin W. Velar motility, velopharyngeal closure and speech proficiency in cartilage pharyngoplasty: The effect of age at surgery. Cleft Palate J 1968; 5:317.

Hardin MA, Lachenbruch PA, Morris HL. Contribution of selected variables to the prediction of speech proficiency for adolescents with cleft lip and palate. Cleft Palate J 1986; 23:10.

Harris J, Cottam P. Phonetic features and phonological features in speech assessment. Br J Disord Commun 1985; 20:61.

Hawkins P. A tutorial comment on Harris and Cottam. Br J Disord Commun 1985; 20:75.

Henningsson EG, Isberg AM. Velopharyngeal movement patterns in patients alternating between oral and glottal articulation: a clinical and cineradiographical study. Cleft Palate J 1986; 23:1.

Hewlett N. Phonological versus phonetic disorders: some suggested modifications to the current use of the distinction. Br J Disord Commun 1985; 20:155.

Hodson BW, Chin C, Redmond B, Simpson R. Phonological evaluation and remediation of speech deviations of a child with a repaired cleft palate: a case study. J Speech Hear Dis 1983; 48:93.

Hubbell RD. Children's language disorders: an integrated approach. Englewood Cliffs: Prentice-Hall, 1981.

Hutchinson JM, Robinson KL, Nerbonne MA. Patterns of nasalance in a sample of normal gerontologic subjects. J Commun Dis 1978; 11:469.

Hutters B, Brondsted K. Strategies in cleft palate speech—with special reference to Danish. Cleft Palate J 1987; 24:126.

Ingram D. Phonological disability in children. New York: Elsevier, 1976.

Isberg A, Henningsson G. Influence of palatal fistulas on velopharyngeal movements: A cineradiographic study. Plast Reconstr Surg 1987; 79:525.

Johnston JR. Generalization: the nature of change. Lang Speech Hear Serv Schools 1988; 19:314.

Jones DL, Folkins JW. The effect of speaking rate on judgments of disordered speech in children with cleft palate. Cleft Palate J 1985; 22:246.

Kagan J, Kearsley RB, Zelazo PR. Infancy: its place in human development. Cambridge, MA: Harvard University Press, 1978.

Karnell MP, Folkins JW, Morris HL. Relationships between the perception of nasalization and speech movements in speakers with cleft palate. J Speech Hear Res 1985; 28:63.

Kawano M, Isshiki N, Harita Y, Tanokuchi F. Laryngeal fricative in cleft palate speech. Acta Otolaryngol (Stockh) 1985; Suppl 419:180.

Kent RD. Contextual facilitation of correct sound production. Lang Speech Hear Serv Schools 1982; 13:66.

Kent RD. Psychobiology of speech development: coemergence of language and a movement system. Am J Physiol 1984; 246: R888-R894.

Kent RD. Developing and disordered speech: strategies for organization. ASHA Reports No. 15:29.

Kent RD. Normal aspects of articulation. In: Bernthal JE, Bankson NW. Articulation and phonological disorders. 2nd ed. Englewood Cliffs: Prentice Hall, 1988.

Klinger H. A palatographic and acoustic study of cleft palate speech. Cleft Palate Bull 1956; 6 (2):10.

Langacker JW. Language and its structure. New York: Harcourt, Brace, World, 1967.

Lass NL, Noll JD. A comparative study of rate characteristics in cleft palate and noncleft palate speakers. Cleft Palate J 1970; 7:275.

Leonard LB. Unusual and subtle phonological behavior in the speech of phonologically disordered children. J Speech Hear Dis 1985; 50:4.

Linville RN. Articulatory events and neuromotor strategies (Letter to the Editor). Cleft Palate J 1984; 21:42.

Locke JL. The inference of speech perception in the phonologically disordered child. Part 1. A rationale, some criteria, the conventional tests. J Speech Hear Dis 1980; 45:431.

Locke JL. Clinical phonology: the explanation and treatment of speech sound disorders. J Speech Hear Dis 1983; 48:339.

Logemann JA. Treatment of articulation disorders in cleft palate children. In: Perkins WH, ed. Phonologic-articulatory disorders. New York: Theime-Stratton, 1983.

Lubker JF. Some teleological considerations of velopharyngeal function. In: Daniloff RG, ed. Articulation assessment & treatment issues. San Diego: College-Hill, 1984.

Lynch JI, Fox DR, Brookshire BL. Phonological proficiency of two cleft palate toddlers with school-age follow-up. J Speech Hear Dis 1983; 48:274.

McDermott RP. A study of /s/ sound production by individuals with cleft palates. Doctoral dissertation. University of Iowa, 1962.

McDonald ET. A deep test of articulation. Pittsburgh: Stanwix House, 1964.

McWilliams BJ. An experimental study of some of the components of intelligibility of the speech of adult cleft palate patients. Doctoral dissertation. University of Pittsburgh, 1953.

McWilliams BJ. Some factors in the intelligibility of cleft palate speech. J Speech Hear Dis 1954; 19:524.

McWilliams BJ. Articulation problems of a group of cleft palate adults. J Speech Hear Res 1958; 1:68

McWilliams BJ. Cleft palate management in England. Speech Path Ther 1960; 3:3.

McWilliams BJ. Cleft palate. In: Shames G, Wiig E, eds. Human communication disorders. Columbus, OH: CE Merrill, 1982.

McWilliams BJ, Matthews HP. A comparison of intelligence and social maturity in children with unilateral complete clefts and those with isolated cleft palates. Cleft Palate J 1979; 16: 363.

McWilliams BJ, Musgrave RH. Diagnosis of speech problems in patients with cleft palate. Br J Commun Disord 1977; Spring:26.

McWilliams BJ, Philips BJ. Audio seminars in speech pathology, velopharyngeal incompetence. Toronto: BC Decker, 1989.

Milisen R. A rationale for articulation disorders. J Speech Hear Dis 1954; Suppl 4:5.

Miller GA. Some preliminaries to psycholinguistics. Am Psychol 1965; 20:15.

Milroy L. Phonological analysis and speech disorders: a comment. Br J Disord Commun 1985; 20:171.

Moll KL. Speech characteristics of individuals with cleft lip and palate. In: Spriestersbach DC, Sherman D, eds. Cleft palate and communication. New York: Academic Press, 1968.

Moller KT, Broen PA, Schwartz RG. Early phonological development. The normal and cleft palate experience. Annual Convention—ASHA New Orleans, 1987. Asha 1987; 49:117.

Moore WH, Sommers RK. Phonetic contexts: their effects on perceived intelligibility in cleft-palate speakers. Folia Phoniatr 1975; 27:410.

Morley ME. Cleft palate and speech. 7th ed. Baltimore: Williams & Wilkins, 1970.

Morris HL, Spriestersbach DC, Darley FL. An articulation test for assessing competency of velopharyngeal closure. J Speech Hear Res 1961; 4:48.

Morris HL. Etiological bases for speech problems. In: Spriestersbach DC, Sherman D, eds. Cleft palate and communication. New York: Academic Press, 1968.

Morris HL. Cleft palate. In: Weston AJ, ed. Communicative disorders: an appraisal. Springfield: CC Thomas, 1972.

Moussett MR, Trichet C. Babbling and phonetic acquisitions after early complete repair of cleft lip and palate. Fifth International Congress on Cleft Palate and Related Craniofacial Abnormalities, Monte Carlo, 1985.

Mowrer DE. Methods of modifying speech behaviors. 2nd ed. Prospect Heights, IL: Waveland, 1982.

Newmeyer FJ. The politics of linguistics. Chicago: The University of Chicago Press, 1986.

O'Gara MM, Logemann JA. Phonetic analyses of the speech development of babies with cleft palate. Cleft Palate J 1988; 25:122.

Olson DA. A descriptive study of the speech development of a group of infants with cleft palate. Doctoral dissertation. Northwestern University, 1965.

Panagos JM. Persistence of the open syllable reinterpreted as a symptom of language disorder. J Speech Hear Dis 1974; 39:23.

Paynter ET, Kinard MW. Perceptual preferences between compensatory articulation and nasal escape of air in children with velopharyngeal incompetence. Cleft Palate J 1979; 16:262.

Paynter ET. Parental and child preference for speech produced by children with velopharyngeal incompetence. Cleft Palate J 1987; 24:112.

Peterson SJ. Nasal emission as a component of the misarticulation on sibilants and affricates. J Speech Hear Dis 1975; 40:106.

Philips BJ, Harrison RJ. Articulation patterns of preschool cleft palate children. Cleft Palate J 1969; 6:245.

Philips BJ, Kent RD. Acoustic-phonetic descriptions of speech production in speakers with cleft palate and other velopharyngeal disorders. Speech Lang Adv Basics Res Pract 1984; 11:113.

Phillips BR. An experimental investigation of the relationship between ratings of speech intelligibility based on auditory and visual cues and on auditory cues alone in a group of cleft palate adults. Masters thesis. University of Pittsburgh, 1954.

Pitzner JC, Morris HL. Articulation skills and adequacy of breath pressure ratios of children with cleft palate. J Speech Hear Dis 1966; 31:26.

Platt LJ, Andrews G, Howie PM. Dysarthria of adult

cerebral palsy: II. Phonemic analysis of articulation errors. J Speech Hear Res 1980; 23:41.

Powers GR. Cinefluorographic investigation of articulatory movements of selected individuals with cleft palate. J Speech Hear Res 1962; 5:62.

Powers G, Erickson CB, Dunn C. Speech analyses of four children with repaired cleft palates. Paper presented at the annual convention of the American Cleft Palate Association. Seattle, Washington, 1984.

Prins D, Bloomer HH. A word intelligibility approach to the study of speech change in oral cleft patients. Cleft Palate J 1965; 2:357.

Prins D, Bloomer HH. Consonant intelligibility: a procedure for evaluating speech in oral cleft subjects. J Speech Hear Res 1968; 11:128.

Pullum GK, Ladusaw WA. Phonetic symbol guide. Chicago: The University of Chicago Press, 1986.

Renfrew CE. Present day problems in cleft palate speech. Logopeden. 1960, June. As cited by: Moll KL. Speech characteristics of individuals with cleft lip and palate. In: Spriestersbach DC, Sherman D, eds Cleft palate and communication. New York: Academic Press, 1968.

Riski JE. Articulation skills and oral-nasal resonance in children with pharyngeal flaps. Cleft Palate J 1979; 16:421.

Riski JE. DeLong E. Articulation development in children with cleft lip/palate. Cleft Palate J 1984; 21:57.

Ross BR, Johnston MC. Cleft Lip and Palate. Baltimore: Williams & Wilkins, 1972.

Schwartz RG. The phonological system. In: Costello J, ed. Speech disorders in children. Boston: College-Hill, 1984.

Shelton RL, Brooks AR, Youngstrom KA. Articulation and patterns of palatopharyngeal closure. J Speech Hear Dis 1964; 29:390.

Shelton RL, McCauley RJ. Use of a hinge-type speech prosthesis. Cleft Palate J 1986; 23:312

Sherman D, Spriestersbach DC, Noll JD. Glottal stops in the speech of children with cleft palates. J Speech Hear Dis 1959; 24:37.

Shontz FC. Research methods in personality. New York: Appleton-Century-Crofts, 1965.

Shriberg LD, Kwiatkowski J. Natural process analysis. New York: John Wiley and Sons, 1980.

Shriberg LD, Kwiatkowski J. Phonological disorders II: A conceptual framework for management. J Speech Hear Dis 1982; 47:256.

Shriberg LD, Kwiatkowski J. A follow-up study of children with phonologic disorders of unknown origin. J Speech Hear Dis 1988; 53:144.

Singh S, Hayden ME, Toombs MS. The role of distinctive features in articulation errors. J Speech Hear Dis 1981; 46:174.

Smith BL. Explaining the development of speech production skills in young children. J Nat Student Speech Lang Hear Assoc 1981; 9:9.

Synder LK, McLean JE. Deficient acquisition strategies: a proposed conceptual framework for analyzing severe language deficiency. Am J Ment Defic 1976; 81:338.

Spriestersbach DC, Curtis JF. Misarticulation and discrimination of speech sounds. Quart J Speech 1951; 37:483.

Spriestersbach DC, Darley FL, Rouse V. Articulation of a group of children with cleft lips and palates. J Speech Hear Dis 1956; 21:436.

Spriestersbach DC, Moll KL, Morris HL. Subject classification and articulation of speakers with cleft palates. J Speech Hear Res 1961; 4:358.

Spriestersbach DC, Powers GR. Articulation skills, velopharyngeal closure, and oral breath pressure of children with cleft palates. J Speech Hear Res 1959; 2:318.

Starr C. A study of some of the characteristics of the speech and speech mechanism of a group of cleft palate children. Doctoral dissertation. Northwestern University, 1956.

Stengelhofen J. The nature and causes of communication problems in cleft palate. In: Stengelhofen J, ed. Cleft palate: the nature and remediation of communication problems. Edinburgh: Churchill-Livingstone, 1989.

Stoel-Gammon C, Dunn C. Normal and disordered phonology in children. Baltimore: University Park Press, 1985.

Subtelny J, Subtelny JD. Intelligibility and associated physiological factors of cleft palate speakers. J Speech Hear Res 1959; 2:353.

Subtelny J, Koepp-Baker H, Subtelny JD. Palatal function and cleft palate speech. J Speech Hear Dis 1961; 26:213.

Subtelny JD, Van Hattum RJ, Myers BA. Ratings and measures of cleft palate speech. Cleft Palate J 1972; 9:18.

Szent-Gyorgi A. Teaching and the expanding knowledge. Science 1964; 146:1278.

Trost-Cardamone JE. Effects of velopharyngeal incompetence on speech. J Childhood Commun Dis 1986; 10:31.

Trost JE. Articulatory additions to the classical descriptions of the speech of persons with cleft palate. Cleft Palate J 1981; 18:193.

Van Demark DR. Misarticulations and listener judgments of the speech of individuals with cleft palates. Cleft Palate J 1964; 1:232.

Van Demark DR. A factor analysis of the speech of children with cleft palate. Cleft Palate J 1966; 3:159.

Van Demark DR. Consistency of articulation of subjects with cleft palate. Cleft Palate J 1969; 6:254.

Van Demark DR. A comparison of articulation abilities and velopharyngeal competency between Danish and Iowa children with cleft palate. Cleft Palate J 1974; 11:463.

Van Demark DR, Morris HL, VandeHaar C. Patterns of articulation abilities in speakers with cleft palate. Cleft Palate J 1979; 16:230.

Van Demark DR, Van Demark AH. Misarticulations of cleft palate children achieving velopharyngeal closure and children with functional speech problems. Cleft Palate J 1967; 4:31.

Waldrop MM. Soar: a unified theory of cognition? Science 1988; 241:296.

Warren DW. Nasal emission of air and velopharyngeal function. Cleft Palate J 1967; 4:148.

Warren DW. Compensatory speech behaviors in individuals with cleft palate: A regulation/control phenomenon? Cleft Palate J 1986; 23:251.

Warren SF. A behavioral approach to language generalization. Lang Speech Hear Serv Schools 1988; 19:292.

Weiss CE, Lillywhite HS, Gordon ME. Clinical management of articulation disorders. St. Louis: CV Mosby, 1980.

Wells CF. Cleft palate and its associated speech disorders. New York: McGraw-Hill, 1971.

Winitz H, Reeds J. Comprehension and problem solving as strategies for language training. The Hague, Paris: Mouton, 1975.

16 | DIAGNOSIS OF LANGUAGE DISORDERS

All children born with clefts or with any other craniofacial malformation should be routinely followed for language development just as they are for hearing, dental problems, facial growth, special pediatric needs, and psychosocial well-being. They are prone to the same developmental problems that may occur in any child, and, in addition, special factors create added risks which should not be ignored. The speech pathologist working with individual children has no foundation upon which to assume that language will be either normal or aberrant although, as we saw earlier, language deficits over a wide range occur more frequently in children with clefts than in noncleft children. For this reason, surveillance is always indicated, with routine testing as a regular part of clinical care and special testing in response to need. Language evaluation must include information about environmental factors, psychosocial, motor, and mental development, and hearing as well as the nature of language behavior.

ENVIRONMENTAL FACTORS

It is important to discover any environmental conditions that may create or maintain a language deficit or be responsible for slow language development. Differential treatment in the family, poor parent-child relationships, child management problems, overprotection, parental anxiety, general health of the child and the family, socioeconomic factors, the parents' marital stability and happiness, the kind of verbal interaction in the family and with the child—any one of these alone or in combination can play a role in influencing language deficiencies and in slowing the process of development or recovery. Thus, the child's environment must be freely explored by conversations with parents and observations of parent-child interactions and of the child's behavior in a variety of contexts.

PSYCHOSOCIAL DEVELOPMENT

Of interest to the speech pathologist are many aspects of psychosocial functioning including the kind of personality the child has, the ease with which he or she accepts change, the kinds of behaviors that seem out of line for chronological age, consistent behaviors of concern to the parents, patterns of behavior about which the parents seem not to be concerned but about which they probably should be, interactions with other family members and peers, response to school and to separation from the parents, sleep habits, eating patterns, ritualistic behaviors that may be present, in short, any factor, positive or negative, that may influence a child's communicative behavior. For example, most children with clefts have somewhat slow onset of speech, and they tend to talk less than other children. However, this is not true for all. Some are linguistically and communicatively precocious; a few will have elective mutism; an occasional child will demonstrate aphasia-like or autistic behavior; and some will have learning disabilities or mental retardation that may affect linguistic and psychosocial functioning. Only the parents can provide the background detail required, and they will do so only if we ask them as part of the case history. We cannot afford to ignore this avenue of exploration.

HEARING EVALUATION

Hearing evaluations are always important for all children, and especially for those who are experiencing language delay. They are essential for children with clefts since, as we have already seen, they all begin life with ear disease and remain at increased risk for conductive hearing losses in the preschool years and even later. Any sign of even a mild hearing loss should be cause for referral to an otolaryngologist for examination and for treatment as indicated. No loss is too minimal to be ignored since it may mean that hearing sensitivity is fluctuating, a condition difficult for any child to deal with. While the evidence is far from clear that these conductive losses are implicated in a major way in language deficits in children with clefts, we do know that such sensory variations do nothing to enhance language development and that, left untreated, they may grow progressively worse. The need for careful audiological assessment, including tympanometry, cannot be overemphasized.

DEVELOPMENTAL EVALUATION

In our zeal to recognize and treat language impairments, we sometimes forget that language in all its forms is a part of the total fabric of human development. If a child's language is not maturing as we would wish, all aspects of development should be assessed. It may be that language is out of keeping with the rest of development or that it is consistent with other developmental characteristics. A 2-year-old doing well in almost every way except language would be a candidate for language management. A 2-year-old showing, in addition, deficits in motor, cognitive, and interpersonal skills might more reasonably be considered for placement in a program designed to stimulate general development including language, even though the outcome of such programs remains speculative.

A word of caution is necessary here. Speech pathologists should be developmental specialists who understand normal development and recognize variations when they occur. Not all young children reach the same developmental milestones at precisely the same ages. Thus, a child who is using little or no expressive language at 18 months may or may not require intervention. This is especially true if the child has had life experiences that may reasonably explain the delay. For exam-

ple, surgery at 12 and 18 months may be incompatible with the onset of speech in some children but not in others. A child who understands appropriately for chronological age but does not talk is different from one who neither talks nor understands. The same may be said for slow acquisition of early motor behaviors. The pieces of the puzzle must fit together in a reasonable way, or the clinician is pursuing the wrong course. Only careful study will provide the evidence needed to decide.

Few speech pathologists are well qualified to administer psychological tests, and some seem not to recognize the importance of these in reaching even tentative conclusions about the nature of language disorders. We think that it is a mistake to attempt language therapy without evaluation of the patient by a competent psychologist experienced in testing young children, especially those with clefts, craniofacial abnormalities, and disordered speech. Significant language impairment usually does not exist as a single, isolated problem.

Of special concern in the developmental evaluation is the administration at appropriate ages of neuropsychological batteries and the neuropsychological interpretation of test findings when that is possible. The need for that was described in Chapter 13.

Neuropsychological testing is not new. It has its roots in the work of early psychologists who tried to devise ways of understanding the effects of neurological impairment on various aspects of mental functioning and sought test data that might be used as evidence of neurological impairment. Scatter across tests, inconsistency in responses such as passing an item at one level and failing the same type of task at a lower level, poor auditory memory span or discrepancies between short-term memory for digits and meaningful material, evidences of poor eye-hand coordination, concreteness, unusual responses to block designs or coding, *significant* discrepancies between verbal and performance measures in *either* direction, and patterns of successes and failures on subtests are all of interest and of concern in any diagnostic effort. Both neurological and psychiatric deficits may be associated with test variations.

We make routine use of the Bayley Scales of Infant Development, the Stanford-Binet, and the various forms of the Wechsler depending upon the age of the child with additional special testing as required.

It is to be remembered that information derived from intelligence and other testing is less reliable in infants and preschool children than it is as they get older. Thus, it is not IQ that best describes a child's level of functioning or his potential. An experienced psychologist will be able to weigh the relevant factors in arriving at a test interpretation that will be most useful in planning treatment, including language and education.

Developmental assessment in conjunction with language testing is mandatory given the serious deficits in the language tests that are available. In our view, students and speech-language pathologists frequently place too much confidence in these tests and fail to recognize the need to look at overall development in children who are at risk for or seem to have language problems. These issues are reviewed in the next section.

LANGUAGE EVALUATION

McCauley and Swisher (1984a) examined 30 language and articulation tests to determine whether or not they met a set of 10 criteria appropriate to norm-referenced tests. The Test of Language Development (TOLD) met eight of the criteria; the Illinois Tests of Psycholinguistic Abilities (ITPA) met five of the 10 criteria; The Peabody Picture Vocabulary Test-R (PPVT-R) met five, while the PPVT met four. Half of the tests met no more than two of the criteria, and six met only one.

Of special interest and concern is the finding that *none* of the tests met the criteria for predictive validity or inter-examiner reliability and only one test met the criteria for test-retest reliability. Normative data were sadly lacking as were item analyses, means and standard deviations, concurrent validity, and description of tester qualifications. Surprisingly, five of the tests did not even provide a description of test procedures.

McCauley and Swisher suggest that test users can reduce the impact of poor test construction by becoming more knowledgeable about psychometric principles and applying them to the tests they use or consider using. If we were to do that, it would be difficult to justify using most of the language tests now available commercially, and it explains why speech-language pathologists dually trained in psychology have taken a general-

ly grim view of using language tests apart from more extensive, valid, and reliable testing.

These authors suggest further that clinical decisions are never properly based on test results alone. Rather, results should be weighed in combination with other kinds of objective and subjective evidence. That, of course, would be the ideal outcome; but sadly, it is, often not the case. We have removed many children with clefts from ill-advised and unneeded language therapy predicated on language tests taken out of context of other developmental information or simply misinterpreted in ways described in a later article by McCauley and Swisher (1984b).

Ideally, speech-language pathologists would also have training in test construction and a solid background in psychology before attempting the awesome task of selecting, using, and interpreting language tests. Since that is not happening, thorough training and clinical practicum in using such instruments as the Vineland Social Maturity Scale and the ITPA, which is far from an easy test to administer, will provide additional evidence against which to evaluate decisions growing out of currently available language tests.

This is not to say that, properly used, language tests are worthless. They can suggest areas that require further exploration and that *may* be in need of treatment if observation and interaction with the child support that conclusion. The clinician should not be surprised, however, if several of these questionable tests yield widely differing results on the same child.

Language assessment of children with clefts is not fundamentally different from that of any other child except that the examiner needs to be especially alerted to the possible low levels of expressivity employed by these children, quite apart from their language capabilities, and to the inhibitions that may mediate between the child and the examiner. Care must be taken to assure that the child can be adequately assessed at the time that has been established. If that does not seem probable, it may be necessary for the examiner to schedule several play sessions with the child before undertaking the actual testing.

With those precautions, the clinician will select those language tests that are appropriate to the age of the child, that explore those aspects of receptive and expressive language that are of particular interest, and with which the clinician is comfortable. In addition, it is to be hoped that the shortcomings of formal language tests will be seriously considered.

Receptive Language

The goal of receptive-language testing is to discover how complicated verbal expression can become before the child ceases to understand it and what, if any, particular forms cause breakdown in performance.

In addition to formal tests of receptive language that are available and that are commonly used, behavioral observations have also been suggested. Leonard (1982) discussed the use of both formal and informal acting-out items in the assessment of receptive language. Bangs (1975) used this technique, and it is often employed in an informal play situation wherein a child is asked to do something such as "put the kitten under the chair." We find that information about this kind of behavior emerges more satisfactorily from psychological tests that have adequate normative data. Beyond that, it is often desirable to explore the various levels of function through informal play designed to elicit specific behaviors of interest.

The outcome of both formal and informal receptive-language testing is closely related to the child's ability and desire to cooperate, to his or her comfort in the testing situation, to the sophistication of the examiner, and to his or her rapport with the child. The speech pathologist who undertakes testing of this sort on an informal basis must be knowledgeable about the levels of difficulty and abstraction of the requests made to the child and must recognize the structural elements involved. For example, when asked to "point to the shoe," the child may do so but then fail to respond to "point to the one you put on your foot," a more abstract task. A speech pathologist once explained to us that the child in question "understood everything," as he had already demonstrated by pointing to the shoe, but that it wasn't "fair" to ask him the more obscure question. She failed to understand the importance of testing to find the limits of receptive abilities, even though we recognize how nearly impossible that task is. When we have finished testing receptive language abilities, we know only what we have been able to judge from overt behavior. While that is not nearly enough, it is the best we have.

Expressive Language

Children fail to acquire and develop the complex use of expressive language at the expected ages for a variety of reasons. One child may have extensive problems encompassing both receptive and expressive language, whereas another will have relatively minor deficits involving only verbal communication. Although neither talks, their clinical pictures differ markedly and so should their treatment. If receptive language is seriously impoverished, there is usually little if any expressive language, although there may be some echolalia. Of course, both receptive and expressive abilities may be impaired.

When some speech is present, language assessment is somewhat easier. The speech pathologist can listen both formally and informally and describe what is heard in objective terms. One rather time-consuming but useful approach is to collect a sample of 50 spontaneous utterances and then analyze their content according to some system of analysis such as the Developmental Sentence Analysis (Lee, 1974), the Sequenced Inventory of Communication Development (Hedrick et al., 1975), or Leonard's Adaptation (1982) of Language Sampling, Analysis and Training (Tyack and Gottsleben, 1974). These analyses are complicated and time-consuming to carry out, but they do, overall, provide what is probably the best information that can be gathered about language usage.

The 50 utterances can also be analyzed for mean length of response (MLR) or mean length of utterance (MLU). This is an important area for investigation because children with clefts appear to have their most significant problems in the amount of verbal output they use. The children, on the average, are only mildly deficient, but some will have significant problems in this regard, and MLR or MLU are techniques of value. The details for arriving at MLR have been well described by Johnson et al. (1952).

A simpler way of testing expressive language is to use some form of sentence imitation. It is generally recognized that it is rare (but by no means impossible) for children to use grammatical forms when imitating sentences if they do not have access to the same forms in their own verbal development. Thus, a number of expressive language tests make use of this principle. The Stephens Oral Language Screening Test (Stephens, 1977) and the Carrow Elicited Language Inventory (1974), among others, use this technique and score the responses for deviations. An example of a child's successful response to, "Robert found a shiny penny," would be an exact repetition of the stimulus sentence. On the other hand, a very young child, or an older child with a language disorder, might say "Robert finded a penny," "Him find penny," or some other structure unique to the child being tested. Short-term memory is, of course, a factor.

A number of language tests investigate both receptive and expressive language either for screening or for diagnostic purposes. There is dissatisfaction with most of the testing tools now available because, in addition to their other problems, they are often too simple to address in any detail the complex issues involved in language disorders. However, they do offer systematic approaches and can be useful in helping the clinician delineate general problems that can then be explored in greater depth.

Because children with clefts may have hearing impairment, negative social-emotional factors, or aberrant mental development, we consider this population to be at increased risk for language problems, especially if they have isolated palatal clefts or any other type of cleft that is associated with other malformations, including syndromes. All children with clefts or other craniofacial malformations should be carefully followed from birth, and developmental and language screening should be routine, with in-depth testing if there is any doubt about the level of functioning. We believe that this should be accomplished in a low-keyed manner as part of routine clinical evaluations and that only such intervention as is clearly clinically indicated should be prescribed. Alternative approaches should often be used with these children, however, and these will be discussed in Chapter 20.

REFERENCES

Bangs TE. Vocabulary comprehension scale. Boston: Teaching Resources, 1975.

Carrow E. Elicited language inventory. Austin, TX: Learning Concepts, 1974.

Hedrick DL, Prather EM, Tobin AR. Sequenced inventory of communication development. Seattle: University of Washington Press, 1975.

Johnson W, Darley FL, Spriesterbach DC. Diagnostic methods in speech pathology. New York: Harper & Row, 1952.

Lee L. Developmental sentence analysis. Evanston, IL: Northwestern University Press, 1974.

Leonard L. Early language development and language disorders. In: Shames GH, Weig EH, eds. Human communication disorders. Columbus: Merrill, 1982.

McCauley RJ, Swisher L. Psychometric review of language and articulation tests for preschool children. J Speech Hear Dis 1984a; 49:34.

McCauley RJ, Swisher L. Use and misuse of norm-referenced tests in clinical assessment: a hypothetical case. J Speech Hear Dis 1984b; 49:338.

Stephens MI. The Stephens oral language screening test. Peninsula, OH: Interim Publishers, 1977.

Tyack D, Gottsleben R. Language sampling, analysis and training. Palo Alto: LCA Consulting Psychologist Press, 1974.

17 | DIAGNOSIS OF DISORDERS OF PHONATION AND RESONANCE

PHONATION DISORDERS

The evidence currently available suggests that certain fundamental diagnostic principles should be followed in determining the nature of phonation disorders in cleft-related problems.

Assessment of Phonation

Examination by the Speech Pathologist

First, the speech pathologist must always listen to the phonatory aspects of voice and decide whether or not a phonation problem is present. If it is not, the course is clear, and no additional attention need be given to this issue. If phonation is not within normal limits, a voice evaluation is in order. For details of how to conduct voice examinations in general the reader is referred to Aronson (1980) and Boone and McFarlane (1988). However, in our experience, the common phonatory deviations associated with velopharyngeal incompetence are those presented in Chapter 14, and those are the deviations that are discussed here.

If it is decided that a phonation disorder is present, a careful history should be taken to discover whether the symptom is of recent origin, is chronic or acute, or is associated with an allergy, upper respiratory infection, or unusual vocal abuse. People who have had voice problems for a long time may not realize it, and their families, accustomed to hearing the speech, may not recognize that there is anything unusual. For this reason, it is necessary to be alert for such statements as, "This is the way I always talk," or "I

don't notice anything different about my voice," or "My voice sounds all right to me." These comments suggest that the phonation is not different from what the patient views as "normal."

If the voice disorder appears to be chronic, a behavioral history is important in order to determine whether there are environmental factors or patterns of vocal abuse that might account for laryngeal hypo- or hyperfunction. Frequent screaming, excessively loud talking, frequent coughing or throat clearing, imitating motor noises, and making animal sounds are activities common among children who develop various types of hyperfunctional phonatory disorders. Although we have no systematic information about these vocal abuses in children with clefts, it is our clinical impression that we fail more often than not to find evidence of such vocal misuse. Nevertheless, the information must be sought and acted upon in those cases where it is appropriate. Speech therapy with the goal of reducing hypernasality may contribute to either hypo- or hyperfunctional disorders.

A second area that should be explored is personality and interpersonal relationships. Phonatory problems with origins in hyperfunction often occur in tense people who are loud and somewhat aggressive. Although such behaviors are not typical of children with clefts, the possibility of their existence outside the clinic should be investigated. The socially reticent, somewhat withdrawn individual may also develop voice problems, which reflect confusion about the need to communicate and the desire to remain quiet.

The third step in the phonation evaluation is to determine the nature of the deviation. We are interested in the appropriateness of vocal pitch,

TABLE 17.1 Sentences for Use in Rating Hypernasality

Sentence	Rationale
Lie low awhile	Vowels uncontaminated by nasals or pressure consonants
Mimi may mop the mall.	Vowels in nasal contexts
The big baby bought a buggy.	Voiced plosive context
Kindly give Kate a key.	Voiceless plosive context
Shelly shows her sheep.	Affricate context
Sissy sees the stars.	/s/ context, most demanding consonant of sibilant family

range, loudness, and rate, and whether the voice is hypo- or hyperfunctional.

A simple system of evaluation that includes these dimensions of voice is the voice profile suggested by Wilson (1971). Figure 17.1 presents a modification of this system. The voice profile provides the clinician with the information required to decide whether the voice is or is not defective and, if defective, what the nature of the problem is. Another approach of interest is the one by Boone (1980) and reproduced by Boone and McFarlane (1988).

Bzoch (1979), in discussing aspirate voices, which resemble our "soft-voice syndrome" and even hoarseness, recommended having the patient sustain the vowels /i/, /a/, and /u/, timing the duration of each production and deciding whether it is normal, aspirate, or hoarse. This is a commonly used technique, and Aronson (1980) considered the sustaining of /a/ to be the single most revealing voice test available. He recommended assessing quality, pitch, loudness, and steadiness using vowel prolongation. Bzoch indicated that subjects with aspirate voices are usually unable to sustain vowels for 10 seconds or more on three trials for each vowel. We are uncertain about how this should be interpreted because data presented by Wilson (1972), adapted from Launer (1971), indicated that girls cannot sustain /a/, /i/, or /u/ for 10 seconds until after age 10, whereas boys sustain vowels, on the average, for 11.4 seconds at age 9 and for only 10.4 seconds at age 10. The standard deviations for girls range from a low of 2.7 at age 11 to a high of 6.2 at age 14 and, for boys, from 4.2 at age 10 to 8.0 at age 17, when the mean is 16.9 seconds. These standard devia-

tions point to considerable variability in the data, and we obviously need to exercise caution in interpreting the duration of vowel prolongation. In addition, it may be influenced by personality characteristics.

Boone (1977) recommended having the patient sustain /s/ and /z/ and determining the length of each. Presumably, when vocal cord pathology is present, the patient may show a differential between the two with /z/ being shorter. However, Rastatter and Hyman (1982) failed to find support for that conclusion in their study of 16 children with vocal cord nodules. They found that *both* /s/ and /z/ were shorter in these children than in normals but that /z/ was longer than /s/. However, /z/ was produced with less consistency than /s/, so Boone's test is still seen as having merit.

As we indicated in Chapter 14, the phonation disorders most likely to be encountered in people with clefts or with velopharyngeal incompetence from other causes include hoarseness and strangled voice, both hyperfunctional voice disorders, and soft-voice syndrome, usually a hypofunctional problem but sometimes associated with elements of laryngeal tension.

The fourth step in the evaluation is to determine whether or not the voice can be modified. For hyperfunctional voice deviations and for pitch problems, the "um-hum" technique (Aronson, 1980) may be tried to see if this easy, natural vocal behavior brings about any change in pitch or increase in clarity. Boone (1977) and Boone and McFarlane (1988) refer to strategies of this type as "facilitating approaches" that are useful in both diagnosis and therapy. Other techniques worth trying include lowering the back of the tongue, increasing or decreasing loudness, chant talk, chewing with phonation, and coupling phonation with a yawn-sigh. We also like to place the patient in a supine position in quiet surroundings and allow him or her to lie quietly breathing in the deeper, more relaxed manner that this position encourages. After 5 or 10 minutes, we introduce very easy conversation. We do not give instructions during this time but speak quietly and gently ourselves, suggesting that this is a restful, lazy time free of all pressures. Other positional alterations may also be tried. Patients sometimes respond by reducing the amount of hyperfunction present in their phonation, which is the goal of any method used. It is important to be flexible and to try several techniques if necessary.

Boone (1977), Boone and McFarlane (1988), and Aronson (1980) discussed "digital manipulation" as a means of testing the influences of musculoskeletal tension on phonation. Aronson felt that *all* patients with voice disorders, regardless of etiology, should be so tested. The goal is to determine: (1) the extent of laryngeal elevation, a condition characteristic of vocal hyperfunction, (2) any pain in response to pressure in the laryngeal area, and (3) the extent of voice improvement following tension reduction. Aronson (1980) provided the following instructions for conducting this examination:

1. Encircle the hyoid bone with the thumb and middle finger, working posteriorly until the tips of the major horns are felt.
2. Exert light pressure with the fingers in a circular motion over the tips of the hyoid bone and ask if the patient feels pain, not just pressure. It is important to watch facial expression for signs of discomfort or pain.
3. Repeat this procedure with the fingers in the thyrohyoid space, beginning from the thyroid notch and working posteriorly.
4. Find the posterior borders for the thyroid cartilage just medial to the sternocleidomastoid muscles and repeat the procedure.
5. With the fingers over the superior borders of the thyroid cartilage, begin to work the larynx gently downward, also moving it laterally at times. Check for a lower laryngeal position by estimating the increased size of the thyrohyoid space.

As the larynx is lowered and relaxation occurs, the patient often demonstrates a dramatic change for the better in voice production. The three parts of the goal stated above are the foundation for evaluating the outcome of digital manipulation.

Attempts at modification of phonation may or may not be successful. If they are successful, therapy without other forms of treatment may reasonably be undertaken but only after the complete diagnostic study has been carried out. If the voice cannot be modified after reasonable attempts have been made, therapy would be inappropriate.

Audiological Evaluation

We recommend that an audiological evaluation be included as part of all voice examinations.

Hearing losses, usually of a conductive nature, occur more frequently in children with clefts than in those without. Conductive losses, when great enough, can be associated with a reduction in loudness as well as with variations in loudness, while sensorineural losses may be accompanied by an increase in loudness (Wilson, 1972). If hearing loss is found, the patient will, of course, be referred to an otologist before any other recommendations are made.

Otolaryngological Examination

If hoarseness or any other condition that may be accompanied by vocal cord pathology is present, it is necessary for the patient to be examined by an otolaryngologist in order to acquire definitive information about the condition of the vocal cords. When hoarseness and a cleft occur together, the chances are that the diagnosis will be bilateral vocal cord nodules or some preliminary condition such as edema or inflammation. Unless the nodules are unusually large, surgery is not likely to be recommended (Aronson, 1980; Boone, 1977; Boone and McFarlane, 1988). Rather, the preferred treatment will undoubtedly be to eliminate the vocal hyperfunction usually associated with nodules.

Instrumental Assessment of Phonation

Whenever possible, it is wise to evaluate various aspects of phonation instrumentally using instruments described in the chapters on instrumentation and voice disorders.

Since several of these evaluational techniques are applicable to both phonation and resonance, this aspect of evaluation is discussed after the diagnosis of resonance disorders has been presented.

RESONANCE DISORDERS

Assessment of Resonance

Moll (1964) made a strong case for the desirability and necessity of making listener judgments the basis of all assessments of speech, including resonance deviations. He suggested that listener judgments provide the only measures that are direct and logically valid, given the basic perceptual nature of speech, and that any instrumental approach to measuring hypernasality, if it is to be useful, must provide reliable data that are closely related to listener judgments. We are in agreement with this position but recognize with others (Bradford et al., 1964; Wells, 1971) that listeners do not always agree on the presence, absence, or amount of nasality in normal speech. The same statement applies to the assessment of other resonance disorders found in speakers with varying degrees of velopharyngeal incompetence. Several methods for assessing these problems are discussed below.

Hypernasality

Rating Scales. Obviously, the easiest and most reliable way of rating a resonance disorder, including hypernasality, is to make a decision that the problem is either present or absent. Bzoch (1979) felt that this is the only reliable decision that can be made in most cases. However, that decision, by itself, is not very useful clinically since it does not discriminate between the nasality that is environmental or idiosyncratic and the nasality that reflects an incompetent valve. The next decision that must be made, then, is whether the speech, in spite of its nasal elements, falls within a normal distribution or whether its characteristics suggest that it is pathological. In order to overcome that problem, many writers have recommended the use of scales designed to provide information about the degree of perceived hypernasality. Needless to say, the more choices listeners have, the harder it is to develop reliability. However, many studies carried out in the past have used rating scales reliably.

Sherman (1954) and Morris et al. (1973) have discussed "equal-appearing-interval" scales, usually containing five, seven, or nine points. On such scales, the uppermost point is indicative of the most severe form of hypernasality. Figure 17.2 provides examples of several different rating scales that may be used among others.

Wilson (1971) also suggested a scale for rating nasal resonance (Fig. 17.3). It follows the same general scheme used in his other scales described in the section on phonation.

Reliability in using scales of these types rests with the rater(s). Many studies have, through training listeners, reported acceptable levels of agreement among listeners (McWilliams, 1954; McWilliams and Philips, 1979). However, rating reliably remains a difficult task and one that has been approached in several different ways. Scales are most reliable when *groups* of listeners participate, and the central tendencies of the pooled ratings are used as the final ratings. This is so because of the wide variations found among raters assessing the same speech sample. This system is not an appropriate clinical tool because it is far too cumbersome, expensive, and time-consuming. A more effective technique that has been successfully used in clinics has speech pathologists first test their reliability against group ratings by listening to and independently rating speech samples previously rated by a group of listeners. They then discuss their ratings, attempting to decide what elements in the speech pattern led them to respond as they did, and gradually they reach agreement on the nature of the speech that is to be associated with a particular point on the scale. Then, if the individual clinicians doing the ratings also agree with each other and frequently reestablish their agreement, they may have confidence in their ratings. All of these steps are necessary in order to ensure that the ratings are reliable. Anyone working with patients who have velopharyngeal incompetence should routinely collect data on interjudge agreement and should establish clinical protocols to ensure that this important aspect is not neglected.

In the clinic at the University of Pittsburgh, all borderline decisions are arrived at by comparing the assessments of two and sometimes three speech pathologists. A promising technique to increase the reliability of ratings is the use of time-expanded speech judgments. Leeper et al. (1980) found that listeners rated hypernasality more severely and slightly more reliably as time expansion increased. This technique may be particularly useful in listening and rating training.

McWilliams and Philips (1979) developed a series of training audiotapes that may be used to help listeners learn to make reliable judgments about hypernasality as well as about other speech attributes discussed throughout this book.

The *validity* of rating scales is also a matter of concern. Listeners have difficulty separating hypernasality from the other speech characteristics associated with velopharyngeal incompetence. The more "other" symptoms, the higher, the ratings of nasality (McWilliams, 1954). Thus, it seems that raters, in reality, rate their global perceptions and are not able to rate the single element of nasality. This always means that ratings, even those on which listeners agree, may be invalid.

Name _____ Birth Date _____ Age _____ Date _____

Severity of Problem:

Normal	Mild		Moderate		Severe	
1	2	3	4	5	6	7

Length of sustained *Ah* in seconds: _____

Deviations in sustained Ah: _____ Tremor; _____ Breaks; _____ Variations in loudness, _____ Pitch, _____ Quality, _____ Steadiness, _____ Other.

Describe deviations: _____

Intensity:
Soft	Normal	Loud
−2	1	+2

Range:
Monotone	Normal	Variable
−2	1	+2

Rate: _____ Constant _____ Variable
Slow	Normal	Fast
−2	1	+2

Pitch:
Low		Normal	High	
−3*	−2	1	+2	+3**

* A female loses sexual identity. ** A males loses sexual identity.

Vocal Cord Function:

Open	Partially open	Cords hypo-adducted	Normal	Cords hyper-adducted	Cords closed
−4	−3	−2	1	+2	+3

Aphonia	Little voice	Breathiness	Tense voice	Spastic dysphonia
−4	−3	−2	+2	+3

Figure 17.1 Evaluation of phonation (a modification of the system suggested by Wilson, 1971.)

A. Resonance: _____ Normal _____ Abnormal

B. If abnormal, is speech excessively _____ Hypernasal; _____ Hyponasal; _____ Both?

C. Four-Point, Equal-Appearing-Intervals Scale for Rating Hypernasality:

	Hypernasality		
1	2	3	4
Normal	Mild	Moderate	Severe

D. Seven-Point, Equal-Appearing-Intervals Scale for Rating Degrees of Nasality:

Within Normal Range Nasality			Hypernasality			
1	2	3	4	5	6	7
Low	Moderate	High	Mild	Moderate	Severe	Very Severe

E. Another Version of a Seven-Point Scale Emphasizing Hypernasality:

Normal	Hypernasality					
	Mild		Moderate		Severe	
1	2	3	4	5	6	7

F. An Eight-Point Scale for Rating Nasal Resonance:

Hypo-nasality	Normal	Hypernasality					
		Mild		Moderate		Severe	
−1	0	1	2	3	4	5	6

G. Scale for Rating Hyponasality:

Hyponasality _____ Absent; _____ Present.

Mild	Moderate	Severe
1	2	3
Nasals lose minimal nasal character.	Nasals lose greater nasal character.	Nasal character absent.

H. Indication of cul-de-sac resonance: Left Nostril: _____ Absent; _____Present.

Right Nostril: _____ Absent; _____Present.

I. Indication of combined hypo-hypernasality: _____ Present; _____ Absent.

Figure 17.2 Methods of rating resonance.

Sherman (1954) theorized that ratings of nasality might be more nearly valid and more reliable if the contaminating cues were eliminated by playing audiotapes backward and having judges rate nasality under that condition. Her hypothesis that backward play would yield more reliable results than forward play was not borne out. However, Sherman concluded that there was evidence that backward play may have greater validity than forward play because certain irrelevant factors are removed from the stimulus material to which the listeners respond, and the spread along the continuum is increased.

Black (1973) showed, however, that backward play of speech alters some characteristics of the signal to a greater extent than it does others. Of interest in the assessment of hypernasality is the finding that vowels are changed more than are such consonants as /k,z,r,s,ʃ/. All but the /r/ are elements of extreme importance when velopharyngeal competence is a factor. In addition, frication was identifiable on backward play. These findings suggested that the backward play of speech samples may be questionable in the rating of hypernasality, and this was the conclusion of Fletcher (1976) as well.

There is modest evidence that speech rated from tape recordings may, in some cases, lead to somewhat different conclusions from those achieved from live ratings (McWilliams and Phil-

Hypernasal

+4 Gereralized nasality with consonant impairment

+3 Nasalization of vowels (consonants may be *slightly* impaired)

+2 Assimilative nasality

1 Normal

−2 Hyponasality

Hyponasal

Figure 17.3 The Wilson scale for rating characteristics of the resonating cavity.

ips, 1979). Thus, if taped samples are to be used for rating hypernasality, it is wise to have data from live ratings as well. If the two do not agree, additional evaluations are in order since questions of validity arise.

The problem of rating hypernasality as a single entity persists. Bzoch (1979), as noted earlier, stated that hypernasality can be reliably rated *only* under conditions of clear phonation and normal articulation. We agree that those conditions make the task easier, but the clinical reality is that hypernasality is one of several characteristics associated with velopharyngeal incompetence, and we have to continue our efforts to make valid and reliable judgments concerning it. Bzoch also recognized this need.

In our view, a rating scale is a useful device provided reliability is consistently monitored and provided speech is heard in a variety of contexts ranging from a sentence containing neither high-pressure consonants nor nasals through one loaded with sibilants. Table 17.1 provides sample sentences and the rationale for each. Note that there is nothing sacred about these particular combinations of words and that other writers suggest other tasks, such as counting from 60 to 100. Concentrate on vowels in these short speech samples and then listen in the same way to conversational speech. Try to discern the influence of consonant context. To begin with, you may wish to experiment with a 4-point scale for rating hypernasality as shown in Figure 17.2. From there, you can move into the expanded scales also shown to provide for more variations in the speech patterns you are rating. Always carry out ratings so that reliability is provided for.

Cul-de-Sac Test. Bzoch (1979) reported an old approach to assessing hypernasality, referring to it as the cul-de-sac test, which he considered the best procedure in a clinical setting. The test, simply stated, is the alternate compressing and releasing of the nares during speech and listening for a shift in resonance when the nares are occluded. If hypernasality is present when the nares are unoccluded, a shift to cul-de-sac resonance will be heard. The short test used by Bzoch is reproduced in Figure 17.4. Ten words or ten vowels are tested. If a shift occurs, the word or vowel is circled. The ratio that eventually emerges provides an index of hypernasality. If all ten words demonstrate a shift, the ratio would be 10:10; if a shift occurs on only two of ten words, the ratio would be expressed as 2:10. Presumably, higher ratios are associated with more consistent or greater degrees of hypernasality. Others ask patients to sustain various vowels while their nostrils are alternately compressed and released. The test is invalidated if hyponasality is present with or without hypernasality or if cul-de-sac resonance is already a characteristic of the speech being tested.

In our clinical experience, we use the cul-de-sac test but do not always find it useful, especially for small children, who sometimes demonstrate a shift even though they do not sound hypernasal in conversational speech and have no unusual behaviors that would tend to invalidate the test. In addition, some children are deeply embarrassed by the procedure. For these reasons, we view the test as one that is sometimes useful but cannot always be relied upon to provide valid data.

Other Resonance Disorders

As was shown in the section on hypernasality, a number of suggested scales rate resonance on a continuum. Our preference is to rate hyperna-

Ask patient to repeat word or vowel with nostrils open and again with nares pinched. Circle words or vowels on which a shift in resonance is heard under the second condition.

A. beet bit bait bet bat
  bought boat boot but Bert

B. /i/ /u/ /i/ /u/ /i/ /u/ /i/ /u/ /i/ /u/
 (Vowel sample recommended for speakers with verbal limitations)

Figure 17.4 The cul-de-sac test for hypernasality (after Bzoch, 1979).

sality separately and then to indicate the presence or absence of other possible features. Figure 17.2 illustrates this approach. Hyponasality, if present, can be rated on a 3-point scale, while cul-de-sac resonance and combined hypo-hypernasality can be evaluated as present or absent. Any person with the latter combination will already have been rated on the two resonance characteristics, and the severity of the cul-de-sac attribute will be reflected in the ratings of hyponasality. It is important to understand that cul-de-sac resonance reflects hypo- or denasality. It is of interest to test the two nostrils separately, since our goal is to determine as much as possible about the characteristics of the nasal resonating system.

INSTRUMENTAL DATA REGARDING PHONATION AND RESONANCE PROBLEMS

It is useful, when possible, to collect objective data about the phonation and resonance deviations that have been identified by perceptual means. Since there is such a close relationship between phonation and resonance disorders in an interactive system influenced by the integrity of the velopharyngeal valve, information derived from different instruments is also interactive. Chapters 11 and 14 discuss some of the available instruments.

As we have seen, respiration is influenced by velopharyngeal incompetence, and it is often helpful to have instrumental evidence of certain aspects of respiration. Boone and McFarlane (1988) present a succint discussion of this topic. They recommend use of the dry spirometer to determine vital capacity, tidal volume, inspiratory reserve, and expiratory reserve. In our own clinics, we often rely on the Respiration Laboratory for determining these measurements on the assumption that experienced technicians who do little else will provide the most reliable data.

Boone and McFarlane also discuss the use of air-flow measurements to determine the volume of air that passes through the glottis in a given period of time. They note that the hypofunctional voice is produced with high flow rates, whereas the hyperfunctional voice is associated with reduced flow rates. They view the Phonatory Function Analyzer and devices incorporating pneumotachometers as useful for deriving this type of information. We routinely utilize pneumotachometers, and these have already been discussed.

As we have seen, pneumotachometers are useful also in determining air-flow pressures and

in indicating discrepancies between oral and nasal measurements. Estimates of the size of the velopharyngeal portal can then be derived. This latter information is of value since both phonation and resonance disorders are associated with inadequate velopharyngeal valving. Of added value are measurements of nasal resistance.

The Visi-Pitch may be used when differences in pitch, loudness, or quality are suspected. The sound spectrograph is also applicable. The electroglottograph mentioned earlier is clinically useful when phonatory variations are perceived. We like to use the instrument when hypernasality is heard even though phonatory variations are not notable. It will often demonstrate that laryngeal adjustments are occurring simultaneously, and this information strengthens the case for clinical management of borderline valving mechanisms.

Tonar and the new Nasometer are also instruments that can be of value in substantiating clinical impressions of resonance disorders. It is likely also that accelerometers will be used with increasing frequency in clinical situations where more sophisticated instruments are not available.

Viewing the larynx by means of the endoscope or stroboscope is of infinite value, since it enables the clinician to observe the characteristics and function of the larynx. Neither of these instruments, however, is a substitute for the others designed to measure specific attributes of speech physiology or of the speech signal.

Related to the instrumental assessment of phonation, the larynx, and resonance is the evaluation of the velopharyngeal valve, which should always be assessed when phonation or resonance problems are noted. This is discussed in detail in Chapters 11 and 19.

INTEGRATION AND INTERPRETATION OF DIAGNOSTIC INFORMATION ABOUT PHONATION AND RESONANCE

Clinical decision making is based largely on the nature and severity of the problem and the potential for a given treatment to be successful in light of underlying etiological factors. Decisions vary from patient to patient and are sometimes influenced by conditions other than the defect itself.

The first step in the process is to decide about the significance of the phonation or resonance problem, or both, in the life of the patient. If the deficit is not associated with pathology that is of concern, if it is so mild as to be almost imperceptible to all but trained listeners, if it is not distressing to the patient and family, and if future goals are unlikely to be affected by the problem, the decision might be not to intervene but instead to watch and wait.

For example, some boys with mild hoarseness, mild hypernasality, or both, may sound better after voice change with puberty. Others may sound worse, and some type of intervention becomes mandatory. All in this group should be taught the nature of vocal hyperfunction, and a program of vocal hygiene should be initiated (Cooper, 1977; Wilson, 1987; Boone and McFarlane, 1988).

On the other hand, some children with interests in dramatics, public speaking, or other careers involving extensive use of the voice, or those with high overall aspirations may, in the presence of mild phonation or resonance symptoms or both, want and require correction of the velopharyngeal valving mechanism and subsequent speech therapy if it is needed.

Individuals with more obvious phonation and resonance deviations should have treatment regardless of their goals and aspirations, provided of course that they are willing.

The presence of hyponasality, cul-de-sac resonance, or a combination of hyper-hyponasality points to increased nasal resistance, often in conjunction with velopharyngeal incompetence. Under all of these conditions, the first recommendation would be to assess the nasal airway and to correct it if possible. After that, it is then necessary to reassess phonation, nasal resonance, and velopharyngeal valving to arrive at a new list of treatment priorities.

Because phonation and resonance problems in patients with clefts, especially in the presence of velopharyngeal incompetence, are complex both in origin and in the systemic interactions which are likely, we warn against speech therapy applied in the absence of the diagnostic data described.

REFERENCES

Aronson AE. Clinical voice disorders. New York: Thieme-Stratton, 1980.

Black JW. The phonemic content of backward-reproduced speech. J Speech Hear Res 1973; 16:165.

Boone DR. The voice and voice therapy. Englewood Cliffs, NJ: Prentice-Hall, 1977.

Boone DR. The Boone voice program for children. Tigard, OR: CC Publications, 1980.

Boone DR. The voice and voice therapy. 3rd ed. Englewood Cliffs, NJ: Prentice-Hall, 1983.

Boone DR, McFarlane S. The voice and voice therapy. 4th ed. Englewood Cliffs, NJ: Prentice-Hall, 1988.

Bradford LF, Brooks AR, Shelton RL. Clinical judgment of hypernasality in cleft palate children. Cleft Palate J 1964; 1:329.

Bzoch KR. Communicative disorders related to cleft lip and palate. 2nd ed. Boston: Little, Brown, 1979.

Cooper M, Cooper MH. Approaches to vocal rehabilitation. Springfield, IL: CC Thomas, 1977.

Fletcher SG. "Nasalance" vs. listener judgments of nasality. Cleft Palate J 1976; 13:31.

Launer PG. Maximum phonation time in children. Unpublished Master's thesis. State University of New York at Buffalo, 1971.

Leeper HA, Nieuwesteeg Y, Bishop L, Lass NJ, Beckwith S. The use of time-expanded speech in judgments of hypernasality. J Commun Dis 1980; 13:335.

McWilliams BJ. Some factors in the intelligibility of cleft palate speech. J Speech Hear Dis 1954; 19:524.

McWilliams BJ, Philips BJ. Velopharyngeal incompetence. Audio Seminars in Speech Pathology. Philadelphia: WB Saunders, 1979.

Moll KL. "Objective" measures of nasality. Cleft Palate J 1964; 1:371.

Morris HL, Shelton RL, McWilliams BJ. Assessment of speech. In: Speech, language, and psychosocial aspects of cleft lip and cleft palate: the state of the art. ASHA Reports, No. 9, 1973.

Rastatter MP, Hyman M. Maximum phoneme duration of /s/ and /z/ by children with vocal nodules. Lang Speech Hear Serv Schools 1982; 13:197.

Sherman D. The merits of backward playing of connected speech in the scaling of voice quality disorders. J Speech Hearing Dis 1954; 19:312.

Wells CG. Cleft Palate and its associated speech disorders. New York: McGraw-Hall, 1971.

Wilson FB. The voice-disordered child. Lang Speech Hear Serv Schools 1971; 2:14.

Wilson DK. Voice problems of children. Baltimore: Williams & Wilkins, 1972, 1979, 1987.

18 | EVALUATION OF ARTICULATION AND PHONOLOGICAL DISORDERS

Although we are considering the evaluation of language, voice, articulation, and the velopharyngeal mechanism each separately, they are closely interrelated. Information from these several components of the overall evaluation must be taken into account in planning a complete treatment program for the patient. Furthermore, the evaluation of the patient is an interdisciplinary effort, and findings contributed by all team members will be used in planning comprehensive service for the patient. The speech pathologist must know about dental, surgical, and other services received by the patient and, certainly, plans for the future. As indicated by Van Demark et al. (1985) and others, evaluation of the relationship between speech and the velopharyngeal mechanism should include a case history, an orofacial examination, and evaluation of articulation and voice quality, including nasality. The findings then contribute to decision making relative to speech therapy and to dental and surgical treatments.

We turn now to the study of the patient's articulation and phonological patterns. Since language, voice, articulation, and velopharyngeal valving are interdependent, information about speech is useful in determining whether patients with cleft palate have velopharyngeal competence, borderline competence, or incompetence. Patients in all of these categories may misarticulate, and decisions about possible articulation therapy require a broad spectrum of information, one aspect of which is knowledge of velopharyngeal status. Patients will differ in their articulation and

phonological patterns, in their treatment needs, and in their response to articulation training. In order to know how best to improve speech, careful evaluation of articulation is imperative. The procedures recommended have much in common with procedures used for articulation and phonological disorders in general, but velopharyngeal disability, oronasal fistulas, maxillary arch collapse, and other physical differences motivate articulatory compensations. Consequently, special attention must be given to how velopharyngeal and other orofacial structures function in speech production.

In this chapter, *speech sound* is used to refer to the speech segments around which evaluation and treatment may be organized. *Speech sound* may refer either to a family of sounds or to a particular sound. The terms *phoneme* and *phone* are also sometimes used. However, *phoneme* is more properly used to refer to an abstract linguistic category (Dinnsen, 1984) rather than to something articulated. *Phone* implies close attention to physiological and acoustical detail. Neither term quite fits the meanings often intended by the speech pathologist.

ARTICULATION TESTING

Bernthal and Bankson (1988) described a four-component battery for study of an individual's speech: articulation tests or inventories, contextual or deep tests, stimulability tests, and connected speech samples. Such a sample represents the patient's speech under different speaking and stimulus conditions. Articulation testing serves various purposes including determination of ability to produce sounds, identification of the relationship between articulation and the speech mechanism that determines the need for altering the mechanism, planning therapy, and evaluating articulation change following any intervention, including speech therapy. The speech sample is studied to obtain information about the child's phonological patterns and production of phonemic contrasts. Additional evaluation purposes will be cited as we progress.

Articulation is usually tested perceptually by listening to and evaluating the individual's speech, and that is the focus here. However, the speech pathologist sometimes uses instrumental analysis of articulation to obtain additional valuable clinical information. (Weismer, 1984). For example, Daniloff et al. (1980) differentiated frontal, lateral, and retracted /s/ distortions by spectrographic analysis.

Speech sounds may be sampled systematically in different contexts and studied under different stimulus conditions such as imitation, picture naming, and reading. Sounds of interest may be assessed in different units including isolation, syllables, words, phrases, sentences, and conversation. Through development of about the first 50 words, children's speech is thought to be organized in word-sized units. As the child's speech becomes more complex, a shift is made to an organization based on systematic sequencing of speech sounds (Schwartz, 1984). The articulation of sounds of interest may be classed as correct or incorrect, scored as substitutions, omissions, distortions, additions, and correct responses, or narrowly transcribed using diacritic symbols to indicate the nature of the misarticulation. In the past few years the field has moved toward much greater use of narrow transcription. The choice of tests and sampling procedures is determined by questions the clinician wishes to answer. For example, does the patient have an articulation or phonological disorder and if so, what is its pattern? Do existing articulation errors reflect velopharyngeal incompetence? Is the patient's misarticulation of sounds from different phonemes consistent or inconsistent? Is the patient stimulable, that is, can correct responses be elicited through imitation or instruction? Do the sound errors fall into patterns that suggest a phonological component to the problem that

should be taken into account to plan efficient therapy? What changes may be expected in the patient's articulation in the future, either with or without some form of intervention? Logemann (1983) recommended giving careful consideration to the child's past and present use of speech at home. Certainly we want to know what concerns the parents, the patient, or both.

Published articulation tests usually consist of stimulus materials for eliciting responses, instructions for administering the test, score sheets for recording evaluations of responses, and information for use in interpreting the responses. However, regardless of the test used, the interaction between the examiner and the patient and the examiner's analysis of the results obtained are critical parts of articulation testing. Articulation tests are valuable if they are used skillfully and cautiously, but they have limitations. While articulation tests are constructed to elicit speech samples that reflect the patient's conversational speech in important ways, the test results are not always representative of articulation in spontaneous speech (Noll, 1970). Shriberg and Kwiatkowski (1982) stated that five articulation tests they had reviewed did not provide adequate sampling of syllable shapes, parts of speech, or morphophonemic markers such as /s-z/ used to signify plurals. For these reasons, test results should be supplemented by recording narrow transcription and analysis of the patient's connected speech.

Winitz (1969) reminded us that the marks we enter on articulation score sheets represent what is in the evaluator's ear or head as well as that which was in the child's mouth. The child may be variable in articulation, and some of that variability may be attributable to interaction between examiner and patient. Similarly, the examiner may be variable in listening or may be unreliable in the decisions he or she makes—at least, some of the time.

Articulation Tests

A number of articulation tests are available for use with all types of patients including those with cleft palate. Some serve a screening function; some are termed diagnostic tests; and some have other special purposes. For example, the Templin-Darley Tests of Articulation (1969) include a 50-item screening test that is used to identify speakers who are in need of more thorough testing as well as a 176-item diagnostic test for more detailed assessment of articulation. From the data collected, the clinician can extract various kinds of information including the consistency with which /s/, /r/, and /l/ are misarticulated. These sounds are at high risk for misarticulation in both those who are physically normal and those who have orofacial abnormalities. The Iowa Pressure Articulation Test, which is used with cleft palate patients or others suspected of having velopharyngeal incompetence, is part of the Templin-Darley, and is described later in this chapter. Paynter (1984) published norms for Spanish-speaking, Mexican-American children imitating words in English from the Templin-Darley Screening Test of Articulation and from the Iowa Pressure Articulation Test.

Among other frequently used articulation tests are the Goldman-Fristoe Articulation Test (1986), the Fisher-Logemann Test of Articulation Competence (1971), and the McDonald Deep Tests of Articulation (1964). The Goldman-Fristoe samples consonant sounds under several stimulus conditions, one of which is story-retelling. Short stories, accompanied by pictures, are read to the child, who is asked to retell the stories with the aid of the pictures. The result is a sample of connected speech that contains consonants of interest. The test also examines consonants in words elicited by naming pictures and in syllables, words, and sentences repeated after the examiner. The Fisher-Logemann Test is distinguished by a system of pattern analysis that utilizes place of articulation, manner of articulation, and voicing features. McDonald (1964) developed tests to sample the patient's articulation of sounds in many contexts in order to discover contexts in which a child correctly produces sounds that are usually misarticulated.

McDonald referred to these tests as deep tests because they sampled speech sounds many times in many environments in a systematic manner. The items in these tests, which take the form of juxtaposed words such as "sheep chain" and "tub sun," sample abutting contexts in a systematic manner even though that combination may not occur in common usage. Items for articulation deep testing may be drawn from drill books that organize sounds according to such variables as context, syllable shape, and stress (Pendergast, 1971; Griffith and Miner, 1979). Also, conversational samples should be studied. In fact, Winitz (1975) recommended that articula-tion testing begin with conversation. Some sounds occur much more frequently in English than do others; conversational sampling may demand stimuli that will encourage the repeated use of less frequently occurring sounds. Correct and incorrect productions of target sounds are then tallied, and a record is kept of specific articulatory details of interest. A tape recorder is helpful, although it should be recognized that slight distortions may be obscured by the tape and that normally-produced sounds may sometimes sound distorted. Use of the recording allows two or more clinicians to evaluate the same responses for purposes of determining their agreement. To meet contemporary standards, information about a specific test should be available, preferably in the test manual. Information is needed about rationale, construction, administration, reliability, validity, and interpretation of results, and probably some other variables as well.

Special Articulation Tests for Patients with Cleft Palate

The Iowa Pressure Articulation Test (IPAT), which is included in the Templin-Darley Tests of Articulation, is composed of 43 fricative, plosive, and affricative sounds identified by Morris et al. (1961) and by others as likely to be misarticulated by persons with poor velopharyngeal closure. That is, the test emphasizes sounds that require the impounding of oral air pressure and is used to identify people who fail to produce velopharyngeal closure adequate for speech. Children with nasal leakage would score poorly on this test as would those who misarticulate sounds from many phonemes for reasons other than velopharyngeal dysfunction. However, children who fail the IPAT because of velopharyngeal dysfunction are likely to produce unique error types that involve nasal emission, lack of oral pressure, and gross substitutions (see Chapter 15 for further discussion). Thus, observations of error type are even more important than test score for differentiating between the disordered articulation associated with past or present velopharyngeal dysfunction and that associated with other origins and patterns. This same statement applies to the results of any articulation test selected.

Van Demark and Swickard (1980) noted that the IPAT contains many consonants that are not developed by 3 and 4 years of age. They concluded that there was a need for a pressure articulation test suitable for use with 3- and 4-year-olds, and suggested a test that emphasized /p/ and /b/ sounds. Those sounds are acquired early, and previous work by Van Demark (1979) had indicated that these sounds had been found useful in discriminating between young children who eventually required secondary palatal surgery and those who did not. The authors developed a set of words and corresponding pictures that were recognized and named by most of the normal children who were studied. Also, these normal children articulated most of the test sounds correctly. This test is directed to the identification of velopharyngeal insufficiency. An individual who fails the test because of reduced intraoral pressure is likely to have velopharyngeal insufficiency. If he fails the test because he does not produce /p/ and /b/, the results are not necessarily indicative of velopharyngeal insufficiency. The person who passes the test may, nonetheless, have nasal air leakage during the production of more demanding speech sounds such as sibilants. Thus, this test can undoubtedly identify children with gross valving problems but may fail to isolate those with marginal incompetence. Obviously, the clinician can informally assess the production of many words containing /p/ and /b/.

Bzoch (1979) constructed an articulation test, for use with patients with cleft palate, which stresses type of articulation error. Its scoring system distinguishes among five articulation error types: nasal emission, distortion, simple substitution, gross substitution, and omission. These errors are considered to fall on a severity continuum in the order presented above with omission representing the most severe type of misarticulation. The test samples fricatives, affricates, and plosives, the sound classes that children with cleft palates are most likely to misarticulate. Bzoch recommended that the clinician administering this test observe the patient's speech visually as well as auditorily. The screening form of the test is shown in Figure 18.1.

The analysis of a conversational sample is essential to a thorough understanding of the articulatory behavior of people with clefts. There are many reasons for variations in articulatory performance between test and conversational conditions. In some cases, the careful articulation of single words or of cued sentences is not possible under the demands of connected discourse. In other cases, improved articulation is possible in conversational contexts, but has not become automatic. The articulation test, therefore, is only one step in assessing articulation.

SOUND ELEMENTS	PLOSIVES	C	I	D	SS	GS	O
/p/	aPPle						
/b/	baBy						
/t/	mounTain						
/d/	canDy						
/k/	chicKen						
/g/	waGon						
	FRICATIVES						
/f/	elePHant						
/v/	shoVel						
/θ/	tooTHbrush						
/ð/	feaTHer						
/s/	biCycle						
/z/	sciSSors						
/ʃ/	diSHes						
	AFFRICATES						
/tʃ/	maTCHes						
/dʒ/	briDGes						
	GLIDES						
/w/	sandWich						
/l/	baLLoons						
/j/	onIons						
/r/	aRRow						
	NASALS						
/m/	haMMer						
/n/	baNana						
/ŋ/	haNGer						
	BLENDS						
/sp/	SPider						
/st/	STar						
/sk/	SKirt						
/sm/	SMoke						
/bl/	BLock						
/kl/	CLown						
/br/	BRoom						
/str/	STRawberries						

ERROR SCORE_____ /30 GS Pattern: Yes___ No___

Figure 18.1 Bzoch Articulation Screening Test.

Scoring the Responses

Scoring articulation responses as correct or incorrect provides only a gross description of speech and offers little help in the consideration of velopharyngeal disability. Classification of errors as substitutions, omissions, and distortions adds little more information.

McWilliams (1979) advised a detailed analysis of each error sound including place and manner of articulation and presence of nasal escape whether visible, audible, or both. Shriberg and Kent (1982) presented a transcription system and taped samples useful in transcribing the speech of patients with cleft palate. Diacritics may be used to indicate the occurrence of nasalization, audible nasal escape, and weak consonants or reduced oral air pressure or intensity. Trost (1981) recommended symbols for compensatory articulations that she identified and described and that have been reviewed in Chapter 15. Additional symbols for articulatory descriptions are provided by Pullum and Ladusaw (1966) (see Fig. 15.2). Listener agreement about narrow transcription is probably poorer than for right-wrong scoring, but more information is obtained. Speech sampling should continue until the clinician has a clear idea of the nature of sound distortions in the patient's speech. Acoustical and aerodynamic analyses of responses can supplement the speech pathologist's ear. Inaudible nasal emission may be detected with a cold mirror; its quantification, like that of audible nasal emission, requires a flow meter.

The clinician scoring articulation responses must first decide whether a particular response was correct or incorrect. If the response was incorrect, the nature of the error should be determined or estimated and transcribed. The speech pathologist may supplement response classification and transcription with descriptions of how the speech mechanism is used in the production of sounds. Examples of possible observations include incomplete bilabial closure, tongue tip deflected into spaces created by missing or misplaced teeth or maxillary collapse, placement of the tongue within or outside the maxillary arch and in or out of contact with lateral teeth for coronal sounds, unusual adjustments of the mandible, or posterior tongue placement for anterior consonants. In short, the articulation errors of subjects with cleft palate should be detailed as thoroughly—and as reliably—as possible. Dental distortions should be delineated, gross substitutions described, and nasalization identified. McWilliams and Philips (1989) urge that inaudible but measureable visible nasal emission be detected. Logemann (1983) recommended giv-

ing special attention to place of articulation and site of oral pathology. She would identify the child's use of various places and manners of articulation with specific interest in tongue movement and size relative to the height and width of the maxilla. Van Demark et al. (1985) recommended study of diadochokinesis (syllable repetition rate) as an index to speech motor control, and they recommend checking for deterioration of articulation, voice, or both with fatigue or stress.

Sometimes clinicians ask patients to repeat responses to allow the clinician additional opportunity for listening, watching, and feeling. A repetition of a questionable response may differ from the original response, and that kind of inconsistency should be noted if possible. The repetition may be better or worse than the original response. Sometimes more deliberate production following a request for repetition results in improved articulation, but it can also result in an excessively forceful and, hence, distorted production. Tests, stimulability techniques, and conversational sampling provide the means to obtain a speech sample from which the individual's sound patterns and capabilities can be identified.

Examiner Reliability and its Clinical Significance

Reliability in articulation testing is an important concern of speech pathologists. Precautions must be taken to ensure that the same standards for evaluation of the response be used from one examination and from one examiner to another. Concern about reliability should extend beyond item agreement to the results of pattern analysis that is conducted after the articulation responses have been obtained from the patient.

Studies with cleft subjects have indicated that the identification of the type of error is considerably less reliable than is scoring the response as correct or incorrect (Philips and Bzoch, 1969; Bzoch, 1979). Articulation judgments of /s/ made from tapes are less likely to be reliable than are live judgments (Stephens and Daniloff, 1977).

The reliability of the ratings of the speech of patients with clefts has also been studied. Moller and Starr (1984) compared speech ratings obtained under three listening conditions: face-to-face with the patient, observing via a mirror and sound system, and listening to tape recordings.

The study was motivated by evidence that data obtained by individual observers sometimes lack reliability. Speech samples from one hundred consecutive patients (age range 2 to 42 years) were rated on eight-point scales for intelligibility, resonance distortion, articulation deviation, voice deviation, and overall speech acceptability. Multiple listeners, including graduate students and speech pathologists, participated. Each underwent listening training. For each measure, data obtained from students correlated highly with that obtained from speech pathologists (for articulation, $r = 0.92$). The speech sample included two or more minutes of conversation, a standard paragraph, selected sentences, counting to ten, and sustained /i/ and /a/ vowels. The authors found no statistically significant difference among the three listening conditions for any measure except voice. They questioned whether a single rating can successfully represent voice quality, which is multidimensional. Speech ratings made by panels of observers trained for the task constitute good data for use in study of patients with cleft palate. There is the difficulty, however, in reliable distinction between oral and nasal distortion from tape-recorded samples.

The determination of tester reliability for research purposes is done in a number of ways. One involves computation of correlation coefficients based on total test scores. If total articulation scores obtained through testing done by two examiners are similar, the resulting correlation will be high, and reliability will appear to be adequate. However, total score agreement can mask disagreements on particular test sounds. Consequently, agreement between observers is often expressed as a percentage of agreement based on an item-by-item analysis. Again, item agreement tends to be lower when the examiners must determine the exact nature of the error than it is when the judgment is only whether the sound is correct or incorrect.

A distinction has been drawn between agreement among observers on all test items (speech sounds) under consideration and observer agreement regarding responses that occur infrequently. For example, agreement may be high on clearly correct or grossly distorted responses but marginal on marginal responses (Byrne et al., 1961). McReynolds and Kearns (1983) and Kearns and Simmons (1988) recommend that observer agreement be identified for the infrequently-occurring responses and that the agreement be tested to determine whether it exceeds that which would be expected on the basis of chance.

Articulation tests are usually administered in a clinic by one examiner rather than by several. Reliability is an issue in this solo testing. The clinician can improve the reliability of his or her articulation testing by recognizing several problems such as anchoring and sequencing effects (Young, 1970). *Anchors* are the standards against which responses are to be judged. In psychophysical scaling, test responses may be compared with a recorded standard. Clinically, the standard is likely to be in the examiner's head, that is, remembered from previous experience. The clinician should strive to maintain a consistent standard or at least to be aware of a shift in the standard against which a patient's articulation is evaluated. For example, when beginning therapy with a patient who severely misarticulates a unit to be trained, the clinician may utilize a lenient standard of acceptability. Then, as articulation improves, the clinician may shift to a more stringent criterion. If this occurs without anyone's knowledge, judgments of articulation made at different times are confounded. It is possible that a shift in criterion could interfere with the patient's response to therapy even if the shift were not recognized by the patient. Such unknown changes in criterion quickly decrease reliability.

Sequencing is the interacting influence of neighboring items. Whether a given sound production is scored as correct or incorrect may be a function of neighboring sounds. If the /s/ sound in a test word follows a very well articulated /s/ in a previous word, the second /s/ might be scored as incorrect, whereas the same response might be scored as correct if it occurred after a poorly articulated /s/. On the other hand, there may also be a tendency to score all productions of a given sound consistent with the scoring on the first production.

We think that the effects of anchoring and sequencing can be tempered by the instructions examiners give themselves. For example, they may arbitrarily decide to score marginal or questionable responses as incorrect. This instruction would be expected to reduce the occurrence of sequencing effects, but it would do so at the cost of sensitivity to marginal articulation which might well be acceptable. Again, the clinician may instruct himself or herself to categorize a response as correct or incorrect and then, if possible, to specify additional information: correct but slightly dentalized; incorrect because of lateral emission; correct in place of articulation but accompanied by audible nasal emission.

Sometimes comparison of articulation judgments by two speech pathologists will show that examiner disagreement was of a semantic rather than a perceptual nature. The two examiners may agree, for example, that the /s/ sounds are slightly dentalized but are free from tongue protrusion. However, one examiner chose to accept those responses as correct, whereas the other classified them as incorrect. Some sounds, particularly sibilants, can be produced with a wide range of behaviors. Judges may have poor item-by-item agreement and yet agree that a certain sound was sometimes correctly articulated and sometimes misarticulated. Disagreement will often involve sounds that fall on or near the boundary between acceptability and unacceptability.

Articulation deep testing and articulation therapy both require the clinician to evaluate a speech sound as it occurs in a series of words or other units. Repeated listening to the same stimulus, and perhaps to very similar stimuli, has been found to result in alterations in perception. This applies to articulation testing in that it has been demonstrated that some persons evaluating repeated productions of a particular consonant classify some as correct and some as incorrect when, unknown to them, they are listening to dubbings of a single utterance (Shelton et al., 1974; Ruscello et al., 1980). When informed of the deception, some listeners express the conviction that the articulation of the target sound differed in correctness from one time to another. Our ears can play tricks on us in different ways. Diedrich and Bangert (1980) found that clinicians who have provided training to misarticulating children are more likely to hear improvement in the articulation of those children than are other clinicians who are equally qualified but who do not know the children. We assume that bias is involved in this occurrence.

The emphasis on correlations between test scores obtained by different examiners and item-by-item percentage of agreement ignores the extent to which different clinicians arrive at similar impressions about the patient's speech and clinical needs. Nasal emission is not necessarily evident on each and every sound. Item-by-item agreement should be supplemented by information about agreement on such things as the presence *at times* of either visible or audible nasal emission. If the two clinicians do not make similar treatment recommendations, they either do not hear the speech the same way or they endorse different treatment rationales. Such differences may be discussed and resolved.

Clinicians may improve interobserver reliability by analyzing live speech samples that are also recorded for repeated study. The recording is used as a referent, and disagreements are discussed and, when possible, resolved.

Validity

Criteria stated in Standards for Educational and Psychological Tests (1985) require that test developers consider validity as well as reliability. Test results can be highly reliable but wrong. Different sorts of validity should be established. It is not sufficient that an articulation test be composed of a set of items that make sense to the test author. Rather it must be demonstrated that clinical decisions based on the test result are appropriate for the patient. A test with predictive validity would allow the clinician to predict the patient's future articulation behavior including response to treatment.

In a sense, articulation is an abstraction, a theoretical construct. Some speech pathologists think of disordered articulation primarily in phonetic terms and some in phonological terms. To the extent that an articulation test is based on a theoretical conceptualization of articulation, test results should be compatible with the theory on which the test was based. Evidence of this sort provides construct validity. Predictive and construct validity are difficult to establish. To the extent that articulation testing has validity, it resides in the expertness of the individual clinician rather than in the test product.

McCauley and Swisher (1984) described a distinction between obtained test scores and estimated true scores. When test reliability data and confidence intervals are utilized, a test score may be interpreted as an index to an estimated true score that could be expected to fall within specified limits at a selected probability level.

McReynolds and Kearns (1983) discussed the social validation not of tests but of experiments. This validity is concerned with whether the results of experimental treatments are seen by patients and others in the natural environment as being of value. Behaviors may be rated for naturalness, and subjects' performance may be compared with that of normal individuals. Experimental findings are considered to have social validity when they effect behavior outside the experimental setting and when the change is pleasing to persons in addition to the experimenter.

Articulation ratings and test results are often not clearly interpretable relative to their relationship to the criteria of naturalness or normality. Invalidity is present when ratings of one characteristic are influenced by another characteristic. The evidence is somewhat ambiguous (Ramig, 1982; Sinko and Hedrick, 1982), but speech ratings may be influenced by facial appearance or vice versa, and ratings of nasality may be influenced by presence of misarticulation. High levels of validity are difficult to obtain, and the validity construct in a sense serves as a reminder of test limitations.

IDENTIFYING ARTICULATION PATTERNS

Information descriptive of the severity of misarticulation is used to decide whether a problem exists and, if so, whether it requires speech therapy or some other kind of management. Number of articulation errors on sounds produced as singles (not members of blends) was found to correlate significantly ($r = 0.78$; $p < 0.01$) with ratings of articulation adequacy (Jordan, 1960), and comparison of the number of correct responses with normative data provides information about the severity of misarticulation and may contribute to decision making. However, such a score does not provide cues about the types of therapy or other interventions that are likely to be beneficial to the patient (Turton, 1973), and it offers no prognostic information.

Information of greater clinical value comes from analysis of the patient's articulation test records to determine which sounds were misarticulated and how they were misarticulated. Were sounds that were usually misarticulated produced correctly during stimulability testing when the patient was asked to attend carefully to the sound before attempting to imitate its production in isolation or perhaps syllables or words? Were the misarticulated sounds produced correctly spontaneously in some contexts, perhaps in consonant clusters? Which of the misarticulated sounds are usually articulated correctly by other persons of the patient's age? Some articulation tests specify procedures to be used to identify pattern information of these kinds.

Responses to articulation tests and the conversational speech sample should be analyzed to obtain an inventory of speech sounds always used correctly and of those sounds that are sometimes or always misarticulated. Information about the nature of distortions should be included in this inventory. Substitution and omission information is utilized in the study of phonological patterns as described below. The articulation inventory may be combined with a place-manner-voice analysis (see below).

Three procedures are used clinically to identify patterns in which different speech sounds share influences that contribute to misarticulation. The procedures are place-manner-voice analysis, distinctive feature analysis, and phonological process analysis. The three procedures are interpreted similarly so far as therapy planning is concerned. If several sounds that are misarticulated share place or manner of articulation or distinctive features or are influenced by the same phonological processes, then therapy may be organized in such a way that treatment that is effective in favorably influencing one or two sounds will also influence the related sounds. In patients with cleft palate and related disorders, the possibility of structural or physiologic constraints must be considered.

Chapter 2 in the handbook by Elbert and Gierut (1986) serves well as a laboratory manual for orientation to traditional articulation analyses, place-manner-voice analysis, distinctive feature analysis, and phonological process (pattern) analysis. Stoel-Gammon and Dunn (1985) wrote that analysis of a child's speech should provide an inventory of the sounds produced, positional and sequential constraints on the production of those sounds, contrastive units present in the child's speech, and comparison of the child's sound system with the adult system. The child's speech is first studied as an independent system and then as it relates to the adult system. These authors determine the phonetic inventory, identify syllable and word shapes that the child uses, and positional and sequential constraints operating in the child's speech. The relational analysis includes identification of phonological processes that are used including those of a presumably idiosyncratic (provisionally unique) nature. Phonemic contrasts and variability in production are also considered. The text by Bernthal and Bankson

(1988) provides a catalog of many published articulatory and phonological analysis materials.

The Fisher-Logemann Tests of Articulation (1971) have a built-in place-manner analysis. A similar analysis procedure described by Turton (1973) (Figure 18.2) may be used with any articulation testing procedure in which the various consonants are sampled several times each. Information gained from the articulation testing is transferred to a grid that classifies sounds according to place and manner of production and voicing. Patterns such as misarticulation of all or most fricatives or linguadental sounds are readily identified.

Distinctive feature analysis provides a means of organizing misarticulated sounds according to shared and unshared features. This information may be taken into account in selecting sounds for training in the hope of encouraging generalization of gains with therapy along feature lines. Distinctive feature usage is sometimes inferred from study of children's substitutions and omissions and comparison of those responses with mature articulation (McReynolds and Engmann (1975). In this procedure, distortions are ignored. However, Weiner and Bernthal (1978) described a procedure whereby the clinician listens for features that contribute to each test sound. The speech clinician analyzing the speech of the patient with cleft palate would obtain distortion information as a part of articulation testing and description.

Phonological Process Analysis

Phonological process analysis constitutes another means of identifying patterns of misarticulation, of arriving at a prognosis, and of organizing therapy to influence the articulation of two or more sounds that share one or more common characteristics. Phonological processes and distinctive features are not independent concepts in that the rules governing some processes are expressed in terms of features (Schane, 1973), and sounds that share distinctive features are likely to be influenced by the same phonological processes.

Phonological processes and rules were introduced in Chapter 15. Articulation is both physiological and linguistic in nature. The study of phonology contributes to our understanding of the sound pattern as part of the speaker's language and its relationship to morphology, syntax, semantics, and pragmatics. It supplements the phonetic information gained by articulation analysis.

Different authors have employed different lists of phonological processes in analyzing disordered articulation. Ingram (1976) used three process categories: syllable structure, assimilation, and substitution. These process constructs are used to explain articulatory behaviors such as deletion of consonants from syllables and clusters, alteration of a sound to resemble a neighboring sound, and replacement of sounds in one phonetic category with sounds from another category. For example, a child may replace fricatives with stops. Use of processes drops out with maturation, and authors have published information relating process usage and age (Grunwell, 1985; Vihman and Greenlee, 1987; Preisser et al., 1988). As introduced in Chapter 15, processes are conceptualized as mediating children's knowledge of the sound system and their sound production. Some authors assume that the child's knowledge is the same as that of adults; others attempt to identify the child's knowledge. When phonological analysis is performed without consideration of the child's underlying phonological knowledge—and this is done commonly—it seems appropriate to speak of phonological patterns rather than processes. Unambiguous information about the child's underlying knowledge is not commonly available. Without it, phonological analysis becomes a search for patterns in articulatory-phonetic data.

D'Antonio and Compton (1977) wrote that techniques of phonological analysis might help in understanding the speech patterns of cleft palate persons, and they suggested a model to explain the sources of articulation errors made by children with cleft palate. The model took both phonetic and phonological influences into account. According to this model, some articulatory errors are purely structural in origin, whereas others are linguistic in nature. The latter may reflect normal developmental patterns or learned deviant phonological rules. Errors in the linguistic category may reflect interaction between physical and linguistic forces, and they may be related to any past or present structural abnormality. As we indicated in Chapter 15, we view phonological process analysis in descriptive terms. Inferring causation from phonological process analysis alone is unwarranted.

Several phonological analysis kits have been published (Compton and Hutton, 1978; Weiner,

	Labial	Labio-dental	Lingua-dental	Lingua-alvoclar	Lingua-palatal	Lingua-velar	Glottal
Nasal	m			n		ŋ	
Plosive	p ⋮ b			t ⋮ d		k ⋮ g	
Fricative		f ⋮ v	θ ⋮ ð	s ⋮ z	ʃ ⋮ ʒ		h
Affricate					tʃ ⋮ dʒ		
Lateral				l			
Semi-vowel	w				r ⋮ j		

Figure 18.2 Form for indicating articulatory place, manner and voicing. Data may be recorded about the occurrence of correct and incorrect responses in each category.

1979, Hodson, 1980; Shriberg and Kwiatkowski, 1980; Ingram 1981; Grunwell 1985; and Kahn and Lewis, 1986). Several are directed to analysis of variables in addition to processes. These materials differ in the processes studied, in the procedures for obtaining speech samples, in the techniques for analysis, and perhaps most importantly, in their theoretical bases. The Kahn-Lewis kit was developed on a psychometric base and may be interpreted as a test. Dinnsen (1984) wrote that an adequate phonological analysis cannot be performed in a mechanical fashion but rather that the clinician should have the capability of adapting the analysis to the child. He noted that many of the analytical procedures that have been published compare the child's pattern with that of the ambient language. He would relate the child's spoken utterances to the child's underlying representations, which may or may not be the same as those used in the child's community. Procedures for generative phonological analysis such as that recommended by Dinnsen (1984) are described by Elbert and Gierut (1986). Phonological analysis contributes to determination of which sounds the child uses in a phonemic fashion—that is with the child's success in using the sound system in the expression of meaning.

McReynolds and Elbert (1981) recommended that we not consider a phonological process to be operative unless we have observed several appropriate contexts in which it occurred. They also listed qualitative criteria that might be applied in identifying the operation of processes: (1) that speech sounds influenced by processes in certain contexts be correctly articulated in contexts where those processes are not operative; (2) that the correctly articulated speech sound serve to establish contrast between minimal pairs, and (3) that the sound not be articulated correctly in contexts where the process is expected to be operative. As phonological process analysis is applied in the evaluation of patients with cleft palate, the speech pathologist must consider whether the analysis employed captures pattern information important to decision-making and whether that information is a valuable addition to that obtained from articulation testing. In a statistical sense, researchers are trying to account for as much variance in the articulation of patients with cleft palate as possible. Measurements based on linguistic concepts are of special interest in that they may account for portions of the variance still to be explained.

Harris and Cottam (1985) used a case study to explicate a two-stage analysis of disordered articulation-phonology. The first stage, a phonetic analysis, showed the sound pattern of the child to include replacement of voiceless plosives with affricates or fricatives and replacement of affricates with fricatives. This pattern was considered to be deviant because in normal development fricatives and affricates are commonly replaced with stops. The authors discussed the child's affrication and fricationalization (spirantization) of stops in terms of an articulatory strength construct whereby the child was unable to produce the vocal tract constrictions needed for resistance to airflow. The second stage of their analysis was phonemic in nature. Distinctive features were employed in the determination of the impact of the phonetic errors on the child's production of phonemic contrasts. The authors concluded that the child had underlying knowledge of the [+ continuant] versus [− continuant] distinction and that the origin of the problem was phonetic rather than phonological.

Identification of children's abstract knowledge of the sound system is important to understanding of disordered articulation-phonology. Some authors infer that knowledge from study of speech production; (Gierut et al., 1987). Elbert (1984) suggested that production of a sound indicates some knowledge of it; hence, stimulability testing provides some information about

knowledge. It doesn't indicate that the child knows when to use a sound that can be produced. However, as Elbert wrote, the first exemplar [repeatable occurrence] of a sound is clinically important. It indicates that an articulatory concept for that phoneme has been established, and this is essential to increased usage of that sound through generalization. Other writers use responses to perceptual tasks to gain information about children's phonological knowledge (Hoffman et al., 1985). The Indiana group (Gierut et al., 1987) has presented somewhat ambiguous evidence that the efficacy of therapy is enhanced when underlying knowledge is taken into account in selecting phonetic targets for therapy. Nonetheless, the assessment of abstract knowledge is a difficult task. The achievement of a satisfactory solution to this measurement problem awaits further research; we will not pursue the matter further in this book.

SPEECH RATINGS

In addition to testing articulation and performing pattern analysis relative to the patient's speech, the speech pathologist often employs rating scales to describe speech and change in speech. For example, The Templin-Darley Tests of Articulation include the following descriptive intelligibility scale: readily intelligible, intelligible if listener knows topic, words intelligible now and then, completely unintelligible.

Subtelny et al. (1972) presented rating scales for use in measuring articulation, intelligibility, nasal emission, and other characteristics of speech as studied in patients with cleft palate. They described their scales as reliable and recommended that they be applied to conversational speech samples. Speech intelligibility ratings were correlated with intelligibility ratings obtained by the write-down technique described in Chapter 15, and a correlation of 0.70 resulted. A modification of the Subtelny intelligibility scales is as follows: (1) normal for age and sex; (2) mild difficulty in understanding, repetition not required; (3) moderate difficulty, repetition required infrequently; (4) marked difficulty, repetition required frequently; and (5) unintelligible even with repetition. For a discussion of the technology of scaling, see Guilford (1954). Another approach is a global rating scale described by McWilliams and Philips (1979) described in Chapter 19 and in Figure 19.1.

PROGNOSIS

Tentative prognostic inferences about the patient's articulation may be drawn from knowledge of developmental misarticulation and from the cleft palate literature. Data about developmental articulation disorders indicates that, although most children who misarticulate in kindergarten will no longer do so by the end of the third grade, certain sound errors are likely to persist. Similarly, young children with cleft palate who misarticulate are likely to improve over time, but certain articulation errors that are heard in some of these children continue. As indicated previously, the percentage of cleft palate children who eventually develop normal articulation is lower than is the percentage for children with developmental articulation disorders. This is logical and expected in view of the anatomical and physiological defects that may also persist in some of these children. Fortunately, differences in sound usage between older persons with clefts and other persons may be small (Karnell and Van Demark, 1986). In this section we review information regarding articulation prediction in persons with developmental disorders and then consider the applicability of that information to cleft palate patients. Consideration is also given to predictive articulation data collected on cleft palate children.

Group Trends

The speech pathologist's predictions of articulation improvement, either spontaneously or with therapy, tend to be based on knowledge of group trends toward mature articulation, stimulability testing, and prediction from gains made in early articulation therapy sessions (Arndt et al., 1971).

Children with developmental articulation disorders, but presumably normal oral structures, are known to improve their articulation without therapy between kindergarten and the end of the third grade. For example, Pendergast et al. (1969) found that 56% of a large group of children with frontal lisps spontaneously corrected their lisps during that time period. Importantly, 44% of the children did not show these changes and they must not be lost sight of. Similarly, the majority of a large group of children in first, second, and third grades studied by Huskey et al. (1973) and Irwin et

al. (1974a, b) spontaneously corrected articulation errors during that period. These children misarticulated one or more sounds at the beginning of the studies. Gains were made on all misarticulated sounds, and the only articulation errors found for some children at the end of the third grade involved /s/, /z/, or /r/. Again those children and those sounds cannot be ignored.

Unfortunately, it is difficult to use group trends like these to identify specific children who cannot be expected to correct their errors completely or in part. Pendergast et al. (1969) used sophisticated multivariate statistical procedures to attempt to predict spontaneous change in noncleft children with frontal lisps. Articulation test items tended to be better predictors than did other measures such as indices to vocabulary, motor skills, and social maturity, but this excellent study did not result in a predictive algorithm for clinical use. Not much is known about identifying those individual patients who are the exceptions to group articulation trends, even though the exceptions may constitute a sizable proportion of the group sampled. Science can predict population effects, but not the future of individuals. Data regarding group trends in articulation change may permit estimates about the number of persons likely to require speech therapy, but they won't help in the identification of individuals who will comprise the group eventually needing therapy.

Some articulation errors are, however, likely to persist. These include lateral lisps (Van Riper and Erickson, 1968) and consistent misarticulation of /r/ (McDonald and McDonald, 1974). Children with vowel and diphthong errors and those with voiced for voiceless substitutions are also poor risks for maturational changes (McWilliams, personal communication). Children with articulation disorders of the kinds just described should be considered for speech therapy.

Cleft palate children who use glottal stops and pharyngeal fricatives may persist in those misarticulation patterns even after improvement in velopharyngeal valving (Bzoch, 1965; Morley, 1970). Sibilant distortions associated with dental differences also seem unlikely to improve spontaneously unless the structural variation is corrected. The longer these errors persist, the more likely they are to continue for children with clefts. The decision to recommend therapy will be based on knowledge of the patterns of the individual patient. When therapy is not scheduled because spontaneous improvement is anticipated, the clinician will test that prediction. Testing will be repeated to identify relatively short term change or its absence.

Stimulability

The speech pathologist sees prognostic value in the difference between the way an individual articulates spontaneously and under what is termed strong auditory-visual stimulation. That is, if an individual articulates a sound correctly in imitation of an examiner who stresses a particular sound and who directs the patient's attention to information regarding place and manner of articulation, then that patient is thought to be able to improve his or her articulation with therapy and perhaps without it. The concept of this "stimulability" as a predictor was first suggested by Milisen (1954) and Snow and Milisen (1954a, b) and was further developed by Carter and Buck (1958). The latter authors developed a predictive articulation test with cut-off scores for use in making articulation predictions. Persons who met the authors' subject selection criteria and whose scores exceeded the cut-off score tended to develop normal articulation without therapy. Unfortunately, from the viewpoint of predicting change in individuals, so did most persons who had lower predictor scores. This same problem exists with other predictive articulation tests that have been published. Weiss et al. (1980) cited evidence that persons who perform well on stimulability measures may not progress rapidly in therapy. However, poor performance on stimulability measures tends to be associated with poor speech improvement. Cleft palate children sometimes succeed in imitating sounds that they are physically unable to maintain in more complex contexts, especially in running speech.

The Miami Imitative Ability Test (Harrison, 1969; Jacobs et al., 1970) was developed for use in a research project intended to evaluate the speech of preschool children with cleft palate. The test samples the subject's ability to imitate lingual and labial placement when producing 24 consonants in CV syllables. Children were instructed to watch and listen as the examiner presented each test syllable three times. After the three presentations, the examiner said, "Now you do it." Each response was scored for placement and acceptability to the examiner's ear.

Harrison (1969) administered both a word articulation test and the Miami Imitative Ability Test to a control group and to 24 preschool cleft palate children who later received stimulation therapy for 12 months. The word articulation test was readministered to each group after the 12 months. Harrison found that the children made greater articulation gains over the course of the study on those sounds on which they were initially stimulable. This was true for both the treated and the untreated subjects. However, the treated subjects made greater articulation gains than did the untreated subjects. Data in the report do not indicate whether sounds in different manner or place categories differed in stimulability. If the sounds on which the subjects were stimulable and on which they improved were a subset of the total set on consonants studied, that information might influence the interpretation of the study. It would be interesting to know how highly Harrison's syllable imitation scores correlated with the difference between his pre- and post-treatment word articulation scores. We have no basis from this or other studies to predict articulation change in individual cleft palate children with or without therapy.

Neither stimulability testing nor other tests provide bases for predicting articulation change in individual children. Stimulability data do contribute to descriptive understanding of the child's articulatory status and capability. Use of stimulability techniques to sample production of target sounds in isolation, syllables, words, and other units can help the clinician to select units for use in therapy. Success at stimulability tasks suggests that the child has the phonetic capability to produce sounds of interest. Failure to use stimulable sounds in spontaneous speech could, however, reflect either phonetic-physiological or phonological variables or both.

Arndt et al. (1971) found gains made by individual subjects in early therapy to provide a better basis for prediction of improvement with therapy than did knowledge of the mean gain made by a group of subjects over the course of the therapy provided them. Research of this sort has not been conducted with cleft palate subjects. However, clinically, information gathered in early treatment sessions is used to plan future speech therapy.

Occasionally, children with clefts are seen whose speech consists primarily of nasal consonants and vowels in the absence of velopharyngeal incompetence. The hypernasality associated with this delay has been termed pseudohypernasality because the speech may improve spontaneously or with therapy (McWilliams, 1980). Sometimes these children are highly stimulable and develop normal articulation, and the hypernasality ceases. Such children are candidates for articulation therapy, and during that therapy continuing assessment of velopharyngeal function for speech should be employed. Children who have few or no consonants in connected discourse, but who are highly stimulable for use of consonants even in complex contexts, are also candidates for therapy. McWilliams (1980) described one such patient. Here the psychodynamics of family interaction required professional attention. The child had no evidence of a velopharyngeal valving deficit. On the other hand, this pattern can also indicate velopharyngeal incompetence.

Unfortunately, we have no regression formulas that allow us to predict the individual's future articulation scores from current measures. We note that predictions based on univariate correlations of much less than 0.90 are likely to make essentially the same predictions for everybody. Prediction of future articulation behavior of cleft palate children is a multivariate task. In addition to articulatory data, the researcher will consider velopharyngeal valving, other intraoral structures and functions including dental variables, hearing, social-emotional development, language status, mental capabilities, and many other variables.

USING ASSESSMENT RESULTS

Once information about articulation has been gathered, the pattern analyzed, the prognosis considered, the speech pathologist interprets the data and information in order to plan appropriate management. The clinician will use knowledge of the speech mechanism, of the child's articulatory pattern, and of speech development to decide if disordered articulation is likely to improve spontaneously, if articulation improvement appears to be contingent upon medical or dental treatments, or if articulation training appears to be warranted. Other decisions, such as need for language training, must also be made.

Articulatory patterns indicative of velopharyngeal insufficiency likely to require surgery or obturation include weakness of pressure consonants, audible nasal emission, and gross substitutions. Dental variables to be considered in interpreting the articulation pattern include irregularity of the cutting edge of the maxillary teeth. Supernumerary teeth, protrusion of the premaxilla, rotation of teeth, and maxillary collapse may distort the cutting edge and also prevent positioning of the tongue within the maxillary arch. The speech clinician must decide whether to attempt articulation therapy before orthodontics is completed. If the clinician waits for that completion, the patient will probably have entered puberty and may have passed through the "sensitive period" during which speech learning is relatively easy. On the other hand, the behavioral modification of articulatory errors related to structural deviations is often difficult or impossible, and speech may improve spontaneously with successful orthodontic correction or midface advancement so that therapy will not be required. The potential for change is always a factor in making recommendations either for or against speech therapy.

Children with cleft palate may have articulation patterns that were acquired when the speech mechanism was defective and that persisted after successful treatment of the mechanism. They may also present errors that are developmental in nature. That is, they may follow the normal developmental sequence but at a slow rate. These children may have the lisps and the problems with /r/ in its several forms observed in some physically normal children. In these cases, therapy may be appropriate. The clinician will decide what articulatory skills should be developed and how the therapy should be carried out. One child may need help in learning to produce some sounds or in the patterning of sounds he can already produce; others may require assistance with both.

Treatment planning is an essential part of the evaluation, and articulation therapy may be initiated with the expectation that dental and surgical treatments may follow. Both treatment and further sound system evaluation may be scheduled in a staged fashion after an initial evaluation (Maxwell and Rockman, 1984; Shelton, 1987). The clinician gathers enough information to initiate therapy but does not spend great amounts of time on analyses that fail to provide information essential to decision making and that may soon be obsolete. That is, the system may change quickly, and therapy may be begun on the basis of an initial sound system assessment, other components of the overall evaluation, and a model of treatment. There are differences of opinion about the depth of phonological analysis that should precede the initiation of articulatory-phonological therapy. However, as therapy continues, the clinician continues to gather and analyze phonetic and phonological information, as well as information about structural and physiologic status. That information, including information about response to treatment, will influence the variety and course of treatments that follow. Therapy sessions will be devoted to multiple goals some of which will probably be phonetic in nature while others are phonological.

One sequence of observations for the articulatory-phonological evaluation and treatment of the patient with cleft palate begins with consideration of information from parent, child, or both and from the referring person. The child is then asked to imitate different passages. The "measure why" passage (Fairbanks, 1960) samples the sounds of English, and the "zoo" passage (Fletcher, 1978) is free from nasal consonants. Fletcher also provides a list of sentences loaded with nasal consonants. Conversational speech is sampled, and the Iowa Pressure Articulation Test may be administered imitatively. The place-manner sheet (Figure 18.2) is used to guide further sampling, and misarticulated sounds are deep tested. This sampling and spontaneous speech are tape recorded, and selected utterances are narrowly transcribed—some live and some from tape. This work, provides a phonetic inventory of which sounds the child is unable to articulate and which are misarticulated even though the child can produce them. Place-manner information is evident on the score sheet, and commonly occurring phonological patterns may be identified (e.g., cluster reduction, stopping, final consonant deletion). Consideration is given to starting places for therapy and to what additional information is needed. If therapy is needed, both phonetic and phonological goals may be selected. Part of each session may be devoted to establishing and extending phonetic skills in different place and manner of articulation categories, and part may be directed to carryover of phonetic skills into automatic speech. This involves modification of the phonological pattern and makes use of contrasts to discourage unwanted homonymy. Parent

monitoring of the child's speech and provision of descriptive feedback, benign misunderstanding by the parents, self-monitoring and planning by the child, and other procedures may be used. Therapy for articulation and phonology is discussed in Chapter 22.

SUMMARY

In articulation evaluation, the speech of the patient with cleft palate is sampled in detail to determine whether or not there is an articulation problem and, if there is, to get a carefully detailed analysis of its nature. The articulation assessment must be reliably performed if it is to support clinical decision-making. Articulation pattern analysis is used to identify place-manner features, other distinctive features, and perhaps phonological processes that may be involved in the patient's misarticulation of two or more sounds. Crude prognostic inferences are drawn from knowledge about the likelihood of articulation change, from stimulability testing, from performance in trial therapy, and from descriptive information about which sounds the patient misarticulates and how these are misarticulated.

The articulation information that is gathered is interpreted relative to other information about the patient—especially to that concerning the speech mechanism and hearing. The available evidence may indicate a need for surgery to improve the velopharyngeal valve or other medical or dental treatment. If articulation therapy is indicated, the diagnostic information will be used to select training goals.

REFERENCES

Arndt WB, Elbert M, Shelton RL. Prediction of articulation improvement with therapy from early lesson sound production task scores. J Speech Hear Res 1971; 14:149.

Bernthal JE, Bankson NW. Articulation and phonological disorders. 2nd ed. Englewood Cliffs: Prentice Hall, 1988.

Byrne MC, Shelton RL, Diedrich WM. Articulatory skill, physical management, and classification of children with cleft palates. J Speech Hear Dis 1961; 26:326.

Bzoch KR. Articulation proficiency and error patterns of preschool cleft palate and normal children. Cleft Palate J 1965; 2:340.

Bzoch KR. Measurement and assessment of categorical aspects of cleft palate speech. In: Bzoch KR, ed. Communicative disorders related to cleft lip and palate. 2nd ed. Boston: Little, Brown, 1979:161.

Carter ET, Buck M. Prognostic testing for functional articulation disorders among children in the first grade. J Speech Hear Dis 1958; 23:124.

Compton AJ, Hutton JS. Compton-Hutton phonological assessment. San Francisco: Carousel House, 1978.

D'Antonio LL, Compton AJ. Generative studies of articulation disorders in cleft palate children. Presented at the Annual Convention, ASHA, Chicago, 1977.

Daniloff RG, Wilcox K, Stephens MI. An acoustic-articulatory description of children's defective /s/ productions. J Commun Dis 1980; 13:347.

Diedrich WM, Bangert J. Articulation learning. Houston: College-Hill, 1980.

Dinnsen DA. Methods and empirical issues in analyzing functional misarticulation. In: Elbert M, Dinnsen D, Weismer G, eds. Phonological theory and the misarticulating child. ASHA Monographs No. 22, 1984:5.

Elbert M. The relationship between normal phonological acquisition and clinical intervention. Speech Language Adv in Basic Res Pract 1984; 10:111.

Elbert M, Gierut JA. Handbook of clinical phonology: approaches to assessments and treatment. San Diego: College-Hill, 1986.

Fairbanks G. Voice and articulation drillbook. 2nd ed. New York: Harper, 1960.

Fisher MB, Logemann JA. The Fisher-Logemann test of articulation competence. New York: Houghton Mifflin, 1971.

Fletcher SG. Diagnosing speech disorders from cleft palate. New York: Grune and Stratton, 1978.

Gierut JA, Elbert M, Dinnsen DA. A functional analysis of phonological knowledge and generalization learning in misarticulating children. J Speech Hear Res 1987; 30:462.

Goldman R, Fristoe M. Goldman-Fristoe articulation test. Circle Pines: American Guidance Services, 1986.

Griffith J, Miner LE. Phonetic context drillbook. Englewood Cliffs: Prentice-Hall, 1979.

Grunwell P. Phonological assessment of child speech (PACS). San Diego: College-Hill, 1985.

Guilford JP. Psychometric methods. 2nd ed. New York: McGraw-Hill, 1954.

Harris J, Cottam P. Phonetic features and phonological features in speech assessment. British J Dis Commun 1985; 20:61.

Harrison RJ. A demonstration project of speech training for the preschool cleft palate child. Final report, Project No. 6-1101 Grant No. OEG-2-6-061101-1553. US Office of Education, Bureau of the Handicapped, HEW, 1969.

Hodson BW. The assessment of phonological processes. Danville: Interstate Press, 1980.

Hoffman PR, Daniloff RS, Bengoa D, Schuckers GH. Misarticulating and normally articulating children's identification and discrimination of synthetic [r] and [w]. J Speech Hear Dis 1985; 50:46.

Huskey R, Knight N, Oltman S, Irwin JV. A longitudinal study of the spontaneous remission of articulatory defects of 1665 school children in grades 1, 2, and 3: Part 1: Reliability. Acta Symbolica 1973; 4:73.

Ingram D. Phonological disability in children. New York: Elsevier, 1976.

Ingram D. Procedures for the phonological analysis of children's language. Baltimore: University Park Press, 1981.

Irwin JV, Huskey R, Knight N, Oltman S. A longitudinal study of the spontaneous remission of articulatory defects of 1665 school children in grades 1, 2, and 3. Part 2: The sample. Acta Symbolica 1974a; 5:1.

Irwin JV, Huskey R, Knight N, Oltman S. A longitudinal study of the spontaneous remission of articulatory defects of 1665 school children in grades 1, 2, and 3. Part 3: The study group. Acta Symbolica 1974b; 5:9.

Jacobs RJ, Philips BJ, Harrison RJ. A stimulability test for cleft-palate children. J Speech Hear Dis 1970; 35:354.

Jordan EP. Articulation test measures and listener ratings of articulation defectiveness. J Speech Hear Res 1960; 3:303.

Kahn ML, Lewis NP. Kahn-Lewis phonological analysis. Circle Pines: American Guidance Service, 1986.

Karnell MP, Van Demark DR. Longitudinal speech performance in patients with cleft palate: Comparisons based on secondary management. Cleft Palate J 1986; 23:278.

Kearns KP, Simmons NN. Interobserver reliability and perceptual ratings: more than meets the ear. J Speech Hear Res 1988; 31:131.

Logemann JA. Treatment of articulatory disorders in cleft palate children. In: Perkins WH, ed. Phonologic-articulatory disorders. New York: Thieme-Stratton 1983:37.

Maxwell EM, Rockman BK. Procedures for linguistic analysis of misarticulated speech. In: Elbert M, Dinnsen DA, Weismer G, eds. Phonological theory and the misarticulating child. Rockville, MD: American Speech-Language-Hearing Assoc. ASHA Monographs 22, 1984:69.

McCauley RJ, Swisher L. Use and misuse of norm-referenced tests in clinical assessment: A hypothetical case. J Speech Hear Dis 1984; 49:338.

McDonald ET. A deep test of articulation. Pittsburgh: Stanwix House, 1964.

McDonald ET, McDonald J. Norms for the screening deep test of articulation based on a longitudinal study of articulation development from beginning kindergarten to beginning third grade. Report regarding project 73024; ESEA Title III grant. 1974.

McReynolds LV, Engmann DL. Distinctive feature analysis of misarticulations. Baltimore: University of Park Press, 1975.

McReynolds LV, Elbert M. Criteria for phonological process analysis. J Speech Hear Dis 1981; 46:197.

McReynolds LV, Kearns KP. Single-subject experimental designs in communicative disorders. Austin, TX: Pro-Ed, 1983.

McWilliams BJ, Philips BJ. Manual, audio seminars in speech pathology, velopharyngeal incompetence. Toronto: BC Decker, 1989.

McWilliams BJ. Cleft palate. In: Shames G, Wiig E, eds. Human communication disorders. Columbus: CE Merrill, 1980.

Milisen R. A rationale for articulation disorders. J Speech Hear Dis 1954; Suppl 4:5.

Moller KT, Starr CD. The effects of listening conditions on speech ratings obtained in a clinical setting. Cleft Palate J 1984; 21:65.

Morris HL, Spriestersbach DC, Darley FL. An articulation test for assessing competency of velopharyngeal closure. J Speech Hear Res 1961; 4:48.

Morley ME. Cleft palate and speech. 7th ed. Baltimore: Williams & Wilkins, 1970.

Noll JD. Articulatory assessment. In: Wertz RT, ed. Speech and the dentofacial complex: the state of the art. ASHA Report No. 5, 1970:283.

Paynter ET. Articulation skills of Spanish-speaking Mexican-American children: normative data. Cleft Palate J 1984; 21:313.

Pendergast K. Building good speech. Pittsburgh: Stanwix House, 1971.

Pendergast K, Dickey SE, Soder AL. A study of protrusional lisps to identify children requiring speech therapy. Final report Project No. 5-0319 Contract No. OE-5-10-180. Office of Education, Bureau of Research, US Department of Health, Education, and Welfare, 1969.

Philips BJ, Bzoch KR. Reliability of judgments of articulation of cleft palate speakers. Cleft Palate J 1969; 6:24.

Preisser DA, Hodson BW, Paden EP. Developmental phonology: 18-29 months. J Speech Hear Dis 1988; 53:125.

Pullum GK, Ladusaw WA. Phonetic symbol guide. Chicago: The University of Chicago Press, 1966.

Ramig LA. Effects of examiner expectancy on speech ratings of individuals with cleft lip and/or palate. Cleft Palate J 1982; 19:270.

Ruscello DM, Lass JJ, Bosch W, Jones C. The verbal transformation effect as studied in judgments of misarticulations. Presented at Annual Convention, ASHA, Detroit, 1980.

Schane SA. Generative Phonology. Englewood Cliffs: Prentice Hall, 1973.

Schwartz RG. The phonologic system: normal acquisition. In: Costello JM, ed. Speech disorders in children: recent advances. San Diego: College-Hill, 1984.

Shelton RL. Review of handbook of clinical phonology: approaches to assessment and treatment. Cleft Palate J 1987; 24:261.

Shelton RL, Johnson A, Arndt WB. Variability in judgments of articulation when observer listens repeatedly to the same phone. Percept Mot Skills 1974; 39:327.

Shriberg LD, Kent RD. Clinical phonetics. New York: Wiley, 1982.

Shriberg LD, Kwiatkowski J. Natural process analysis (NPA): a procedure for phonological analysis of continuous speech samples. New York: Wiley, 1980.

Shriberg LD, Kwiatkowski J. Phonological disorders II: A conceptual framework for management. J Speech Hear Dis 1982; 47:242.

Sinko GR, Hedrick DL. The interrelationships between ratings of speech and facial acceptability in persons with cleft palate. J Speech Hear Res 1982; 25:402.

Snow K, Milisen R. The influence of oral versus pictorial presentation upon articulation testing results. J Speech Hear Dis 1954a; Suppl 4:29.

Snow K, Milisen R. Spontaneous improvement in articulation as related to differential responses to oral and picture articulation tests. J Speech Hear Dis 1954b; Suppl 4:45.

Standards for educational & psychological tests. Washington: American Psychological Assoc, 1985.

Stephens MI, Daniloff R. A methodological study of factors affecting the judgment of misarticulated /s/. J Commun Dis 1977; 10:207.

Stoel-Gammon C, Dunn C. Normal and disordered phonology in children. Baltimore: University Park Press, 1985.

Subtelny JD, Van Hattum RJ, Myers BB. Ratings and measures of cleft palate speech. Cleft Palate J 1972; 9:18.

Templin MC, Darley FL. The Templin-Darley tests of articulation. 2nd ed. Iowa City: Bureau of Educational Research and Service, University of Iowa, 1969.

Trost JE. Articulatory additions to the classical description of the speech of persons with cleft palate. Cleft Palate J 1981; 18:193.

Turton LJ. Diagnostic implications of articulation testing. In: Wolfe WD, Goulding DJ, eds. Articulation and learning: new dimensions in research, diagnostics, and therapy. Springfield: CC Thomas, 1973.

Van Demark DR. Predictability of velopharyngeal competency. Cleft Palate J 1979; 16:429.

Van Demark D, Bzoch K, Daly D, Fletcher S, McWilliams BJ, Pannbacker M, Weinberg B. Methods of assessing speech in relation to velopharyngeal function. Cleft Palate J 1985; 22:281.

Van Demark DR, Swickard SL. A pre-school articulation test to assess velopharyngeal competency: normative data. Cleft Palate J 1980; 17:175.

Van Riper C, Erickson RL. Predictive screening test of articulation. Kalamazoo: Continuing Education Office, Western Michigan University, 1968.

Vihman MM, Greenlee M. Individual differences in phonological development: ages one and three years. J Speech Hear Res 1987; 30:503.

Weiner FF, Bernthal J. Articulation feature assessment. In: Singh S, Lynch J, eds. Diagnostic procedures in hearing, language and speech. Baltimore: University Park Press, 1978.

Weiner FF. Phonological process analysis. Baltimore: University Park Press, 1979.

Weismer G. Acoustic analysis strategies for the refinement of phonological analysis. In: Elbert M, Dinnsen DA, Weismer G, eds. Phonological theory and the misarticulating child. Rockville MD: American Speech-Language-Hearing Assoc. ASHA Monographs No. 22, 1984:30.

Weiss CE, Lillywhite HS, Gordon ME. Clinical management of articulation disorders. St. Louis: CV Mosby, 1980.

Winitz H. Articulatory acquisition and behavior. New York: Appleton-Century-Crofts, 1969.

Winitz H. From syllable to conversation. Baltimore: University Park Press, 1975.

Young MA. Anchoring and sequence effects for the category scaling of stuttering severity. J Speech Hear Res 1970; 13:360.

19 | DIAGNOSIS OF VELOPHARYNGEAL INCOMPETENCE

This chapter concerns the evaluation of velopharyngeal valving by ear and by instrument. This evaluation is difficult because valving success is a function of structure, including its innervation and the use the patient makes of it. It is fairly easy to determine that an individual failed to close the velopharyngeal port during a particular act; it is often difficult to know if that lack of closure reflected a poor mechanism or failure to make good use of a satisfactory mechanism.

Evaluation involves the collection of data and their use in answering questions and formulating hypotheses. Did the patient produce velopharyngeal closure? If closure was achieved only intermittently, in what contexts was the closure achieved? What patterns of velopharyngeal movements did the patient use? Is there reason to think the patient has the capability of improving the velopharyngeal closure pattern with the mechanism he or she has?

Evaluation may proceed in hierarchical fashion. The answer to one question determines the next step. If perceptual assessment of speech indicates that speech is indistinguishable from normal, there is no reason to proceed further. If speech is marked by symptoms of velopharyngeal disability—hypernasality, audible nasal emission, weak obstruents—then additional data are needed. History is important. What prior treatment has the patient received and when? Has the speech pattern been constant for some time or has it been improving or deteriorating? How old is the patient? What is his or her status on other variables that relate to speech (e.g., hearing, language). Van Demark et al. (1985) outlined the overall assessment of the patient including history, voice and articulation, and orofacial mechanism.

The perceptual analysis of the individual's speech will involve narrow phonetic transcription and a search for orderly patterns (see Chapter 15).

Instrumental analysis will provide information about nasal pathway obstruction, movement of velum and pharyngeal walls, area of the narrowest velopharyngeal constriction during /p/, nasal air leakage during other obstruents, timing coordination of velopharyngeal and other speech movements and nasalance (Chapter 11). Inconsistent closure in a random pattern is possible but unlikely. The data collected will be used to formulate hypotheses about possible treatment courses. If speech is strongly degraded by long-standing, consistent and substantial failure to close the velopharyngeal port, then surgical or prosthodontic treatment is the logical course. Success of such treatment will not necessarily result in speech improvement. Some patients will persist in presurgical speech patterns—such as posterior articulatory placements—even after successful surgery. Those persons will need speech therapy to learn new articulatory patterns.

Quality of speech and quality of velopharyngeal valving may each fall on a continuum from normal to poor. It is important to know, for example, that one person presents a severe speech problem and a moderate valving problem and another presents mild problems in each area. Many patterns exist, and they should be identified to permit planning suitable to the individual. This contrasts with the practice of administering of a trial period of unspecified speech therapy to many patients as a precursor to secondary velopharyngeal closure.

In the last analysis, clinical decisions are made on the basis of the overall pattern of information available for each individual patient. Goals include providing the patient with the needed treatments, including surgery and speech therapy, and avoidance of unnecessary or ineffective treatments. The delivery of any unneeded or ineffective treatment is a serious error and a disservice to the individual patient and to society. The stakes in this work are high. Clinical judgment is fundamental to the diagnostic process. That judgment rests on the informed use of a variety of information. No algorithms are available that permit decision making from data by rule, and we can't solve all problems.

EVALUATION OF THE VELOPHARYNGEAL MECHANISM FOR SPEECH

Evaluation of the velopharyngeal mechanism for speech may be regarded as a hierarchical function beginning with speech itself and ending with the interpretation of data derived from instrumental evaluation. Speech assessment has been discussed in previous chapters; here we will present information about assessment of the velopharyngeal valve. The discussion that follows by necessity reflects our personal experiences, biases, interpretations of available data, and, to a very large extent, our work settings.

Information gained from the evaluation of voice, resonance, and articulation will influence the decision to evaluate velopharyngeal function for speech. The articulation and voice evaluations (Chapters 17 and 18) that are part of the study of the patient with cleft palate should have identified any existing speech characteristics associated with velopharyngeal incompetence. The speech symptoms include nasal emission, weak pressure consonants, hypernasality, and sometimes, gross articulatory substitutions. Also obstruents may be stronger with the nares closed than open. Procedures are needed that help the clinician to elicit the patient's best velopharyngeal performance. Performance may vary with context, prosody (including intensity), feedback, imitation, and other variables. If speech symptoms of velopharyngeal incompetence are present, the speech mechanism should usually be studied further by instrumental means. Instrumental assessment should be structured to include study of performance variability identified during speech assessment.

A global rating scale (Figure 19.1) developed by McWilliams and Philips (1979) and by McWilliams et al. (1981) is a useful tool for drawing together speech data to make an inference about the adequacy of velopharyngeal function. Research published by these authors indicated that ratings based on the scale agree well with ratings based on multiview videofluoroscopic records. McWilliams and Philips (1979) suggest that persons whose speech ratings total 7 or higher probably present velopharyngeal incompetence. The further study of those patients by intraoral inspection and instrumental means is recommended. Those with scores between 3 and 6 also require further investigation.

Intraoral Inspection of the Speech Mechanism

The speech pathologist evaluating the velopharyngeal mechanism often uses check lists and rating scales to ensure systematic study of the speech mechanism (Spriestersbach and Darley, 1978; Bateman and Mason, 1984; Dworkin and Cullata, 1985; St. Louis and Ruscello, 1987). These tools will guide the examiner in the observation of lips, dentition, maxillary arch width, occlusion, tongue, pillars of the fauces, tonsils, hard palate, soft palate, uvula, and pharyngeal walls. To the extent possible, these structures should be observed and described as they function in speech.

There are certain phenomena that the clinician should watch for in the assessment of a patient with suspected velopharyngeal insufficiency. If the individual has a cleft palate, how extensive is it? The speech pathologist can make limited observations of the rate, extent, and direction of movement of the velum and portions of the pharyngeal walls during sustained phonation or gag. However, the information derived from observation has little value in predicting velopharyngeal closure during connected speech except in cases of severe incompetence caused by very short, scarred immobile palates.

As indicated in Chapter 4, an oronasal fistula or an unrepaired opening in the hard palate may result in nasalization of speech. The possibility of submucous cleft palate or other congenital palatal defect should be considered when speech is nasalized but there is no cleft palate or history of one. The speech pathologist must be aware that velopharyngeal insufficiency may have anatomical or physiological origins that are not evident on intraoral inspection. Those physical defects may influence velar length, palatal elevation, movement of the pharyngeal walls, and hence velopharyngeal valving.

	Value
Nasal Emission	
Inconsistent, visible	_____ 1
Consistent, visible	_____ 2
Audible	_____ 2
Nasal turbulence	_____ 2
Facial grimace	_____ 2
Nasal resonance	
Mild hypernasality	_____ 1
Moderate hypernasality	_____ 2
Severe hypernasality	_____ 3
Hypo-hyper nasality	_____ 2
Cul-de-sac resonance	_____ 2
Hyponasality	_____ 0
Phonation	
Mild hoarseness	_____ 1
Moderate hoarseness	_____ 2
Severe hoarseness	_____ 3
Reduced loudness	_____ 2
Strangled voice	_____ 2
Articulation	
Omission of fricatives or plosives	_____ 1
Reduced intraoral pressure of fricatives	_____ 2
Lingual-palatal sibilants	_____ 2
Omission of fricatives with hard glottal attack on vowels	_____ 3
Reduced intraoral pressure on plosives	_____ 3
Pharyngeal fricatives, snorts, inhalation or exhalation substitutions	_____ 3
Glottal stops	_____ 3
Total	_____
	_____

Best estimate of efficiency of velopharyngeal valving mechanism using total (cumulative) score:

0	_____ Competent
1–2	_____ Competent to borderline competent
3–6	_____ Borderline to borderline incompetent
7+	_____ Incompetent

Figure 19.1   Weighted values for speech symptoms associated with velopharyngeal incompetence. (From: Cleft Palate-Craniofacial Center, University of Pittsburgh.)

There are two levels of evaluation of the velopharyngeal mechanism: screening and definitive. A screening evaluation may be done by the speech pathologist in general practice for the purpose of deciding whether to provide trial speech therapy or whether to refer the patient for more comprehensive study. A definitive evaluation is made by the speech pathologist working with a special management team. The major difference between the two speech pathologists is their training in disorders of this type, the array of diagnostic tools available for their use, and their experience in interpreting findings and conducting treatment.

Screening Devices

Speech clinicians have long used simple devices to supplement the ear when studying suspected velopharyngeal incompetence. Condensation on a cold mirror held under the nose will show nasal emission not easily detected by listening. This is useful clinically, although it is imprecise. Obviously, it does not quantify air pressure or air flow, and it is sometimes difficult to differentiate between abnormal air leakage and normal nasal exhalation.

Other devices with similar purposes and similar limitations are the listening tube (Blakeley, 1972) and plastic "scopes" that resemble water manometers. The listening tube is a catheter with a nasal olive in each end, one for the patient's nose and one for the examiner's ear. The scopes consist of glass or plastic tubing containing a float or piston that is displaced by nasal emission of air. These devices supplement the clinician's ear in the evaluation of velopharyngeal function. However, as Glaser and Shprintzen (1979) noted, they do not provide information about the size of the orifice responsible for the nasal emission or the utterance segment associated with nasal air leakage.

A procedure sometimes used for screening potential velopharyngeal closure is to have the patient puff the cheeks while the tongue is protruded, the modified "tongue-anchor technique" of Fox and Johns (1970). The person with an inadequate mechanism may fail the test, but it may not detect borderline problems.

Water manometers coupled to the nares by means of nasal olives have been used to measure nasal air pressure during speech (Hess and McDonald, 1960; Shelton et al., 1965). Hess (1976) attempted to increase the sensitivity of the U-tube water manometer for use in the assessment of velopharyngeal closure. Although the water manometer measures nasal air pressures during speech, it does not provide information about the area of velopharyngeal opening or the precise context in which leakage occurs.

As was reported in Chapter 11, oral-nasal differential pressure during /p/ in *hamper* functions as a screening procedure in the identification of patients who need thorough assessment of the velopharyngeal mechanism.

Manometers in the form of pressure gauges have been used in the diagnosis of velopharyngeal competence (Pitzner and Morris, 1966). Intraoral air pressure is measured as the patient blows into the instrument. Sucking pressures are sometimes used in place of blowing pressures. The measure is more stable when a systematic leak or bleed is introduced into the system. A ratio is computed between pressures recorded with the nares open and with them closed. If the oral air pressure obtained with the nares closed is greater than that obtained with them open, then, presumably, the velopharyngeal mechanism was not closed during the blowing act. The manometric ratio is at best an imprecise indicator of velopharyngeal function during speech and is best used, if at all, as a screening tool.

Warren (1979) reported that measurement of oral-nasal differential pressure is a suitable means for screening velopharyngeal competence. Most patients with differential pressures greater than 3.0 cm of water pressure (H_2O) presented velopharyngeal areas of 10 mm^2 or less which is considered to be adequate. Most patients with differential pressures less than 1.0 cm H_2O presented areas greater than 20 mm^2, which is considered to be inadequate. Persons with intermediate differential air pressure were also intermediate in velopharyngeal area and were considered borderline in velopharyngeal competence. These findings were confirmed by Morr et al. (1989) who remind us that the differential air pressure is only a screening measure to be used in the selection of individuals for more extensive assessment of velopharyngeal function. The /p/ in *hamper* is often used in aerodynamic screening of velopharyngeal competence.

Laine et al. (1988b) reported that measurement of nasal air flow also serves as a fairly accurate predictor of velopharyngeal competence. Their data indicate that 96% of patients who produced less than 125 cc per second of nasal air flow during /p/ in *hamper* had velopharyngeal areas of less than 10 mm^2 during that utterance whereas 90% of subjects with 125 cc per sec or more flow had areas greater than 10 mm^2. Velopharyngeal areas less than 10 mm^2 are aeromechanically adequate but in some cases may be accompanied by symptoms of cleft palate speech— especially if the tongue is humped or the oral port opening is reduced.

Cephalometric radiographs have been widely used in the evaluation of cleft palate patients. They usually involve midsagittal views of the velopharyngeal mechanism during the production of sustained consonants or vowels. Films made in cervical extension may show velopharyngeal openings missed when the patient is studied in upright posture (McWilliams, 1980). Velopharyngeal information illustrated in still radiographs will often not reflect phenomena that can be identified in motion studies. When the balance between hazard and benefit is considered, motion radiographic studies are strongly preferred over use of still radiographs. However, sometimes cephalometric studies conducted for orthodontic purposes can be structured to include speech observations that contribute to the screening function. Graber et al. (1959) tape recorded the test utterance and the sound of the x-ray machine during the exposure of the cephalometric film. They then listened to the tape to make certain that the test sound was indeed produced during the film exposure. Bateman and Mason (1984) described the cephalometric radiographic analysis of the speech mechanism.

The question arises as to whether manometers, mirrors, and simple flow detectors should be employed in clinical work when better tools are available. Some screening devices can supplement the clinician's auditory evaluation and can help the clinician make decisions about referring children to cleft palate centers. However, the results of such assessment must always be regarded with caution. It is important to rely on speech characteristics as grounds for referral when disagreement exists between patient speech and these screening instruments.

Definitive Instruments

Definitive assessment of velopharyngeal function for speech requires some combination of fluoroscopy, endoscopy, and aeromechanical instrumentation.

Motion Fluoroscopy

Teams serving patients with clefts differ in viewpoint regarding cine- or videofluorographic assessment of velopharyngeal function. Some assert that it is indispensible; some use it occasionally; others don't use it. There is agreement that the most comprehensive information is obtained when radiographic studies of the velopharyngeal mechanism include three views: mid-sagittal, frontal, and base or its equivalent (see Chapter 11). These views provide information about movement of the velum and posterior pharyngeal wall, the lateral pharyngeal walls, and the movements of walls and velum together from a transverse perspective. The latter provides information about the sphincteric function of the velum and walls as

they work together. If the radiographic record is to be analyzed by inspection and psychophysical scaling rather than by use of frame-by-frame measurements, then videofluorographic recording should be used rather than cinefluorographic filming. The radiation exposure is substantially less (see Chapter 11).

The use of fluoroscopy in the evaluation of the velopharyngeal mechanism during speech requires team work between the radiologist and the speech pathologist. Information gathered by the speech pathologist is used in planning the fluoroscopic procedure, which the radiologist performs. The speech pathologist should arrange to elicit speech responses from the patient during the study.

No standard passage has been adopted for use in videofluoroscopic studies. Speech sampling tends to emphasize plosive, affricate, and fricative consonants, which are particularly dependent upon velopharyngeal closure because they require intraoral air pressure. The study may be planned to answer specific questions that arise during speech evaluation. For example, does the patient show palatal surrender by moving away from closure during /s/ sounds? Does the velum remain elevated during nasal consonants? Does the tongue appear to support the velum or to fill space between the velum and the pharyngeal walls? Does the patient achieve closure, but not until after speech onset? Is closure achieved but lost prematurely? Does the velopharyngeal port open slightly as the tongue moves downward as for low vowels? Is the velopharyngeal port closed when the patient speaks in an upright posture but not when the speaker talks while in cervical extension? Does the patient achieve closure during nonspeech acts such as blowing and whistling but not during speech? Does tongue posture appear to direct air and sound streams into the nasal passages? The behaviors selected for study should be sufficient to make the clinical decisions that are needed. However, the study should be no more comprehensive than is necessary to answer the questions at hand.

Aerodynamic Measures

In the evaluation of patients with cleft palate, the pressure-flow instrumentation described in Chapter 11 is used primarily to identify the narrowest cross-sectional areas of the nasal valve and of the velopharyngeal valve. The nasal valve is studied during nasal breathing and the velopharyngeal valve during /p/ in nasal and non-nasal contexts.

Nasal pathway obstruction can confound aerodynamic estimates of velopharyngeal area and may lead to incorrect treatment decisions. Therefore, it should be identified. Furthermore, in recent years clinicians and investigators have become increasingly aware of the danger of nasal pathway obstruction in patients with clefts because of either deformity at birth or velopharyngeal or nasal surgery, or some combination (Hairfield and Warren, 1989). A patient may present a small nasal airway because of septal deformities, vomerine spurs, turbinate and mucosa hypertrophy, atresia of the nostrils, maxillary growth deficits, or a combination. Pharyngeal flaps and cosmetic surgery for the nose may also increase nasal pathway resistance. Hairfield and Warren (1989) noted that to achieve symmetry of the patient's nose, the surgeon may reduce the size of the naris on the normal side. The symmetrical but small nares may not permit normal nasal breathing. Argamaso (1986) wrote that patients with a history of apneic spells should be studied for abnormalities in the upper airway. He stated that patients with Treacher Collins syndrome, Pierre Robin sequence, and the velo-cardio-facial syndrome are at special airway risk because of the occurrence of a narrow hypopharynx and acutely angulated basicranium in those conditions. Riski (1988) reviewed variables that influence nasal pathway patency and with it resistance to air flow. Patency is cyclic and thus requires repeated measurement. It is influenced by body position (upright, supine), temperature, exercise, medication, and nasal hygiene.

The speech clinician may also measure nasal air flow as a means of identifying nasal escape during obstruents and the Zoo passage. The Zoo passage is free from nasal consonants (Fletcher, 1978). This does not permit estimation of area of the velopharyngeal opening, but it does provide information about the patient's pattern of velopharyngeal function. Nasal air flow during an obstruent indicates that it was made with the velopharyngeal port open, but the flow is also influenced by other variables (Chapter 11). Nasal air flow during nasal breathing and nasal consonants indicates that the nasal passages are not completely obstructed. However, estimation of the minimal area of the nasal valve requires measurement of flow through the valve and of pressure drop across it—as for estimation of velopharyngeal area (see Chapter 11).

Pressure-flow instrumentation may also be used to identify intraoral air pressure during obstruent production. Laine et al. (1988a) reported that only 45% of a group of patients with velopharyngeal areas equal to or greater than 20 mm^2 produced less than 3.0 cm H_2O of intraoral air pressure during the /p/ in *hamper*. Thus, patients tend to maintain intraoral air pressure that is at least minimally adequate for production of obstruents (Dalston et al, 1988).

A number of procedural issues should be considered in the interpretation of pressure-flow data. The importance of calibration and informed use of the equipment was cited in Chapter 11. Children as young as 3 years of age often participate in pressure-flow testing. Young children should be introduced to the pressure and flow sensing tubing before they are shown the remainder of the apparatus. Small amounts of nasal air flow are probably not clinically significant. Small flow traces will be recorded if the pressure transducer used to measure flow is unbalanced. Thompson and Hixon (1979), in a study of normal subjects, scored as zero nasal flows less than 5 cc per second. Nasal exhalation at the end of an utterance is normal and should not be interpreted as a sign of velopharyngeal disability. Small amounts of nasal air flow during pressure consonants adjacent to nasal consonants are of little clinical significance if they are not audible. Kunzel (1977) described nasally released stops. These occur when an individual saying a word like *cup* impounds air for the /p/ and then releases it through the nose. This is common in normal speech; the stops involved are sometimes described as unreleased. Small amounts of nasal air flow are sometimes observed as the velum elevates, even though the velopharyngeal port is closed (Lubker and Moll, 1965), because movement of the velum displaces air from the nasal chambers.

Velopharyngeal disability sometimes takes the form of failure to achieve or maintain closure in a normal timing sequence. Either slowness in the achievement of closure or early onset of velopharyngeal opening movements may cause hypernasality or audible nasal emission of air. Warren et al. (1985) used their pressure-flow equipment to quantify temporal patterns of velopharyngeal closure. During normal production of *hamper*, intraoral air pressure begins to build for

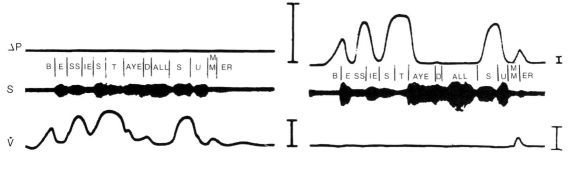

Pressure Cal.=20 mm H$_2$O   Flow Cal.=250 cc/sec

Figure 19.2 *A.* Patterns of low oral-nasal ΔP and high nasal flow without appliance. *B.* Insertion of appliance results in a more adequate pressure-flow pattern. Voice quality, however, was judged to be denasal, indicating the need for reduction in speech bulb size. (From Warren DW. Velopharyngeal orifice size and upper pharyngeal pressure-flow patterns in cleft palate speech: a preliminary study. Plast Reconstr Surg 1964; 34:15.)

the /p/ as nasal air flow for the /m/ falls. The pressure peak occurs after nasal flow has stopped. The patient with velopharyngeal incompetence shows substantial nasal air flow at the same time peak intraoral air pressure is achieved. Warren et al. illustrate several timing patterns. Dalston and Warren (1986) in interpreting the 1985 timing study indicated that closure timing differentiates between borderline patients with low ratings of hypernasality and borderline patients with high nasality ratings. Those in the first group were similar in timing to the normal subjects, whereas those with high nasality ratings were similar in closure timing to subjects with velopharyngeal inadequacy.

Pressure-flow data are useful in obturator fitting (Lubker and Schweiger, 1969). Figure 19.2 shows oral-nasal differential (Δ) air pressure, oscilloscopic, and nasal flow patterns for an individual without and then with an obturator. Without the appliance, ΔP is low and nasal flow high; with the appliance the reverse pattern— which is normal—is seen.

Bless et al. (1979) developed a procedure for evaluating the impact of oronasal fistulas on pressure-flow measures. Data are taken with the fistula open and with it covered by a small prosthesis. If oral air pressures are greater and nasal flows are less with the fistula closed than open, then it is evident that the fistula contributes to nasal air flow. Reduction but not elimination of

nasal flow with closure of the fistula indicates that another source of nasal air escape is present, perhaps an open velopharyngeal port, a second fistula, or an inadequate seal in the plugging of the first fistula.

Endoscopy

As indicated in Chapter 11, oral and nasal endoscopy are available for study of the velopharyngeal mechanism, but nasendoscopy is preferred for most purposes. Good endoscopic evaluation includes videorecording which permits essential repeated study of the velopharyngeal image. As in radiographic examination, the speech sample studied should be suitable to help answer questions that arose during the speech evaluation. Clinicians sometimes select a sample for use in all or most recordings and supplement it with material appropriate to the individual.

Positioning of the endoscope to obtain a complete view of velum and pharyngeal walls is essential, and the valve may be inspected at different levels (Shprintzen, 1989). Presumably movements unobserved through a scope positioned above the entrance to the velopharyngeal port may be identified when the scope is moved into and through the port. The presence of a scope, or other clinical tool, may influence the patient's performance.

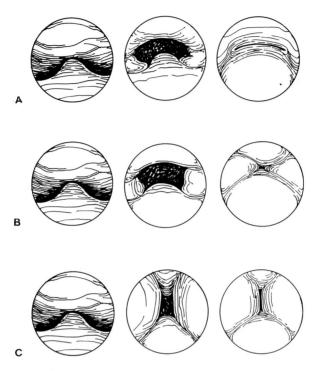

Figure 19.3 The velopharyngeal valve as seen on nasopharyngoscopy at rest and during partial and complete closure. The posterior pharyngeal wall and adenoid tissue are at the top of the circle and the soft palate is at the bottom. *A*. Coronal pattern; *B*. Circular patterns; *C*. Sagittal pattern. (From Witzel MA, Posnick JC. Patterns and location of velopharyngeal valving problems: atypical findings on video nasopharyngoscopy. Cleft Palate J 1989; 26:63–67.)

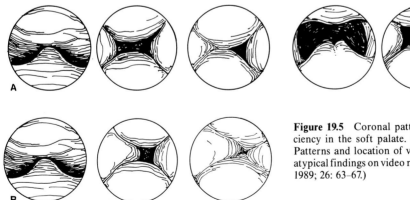

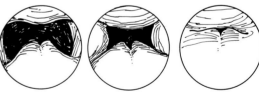

Figure 19.5 Coronal pattern valving with a midline deficiency in the soft palate. (From Witzel MA, Posnick JC. Patterns and location of velopharyngeal valving problems: atypical findings on video nasopharyngoscopy. Cleft Palate J 1989; 26: 63–67.)

Figure 19.4 Asymmetrical VP valving with a lateral gap. *A*. Coronal pattern; *B*. Circular pattern. (From Witzel MA, Posnick JC. Patterns and location of velopharyngeal valving problems: atypical findings on video nasopharyngoscopy. Cleft Palate J 1989; 26: 63–67.)

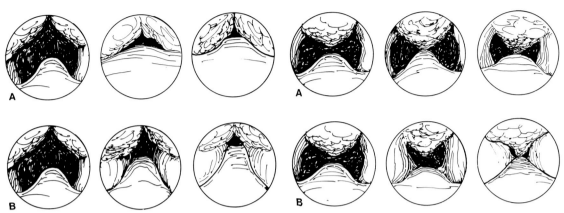

Figure 19.6 VP valving with a midline indentation in the adenoid tissue. *A.* Coronal pattern; *B.* Circular pattern. (From Witzel MA, Posnick JC. Patterns and location of velopharyngeal valving problems: atypical findings on video nasopharyngoscopy. Cleft Palate J 1989; 26: 63–67.)

Figure 19.8 VP valving with a midline projection of the adenoid tissue. *A.* Coronal pattern; *B.* Circular pattern. (From Witzel MA, Posnick JC. Patterns and location of velopharyngeal valving problems: atypical findings on video nasopharyngoscopy. Cleft Palate J 1989; 26: 63–67.)

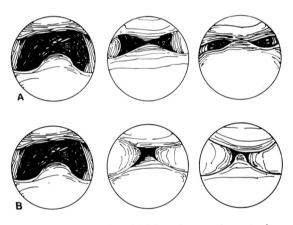

Figure 19.7 VP valving with bilateral gaps and a protrusive border of the soft palate or musculus uvulae. *A.*Coronal pattern; *B.* Circular pattern. (From Witzel MA, Posnick JC. Patterns and location of velopharyngeal valving problems: atypical findings on video nasopharyngoscopy. Cleft Palate J 1989; 26: 63–67.)

A key feature of endoscopic and other instrumental examinations is the extraction of information from recordings in a way that is as free as possible from clinician biases. Paradoxically, at the same time, knowledge of possible velopharyngeal closure patterns, such as those described and illustrated by Witzel and Posnik (1989) (Figs. 19.3–19.8) helps prepare the clinician for informed study of the recorded endoscopic image. Again, scaling routines may be helpful. Independent study of recordings by qualified but independent observers serves to establish the reliability of the assessment—when the observers' findings agree.

Figure 19.3 from Witzel and Posnick shows three patterns of movement toward velopharyngeal closure: coronal, where most of the movement is contributed by the velum; circular, in which both the velum and the lateral pharyngeal walls are active; and sagittal, in which the lateral pharyngeal walls are the most active. Similar patterns have been identified by other authors through baseview videofluorography (Chapters 11 and 12). A given individual may show a distinctive closure pattern, and closure movements may change with speech context and prosody. Later figures in the Witzel and Posnick series show failure of velopharyngeal closure in a variety of patterns.

Endoscopy has been used in the fitting of obturators. Riski et al. (1989) used a nasal scope in combination with aerodynamics. The latter was used to measure area of velopharyngeal constriction during / p / and nasal pathway patency during breathing. Charles U. Kastner (personal communication) found oral endoscopes useful in observation of the relationship between obturator materials and velopharyngeal structures.

Nasometry

Nasometric measures are likely to be interpreted as evidence of velopharyngeal competence. In an exploratory study, Dalston, et al. (1989) stated that individuals with nasalance values of

32% or less tended to fall into an adequate velopharyngeal category as determined aerodynamically. However, they found a correlation of only 0.73 between pressure-flow estimates of velopharyngeal opening during *papa* and nasalance during the Zoo passage. As we indicated in the instrumentation chapter, variables in addition to velopharyngeal opening contribute to high nasalance readings. Consequently, we find this instrument of interest in the study of hypernasality and in the overall evaluation of the patient but not as a device for evaluation of velopharyngeal competence. Dalston et al. found nasalance values from 26 through 39 to be associated with normal nasality to mild hypernasality. Nasalance greater than 40 was associated with moderate to severe hypernasality ratings.

Interpretation of Data

As stated earlier, clinical work with patients with clefts is directed to planning to meet the needs of the individual. Nonetheless, it is convenient to discuss categories into which patients may fit. Trost-Cardamone (l989) used the broad category velopharyngeal inadequacy as a cover term to subsume insufficiency which is structural, incompetence which is neurogenic, and mislearning which involves misuse of available mechanism. A given pattern of velopharyngeal movement could involve interaction among structure, innervation, and learning. As a result of compensatory movements, an individual with a velopharyngeal structural defect could present velopharyngeal competence (Folkins, 1988). Folkins noted that a set of categories won't be satisfactory for all patients, and he observed that individuals should be free to use terms as they see fit so long as their meanings are clear. Here for purposes of discussion, we consider the placement of patients into one of at least three categories: velopharyngeal competence (VPC), borderline velopharyngeal competence/incompetence (BVP), or velopharyngeal incompetence (VPI). The characteristics of each category are described as we proceed.

Velopharyngeal Incompetence

We consider VPI first because in many ways the clinical findings for this group are distinct and easily recognized. The key speech finding is nasalization which includes nasal emission during obstruents and hypernasality. The consonants are likely to be weak in terms of intraoral air pressure, and they may be distorted by compensatory articulation such as glottal stops and pharyngeal fricatives. Hypernasality is consistent, even though it may not be severe in some patients. Patients in this category are not stimulable to oral speech by auditory-visual assistance from the examiner. These patients may or may not show nares constriction or facial grimacing during speech. Information relative to this classification is summarized in the earlier section on global speech ratings.

Evaluation of the speech mechanism may yield one or a combination of several findings. There may be an open cleft palate, a residual anterior cleft palate, or a large palatal fistula perhaps resulting from surgical breakdown. The patient may have a pharyngeal flap or an obturator that is unsatisfactory, a surgically repaired cleft palate that is not functionally adequate, or a congenitally incompetent velopharyngeal valving mechanism that looks normal.

Fluoroscopic and endoscopic studies consistently show velopharyngeal openings even though the velum and lateral walls may move substantially. Aerodynamic procedures show consistently high nasal air flow, low oral air pressure, and large velopharyngeal areas.

Trial speech therapy for these patients is a questionable practice. Therapy will not eliminate the nasalization because the velopharyngeal mechanism is structurally deficient. There are other goals of therapy, of course, such as articulatory placement instruction, that may be appropriate. However, if normal oral speech is the objective, physical management such as a pharyngeal flap, which is the most common choice, or a prosthetic speech aid will be required. Surgical modification of an existing flap or alteration of an obturator may also be undertaken. Sometimes obturators or prostheses are used to supplement flaps.

Velopharyngeal Competence

The identifying characteristic of VPC patients is that they clearly show either normal oral dynamics of speech production and oral voice quality or demonstrate the ready physiological potential to do so. In the first case, there is no undesirable nasalization, no nares constriction, and no unusual nasal air flow during speech. Oral air pressure is normal, and there is no instrumental evidence of velopharyngeal openings where they do not belong during speech. The speech pathologist may find articulation errors, but they are usually oral distortions related to dental deformities or immature articulatory patterns similar to those of many noncleft children. Some patients with clefts do persist in use of gross substitutions after velopharyngeal competence has been established.

Unachieved potential for oral speech is evident when, there is nasalization of only a few sounds. For example, /s/ and /z/ may be directed nasally and all other sounds orally. This has been given several names, among them *phoneme-specific nasal emission*. Hypernasality is not a problem, and the patient may be stimulable for oral production of the nasalized consonants—particularly if he or she thinks a new sound that is not the target sound is being produced. We presume that this misarticulation has been learned.

Borderline Velopharyngeal Competence/Incompetence (BVP)

The BVP is difficult to describe because there is considerable variation among these patients, and individuals present complex patterns (Morris 1972; 1984). Contextual effects are strong in some individuals. For example, in the clinic the presence of nasal consonants in a speech task seems to cause far more assimilative nasalization in some of these persons than in those with competence. Presumably the borderline mechanism cannot cope effectively with the demands placed on it by nasal sounds. More information about this finding is needed. These individuals may also have consistent speech problems, including nasal escape, hoarseness, and mild hypernasality (McWilliams and Philips, 1979; McWilliams et al. 1981). Some of these patients may speak normally except when they are fatigued or under stress. Thus, the clinician must take the speaking situation into account to understand these patients.

Some patients, mostly young children, show nasalized speech during the speech examination but produce oral speech upon stimulation. Instrumental findings will vary depending on whether the individual delivers representative speech or the best speech of which he or she is capable. Some individuals fail to make good use of a competent mechanism during spontaneous speech. Others may use the mechanism during stimulability testing in a fashion that they are not physically capable of maintaining in spontaneous speech. Time and repeated observation may permit the clinician to arrive at a decision about the velopharyngeal competence of these individuals. Until that time, they can be considered members of the BVP category. Van Demark et al. (1988) reported evidence that some patients slip into incompetence after several years in a borderline category. This is one reason for periodic assessment of the patient by members of the cleft palate team.

Individuals with velopharyngeal timing disorders—those who are slow in achieving closure, too quick to open the port, or do both—may be considered to present borderline velopharyngeal incompetence. Decisions about physical management for patients who have true timing problems are sometimes difficult to make. A pharyngeal flap will reduce the size of the velopharyngeal opening, perhaps making it easier to compensate for a timing disorder during connected speech. An obturator sometimes will serve the same purpose and may be later set aside if it is successful in changing valving behavior. However, neither a flap nor an obturator will remedy impairment of velar timing itself and so cannot be expected to eliminate the nasalization disorder except, in some patients by obstruction of the velopharyngeal port. A patient whose palate never moved at all with a prosthetic appliance in his mouth found that it moved inconsistently when the appliance was removed. He later had a pharyngeal flap, which caused remarkable improvement.

Morris (1972; 1984) attempted to account for variability among and within BVP subjects by hypothesizing that there are two subgroups. His almost-but-not-quite (ABNQ) subgroup resembles VPI patients except that the extent of the incompetence is very small but highly consistent. Oral examination findings are essentially negative. Usually there is no nares constriction. Radiographic and endoscopic measures may indicate a small velopharyngeal opening or, as indicated above, they may also very occasionally indicate velopharyngeal closure just barely achieved. Timing of velopharyngeal movements is not a problem.

The underlying assumption with ABNQ patients is that there is a small but significant structural deficiency in the velopharyngeal mechanism. Perhaps it is a short palate, an unusually deep nasopharynx, or both. The consistency of the nasalization suggests that timing patterns are not impaired.

Speech therapy is generally not productive, but it may be undertaken as a diagnostic procedure for a short period of time, usually not more than 3 months, after which reassessment should take place. Longitudinal observation without therapy is another option for gathering information. The decision for physical management rests on whether or not the extent of the disorder is sufficient to warrant such intervention. The patient or the parents are the ones to make this decision, and it usually is based on social, educational, and vocational considerations.

Morris (1972) labeled the second marginal subgroup as sometimes-but-not-always (SBNA) to indicate the high degree of inconsistency in velopharyngeal function that they demonstrate. Diagnostically, these patients resemble patients who are competent but who nasalize speech because of a failure to employ a mechanism that is competent. That is, they demonstrate adequate velopharyngeal ability during some tasks but not in others. During speech tasks and radiographic, endoscopic, or aerodynamic measures that use single-word or consonant-vowel tasks, adequate velopharyngeal function is often found. However, in connected speech, especially when there are many nasals, velopharyngeal dysfunction is indicated.

An attractive hypothesis about this subgroup of patients is that they present an impairment of velopharyngeal timing. Hardy (1961) suggested that a timing problem is involved in the velopharyngeal dysfunction observed in some cerebral palsy patients. Perhaps SBNA patients also have a minimal dysarthria of the velopharyngeal mechanism. This neurological problem, if it exists, could have accompanied the cleft palate, it could be the result of the cleft palate, or it could be the result of palatal surgery.

The SBNA subgroup, like the ABNQ subgroup, typically does not respond well to speech therapy. The speech pathologist is tempted to continue treatment for long periods of time in the hope of helping the patient generalize to connected speech the velopharyngeal function demonstrated in isolated tasks. Such generalization is probably impossible, and therapy will not be successful in that respect. The speech pathologist in general practice must avoid extensive speech therapy for this patient; rather, the patient should

be referred to a specialty team for further evaluation. Information about the therapy and its result is important information for the speech pathologist on the specialty team.

Several studies have been reported that were designed to describe further the borderline or marginal competence group and the mechanisms underlying the condition (Karnell et al., 1985; Jones and Folkins, 1985; Hardin et al., 1986; Jones et al., in preparation). The findings from this work emphasize the variability in performance of the patients in this category. In particular, the data from the study by Jones et al. (in preparation) emphasize the probable importance of phonetic context in this variability.

Sometimes parents of children with BVP, or the patients themselves, are sufficiently concerned about the speech disorder to seek speech therapy and the advice of a specialty team, but then are reluctant to agree to surgery. That is probably because, in their opinion, the extent of the disorder is not sufficient to warrant surgical intervention. The decision is theirs to make and must be respected. However, the speech pathologist must often withdraw from the case when it has been determined that all possible gains have been made with the existing mechanism. As the care of infants with clefts improves, increasing numbers of patients have either competent or borderline mechanisms, and so this is a problem of no small proportions.

DISCUSSION

We want to emphasize our conviction that it is the role of the speech pathologist to judge the adequacy of velopharyngeal function for speech production. This is done in collaboration with other professionals who also provide valuable information about the mechanism and its function and suggest alternatives for management. If physical management is chosen as the preferred method of treatment the surgeon or the dentist is legally and ethically accountable to the patient and family for proper treatment and must always have the last word about whether or not to perform the surgery or construct the prosthesis. However, it is the speech pathologist who decides whether or not the proposed physical management is indicated for speech improvement.

As we have indicated throughout this discussion, we must be careful about using speech information for evaluating velopharyngeal function, because speech is influenced by so many factors. However, speech information is relevant if the focus is on error type with recognition of errors that involve nasalization, the extent to which such errors are inconsistent, and their stimulability from nasal to oral.

The interpretations drawn here are based on study of a broad literature, theoretical viewpoints regarding measurement and what patients can achieve through learning, and clinical experience. Bias is a factor here as it is in other clinical decision making. The best way to avoid bias in working with patients is through in-depth study of the patients with the best available tools and through open communication with highly competent colleagues from the several disciplines that serve patients with clefts.

A key test of any measurement or evaluation system is the prediction of future events, including speech change, whether spontaneous or in response to treatment. Little has been done to test predictions of speech change in patients with cleft palate who are undergoing speech training, surgery, prosthodontics, or any combination of these. Some predictive research about surgery for these patients is available, but has been retrospective in nature and has not utilized the definitive evaluation procedures discussed above (Van Demark et al., 1975; Van Demark and Morris, 1977; Van Demark, 1979). The evaluation tools that have been discussed are also appropriate for assessing changes in speech and velopharyngeal function in response to therapy and to surgical and dental treatments. Prospective research predictive of treatment outcome is needed. It is difficult to accomplish because many variables in addition to treatment influence the results. For example, patients with different characteristics respond differently to a given treatment, and measurement error is not unknown. Two clinicians may differ in the skill with which they use a particular technique. These confounding variables are difficult to control experimentally, but the development of well-founded treatments depends upon sound treatment research. Although we have used three classifications of velopharyngeal function in our discussion, in actual fact, patients show a range of velopharyngeal closure from competence through borderline and mild, moderate, or severe incompetence, with orifice area

ranging from 1 mm^2 through 20 + mm^2. Within patients, area of velopharyngeal opening during obstruents is variable. Closure problems exist on a wide continuum. Physical management is dichotomous in that surgery or obturation is either done or it is not. However, in actual practice, there is great variation in surgical technique, in the skill of surgeons, in techniques used for construction of obturators, in the skill of prosthodontists, and in the responsiveness of patients. It seems likely that, as we learn more about both velopharyngeal function and physical management, we can be more careful in matching the disorder to its physical management. Indeed, more successful efforts are being made in that direction. Such effort characterizes responsible professions.

As we have indicated, clinicians hold different opinions about how strongly they would urge the patient with a borderline problem to undergo surgery. We advocate sharing with the patient the information that has been gathered and our estimate of the probable outcome of different courses of action. When our experience tells us that one approach has a better chance of success than another, we must be open and honest about what we feel to be the best choice. The patient and family can then participate in the decision.

The evaluation procedures described may also lead to a decision to offer speech therapy, but they do not provide a basis for a precise prescription of therapy. The velopharyngeal mechanism may be adequate, but the patient may be in need of articulation or voice therapy. If the velopharyngeal valve is incompetent or of borderline efficiency, the issue of improving velopharyngeal function through behavioral therapy arises. Such therapy is controversial at best, and we are skeptical of this approach unless there is evidence that the patient is not using clearly available potential for achieving velopharyngeal closure in speech. Here, the velopharyngeal movement pattern made by the patient must be considered. Some surgeons and speech pathologists expect speech therapy to develop velopharyngeal function, and even velopharyngeal structure, thereby reducing the frequency of secondary surgery. Still others conceptualize therapy in terms of what the patient can learn to accomplish with the existing mechanism. Systems of speech therapy for improving velopharyngeal function and what can be expected from them is discussed in Chapter 23.

REFERENCES

Argamaso RV. Physical management of velopharyngeal incompetence. J Child Commun Dis 1986; 10:67.

Bateman HE, Mason RM. Applied anatomy and physiology of the speech and hearing mechanism. Springfield: CC Thomas, 1984.

Blakeley RW. The practice of speech pathology: a clinical diary. Springfield: CC Thomas, 1972.

Bless D, Ewanowski SJ, Dibbell D. A longitudinal analysis of speech and aerodynamic patterns produced by children with cleft palate. Annual Meeting of the American Cleft Palate Association, San Diego, 1979.

Dalston RM, Warren DW. Comparison of Tonar II, pressure flow, and listener judgments of hypernasality in the assessment of velopharyngeal function. Cleft Palate J 1986; 23:103.

Dalston RM, Dalston ET, Warren DW. Clinical assessment utilizing nasometry, pressure-flow and clinical ratings: a preliminary comparison. Annual Meeting of the American Cleft Palate-Craniofacial Association, San Francisco, 1989.

Dalston RM, Warren DW, Morr KE, Smith LR. Intraoral pressure and its relationship to velopharyngeal inadequacy. Cleft Palate J 1988; 25:210–219.

Dworkin J, Cullata R. Dworkin-Cullata oral mechanism exam. Nicholasville, KY: Edgewood Press, 1985.

Fletcher SG. Diagnosing speech disorders from cleft palate. New York: Grune and Stratton, 1978.

Folkins JW. Velopharyngeal nomenclature: incompetence, inadequacy, insufficiency, and dysfunction. Cleft Palate J 1988; 25:413.

Fox D, Johns D. Predicting velopharyngeal closure with a modified tongue-anchor technique. J Speech Hear Dis 1970; 35:248.

Glaser ER, Shprintzen RJ. A review of See-Scape: instrument and manual. Cleft Palate J 1979; 16:213.

Graber TM. Bzoch KR, Aoba T. A functional study of the palatal and pharyngeal structures. Angl Orthod 1959; 29:30.

Hairfield WM, Warren DW, Hinton VA, Seaton DL. Inspiratory and expiratory effects of nasal breathing. Cleft Palate J 1987; 24:183.

Hairfield WM, Warren DW. Dimensions of the cleft nasal airway in adults: A comparison with subjects without cleft. Cleft Palate J 1989; 26:9.

Hardin MA, Morris HL, Van Demark DR. A study of cleft palate speakers with marginal velopharyngeal competence. J Commun Dis 1986; 19:461.

Hess DA. A new experimental approach to assessment of velopharyngeal adequacy: mnemometric blend testing. J Speech Hear Res 1976; 41:427.

Hardy J. Intraoral breath pressure in cerebral palsy. J Speech Hear Dis 1961; 26:309.

Hess DA, McDonald ET. Consonantal nasal pressure in cleft palate speakers. J Speech Hear Res 1960; 3:201.

Jones DL, Folkins JW. Effect of speaking rate on judgments of disordered speech in children with cleft palate. Cleft Palate J 1985; 22:246.

Jones DL, Folkins JW, Morris HL. Speech production time and judgments of disordered nasalization in speakers with cleft palate, in preparation.

Karnell MP, Folkins JW, Morris HL. Relationships between the perception of nasalization and speech movements in speakers with cleft palate. J Speech Hear Res 1985; 28:73.

Kunzel HJ. Some observations on velar movement in plosives. Phonetica 1977; 36:384.

Laine T, Warren DW, Dalston RM, Hairfield MW, Morr KE. Intraoral pressure, nasal pressure and airflow rate in cleft palate speech. J Speech Hear Res 1988a; 31:432.

Laine T, Warren DW, Dalston RM, Morr KE. Screening of velopharyngeal closure based on nasal airflow rate measurements. Cleft Palate J 1988b; 25:220.

Lubker JF, Moll KL. Simultaneous oral-nasal air flow measurements and cinefluoroscopic observations during speech production. Cleft Palate J 1965; 2:257.

Lubker JF, Schweiger JW. Nasal airflow as an index of success of prosthetic management of cleft palate. J Dent Res 1969; 48:368.

McWilliams BJ. Communication disorders associated with cleft palate. In: Van Hattum RJ, ed. Communicative disorders, an introduction. New York: Macmillan, 1980.

McWilliams BJ, Glaser ER, Philips BJ, Lawrence C, Lavorato AS, Beery QC, Skolnick ML. A comparative study of four methods of evaluating velopharyngeal adequacy. Plast Reconstr Surg 1981; 68:1.

McWilliams BJ, Philips BJ. Velopharyngeal incompetence; Audio Seminars in Speech Pathology. Philadelphia: WB Saunders, 1979.

Morr KE, Warren DW, Dalston RM, Smith LR. Screening of velopharyngeal inadequacy by differential pressure measurements. Cleft Palate J 1989; 26:42.

Morris HL. Cleft palate. In: Weston AJ, ed. Communicative disorders. Springfield: CC Thomas, 1972:128.

Morris HL. Types of velopharyngeal incompetence. In: Winitz H, ed. Treating articulation disorders—for clinicians by clinicians. Austin, TX: Pro-ed, 1984.

Pitzner JC, Morris HL. Articulation skills and adequacy of breath pressure ratios of children with cleft palate. J Speech Hear Dis 1966; 31:26.

Riski JE. Nasal airway interference: considerations for evaluation. Internat J Orofac Myol 1988; 14:11.

Riski JE, Hoke JA, Dolan EA. The role of pressure flow and endoscopic assessment in successful palatal obturator revision. Cleft Palate J 1989; 26:56.

Shelton RL, Brooks AR, Youngstrom KA. Clinical assessment of palatopharyngeal closure. J Speech Hear Dis 1965; 30:37.

Shprintzen RJ. Nasopharyngoscopy. In: Bzoch KR, ed. Communicative disorders related to cleft lip and palate. 3rd ed. Boston: College-Hill, 1989.

Spriestersbach DC, Darley F. Diagnostic methods in speech pathology. New York: Harper & Row, 1978.

St. Louis KO, Ruscello DM. The oral speech mechanism screening examination. 2nd ed. Baltimore: University Park Press, 1987.

Thompson AE, Hixon TJ. Nasal air flow during normal speech production. Cleft Palate J 1979; 16:412.

Trost-Cardamone JE. Coming to terms with VPI: A response to Loney and Bloem. Cleft Palate J 1989; 26:68.

Van Demark DR. Predictability of velopharyngeal competency. Cleft Palate J 1979; 16:429.

Van Demark D, Bzoch K, Daly D, Fletcher S, McWilliams BJ, Pannbacker M, Weinberg B. Methods of assessing speech in relation to velopharyngeal function. Cleft Palate J 1985; 22:281.

Van Demark DR, Hardin MA, Morris HL. Assessment of

velopharyngeal competence: a long-term process. Cleft Palate J 1988; 25:362.

Van Demark DR, Kuehn DP, Tharp RF. Prediction of velopharyngeal competency. Cleft Palate J 1975; 12:5.

Van Demark DR, Morris HL. A preliminary study of the predictive value of the IPAT. Cleft Palate J 1977; 14:124.

Warren DW. Velopharyngeal orifice-size and upper pharyngeal pressure-flow patterns in cleft palate speech: a preliminary study. Plast Reconstr Surg 1964; 34:15.

Warren DW. PERCI: a method for rating palatal efficiency. Cleft Palate J 1979; 16:279.

Warren DW, Dalston RM, Trier WC, Holder MB. A pressure-flow technique for quantifying temporal patterns of palatopharyngeal closure. Cleft Palate J 1985; 22:11.

Witzel MA, Posnick JC. Patterns and location of velopharyngeal valving problems: atypical findings on video nasopharyngoscopy. Cleft Palate J 1989; 26:63.

20 | TREATMENT OF LANGUAGE DISORDERS

As we have seen, language assessment of children with clefts is not different from language assessment of other young children. The clinician uses those techniques with which he or she is most comfortable and is likely to find a slight delay in expressive abilities in very young children. Since these mild delays are often found in children with clefts, the speech pathologist should not be unduly concerned and should refrain from alarming parents unnecessarily. This does not mean that the clinician cannot or should not act to minimize any deficits that exist as early as possible. It does mean that it is unwise to adopt a blanket attitude that all children with clefts require language therapy. Those with significant problems require active intervention of the type provided for children without clefts.

A THERAPEUTIC PHILOSOPHY

It is our philosophy that therapy should depend upon and begin with careful longitudinal assessments beginning at birth and continuing in a quiet way for as long as they are indicated. In this way, parents can be provided with easy and ongoing guidance. When help is given with early feeding problems, assistance is also being rendered to the speech mechanism and to the social interaction between mother and child. When the mother is encouraged to start solid foods at ages compatible with those of children who do not have clefts or to enter into verbal play early in the child's life, language intervention is underway. No known therapy can substitute for careful encouragement to permit the baby to do what is emerging within his or her span of capabilities.

The parents can be directed to encourage activities appropriate to the baby's developmental level. It is wiser for the clinician to mention that the baby seems ready to play peek-a-boo and then play the game with both parents and child than it is to try to introduce formal language therapy when the child is 2½ or 3 years old, although it is recognized that some children will need that as well.

If a longitudinal approach is taken, it is not necessary to sit down with the parents to explain in detail the nature of their child's problem. The parents, the child, and the clinician, working together, come to a mutual understanding of the child's particular rate of development and of particular deficits that may require special attention. Certainly this kind of program requires careful follow-up on a regular basis so that special ingredients can be added as they are required with full parental understanding and cooperation. This is the ideal approach to management and is possible in the programs offered by most interdisciplinary treatment teams, since routine follow-along care is usually provided. Even when the ideal is not realized in real life, language intervention must be handled in as natural a manner as possible so that the parents can be partners in the treatment rather than adversaries. Hahn (1971, 1979) put this very well:

Unless such involvement is started early, parents may shift responsibility to the professionals, dutifully following the time tables for closure of the lip, closure of the palate, care of the ears and teeth, orthodontic correction, prosthodontic appliances, and possibly secondary surgical procedures. The ability to speak effectively is then treated as an after-effect of the physical remediation.

Down this road lies linguistic disaster!

Since many children with clefts appear eventually to have expressive deficits reflected most often in reduced verbal output, it is essential that longitudinal attention to speech and language development include providing opportunities and stimulation for the child to express ideas and feelings. This means that the parents must, from the beginning, assume a communicative attitude toward the child, talk about the events and experiences of daily living, encourage and reward responses appropriate to the baby's developmental level, allow time for the infant's independent vocal play, use parallel talk, put the child's activities into a verbal context, and continue in such activities even if the baby's responses are more limited than they would like. Parents must expect that their baby will be a verbal, communicative human being, and they must know and believe that the cleft is not a reason for a child's failure to enjoy the process of communicating with others. Most of all, they must not discourage speech because they think that all surgery should be completed before the child is finally given permission to talk.

Parents nurtured in this way will read to their children and listen while their children "read" to them. They will learn to be good listeners and will recognize the benefits of broadening the baby's life experiences, of creating opportunities for peer interaction, of helping the child become independent, of viewing nursery school as a desirable and rewarding step toward becoming a person who knows no barriers to verbal sharing.

THERAPY FOR INFANTS AND PRESCHOOL CHILDREN

Hahn (1971, 1979) recommended a four-pronged approach to language management of children with clefts. In her system, the first encounter comes with the parents during their child's early infancy. This session is designed to help the parents understand the structure of the normal speech mechanism and its function and the way in which their child differs from children who do not have clefts. The parents also learn about normal speech and language development and are encouraged to enter into vocal play with their infant. Hahn stresses the speech pathologist's role in demonstrating vocal play and interaction with the baby. The importance of allowing the infant time to experiment independently is also emphasized as is the importance of the parents' use of single words that occur frequently in the child's environment, a method of stimulating cognitive development. The parents are encouraged to produce these words strongly, clearly, and repetitiously in the baby's hearing. At the end of the first session, the parents are urged to begin verbal stimulation immediately and are informed that they will continue to receive assistance and support from the speech pathologist in future sessions.

Hahn suggested that the second session with the parents occur when the infant is between 7 and 12 months of age. The clinician again instructs the parents about how to proceed when they are working on their own. This phase of stimulation includes attention to single key words presented and stressed in the context of questions and simple statements. The importance of increasing experiential opportunities is discussed, along with use of vocabulary that matches experiences, again emphasizing cognitive development. During this second visit, which in many centers would almost immediately precede the surgical closure of the palate, the speech pathologist begins to discuss the probable effects of palatal closure on the speech structures and their function.

At the third session, occurring 6 to 8 weeks after surgical closure of the palate, the speech pathologist begins to select objects for the parents to use in stimulating the child to develop initial consonants, particularly, according to Hahn (1971, 1979) /k/ and /g/. In fact, the accurate production of most consonants can be stimulated, and the parents can be instructed to guard against the appearance of extra tension and facial grimacing. (Lip surgery is done at very early ages; this schedule would have to be altered to be consistent with the child's developmental age.)

When the child starts to use single words, the parents should understand the importance of stimulating two-word combinations and of using simple sentences in their conversations with the child. In Hahn's system, as the child responds and uses spontaneous communicative behaviors, the parents are encouraged to offer rewards such as words of approval, candy, or kisses. We prefer strategies of social reinforcement because they seem more conducive to the development of positive communicative attitudes.

This system of management includes another session before the child is 3½ years of age. The exact timing depends upon the speech pathologist's assessment of the parents' eagerness to continue the home program and of the developmental level of the preschooler. At this time the importance of peer-group interaction is stressed along with the necessity for helping the child understand the nature of the physical impairment. The child should also be placed under the supervision of a speech pathologist for direct therapy if there are indicators of need.

Hahn is careful to point out that not all parents are emotionally equipped to help their children in the way she recommends. Some are too aggressive and create emotional problems for the child. Others may be uncomfortable entering into such behavior. These parents will obviously need more counseling and more direct help from the speech pathologist, as may the child.

This stimulation protocol is based upon normal patterns of development in young children, and an effort is made to help the child with a cleft parallel those milestones. It seems important to us to remember that many children with clefts do not develop speech problems and do well with language and speech behavior in the early years of their lives. For this reason, care should be taken that the parents are not somehow taught to expect that their child will be communicatively handicapped. This attitude can be detrimental to good speech and language development. Rather, we believe that the parents should be assured that they are being helped to do well what all parents need to do with their infants and young children. We also favor more frequent contacts with the speech pathologist in these early months and years than Hahn prescribed.

Philips (1971, 1979) also presented a useful system for stimulating syntactic and phonological development in infants with cleft palate. She listed her purposes as follows:

1. To develop the child's confidence in his ability to achieve intelligible verbal communication.

2. To allay parental anxiety concerning the child's development of verbal communication.

3. To encourage development of communication skills to the maximum of the child's potential.

4. To minimize or prevent the development of undesirable compensatory articulation and voice problems when physical inadequacies interfere with the normal development of speech skills.

5. To determine velopharyngeal competence for oral communication as early as possible.

She recommended that these goals be achieved through informal sessions, preferably short ones, with the child and parents. In the beginning these sessions should probably be individual, since young children often do not interact well together. The activities selected should be oriented toward the developmental level of the child, and the participating adults should be highly accepting of the communication attempts of the child. Having the child participate, together with one or both parents, will give the child a greater sense of security and will help to train the parents to use the techniques being demonstrated.

This stimulation program, like that of Hahn, is based on the hypothesis that delay in the development of both receptive and expressive language is frequently the result of deprivation of normal stimulation. It should be pointed out that this assumption of limited stimulation is sometimes not warranted, but that does not rule out the potential advantages of the program outlined. Some infants appear to require increased, perhaps simplified, stimulation. While they may not be deprived in the usual sense, their physical disadvantage may increase their requirements. Some, of course, are genuinely in need of verbal stimulation, which the parents may not be providing.

Like Hahn, Philips suggested naming objects in the environment, accepting the child's attempts to reproduce words, responding in a rewarding manner to the child's attempts to use speech, and reinforcing these attempts by having the adult model the word or words in a meaningful context.

Early in Philips's program, the child is encouraged to produce those phonemes that can be produced successfully, even with an open palate. The examples given were /h/, /w/, and /m/. Philips suggested that, if there is velopharyngeal incompetence, then it is possible to stress placement for certain sounds so that gross articulatory disorders do not develop. In this case, correct placement would be rewarded without penalty for loss of air through the nasal passages. If it is possible for the appropriate amount of intraoral pressure to be impounded, it is then desirable to provide auditory, visual, and tactile stimulation for correct production of the other features of the phonemes being encouraged. This phase is, as in any therapy program, followed by work to develop carryover into social situations.

Neither this system nor Hahn's is unique to the child with a cleft but is designed to take advantage of the period of greatest flexibility in linguistic development and to minimize the language delays that have been found in children with clefts. Neither of the systems is based upon data other than clinical experience. However, both have face validity, and both rely upon information available about early childhood development. They appear to be sensible and practical approaches as long as the speech pathologist uses them conservatively as the authors intended.

Brookshire et al. (1980) published a 123-page book devoted to a combined clinician-parent approach to the systematic stimulation of speech development, cognition, language comprehension and expression, and pragmatics in children with cleft palates. Part I of their program first relates to speech and is divided into six levels, each encompassing 6 months beginning from birth to 6 months and ending with 30 to 36 months. Each level contains from three to six objectives with a rationale for each, suggested activities and materials, and criteria for assessing either the need for or the success of the program designed to accomplish the specific objective. Cognition is presented in a similar manner except that the rationale for the suggested activities is not included. Comprehension and expression of language and pragmatics are similarly discussed in separate sections. Part II consists of informational material for parents on a wide variety of subjects including the nature of the cleft palate team, feeding, surgery, hearing, language, and speech, to name a few.

This developmentally oriented program, which incorporates many of the ideas presented in the foregoing sections, has the advantage of having been field tested in order to determine its utility both in the clinic and at home. Parents demonstrated their work with their children, kept diaries of observations and questions, and had access to videotapes of their sessions with their children. In short, they underwent active training geared to make them effective infant stimulators.

Lynch (1986) noted that there are three types of infant programs that have been most commonly used with high-risk infants. They include those that are home-based with the infant specialist going to the home to work with the mother (or other caregivers) and the child; those where the

mother (or other care provider) brings the child to the center for participation in the developmental program; and those that incorporate both the home and the center. Any one of these models can be effective, but combining the home and center approaches has the advantage of providing opportunities for the clinician to become acquainted with the child's daily environment and for the parent and child to expand their experience outside the home.

Lynch suggests that any program of this type must provide assistance and support for the parents, taking into account both their strengths and their weaknesses; must involve the child and the parent or parents in order to encourage reciprocal communications on both verbal and nonverbal levels with awareness of the need for shared participation; should incorporate prespeech activities appropriate to the age of the child; should be based on "gentle" intervention that is play-centered, encourages the child to initiate interaction with others, and fosters the development of imagination and creativity; and should provide for consistent monitoring by the speech-language pathologist so that any factors that may negatively influence language development can be minimized.

Philips (1987) discussed early management of young children with clefts and presented three levels of intervention. The first level stresses parent education and encompasses the first 12 to 18 months of the child's life. The second is introduced when the child seems ready, usually between 12 and 18 months, and incorporates both speech and language stimulation. The third level, beginning at about 30 months, introduces active intervention of a therapeutic nature. Philips stressed the importance of allowing the child's own development to dictate the need for these strategies and the age at which they should be introduced. Some children will progress well and will require only careful and consistent monitoring without special programming.

Witzel and McWilliams (1977), concerned about the effects of mothers providing more negative than positive feedback to their young children with clefts, developed a 13-week group program for five preschool children with language delay and four mothers. (One declined the training for herself.) During the program each mother interacted with a child other than her own and was taught to assess her verbal behavior using a scale developed by Kasprisin-Burrelli et al. (1972). The categories used in this interactional analysis include statements and questions that have positive value for the child and those that have negative implications. For example, when a child volunteers that he was yelled at in school, a positive response would be, "You must have felt really bad when that happened," while a negative response would be, "You must have been bad or you wouldn't have been yelled at."

The mothers in this program increased their positive verbal behavior significantly, ranging from 16% to 25%. The mothers' comments about the experience were most revealing. "It has taught me to listen more closely to my children," "It's amazing how you can stimulate them to talk by the way you talk to them," are examples.

This type of program is different from those described earlier in that it has a specific focus even as it enters into the more generalized procedures of the other plans. This strategy is useful in research and in changing specific behaviors that are thought to be influential in maintaining language problems.

All of these programs attempt to encourage the achievement of normal developmental landmarks in children born with clefts. They all include stimulation and play activities in which parents may engage with their infants and young children. The presentation of precise instructions and demonstrations is a means of helping parents realize the importance of early interaction with their infants and preschoolers. On the other hand, in an already anxiety-laden situation, the speech pathologist must be alert to the possibility that intervention of this type might, in some cases, trigger or intensify fears detrimental to the parents and to their child. It is important to exercise caution in order to avoid undesirable sequelae.

Akin to this warning is one concerning parents and babies who are doing well on their own. Their behavior may profitably be reinforced, but there is no need to intervene when things are progressing satisfactorily. It is as important to know when to keep hands off as it is to know when and how to render assistance. A third word or warning has to do with the thin line between helping parents and children live together happily and communicatively, with the parents and child deriving joy from their mutual interaction, and turning the parents into pseudo-speech pathologists who feel compelled to sit down with their child and go at him or her like drill sergeants. Let's

encourage parents to be good parents and enjoy the process.

Capitalizing on Normal Childhood Experiences

You will recall from the information presented in Chapters 8 and 9 that children and adults with clefts are often somewhat inhibited, are less verbal than their noncleft peers, and demonstrate mild deficits in some aspects of language development, especially in expression. Since that is the case, it is logical to try to prevent those developmental variations by encouraging children with clefts in as many normal experiences as possible, particularly those that are likely to enhance independence, contribute to a positive self image, encourage social interaction, and promote language usage. Two such approaches are described below.

Preschool Programs

The programs outlined in the previous sections are intended to encourage pleasure in verbal expression, which implies that social development is consistent with developmental age and is sufficiently robust to provide the impetus for interpersonal relationships and interest in communicating with peers. Preschool experience is one way of enhancing cognitive, social, creative, and communicative development in a normal, nonclinical atmosphere that captures the child's natural curiosity, helps to expand horizons, and encourages independence, peer interaction, and the strengthening of self image. Since our goal always is to stress the child's strengths and normality while acting to minimize and reduce weaknesses, the preschool is often a wiser choice than active therapy (see Figs. 20.1, 20.2).

Some children with mild lags in sensory-motor and language development have made significant gains in Montessori preschools, where children are helped to participate in developmentally appropriate activities geared to stimulate sensory-motor capacities.

The preschool is not appropriate for children who demonstrate significant deficiencies in several areas. They require special intervention and specific attention, as do all children with major

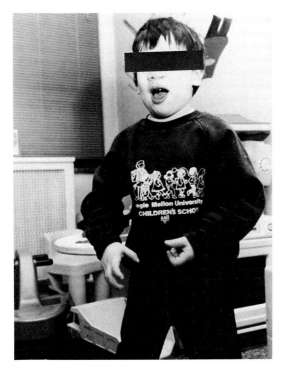

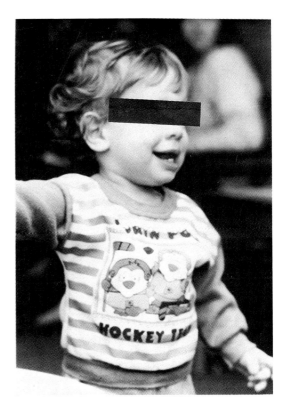

Figure 20.1 This boy proudly wears his preschool shirt.

deficits. However, if mental development and receptive language development are within or close to normal limits but expressive language is reduced, preschool experience often leads to dramatic improvement.

Creative Dramatics

Irwin and McWilliams (1974) reported the effects of creative dramatics on the verbal expression of young language-delayed children with clefts. Creative dramatics, a group activity described by Ward (1957), places a high value on verbal expression in a relaxed, supportive, enjoyable atmosphere. Eleven children between 3 and 6 years of age participated in 32 weekly 2-hour sessions, each conducted by a specialist with background in child development and psychiatry. The first 10 sessions provided for dramatic play, rhythmic activities, and pantomime. Fourteen sessions were then devoted to acting out structured material; in the final eight sessions, the children verbalized fantasies, original stories, and

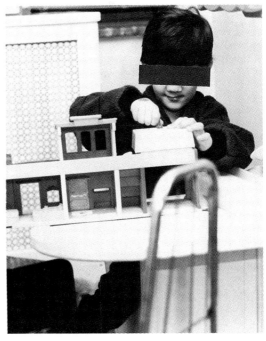

Figure 20.2 A and B. Even informal play in the clinical waiting room has interactional benefits.

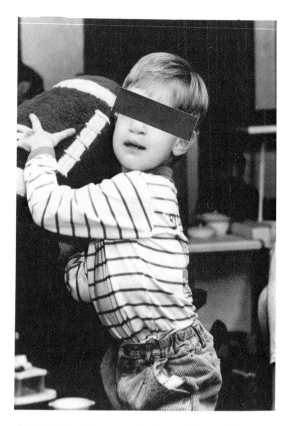

Figure 20.2 C. Informal play in the clinical waiting room.

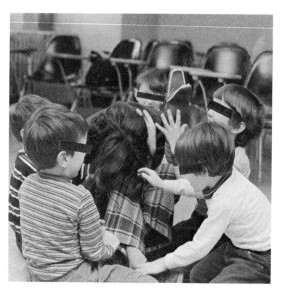

Figure 20.3 Children with clefts enjoying a creative-dramatics session with a sensitive, responsive leader.

fears. The final sessions were not planned but developed spontaneously. At least one observer was present at each session to compile written records of the children's behavior including role selections, pantomime, language use, and speech. The observers rated each child's participation in pantomime, role playing, and speech and language behavior on five-point scales ranging from no participation to superior performance. Reliability for scale usage was acceptable.

The children's ratings for pantomime, role playing, and speech and language improved significantly from one phase of the program to the next. Observers' narratives indicated that the children moved from verbal behavior marked by single words or short phrases to verbal output that was considerably more frequent, complex, and spontaneous. Behavior and speech appeared to change together (see Fig. 20.3).

The final eight sessions were dominated by rushes of verbal expression incorporating a great deal of psychodynamic information. The following is an example of the original stories the children told:

There was a grandma who got sick and had to go to the hospital for 6 weeks. She had the flu, diarrhea, and the measles. Mother comes in and calls, "Grandma," but she can't find her. Finally, she looks under the bed and finds her. "Don't do that again," Mother says, and she's very mad. Then Grandma gets out of bed and hides. "Oh, no, not again," Mother says. And then the Mother calls, "Doctors, nurses, get your guns." And they all get their guns and hunt for Grandma. And then, guess what? They find her under the desk. "If you do that again, I'm going to shoot you. Now don't do that again," Mother tells her. And then the nurse gives her a shot and says, "If Grandma has a baby, throw it out the window. She may not have a baby unless she wants a baby." And sure enough, she has a baby (pretends to take baby and throw it out the window) *and then grandma gets blind and can't see, and then they put up the venetian blinds and she can see again.*

All this from a child who said almost nothing at the start of the sessions!

Creative dramatics is a useful, fun-filled activity that has potential for increasing the verbal

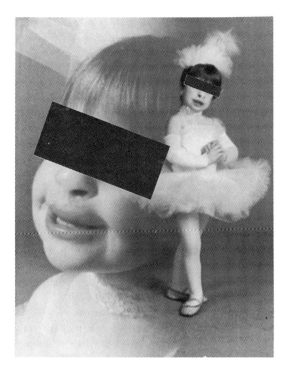

Figure 20.4 This little girl feels like the star she really is.

output of children whose major language problems are related to the amount of verbal output rather than to specific language deficits.

MANAGING CHILDREN AT HIGH RISK FOR LANGUAGE AND DEVELOPMENTAL DEFICITS

The foregoing sections of this chapter are intended to focus on cleft children who have the mild delays that have been discussed in detail in Chapters 8 and 13. As those chapters also indicate, some children are at much higher risk for significant developmental variations, and their overall development should always receive extra scrutiny. Speech-language pathologists should recognize the value of total assessment of the baby and of careful, realistic parental counseling carried out by someone thoroughly knowledgeable about evaluating infants and interpreting test results. Too many parents are needlessly upset and too many inappropriately reassured.

All children with clefts associated with syndromes or other malformations may require intervention beyond what has just been described.

Children with isolated palatal clefts and no other birth defects are also at a somewhat increased risk and should be assessed. In this latter group, there will be a higher occurrence of significant developmental delays, but there will also be more children who are developing at an accelerated rate. It is important to provide extra assistance to those who require it, but it is also essential to identify those who should be encouraged to take their places as early as possible among children like themselves. In those cases, the cleft and its ramifications can often be minimized and should be.

Infant Programs

For those who are experiencing significant developmental delays, the programming described previously for infants can be introduced. As with any child, suggestions given to parents should relate to developmental rather than to chronological age. Parents will undoubtedly realize that their children are not doing the things that are expected, and this increases their anxiety and their counseling needs on an ongoing basis. For these reasons, it is usually desirable that intervention programs for such infants be more intensive than they are for babies who are doing well and that more of the activity be centered in the home, where a specialist in infant development visits on a regular basis.

These programs are usually broadly based and include motor, sensory, cognitive, social, language, and speech training introduced at appropriate levels as the child is ready to participate. Public schools are now mandated to offer such services when children have been identified as having significant developmental deficits. The Easter Seal Society, United Cerebral Palsy, Association for Retarded Citizens, the American Association for Children with Learning Disabilities, some hospitals, other community agencies, and cleft palate programs participate and cooperate with each other to provide a unified approach to each child's special needs.

The Preschool Child

As children grow older, their needs change; and it is desirable to find appropriate preschool placements for them. Those who can function in a normal program should have that opportunity, while those who still need special assistance can find places in special settings offered by the same agencies that provide programs for high-risk infants.

These schools have the same goals as preschools for normal children but are treatment-oriented and offer language, speech, occupational, and physical therapy when they are necessary. Language therapy for children with clefts and other special needs is not different from the various forms of language therapy that are available to language-impaired children who do not have clefts. There is a vast and ever-growing body of literature on this topic, and it is not necessary that it be reviewed here. It is important, however, to recognize that significant language problems complicate the management of the cleft and the other way around. Neither can be ignored, and total treatment planning is mandatory.

Educational Planning

If there is any question at all about development, language functioning, or learning disabilities, children should be reassessed as they approach school age so that appropriate school experiences can be provided. Preventing educational failures, if possible, is preferred to dealing with them after they have occurred and is usually more productive.

Sometimes delaying entrance to kindergarten in favor of an added year in preschool, having access to a pre-first grade or repeating kindergarten, arranging for instruction that takes learning disabilities into account from the very beginning, and continuing with language intervention can eventually minimize any special deficits in these areas. If that is not possible, the child can at least be given all the special aids he requires to reach his fullest potential. Too often these children are well along in school before there is any understanding of their deficits.

It is necessary to realize here that these deficiencies may sometimes be innate to the child, may be the result of a combination of environmental influences interacting with predisposing factors in the child, or may spring primarily from psychological stresses that should be considered in providing treatment, which is sometimes most effectively conducted by a child psychiatrist or a psychologist who has special skills in dealing with educationally fragile children. Almost all problems of this type can be solved within limits if appropriate steps are taken first rather than last.

Not all children with clefts will be able to perform well in some of these areas, and those limitations will have to be taken into account in assessing progress. It is possible, however, to guide children so that they are able to accept and value themselves and can be accepted by others without having to strive to become somebody else or to achieve the impossible. Happy children with certain deficits, which they understand and can live with, are able to make the best possible use of the abilities they have. Unhappy children who strive to achieve beyond their own capacities are never able to reach their full potential.

THE SPEECH PATHOLOGIST IN RELATION TO SPECIAL PROGRAMS

The speech pathologist responsible for the care of a child who is referred to some special program for a particular purpose does not relinquish all responsibility. Rather, he or she coordinates all of the services the child is receiving—or knows that someone else is doing so, follows development closely to be sure that the plan is progressing as expected, and continues to assess the child at regular intervals and to modify the plan if necessary. This, of course, is done with the cooperation and knowledge of everyone else involved. Sometimes someone else in the cleft palate clinic has that assignment, but it is often a speech pathologist.

SUMMARY

In this chapter, we have focused on the special but relatively mild language delays that affect the majority of children with clefts. We have stressed the desirability of early intervention when it is indicated and of recognizing the child who does not require special assistance. Keeping the child's life as close to normal as possible, while providing experiences that will aid in increasing verbal output and in enhancing the pleasure that is derived from communication with others are major goals.

When more profound language problems occur, as they sometimes do, especially in children with other birth defects or isolated palatal clefts, more special programming is likely to be required beginning in infancy and extending into the school years. The goal in these cases is to minimize the effects of language and learning disabilities so that the child's life may be satisfying and rewarding.

REFERENCES

Brookshire BL, Lynch JI, Fox DR. A parent-child cleft palate curriculum, developing speech and language. Tigard, OR: CC Publications, 1980.

Hahn E. Directed home training program for infants with cleft lip and palate. In: Grabb WC, Rosenstein SW, Bzoch KR, eds. Cleft lip and palate. Boston: Little, Brown, 1971:830, and In: Bzoch KR, ed. Communicative disorders related to cleft lip and palate. Boston: Little, Brown, 1979.

Irwin EC, McWilliams BJ. Play therapy for children with cleft palates. Children Today 1974; 3:18.

Kasprisin-Burrelli A, Egolf DB, Thames TH. A comparison of parental verbal behavior with stuttering and nonstuttering children. J Com Dis 1972; 5:335.

Lynch JL. Language of cleft infants: lessening the delay through programming. In: McWilliams BJ, ed. Seminars in Speech and Language. Current methods of assessing and treating children with cleft palates, 1986; 7:255.

Philips BJ. Stimulating syntactic and phonological development in infants with cleft palate. In: Grabb WC, Rosenstein SW, Bzoch KR, eds. Cleft lip and palate. Boston: Little, Brown, 1971:835, and In: Bzoch KR, ed. Communicative disorders related to cleft lip and palate. Boston: Little, Brown, 1979.

Philips BJ. Early speech management. Conference on Current State of the Art in Cleft Palate, University of Iowa, 1987; (in press).

Ward W. Playmaking with children. New York: Appleton, Century, Crofts, 1957.

Witzel MA, McWilliams BJ. The effect of training procedures on mother-to-child verbal statements. Hum Commun 1977, Spring:7.

21 | TREATMENT OF DISORDERS OF PHONATION AND RESONANCE

In this chapter we discuss the advantages and disadvantages of therapy to improve problems of phonation and resonance. Research evidence, when available, is presented along with information derived from clinical experience. Therapeutic approaches and the indicators for their use are included as well.

PHONATION THERAPY

We know of no research that has been carried out to assess the results of therapy in children or adults with the phonation problems sometimes secondary to aberrant velopharyngeal valving. Nor do we have all the information required to discriminate between patients whose phonation problems are primarily the result of behaviors adopted to compensate for valving deficits and those who have phonation problems because of the hypertensive laryngeal function frequently found in children who do not have valving problems. That distinction is important because it helps us make the decision to correct a borderline valve in order to improve phonation. In cases of overt velopharyngeal incompetence, the course is clear; we correct the valve. In some cases, however, the evidence is equivocal. Vocal abuse may spring from causes other than velopharyngeal valving deficits or phonation problems remain after the valve has been corrected. Speech therapy, at least on a trial basis, is indicated under these circumstances.

When phonation therapy of this type is planned, it does not differ appreciably from the therapies described in any standard text for people who do not have clefts (Wilson, 1972; Cooper and Cooper, 1977; Boone, 1977, 1983; Aronson, 1980; Boone and McFarlane, 1988).

Procedures used in therapy are based largely on clinical experience and have been demonstrated to be effective in at least some patients. There are few data to support the efficacy of any one technique as compared to another. Certainly, there are no data available for the response of subjects with clefts to phonation therapy. However, as more and more people with borderline valving abilities are studied, more and more phonation problems are identified, and the need to attempt therapy and to study the origins of the defects is intensified.

Here we discuss therapeutic procedures that we use from time to time in our own clinical settings. We offer them cautiously and recommend that they be applied in a diagnostic sense. If phonation improves without undue sacrifices in other aspects of speech, that is all to the good. If it does not improve or if other speech symptoms are intensified, the therapy will at least have served the purpose of shedding additional light on the efficiency of velopharyngeal valving.

Underlying Principles

An underlying principle of all phonation therapy for those with clefts is that it should not be directed to the elimination of nasal escape and hypernasality since attempts to compensate for those features in speech may have contributed to the phonation problem in the first place.

A second principle is that patients with clefts (particularly children) who have phonation problems require longitudinal follow-along because some may improve as they get older; a few may deteriorate as they grow and their valving mechanisms become somewhat less efficient; and some are likely to stay about the same. We must know what is occurring even after therapy has been completed.

Therapy for Vocal Cord Nodules

Vocal cord nodules are the most common finding when children with clefts who demonstrate hoarseness are examined by laryngoscopy. If, as is generally believed, vocal cord nodules are the result of vocal hyperfunction, including hard glottal attack, it is obviously necessary to reduce tension in the respiratory muscles and vocal tract during speech. What is said about accomplishing this applies to other hyperfunctional disorders as well.

If we are successful in eliminating unwanted vocal stress, the result may well be increased nasal emission, increased perception of hypernasality, and reduced loudness. Thus, this treatment may assist with phonation problems but may reveal other aspects of the speech pattern also related to velopharyngeal incompetence. When this occurs, the clinician should recognize that compensatory laryngeal maneuvers secondary to velopharyngeal incompetence have masked symptoms that are now apparent.

It is our philosophy that the communication potential of patients with velopharyngeal incompetence is better if negative compensatory behaviors can be reduced to a minimum. If this attitude is not shared by the patient, phonation therapy will fail. The patient must want to change and must cooperate in therapy. Careful counseling about the nature of the voice disorder, the reasons for altering vocal behavior, the mechanisms for accomplishing it, and the pros and cons of improving phonation is mandatory in this type of therapy. Self-concept is intimately tied to the image the voice projects. Changing from one voice to another can be frightening, embarrassing, threatening, and personally invasive. A 9-year-old girl summed up her feelings when she said, "Oh, I can do it, but I'm not going to at school. Do you think I want people to think I'm crazy or something?" A young man acknowledged two lives, one in a distant city where he worked and used his new voice and another at home with his family where he used his old voice. A woman was afraid that, if her phonation improved, she would receive less attention from her husband. The feelings, the secondary gains, and the uncertainties contrive to defeat therapy in some cases. When you add the possibility that hypernasality will increase, the resistance demonstrated by some patients is not surprising.

It is obvious that counseling must always be a part of therapy if it is to succeed. In some cases, tensions will be sufficiently intense to warrant intervention by a psychotherapist working in conjunction with the speech pathologist. Usually, however, the speech pathologist is equipped to carry out the required counseling.

Providing Information about Voice

The therapy program begins with helping the parents and, when indicated, the child to understand how voice is produced and why the phonation habits being used are harmful to the vocal cords (Wilson, 1972; Aronson, 1980; and Boone, 1977, 1983; Boone and McFarlane, 1988). Even very young children can be shown diagrams, pictures, and models that will help in this regard, but explanations must be at the child's level. With a 4-year-old we used drawings and stories, and he colored vocal cords red and inflamed with nodules to represent his own cords. Boone (1980, 1983) described a program for accomplishing this goal of developing cognitive awareness in children.

Indirect Therapy for Hyperfunctional Voice

After there is some awareness of the nature of the problem, we try to identify the conditions in the environment that may be contributing to vocal hyperfunction and either change them or help the child understand how to cope with them without increased tension (Moore, 1971). For example, the aforementioned 4-year-old was the youngest of three boys in a highly verbal, high-powered family. He often yelled to make his older brothers pay attention to what he had to say. The mother worked with the older children to enlist their cooperation in reducing the cleft child's need to struggle for his share of talking time, and we helped by having the older boys attend a session or two with their younger brother. During one of these, our patient allied himself with the speech pathologist by putting his chair beside hers and facing his brothers across the table. He then spontaneously showed them pictures of vocal cords and explained what had happened to his and why. The older boys responded by saying that they also did a lot of screaming. The mother was not present for this exchange, but the boys were eager to bring to her attention their new-found insights. This is an example of the exciting events that can be associated with this type of therapy—even though changing long-standing family behavior is a difficult, often impossible, task.

In another family, it became apparent that the father was a loud, dominating speaker and that the whole family followed suit. In another, a family pattern of yelling at each other from all parts of the house had been established. These environmental factors should be changed for the vocal health of the entire family.

We also work with the parents and with the child to eliminate any unusual, damaging, vocal behaviors in which he or she may be engaging. The child who colored vocal cords also made little popping and buzzing noises in the larynx almost constantly. He was masterful in the variety of sounds he could create and in the places he used them to advantage in his play. These had to be eliminated along with loud crying and screaming when his older brothers got in his way. There was so much of this behavior and he was so young that it took time and hard work to change those vocal habits. At home, the crying behavior was charted in half-day segments, and a reinforcement system was used to reward him for the periods when there was no crying and to penalize him for the times when there was crying. His understanding of the therapeutic system was crucial. The laryngeal noises were first worked on in the clinic, and alternate methods of expression were taught. Then a home program was initiated to monitor those behaviors.

For older children, Boone's (1977, 1980, 1983; Boone and McFarlane, 1988) "tally method" is helpful. He states that the importance of this approach cannot be overestimated in eliminating vocal abuse in children. He gives an example of the yelling incidents tallied by an 11-year-old boy (Fig. 21.1). It is obvious that this boy yelled 18 times on day 1 and not at all on day 10. This approach is also effective with adults, who sometimes respond remarkably quickly. An adult counted 15 events of throat clearing in the first hour of charting. Awareness of this behavior led him to reduce throat clearing to two or three times per hour thereafter. That was quite a feat because he suffered from dry throat and allergies, which also had to be treated. His work was also vocally demanding, and he learned to alternate vocal rest with his frequent public appearances. Easier vocal attack was also accomplished. His vocal cord

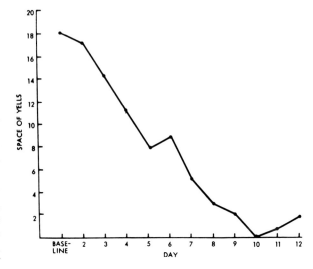

Figure 21.1 Chart of an 11-year-old boy's daily tally of his yelling over a 12-day period. On the first day, a baseline count of 18 yells was tallied. The general overall contour of the curve shows a marked decrement in the amount of yelling recorded. (From Boone D. The voice and voice therapy. 3rd ed. Englewood Cliffs, NJ: Prentice-Hall, 1977.)

nodules cleared up within four months. When his hoarseness recurred 4 years later, it was tempting to rely on past history and treat the symptoms again. Fortunately, that was not done. He saw an otolaryngologist and subsequently had surgery to remove a malignant vocal-cord tumor.

In addition to these approaches, we provide the parents with two pages of suggestions for vocal conservation or vocal hygiene. These include such things as turning off the radio or television while attempting to talk; using a bell or whistle instead of yelling at someone outdoors or in another room; avoiding having the whole family talk at once; engaging in quiet, easy speech within the family; learning to stamp feet or clap hands instead of cheering at sports events; touching the shoulder of another person to attract attention, especially when a number of people are present, and talking directly to people with hearing losses. Parents are encouraged to help their vocally impaired children minimize crying episodes and to teach them alternate means of expression.

These techniques do not represent formal therapy but can be used successfully, sometimes in combination with formal therapy, to eliminate major sources of vocal stress. In children with velopharyngeal valving problems, more direct voice therapy is often indicated.

Direct Therapy for Hyperfunctional Voice

When vocal hyperfunction has been adopted to compensate for valving deficits, it is wise to consider teaching and habituating an easier way of talking. Aronson (1980) recommended, in addition to the informational phase described above, two other phases of therapy: auditory discrimination and voice production.

Auditory Discrimination

In this phase, the child learns to hear differences between his or her voice and the voices of children who do not have vocal cord nodules and between his or her best and poorest vocal attempts. Many writers have stressed the importance of this type of training (Moore, 1971; Wilson, 1972; Boone, 1977, 1980; Boone and McFarlane, 1988).

Voice Production

Aronson indicated that training the child to reduce vocal loudness (often not a problem in children with velopharyngeal valving deficits) and hard glottal attacks is central to voice therapy. Others agree (Murphy, 1964; Boone, 1977; Boone and McFarlane, 1988). We believe that reducing glottal attack is almost always indicated in cleft children who have valving problems. Hard glottal attack is not to be confused with glottal stops substituted for plosives and used as alternative articulatory gestures. Hard glottal attack is initiating speech using hypertensive vocal cord adduction.

During this phase, the patient is taught to initiate words beginning with vowels by using a very easy, gentle attack. This can be introduced by going from an /h/ into the vowel. This breathy attack can be felt, and the child can be taught to sense the relaxed phonation that results. Boone (1983) even resorts to a whisper in order to get an easy attack and then blends that into soft phonation.

We sometimes begin by placing the child in a supine position to relax the respiration system and vocal tract. We add phonation from that position and encourage similar activity at home

four or five times a day. Boone (1983) stressed the usefulness of such instruments as the Visi-Pitch (1980) and the voice monitor (1977) for visual display of hard glottal attack and for comparative purposes as well. After easy phonation is possible on vowels and words beginning with vowels, we attempt words beginning with consonants and initiate them with /h/, which is gradually faded as easy initiation of individual words becomes possible. We then progress to two-word combinations, longer phrases, sentences, paragraphs, and finally to conversational speech.

Self-monitoring is stressed throughout therapy, and a tape recorder is often indicated. Wilson (1972) warned of the dangers associated with this. Some children will be upset when they hear their voices for the first time, especially if the voice problem is severe. He suggested not using the recorder during the first therapy session or until adequate preparation has taken place. We agree with Wilson (1972), who pointed out that operant programs may be useful in therapy. He stressed the need to use shaping procedures, realizing that the target behavior is usually reached by a series of approximations. This type of therapy begins where the patient is and moves in small reinforced steps toward the goal.

Aronson (1980) included in the voice-production phase the discussion of personal and family problems. We mention it here with the admonition that, if there are significant problems of this sort, they should be an ongoing part of all therapy as should efforts to eliminate or minimize such conditions.

Habituating the New Voice

Wilson (1972) recommended the use of negative practice for carryover training of children with phonation problems including vocal cord nodules. In order to accomplish that, he presented side-by-side pictures of liked and disliked items. The child was asked to produce the name of the disliked object in a hard, forceful, explosive manner, whereas the name of the preferred object was spoken in an easy, smooth way. He then used more subtle forms of negative practice, moving from the severe form of glottal attack to moderate, mild, and normal. Wilson's contention was that this approach helps the child realize that he or she has control over phonation and has the capability of speaking at will without tension. Boone (1977) agreed that negative practice is beneficial.

Wilson divided carryover training into two phases—limited and overall habituation. In limited habituation, the child first uses the new pattern only with the speech pathologist and then in highly prescribed situations outside the clinic. During the latter activity, a prearranged monitor should be available to assess the nature of the phonation since the child may not be able to judge adequately in the new environment.

In overall habituation, the child is expected to use the new voice during entire therapy sessions, then in specific classes at school, during certain hours at home, and in predetermined social situations. The times and occasions are gradually extended until the child and those close to him report that the new voice is consistent.

In this discussion, we have stressed work with children. However, therapy for adolescents and adults with vocal-cord nodules is carried out in much the same way, with appropriate changes in the nature of the activities.

This type of therapy is indicated even if hypernasality is increased. If that occurs, consideration should be given to improving the velopharyngeal valve.

Direct Therapy for Soft-Voice Syndrome

This disorder is rather tricky to approach clinically because of the danger of creating vocal hyperfunction. Some problems of reduced loudness originate because of prolonged hyperfunction resulting eventually in the breakdown of glottal surfaces as in nodules (Boone and McFarlane, 1988). However, Boone (1977) and Boone and McFarlane (1988) suggested that attempts to increase loudness (in hypernasal speakers) are sometimes appropriate. Boone also noted that attempts to increase loudness are inappropriate if the symptoms arise out of general physical weakness or a severe personality problem. We would add known velopharyngeal incompetence. However, in cases where borderline valving abilities are implicated, we attempt therapy very cautiously and discontinue it at the first sign of vocal hyperfunction or increased hypernasality.

This type of therapy demands developing an awareness on the patient's part of the nature of the voice problem and of what it communicates to other people. Boone (1977) and Boone and McFarlane (1988) recommended experimenting with pitch to see if a level can be found at which an easy, louder voice can be produced. When that pitch is found and loudness is increased, self-monitoring with a tape recorder becomes important. Much practice is necessary. At first, reading materials can be used with a gradual shift into simple spontaneous speech and then conversation.

Boone (1977) and Boone and McFarlane (1988) stated that respiration training is sometimes indicated, and again we experiment with increasing loudness from a supine position. If that is effective, we institute several practice periods daily of talking in that position. Boone and Boone and McFarlane also recommended the pushing approach which Froeschels et al. (1955) developed to treat palatal paralysis. In this technique, phonation is coordinated with simultaneous movement of the arms. Froeschels et al. described the process in these words:

> The patient is first instructed to raise his fists to his chest and to push his arms down in one quick, elastic sweep. During the downward swing of the arms, the fingers should not open. When the arm movements are completed, the palms should land at the front of the thigh.

When this can be accomplished easily, the patient is instructed to say "ah" just as he begins to push his arms down. Other vowel sounds are used alternately, and syllables and monosyllabic words are gradually added. Froeschels et al. recommended that an exercise cycle consist of 10 pushes at a time and that a cycle be completed every half hour for the first few days and every hour for the remaining days of the first week. The patient is gradually introduced to phonation without pushing but is instructed to think of pushing as phonation takes place. Carryover is initiated as in all other forms of voice therapy. It is not usually necessary to resort to this technique, however, as loudness can usually be increased without it if proper attention is paid to velopharyngeal valving.

Another technique that is commonly used and that we like for some patients is the introduction of a masking noise as competition to the feedback that the patient gets from his or her own voice. The masking sound can be white noise, a pure tone, almost anything as long as it is loud enough to compete with the patient's speech. We especially like Boone's protocol:

1. Tape record the patient as he or she reads a passage of about 100 words.

2. At word 30, introduce the competing sound; the patient's voice should get louder.

3. Remove the masking sound at about the 50th word; the patient's voice will probably get softer.

4. Alternate sound and silence at 15-word intervals for the reading of the rest of the passage.

5. Have the patient listen to the recording.

6. Ask the patient to match his loudness levels.

We repeat the process instructing the patient to maintain the loudness level when the masking is withdrawn.

Training in auditory discrimination is mandatory throughout therapy for loudness problems, and carryover or habituation practice must be a part of the plan. Both are conducted in much the same way as for vocal cord nodules.

We should point out that not all loudness problems require therapy that is this extensive. If the patient can increase loudness easily and at will, we work on habituation immediately. It is important to remember that some patients with reduced loudness will be *unable* to change until velopharyngeal valving is improved or will do so at the price of increasing vocal hyperfunction.

Aspirate Voice Quality

The approaches to this problem are much like those for loudness disorders. Breathy voices are sometimes associated with vocal hypofunction, and the goal is to increase tension to an optimal level so that the vocal cords are more completely adducted during phonation. The key word is *optimal*. We must be very careful to avoid vocal hyperfunction and to distinguish aspirate quality that has its origins in hyperfunction. The pushing method is again recommended and may be indicated in severe cases. In less severe cases, increasing loudness may be all that is required.

Summary of Phonation Disorders

All of these phonation disorders are compensatory behaviors when they are associated with velopharyngeal incompetence or borderline valving. Thus, therapy for changing any one of them

may result in an increase in hypernasality and nasal escape. This should be carefully monitored and the therapy stopped if it occurs. The exception is when vocal-cord nodules are present, and the goal is necessarily to reduce hyperfunction.

Voice therapy may help to confirm the need for correction of the velopharyngeal valve in borderline cases, or it may assist in deciding to postpone such surgery. We urge speech pathologists to refrain from undertaking phonation therapy in cases with unequivocal velopharyngeal incompetence and to recognize that such therapy does not address the major component in the communication problem.

SPEECH THERAPY FOR DISORDERS OF RESONANCE

Hypernasality

Therapy for hypernasality has been undertaken for many years (Young, 1928). The results, however, have been generally disappointing because the origin of the problem is usually a defective velopharyngeal valve, and speech therapy has nothing to offer for correction of that deficit. However, we discuss here the information that is available. Such therapy is based on the underlying assumption that, if hypernasality is modified, velopharyngeal closure is improved. However, the therapy itself treats the hypernasality rather than velopharyngeal closure.

Much of the therapy recommended for hypernasality has to do with directing the air stream through the oral rather than the nasal cavities and attempting to eliminate hypernasal components. We are fearful of this type of therapy if it is used without due regard for the possibility of velopharyngeal incompetence. We are concerned because the attempt to produce speech free of hypernasal characteristics may well result in elevation of the larynx and in vocal hyperfunction leading to phonation disorders. For therapy to be undertaken at all, there should be clear evidence that the patient is capable of achieving velopharyngeal closure. Therapy of this type is contraindicated for those who do not have demonstrable ability to achieve closure.

Morley (1970) recommended against therapy until after surgery and then only if it is absolutely necessary. She noted that velopharyngeal function may improve spontaneously for as long as 8 months following surgery. We have seen improvement continue for as long as a year. We watch for a plateau to occur before deciding that no additional improvement is probable. In any event, we do not recommend any speech therapy for at least 3 months postoperatively because tissues remain edematous and stiff for at least that long. However, the decision to attempt speech therapy is sometimes made on the basis of clinical evidence that improvement is at least possible without further surgical or prosthetic intervention.

Consistent with Boone's earlier emphasis on the use of facilitating techniques, Boone and McFarlane (1988), discuss nine therapeutic approaches for treating hypernasality. Although they overlap with other methods that we consider here, it is useful to lay them out as a group. They include: (1) experimenting with increased loudness; (2) ear training to assist with discrimination between oral and nasal resonance; (4) evaluating the effects of lowering the speaker's pitch; (5) explaining the nature of the problem so that the speaker understands clearly what is to be modified; (6) providing as much auditory and kinesthetic feedback as possible from nasal and oral resonance; (7) developing increased oral opening in cases where the oral port is restricted; (8) assessing the positive or negative effects of placing the voice by focusing on the facial mask; and (9) training respiration to increase loudness.

Most of the therapeutic approaches that are described here make use of one or more of these facilitating techniques.

Some Traditional Techniques

Morley (1970 is a pioneer speech pathologist who devoted most of her long and distinguished professional career to the cleft problem. In the seventh edition of her classic book, *Cleft Palate and Speech*, she recommended that articulation with the nares occluded be attempted. Various techniques for achieving nostril closure have been suggested including finger pinching, nose clips, and cotton balls soaked in petroleum jelly (Westlake and Rutherford, 1966). This approach assumes that the need for compensatory lingual gestures intended to reduce nasal air leakage is eliminated or minimized. However, we must remember that, when there is velopharyngeal incompetence, closing the airway at its point of exit creates a cul-de-sac that may change but not

eliminate oral-pressure drops. It may, in some cases, also result in palatal surrender or abandonment of attempts to achieve velopharyngeal closure.

Most of Morley's excellent therapeutic ideas were designed to improve velopharyngeal function, and those approaches are discussed in Chapter 22.

Wells (1971) also attended to the velopharyngeal valve, but stressed speech activities designed to create oral articulation. Among the suggestions was quick inhalation through the mouth followed by immediate production of a single sound or short, meaningful sound combination. Wells suggested that the immediacy of the reversal of the airstream, from intake to output, may permit the maintenance of closure established for inhalation. There are no data on the results of this procedure.

Wilson (1972) emphasized reducing oral breath pressure on fricatives and stop consonants. He suggested that teaching children to use loose contacts of the articulators allows for greater oral air flow and thus a reduction in hypernasality. This is one approach to the problem that would not be vocally damaging even if it did not successfully eliminate the hypernasality. He also encouraged discrimination training, which is always essential in any approach to reducing hypernasality and nasal air flow—or in any other type of therapy for communication disorders.

Discrimination training was also stressed by Fisher (1975) for the patient who can produce oral speech but does not habitually do so in conversation. Her plan involves the use of contrasts. First, isolated vowels, then meaningful words, then sentences are produced with and without hypernasality. This is done to develop auditory discrimination and self-monitoring and to increase control over speech production. The rate of alternation is increased as the patient's reliability increases. This is, of course, negative practice.

A second technique that Fisher reported is the "pull out" exercise. It starts with the production of a highly nasalized word such as "house." The patient attempts to "pull out" of the nasalization on each of 10 trials. The goal is to pull out as early in the sequence as possible and to work to improve the performance. This technique depends upon clinician feedback and self-monitoring. It is recommended especially during the carryover stages of therapy when occasional, individual words or phrases are nasalized either in reading or connected discourse.

Both of these procedures are directed toward habituating velopharyngeal closure through modifying speech in patients who achieve closure inconsistently. Although there are no data offered in support of these techniques, they have face validity if they are used for the implied intent.

It is relevant to this discussion for the reader to know that the clinical strategies just presented, and hundreds more like them in the literature, have not been proven to be efficacious in eliminating hypernasality in numbers of patients with known velopharyngeal-valving characteristics. Some of these techniques are successful in individual cases, and the speech pathologist, understandably exuberant, comes to believe erroneously that they will be effective in treating hypernasality in general. Experienced speech pathologists are usually well aware of the circumstances in which the techniques will succeed or fail.

Programs Related to Phonetic Contexts

Lang (1974) developed and tested a program designed to eliminate hypernasality. Sommers (1983) said that it was based on the assumption that there is a hierarchy for degree of perceived nasality for both consonants and vowels (Moore and Sommers, 1973, 1975). According to Lang, vowels, from least to most nasal, are $/ɔ/$, $/a/$, $/ɛ/$, $/æ/$, $/u/$, and $/i/$. Consonants, in the same order, are glides and glottal fricatives, except $/z/$, plosives, fricatives, affricatives, and $/z/$. This latter part of the hierarchy is difficult to understand since $/s/$ has been found in many studies to be most difficult for speakers with cleft palates. (See Chapter 15.)

Lang's therapy is summarized in Figure 21.2. The program is highly specific and quite rigid in that 100% nasal-free speech must be produced at each level before moving to the next. Careful programming has also been developed to ensure self-monitoring at 100% agreement with the speech pathologist. Lang tested this program with 11 children from 9 to 13 years of age at an 8-week summer camp at Duke University. All subjects had repaired cleft palates, and hypernasality was present in their spontaneous speech. No information was provided about velopharyngeal valving, although reference was made to valving in the results. One child "whose velopharyngeal valving was very poor" successfully completed only step 1 of the program; three completed step 2, three step 4, one step 5, and two step 9. Lang thought that the

children's progress was "directly related to their degrees of velopharyngeal competence" (Sommers, 1983). Another way to put it is that the lack of significant progress for most of the children during 8 weeks of intensive therapy was related to their *incompetence*.

This program is useful in diagnostic therapy because it is quite specific and permits the speech pathologist to determine the level of speech complexity possible for the patient and the level at which a plateau is reached, indicating the need for further physical restoration of the velopharyngeal valve. Such heroic measures are, however, not usually required.

Biofeedback Methods

Early therapy often included the use of simple feedback displays to give information to the patient about the success or failure of his or her efforts to control nasal air flow during speech. For example, condensation of moisture on cold mirrors and the flickering of candle flames were used to show patients when nasal emission was present.

One of the first reports in the literature was of an attempt to test the use of instrumental data for the monitoring of speech. In this landmark study, Masland (1946) coupled a pneumoscope to the nose and mouth of the patient and used the device in conjunction with a kymograph to record and display oral and nasal air pressures. In this way he studied four patients who wore prosthetic speech appliances. The goal was for them to learn to eliminate air flow by closing the velopharyngeal sphincter against the pharyngeal segments of the appliances. The patients were to accomplish this by monitoring their pressure traces during the production of consonant-vowel syllables. Two subjects eliminated nasal air leakage on oral consonants, and two reduced the frequency of leakage. An approach of this type seems reasonable under the circumstances reported. Valving itself, was not studied.

Tonar, described in Chapter 11, was introduced by Fletcher (1970). In 1978, he used the term "nasalance" when discussing hypernasality and recommended that his new instrument, Tonar II, be used for "biometric shaping of nasalance." Tonar provides a reinforcement display that permits the clinician and the patient to see the percentage of nasalance in both analog and digital form. The speech pathologist can manipulate a

1. Correct production of the following vowels. Practice in the order listed.
/ɔ/, /ɑ/, /ɛ/, /æ/, /u/, /i/
2. Correct production of VCV combinations utilizing each vowel (from least to most nasal) in combination with each consonant (from least to most nasal).
3. Correct production of CVC combinations utilizing each vowel (from least to most nasal) in combination with each consonant (from least to most nasal).
4. Correct production of the varied vowel and consonant combinations (from least to most nasal) in the initial and final positions of monosyllabic words.
5. Correct production of the varied vowel and consonant combinations (from least to most nasal) in bysllabic words.
6. Correct production of the ten short phrases and sentences loaded with the following phonemes in combination with all of the vowels:
/r/, /w/, /h/, /l/, and /j/
7. Correct production of ten short phrases and sentences loaded with the following consonants in combination with all of the vowels:
/t/, /p/, /k/, /g/, /b/, /d/
8. Correct production of ten short phrases and sentences loaded with the following consonants in combination with all of the vowels:
/v/, /f/, /ð/, /θ/, /s/
9. Correct production of ten short phrases and sentences loaded with the following consonants in combination with all of the vowels:
/dʒ/, /ʒ/, /ʊ/, /ʃ/, /z/
10. Correct production of all consonant and vowel combinations in long sentences.
11. Correct production of all consonant and vowel combinations while reading a short paragraph. (If the child does not read, poems or nursery rhymes can be substituted at this step.)
12. Correct production of all consonant and vowel combinations in a structured conversational task.
13. Correct production of all vowel and consonant combinations in a spontaneous conversational task.

Figure 21.2 Thirteen steps for the elimination of hypernasality in phonetic contexts. (From Sommers RK. Articulation disorders. Englewood Cliffs, NJ: Prentice-Hall, 1983.)

goal-ratio dial on the instrument panel so that an actual utterance can be compared with a stated goal. A success counter permits easy record keeping. The speaker is notified of successes by activation of a light on the reinforcement panel.

In a therapy program utilizing Tonar, Fletcher created two sets of sentences, each with five subsets containing 20 sentences. The first stresses low and middle vowels in combination with consonants ordered from least to most difficult. The second set includes high and middle vowels, again in combination with consonants ordered from least to most difficult for speakers with velopharyngeal incompetence.

Fletcher tested his highly specific program on 19 children with hypernasality and a nasalance level averaging 40%. The program was individual and intensive, and each child participated in 13 sessions over a period of a week, with each session lasting from 20 to 30 minutes. The protocol demanded that each child read the prescribed sentences into the sound separator with the goal of demonstrating less nasalance than that shown on the goal-ratio dial. When that was accomplished, lights were activated on the reinforcement panel. Criteria for moving from one task to another were strictly specified, and each child was to try to achieve nasalance of 15% or less and complete at least 5 sessions on the initial set.

Fletcher found great variability in nasalance modification, as would be expected. Eight of the 19 subjects met the 85% success criterion of 15% or less nasalance on at least two subsets of sentences and were able to maintain that level. Five were successful on one or more subsets but could not maintain the performance. Five showed some reduction in nasalance but were highly erratic, and maintenance was very poor. One subject did not modify the nasalance percentage, and surgical or prosthetic intervention was recommended.

Our interpretation of the foregoing data would be that the eight subjects who completed two subtests may still have had velopharyngeal incompetence and that the rest of the subjects are highly suspect. However, this is not a reflection on Tonar II or on the program. It is evidence that criteria for determining the wisdom of using this program are yet to be established. Fletcher himself was well aware of that need. As noted earlier, the nasometer is a new development in this technology.

It is our belief that the system might be successful with individuals who can achieve velopharyngeal closure but who do so inconsistently or who have only minimal evidences of velopharyngeal incompetence. We would not recommend it for those with unequivocal incompetence any more than we would recommend any other system of therapy.

Speech pathologists should be aware that Tonar II and the nasometer are expensive, bulky, and technically demanding. Nevertheless, they are impressive instruments and represent a unique contribution to both clinical and research methodologies.

The whistling-blowing technique, a therapy intended to develop velopharyngeal closure during speech from velopharyngeal closure demonstrated during blowing or whistling, was described and evaluated by Shprintzen et al. (1975). Previously, Shprintzen et al. (1974) had suggested that speech, blowing, and whistling share a similar pattern of closure as observed in frontal, sagittal, and baseview cinefluoroscopy. They speculated that failure to close consistently on speech tasks represented, in some cases, an error in learning and that closure during speech could be conditioned if it were already present in blowing or whistling. In order to achieve their goal, they worked directly on speech rather than on valving.

Four subjects were studied; they were 4, 6, 10, and 19 years of age. Two had normal places of articulation. A third omitted sibilants, and another was hypernasal and had a facial grimace, glottal stops, and distortions of /s/ and /z/. For each subject, the authors reported the frequency of occurrence of nasal emission during passages studied and the percentage of speaking time during which nasal emission was evident. Nasal emission was studied with a scape-scope.

The treatment described is highly specific and must be administered more than once a week, the authors said, to avoid spontaneous extinction of temporarily learned behavior. The general steps in the procedure are:

1. Teach simultaneous blowing or whistling and phonation.
2. Test for nasal airflow and reinforce when it is not present. Keep repeating until phonation accompanied by whistling or blowing is consistently free of nasal escape.
3. Continue phonation without blowing or whistling until it is free of nasal escape.
4. Produce vowel /i/ or /u/ with blowing or whistling and reinforce nasal-free productions until they are consistent.
5. Eliminate whistling or blowing and produce the vowel by itself until 95% success is achieved. Each time nasal emission is found on any step, the patient returns to the blowing or whistling protocol.
6. Incorporate non-nasal consonants with vowels to form monosyllables / pit, sit/.
7. Develop self-monitoring and use of self-operants.
8. Move from a series of emission-free monosyllables to short sentences, then to longer sentences and conversation.

Initially, all satisfactory responses were reinforced. However, as a child progressed, the schedule of reinforcement and punishment was altered. During the training, each subject was asked to sense his or her performance kinesthetically or auditorily. In time, the use of the scape-scope was discontinued in favor of auditory monitoring by the clinician and patient. Thus, discrimination training is also an important element in this protocol.

All four subjects improved their velopharyngeal function as indicated by videofluoroscopy and by evidence of reduced nasal air leakage. One subject, an individual with hearing loss, retained mild hypernasality and nasal snorting. The other 3 subjects developed essentially normal speech. Treatment lasted from 22 sessions over a period of 13 weeks to 36 sessions over 15 weeks.

Once again, this is a system of therapy that has had some success in carefully controlled and evaluated trials. However, it is our belief that the criteria for using the protocol should be investigated in larger numbers of subjects. We have had success in reducing but not eliminating hypernasality with the program. We suspect that its predictive value would be enhanced by adding to the criteria the achievement of velopharyngeal closure on some speech tasks. It would be of interest to know the extent to which the four subjects in the original study did indeed close on some speech tasks even though they did not close consistently. Two of the subjects had had pharyngeal flaps before the study was begun and so, presumably, had the potential to achieve closure. One had postadenoidectomy velopharyngeal incompetence complicated by a severe hearing loss in one ear and a moderate loss in the other. Only one subject, a 4-year-old, had a repaired cleft with no other surgery, and he achieved touch closure during speech.

It is clear that this program, a creative and innovative one, has promise but probably only for subjects who are inconsistent in closure for speech or who have minimal orifice areas yet to be specified.

The accelerometer was used by Nickerson et al. (1976) in biofeedback training intended to reduce nasalization in the speech of hearing-impaired children. It was used with other devices in a computer-based system designed to display nasalization when it exceeded a specific value.

Measurement and manipulation of nasalization in the hearing impaired and in individuals with cleft palate are two different matters. The person with a significant hearing loss fails to use a velopharyngeal mechanism that is usually structurally and functionally adequate. The failure to use the mechanism optimally results from lack of feedback. Most speakers with cleft palates, on the other hand, obtain auditory feedback that is adequate. Thus, failure to achieve closure is likely to be the result of structural or functional deficiency or both.

Nevertheless, for some inconsistent speakers and for those believed to have potential for improving speech without changing the dynamics of the velopharyngeal valve, accelerometers may be profitably used.

Feed-back filtering was used by Garber and Moller (1979). They asked whether 10 normal and 10 mildly hypernasal speakers would alter their nasality when hearing their speech low-pass filtered with cut-off frequencies of 1000, 500, and 300 Hz and high-pass filtered with cut-off frequencies of 500, 1000 and 2000 Hz. Their measurements of nasality were made with a miniature accelerometer attached to the side of the nose. Both groups of speakers significantly reduced nasality with low-pass filtering at a cutoff of 300 Hz. Garber and Moller interpreted their results to mean that nasality is under conscious control and that the subjects, upon hearing increased nasality in their speech, attempted to compensate for it. The differences were quite small, however, and the authors were not prepared to say that they were also clinically significant. They concluded that more research is necessary before filtering can be used as a therapy tool. This work points to challenging possibilities in the future. Horii and Monroe (1983), writing about the HONC, previously discussed, suggested its use for therapeutic as well as for diagnostic purposes. Feedback could be provided by using two sets of nasal-to-voice pick-up systems, one for the clinician and the other for the hypernasal speaker. These systems would be combined with a dual-channel storage oscilloscope permitting traces from the speech of the clinician and of the patient. These can be used for comparative purposes. Both auditory and visual feedback are provided. The usefulness of the system as a therapy technique is still to be proven.

Other methods of providing biofeedback will be discussed in Chapter 23 as they relate to therapy for improving velopharyngeal valving.

Summary of Hypernasality

All in all, speech therapy for improving hypernasality does not appear to us to be warranted in many cases. It may be helpful for those borderline speakers for whom surgical treatment or prosthetics is either unwarranted or unwanted, for those patients who have had pharyngeal flaps, or for those for whom appliances have been made and who need to learn efficient use of the new mechanism.

Again, we warn against these therapeutic approaches with individuals with velopharyngeal incompetence. Their efforts to eliminate hypernasality may result in phonatory disturbances that complicate their problems.

Hyponasality and Cul-de-Sac Resonance

Neither hyponasality nor cul-de-sac resonance can be successfully treated by speech therapy as long as there is resistance in the system. It should be understood, however, that eliminating airway obstruction in the nasopharynx and in the nasal passages may have the immediate effect of increasing hypernasality if a defective velopharyngeal valve is also present. On the other hand, in some cases with only slight incompetence, speech may be greatly improved by the elimination of nasal turbulence created by high intranasal resistance or by the emergence of more acceptable nasal characteristics in the speech pattern.

The exception to this is functional hyponasality, which is rarely seen. Boone and McFarlane (1988) discuss the possibility that denasal resonance may originally have had a physical cause which no longer exists and that the hyponasality remains as a habit or "set." When that occurs, they help the patient to understand the nature of the problem and stress the nasal components in therapy (Boone, 1983); introduce ear training with stress on discrimination; and provide sensory feedback on the differences between oral and nasal sounds. Both Boone and McFarlane (1988) and Wilson (1972) recommend the introduction of humming as a means of getting nasal productions and of providing tactile and auditory feedback about the differences between oral and nasal resonance. Intensive carryover programming is essential.

We know of no evidence of the success or failure of therapy for these rare problems of hyponasality in the absence of increased nasal resistance. We recommend, however, that careful evaluations of the nasal airways be carried out before deciding that hyponasality exists on a functional basis.

CONCLUDING STATEMENT ABOUT SPEECH THERAPY FOR VOICE DISORDERS

Speech therapy for resonance and phonation problems can be discouraging for speech pathologists and patients alike. A wise clinician recognizes this and understands that physical and physiological limitations can defeat the best therapy plan that can be devised. Remember to "think sphincter" (Skolnick, 1973) and undertake therapy only when valving competence or potential for competence can be demonstrated.

REFERENCES

Aronson AE. Clinical voice disorders. New York: Thieme-Stratton, 1980.

Boone DR. The voice and voice therapy. 2nd ed. Englewood Cliffs, NJ: Prentice-Hall, 1977.

Boone DR. The Boone voice program for children. Tigard, OR: CC Publications, 1980.

Boone DR. The voice and voice therapy. 3rd ed. Englewood Cliffs, NJ: Prentice-Hall, 1983.

Boone DR, McFarlane SC. The voice and voice therapy. 4th ed. Englewood Cliffs, NJ: Prentice-Hall, 1988.

Cooper M, Cooper MH, eds. Approaches to vocal rehabilitation. Springfield, IL: CC Thomas, 1977.

Fisher HB. Improving voice and articulation. Boston: Houghton Mifflin, 1975.

Fletcher SG. Diagnosing speech disorders from cleft palate. New York: Grune and Stratton, 1978.

Froeschels E, Rostein S, Weiss DA. A method of therapy for paralytic conditions of the mechanisms of phonation, respiration, and glutination. J Speech Hear Dis 1955; 20:365.

Garber SR, Moller KT. The effects of feedback filtering on nasalization in normal and hypernasal speakers. J Speech Hear Res 1979; 22:321.

Horii Y, Monroe N. Auditory and visual feedback of nasalization using a modified accelerometric method. J Speech Hear Res 1983; 26:472.

Lang M. Program for the elimination of hypernasality. Unpublished manuscript, Kent State University, 1974.

Masland MW. Testing and correcting cleft palate speech. J Speech Hear Dis 1946; 11:309.

Moore GP. Organic voice disorders. Foundations of Speech Pathology Series. Englewood Cliffs, NJ: Prentice-Hall, 1971.

Moore WH, Sommers RK. Phonetic contexts: their effects on perceived nasality in cleft palate speakers. Cleft Palate J 1973; 10:72.

Moore WH, Sommers RK. Phonetic contexts: their effects on perceived intelligibility in cleft palate speakers. Folia Phoniatr 1975; 27:410.

Morley ME. Cleft Palate and Speech. 7th ed. Baltimore: Williams & Wilkins, 1970.

Murphy AT. Functional voice disorders. Englewood Cliffs, NJ: Prentice-Hall, 1964.

Nickerson R, Kalikow D, Stevens K. Computer-aided speech training for the deaf. J Speech Hear Dis 1976; 41:120.

Shprintzen RJ, Lencione RM, McCall GN, Skolnick ML. A three dimensional cinefluoroscopic analysis of velopharyngeal closure during speech and non-speech activities in normals. Cleft Palate J 1974; 11:412.

Shprintzen RM, McCall GN, Skolnick ML. A new therapeutic technique for the treatment of velopharyngeal incompetence. J Speech Hear Dis 1975; 40:69.

Skolnick ML, McCall GN. The sphincteric mechanism of velopharyngeal closure. A 25-minute sound movie. May, 1973.

Sommers RK. Articulation disorders. Englewood Cliffs, NJ: Prentice-Hall, 1983.

Visi-Pitch. Pinebrook, NJ: Kay Electronics Corp, 1980.

Voice Monitor. Hollins, Virginia: Communications Research Unit, Hollins College, 1977.

Wells CC. Cleft palate and its associated speech disorders. New York: McGraw-Hill, 1971.

Westlake H, Rutherford D. Cleft palate. Englewood Cliffs, NJ: Prentice-Hall, 1966.

Wilson DK. Voice problems in children. Baltimore: Williams & Wilkins, 1972.

Young EH. Overcoming cleft palate speech. Minneapolis: The Hill-Young School, 1928.

22 | TREATMENT OF ARTICULATORY AND PHONOLOGICAL DISORDERS

Articulatory and phonological therapy is a key speech pathology service for those patients with cleft palate who misarticulate. This training is appropriate for misarticulating patients who have established velopharyngeal competence and for some patients who present marginal or questionable velopharyngeal incompetence. While much research has been directed to the evaluation of velopharyngeal function for speech, the empirical research literature on articulation training for patients with cleft palate is scanty. Fortunately, practices, theory and data regarding speech training for children with developmental articulatory and phonological disorders appear to be relevant to the sound system disorders associated with cleft palate. This chapter includes a review of clinical opinion about articulation therapy for patients with cleft palate, data relative to the effectiveness of articulation therapy for these patients, and theoretical bases for articulation therapy. Clinical recommendations are made, and assessment of therapy effectiveness is discussed.

Articulation therapy may be conducted as an extension of the evaluation process; responses to diagnostic therapy may suggest termination of that therapy in favor of medical or dental treatment. Therapy may also be delivered on a continuing basis to correct existing disordered articulation and phonology. This consideration of therapy is directed to patients with velopharyngeal competence or a close approximation of competence. Exceptions will be identified as such. The services described are usually offered to children.

A REVIEW OF CLINICAL PRACTICES

Over the years a number of speech pathologists have written about therapeutic procedures

for patients with cleft palate. Early descriptions included activities for improvement of velopharyngeal function, articulation, hypernasality, and other variables that are dealt with separately in this book. Early descriptions of therapy often failed to consider the high failure rate associated with therapy directed to patients with velopharyngeal insufficiency. However, the best of the early work, such as that of Berry (1928) was insightful and anticipated the findings of later research.

Huber (1957) was one of the first to place emphasis on articulation therapy. She advocated teaching the child or adult appropriate placement and to progress from simple to more complex phonetic practice material. She felt that, to a degree, unwanted compensatory articulations were established through reinforcement and that they could be prevented by the withholding of reinforcement. Huber criticized the then-popular use of nonspeech, blowing exercises to "strengthen" the palate. She also criticized the emphasis placed by some upon socialization and psychological therapies as a means of improving the patient's speech. Encouragement of language use in social contexts and psychotherapy are not a means of training articulation. However, they may be important components in a total habilitation program.

Smith (1969) would not teach articulation to children whose language is very immature. She wrote that oral communication should be established before articulation is corrected or taught. Also, she would not provide articulation therapy at a time when a child is reacting emotionally to his or her speech. In her opinion, feedback about speech behaviors that need alteration can increase a child's emotional reactions to speech. Smith would have us remember that we want the children we serve to develop and maintain positive self-images and that self-image is reflected in how freely the child uses verbal expression. Sometimes, however, helping the child know that better speech is possible is a positive experience. Decisions of this sort should be made on an individual basis, and therapy with a poor outlook should not be attempted if other measures can be taken to help solve the patient's problem.

Hahn (1958, 1960, 1989) introduced a language-communication component to speech therapy for preschool patients with cleft palate. Its purpose is to facilitate speech while the child and speech pathologist play together and talk about a shared activity. The clinician may provide articulatory stimulation by restating words the child misarticulated and slightly emphasizing a target sound. The clinician may expand on the child's speech to encourage vocabulary containing target sounds. However, as rapport is established through this indirect speech work, more direct methods of articulation therapy may be introduced if appropriate. Use is not made of "...part processes such as production and drill on single sounds" (Hahn, 1958). Hahn (1989) would provide the parents of cleft palate preschool children with information about the structure and function of the speech mechanism and related oral conditions and the impact of those disabilities on speech production. She indicated that, from information gained by testing the child, the speech pathologist can instruct the parents about speech problems that may appear, what can be done about them, and how the parents can participate in the child's speech development. The information is also used to plan therapy to be delivered by the clinician if necessary.

Rather than developing a universal set of recommendations to be used with the parents of all children, Hahn (1989) stated principles for giving parents information pertinent to the speech patterns of their child. She discussed guidance for the parents to help them provide a home environment that encourages speech but discourages glottal or pharyngeal substitutions or effortful, tense use of the speech mechanism. Parents may erroneously expect perfect speech to follow immediately after surgical or dental procedures. The speech pathologist can help the parents to understand that the child needs time and perhaps help in learning to use the altered mechanism for speech production. McWilliams (1956) described two ways in which the home environment is important to the speech development of the child with cleft palate. First, a loving, accepting home environment that supports emotional well-being and a good self-image contributes to language development. Second, the parents can encourage articulation development by talking and reading to the child slightly stressing selected consonants and by showing pleasure at the child's early speech attempts.

Philips (1979) described a speech stimulation program for preschool children with cleft palate that was intended to develop the confidence of both the child and the parents in the child's ability to have intelligible verbal communication. The program was designed to stimulate better speech and to prevent undesirable compensatory articulation and voice patterns. Philips stated that the services offered the children and their parents through use of this program were intended to be developmental rather than remedial. She urged the speech pathologist to stimulate and facilitate the speech development processes operative in young children. Relative to articulation, Philips encouraged the use in communication of sounds the child can produce correctly and, to the extent possible, the teaching of correct articulatory placement even though velopharyngeal function may be insufficient. She also considered the development of compensatory speech such as easy phonation and articulation and perhaps a slightly slow speech rate. These techniques must be tailored to the individual child. Philips recommended that the mother be present during therapy, noting that separation of the mother and the child may reduce adaptive behavior on the part of the child. An important goal is to teach the mother of the preschool child to be a good observer and a good facilitator of speech and communication. Her participation in therapy can resolve concerns she may have and increase her ability to help in therapy, especially in generalization.

Morley (1970) listed four goals of speech therapy for persons with clefts: (1) teaching correct, that is oral, direction of the breath stream for the purpose of learning to use the palatal and pharyngeal muscles to control the velopharyngeal sphincter; (2) coordinating the neuromuscular control of the velopharyngeal muscles with other articulatory muscles; (3) teaching correct articulation of all consonants and vowels and the ability to use those sounds in all positions in words and in blends as well; and (4) introducing the newly learned sounds into speech and establishing the unconscious use of new and correct habits of articulation. Morley organized articulation training according to principles of motor learning, which involve inhibition of faulty articulation patterns already developed, facilitation of required movements, association of the new movements with auditory, kinesthetic, and touch-pressure feedback, and stabilization of the new performance at an automatic level. She would do little for the child under 4 years of age except attempt to teach oral direction of the air stream. She reported that children with cleft palate at 4 years of age tend readily to incorporate into their speech those sounds that they are taught in therapy.

Morley indicated that persons with correct place of articulation but nasalization should not receive speech therapy until after surgery and that then they either might not need it or they might need assistance with oral direction of the breath stream. She would teach place of articulation skills to children with glottal and pharyngeal substitutions and other articulatory errors even though they also presented nasal emission and nasopharyngeal snorts. She would do this with the nares closed. Morley advocated group therapy to allow the child to realize that he or she is not the only person with cleft palate and disordered speech. Group therapy permits the child to learn that speech can be unintelligible and hence in need of change and to observe that persons with speech disorder do improve. She wrote that the techniques used in therapy do not vary to any great extent with the age of the patient, but the language used to present the therapy is adapted to the patient.

Morley (1970) would work to avoid the tension that is associated with glottal and pharyngeal substitutions. The child may be asked to produce vocalizations that are free from gross substitutions. For example, he or she can be asked to hum and then to glide into different vowels. Laryngeal tension is to be avoided. It can be monitored by palpation and introspection. Another technique is to use whispered vowels to which consonants—initially /h/ and /m/—are gradually added. Next, progress to combinations involving voiceless consonants. When they are easily produced, voiced consonants can be introduced.

For /p/ production, Morley recommended filling the mouth with air, with the lips closed but not tense, and then releasing the air abruptly. Morley encouraged the production of sibilants from a whistly activity. She also used modification of one existing sound in order to develop another. Thus, she begins with what the child can do and moves in easy steps to what initially would have been difficult. Indeed, as a general guide for therapy, begin where the child is and progress to whatever level of complexity the child can achieve and maintain.

Morley's therapy decisions were made with recognition of the limitations imposed by any existing velopharyngeal incompetence. The child with velopharyngeal incompetence who learns correct place of articulation may avoid use of gross articulatory substitutions. However, even after normal place of articulation is achieved, speech will be marked by insufficient intraoral air pressure and nasal emission until the velopharyngeal deficit is treated. Instruction directed to oral emission of the air stream is particularly important for the patient who continues to direct the air stream nasally after surgery has provided a velopharyngeal mechanism capable of closure for speech. We note that in her own clinical practice, Morley rarely found it necessary to do speech therapy with any of her patients since they developed such excellent spontaneous speech. She referred to her role as purely evaluative (McWilliams, personal communication).

The use of fingers, nose clips, and cotton balls containing petroleum jelly for the purpose of closing the nares during articulation instruction for persons with velopharyngeal incompetence was described by Westlake and Rutherford (1966). This practice is controversial. It is appealing in that it should eliminate any need for lingual gestures intended to compensate for nasal air leakage. On the other hand, it may encourage the child to abandon use of the velopharyngeal mechanism. There is videofluorographic evidence that some persons reduce velopharyngeal motion during blowing as compared to speech when the act is performed with the nares closed (McWilliams and Bradley, 1964). Many children with marginal velopharyngeal function improve place of articulation without use of nares occlusion even though there is still nasalization.

Trost (1981) emphasized the change from posterior to anterior placement for treatment of articulatory movements regarded as compensatory. She thinks that an auditory model by itself is insufficient for that purpose, and she advocates use of visual information to explain the desired placement and to contrast it with the faulty placement that is in use. A paired stimulus procedure may also be helpful wherein anterior sounds that are properly placed are paired with anterior sounds that are replaced by compensatory articulations. Generalization to anterior placement may occur. School age children may be able to understand and deliberately strive for anterior placement.

Bzoch (1989), Morris (1989) and McWilliams (1966, 1980) advocates that articulation therapy for persons with cleft palate should be based on detailed observation and description of the patient's speech. Bzoch uses articulation tests to identify misarticulation and instrumental analysis of speech behavior to explore that articulation. He stated that the effectiveness of speech therapy for persons with clefts is reduced if the service is offered too late, if it involves focus on a single sound until that sound is mastered, and if it stresses ear training but not speech production. Morris observed that articulatory pattern information is more important than total test scores and their comparison with norms. He suggested utilizing information regarding type of articulation error, consistency of error, and stimulability in planning articulation therapy. He would conduct trial therapy to determine if the individual has the potential to improve articulation with training.

In a description of speech therapy for children with cleft palate, Logemann (1983) advocated the integration of surgery, prosthodontics, and speech therapy at the earliest possible time. She would help infants to acquire a normal sound system and normal language. To achieve this, the clinician would work with parents, and the child would be placed in either a speech/language play program or in a speech/language therapy program. Her goals for children in the 2 to 5 year age range are to establish a variety of articulatory placements if those placements were lacking and if the velopharyngeal mechanism had been treated. Children with nasal escape can be taught placement for the three nasal consonants. She discussed use of tactile cues in teaching articulatory placement to children over 5 years of age.

Logemann's experience reminds us that tactile cues and instruction may be used to help a child position the tongue within the maxillary arch, thus directing the air stream centrally rather than laterally, and that such placement may be helpful to persons learning vowel and consonant /r/ sounds (Gerber, 1973). The use of motokinesthetic cues in speech therapy was very much in vogue in the 1930s and 1940s. An extensive description of such procedures was provided by Vaughan and Clark (1979). They described sensory guides that can be formed from orthodontic wire and dental floss and used to provide placement cues. Work with parents has been discussed in detail by numerous authors (Hubbell, 1981; Hanson, 1983; Shelton and Johnson, 1984).

Hoch et al. (1986) described articulation therapy directed toward elimination of posterior placement of consonants and of glottalization. They cited observations which indicated that elimination of glottal stops was associated with increase in velopharyngeal closure movements. To disrupt glottalization, Hoch et al. use an easy whisper technique. That includes a combination of slighting and heavy aspiration of voiceless stops. Henningsson and Isberg (1986) also report that some individuals seem to surrender velopharyngeal closure movements when substituting glottal stops for other obstruents. Certainly it is the case that pharyngeal flap surgery, for example, should never be performed when the patient shows only glottal and pharyngeal speech articulation. That is because these articulation patterns do not give information about velopharyngeal status. Any such patient must have speech therapy first to teach appropriate placement for plosives and fricatives in order to assess adequacy of speech aerodynamics.

In this regard, comment is needed to indicate some differences in planning therapy for children and for adults. Since adults have in most instances used the faulty articulatory patterns throughout life, their speech patterns are more automatic and more resistant to change. For that reason, they frequently require more assistance and more practice. Even with such attention, change is difficult to achieve. For example, in our personal experience, we have attempted unsuccessfully to treat cleft palate adults who have habitually used glottal stops for back plosives.

Westlake and Rutherford (1966) made a number of suggestions regarding articulation therapy for the older cleft palate child and the adult. They would decrease the noticeability of incorrectly articulated sounds by attention to the effort and timing with which those sounds are produced. They indicated that speech training for this group should be intensive in terms of the frequency and duration of session. While they would attempt to minimize the impact of some physiological deficits on articulation, they recognized the limitations those deficits placed on prognosis for speech improvement.

A REVIEW OF THE EFFECTIVENESS OF ARTICULATION THERAPY

Empirical evidence regarding the effectiveness of articulation therapy for patients with cleft palate is limited in both quantity and design. Experimental control is often less than desirable, and the velopharyngeal status of the subjects is often not clearly described. Treatment studies are often directed to limited goals and do not permit definitive statements about the value of complex treatments delivered to patients over prolonged periods. However, descriptive information in the literature suggests that children with cleft palate who have received speech training tend to speak better than those who have not (Van Demark and Hardin, 1986).

Prins and Bloomer (1965) reported that 10 persons with surgically repaired cleft palates or velopharyngeal insufficiency improved their scores on a word intelligibility measure during the time they were enrolled in an 8-week, intensive, residential speech program. Group and individual treatment was provided; it included efforts to improve articulation placement, to encourage oral direction of the air stream during speech, and to increase palatopharyngeal function. However, there is little direct evidence that the therapy program resolved social speech patterns.

Chisum et al.(1969) evaluated articulation therapy delivered to children who had hypernasality, audible nasal emission, or both, and who were thought to be borderline velopharyngeal competent. To serve as a subject, an individual was required to have articulation errors on at least three different speech sounds. The experimental subjects, who ranged in age from 6 to 12 years, received 30-minute therapy sessions twice each week. Each subject was seen individually over a mean period of 7.2 months and was taught to produce sounds in isolation and then in nonsense syllables, words, sentences, and conversation. The experimental subjects improved their articulation

to a greater extent than did the control subjects, and the difference was statistically significant. The gains were made primarily on fricatives, which were the sounds stressed in the training, but the subjects' articulation disorders were not all eliminated. The design of the study does not allow any inferences regarding which treatment procedures contributed to the gains made.

Harrison (1969) evaluated a language and speech stimulation program devised for preschool children with cleft palate. In the study by Harrison, subjects with velopharyngeal incompetence and their mothers were taught to accept nasal air flow in the production of speech sounds. The stimulation procedures used were directed to consonant placement regardless of the child's ability to imitate a particular sound. Articulation was tested with the Miami Imitative Ability Test, and the Bzoch Error Pattern Articulation Test, which samples 24 consonants in 100 test items. Both experimental and control subjects made gains on each test, but the experimental group made the greater gains. The difference in gain was statistically significant for the Bzoch test; statistical significance was not mentioned for the Miami test.

Philips and Harrison (1969) interpreted their data to indicate that their stimulation program was beneficial to their subjects. Harrison (1969) thought the gains might have been greater had the stimulation been directed to sounds the children could imitate. However, it is also possible that training directed to sounds the children could not imitate may have helped to make the necessary articulation gestures available for incorporation into the children's phonology.

Schendel and Bzoch (1970) described an intensive summer residential speech therapy program. The program was intended to apply principles of learning and to provide an atmosphere conducive to learning. The authors used a case study format to describe gains made by their patients. No experimental control features were employed, but if one accepts the assumption that the speech of the children would have been stable without therapy for the time of the program, then the evidence presented is favorable to articulation therapy for children with clefts. The lack of control makes it impossible to conclude that any particular treatment procedure used was especially effective. The data presented indicated that the children reduced the number of sounds misarticulated on an articulation test and also that they reduced the severity of the articulation errors that persisted. This was true even of children with velopharyngeal incompetence. These gains were maintained, but the treatment was not effective in the elimination of hypernasality. Some of the subjects might have made greater gains had surgery or obturation preceded the speech therapy.

Van Demark (1974) described from tape recordings the articulation of two groups of Danish children. The recordings had been made when the subjects averaged 63.4 months of age and again when they averaged 82.9 months. In the interim, one group had received unspecified speech therapy. Subjects who demonstrated evidence of velopharyngeal closure, marginal closure, or velopharyngeal incompetence were identified in each group. The occurrence of all types of articulation errors, especially sound omissions, decreased in the children who received therapy. Of the subjects who received therapy, those who were judged to have velopharyngeal closure made greater gains than those with marginal or incompetent closure. Of the children with marginal closure, those who received speech therapy made articulation gains, whereas children not in therapy did not. This study demonstrated that a group of children with cleft palate improved their articulation during a period in which speech therapy was provided. Although the articulation changes cannot be clearly attributed to the therapy, the data reported indicate a positive result from speech therapy. They do not indicate that all speech problems related to velopharyngeal incompetence can be eliminated through speech therapy.

Shelton and Ruscello (1979) reported descriptive information regarding the responses of patients with cleft palate or velopharyngeal valving disabilities to articulation training, to biofeedback intended to influence velopharyngeal function, or to a combination of these two procedures. No experimental control was claimed for observations reported. Articulation training involved placement procedures, imitation practice, and reinforcement of correct responses. Subjects with presumed borderline velopharyngeal incompetence, as evidenced by nasal airflow during some but not all pressure consonants, made articulation gains with training. For example, a 7-year-old girl produced /s/, and other sounds posteriorly and consistently emitted air nasally during obstruents. The nasal air flow was usually less than 80 cc per second. She corrected her articulation faults and

later established normal articulation. Two children who accompanied oral sounds with nasal fricative and affricate noises eliminated these distracting speech faults.

Two children were provided with articulation training during their third through their fifth years. When therapy was started, their speech was unintelligible and their velopharyngeal competence was not clearly identified. Although each child underwent pharyngeal flap surgery during the treatment period—at the recommendation of the speech clinicians—each made substantial articulation gains prior to surgery. In particular, they added stops and fricatives to their limited phonetic inventories. Each continued to leak air nasally for months after the pharyngeal flaps. With continued training, each developed normally intelligible speech. One continued to present slight hypernasality and measurable nasal air leakage; the other presented moderate oral distortions of /s/. He presented malocclusion associated with his bilateral, complete cleft. The boy's father stated that, given a mustache in adulthood, the boy would be indistinguishable from persons born without cleft palates.

The descriptions by Shelton and Ruscello suggested that therapy can substantially improve articulation in selected patients with borderline velopharyngeal insufficiency. Some of their patients presented slight insufficiency; in some cases the patient's parents did not consider the speech symptoms to be sufficiently severe to warrant surgery. Other patients, prior to therapy, may not have made full use of their potential for velopharyngeal closure during speech. Agreement regarding a definition of such potential is elusive. Some of the patients observed by Shelton and Ruscello continued to leak air nasally for long periods of time after secondary velopharyngeal surgery. In some patients, that leakage eventually diminished greatly or disappeared; presumably, these patients unconsciously discovered use of the reconstructed velopharyngeal valving mechanism. Perhaps speech therapy directed to articulation skills contributes to such learning. If nasal air leakage continues after secondary velopharyngeal surgery, it is inappropriate to ask the surgeon to perform additional surgery until at least 1 year has elapsed to allow the patient the opportunity to learn to use the new mechanism.

Hodson et al. (1983) reported a case study wherein therapy oriented to elimination of phonological patterns was given to a 5-year-old child with cleft palate. Cephalometric radiographs and phonetic pattern indicated that the child's velopharyngeal mechanism was competent. The child received therapy from the authors and from a school clinician simultaneously, and an older sibling was instructed to present word lists at home for the child to listen to and repeat. The therapy delivered by the authors was organized into four cycles. Each cycle focused on a particular phonological pattern and included work on several sounds involved in the pattern. The authors reported that the boy received approximately 65 hours of remediation at their university clinic over a period of 13 months. Sessions were 60 to 90 minutes in duration. The boy established use of prevocalic voiceless single obstruents, stridents, velars, consonant clusters, and liquids, and "generally intelligible" speech was established and maintained.

Albery and Enderby (1984) compared the effectiveness of speech therapy delivered on two schedules: an intensive 6-week course and weekly. The children in the intensive group resided in a hospital during the week for the therapy period. The comparison children received therapy from the home therapist. All subjects had velopharyngeal competence or near competence as evidenced by freedom from hypernasality and little or no nasal escape as measured by nasal anemometry; most had repaired cleft palate or submucous cleft palate, but a few presented corrected pharyngeal disproportion or palatal incoordination. Children were assigned to the two groups by random method, and the mean age of children in each group was 8.7 years. Members of the two groups were assessed 1 month before treatment, immediately before treatment, immediately post-treatment, and at 6-month intervals after treatment, through 2 years post-treatment. Children in intensive therapy were taught consonants in isolation, syllables, words, sentences, and everyday speech. Little time was spent on auditory discrimination training. Except for the pretreatment data, the group receiving the intensive therapy was superior to the comparison group at each assessment on both the Edinburgh Articulation Test and the Frenchay Articulation Test. In each group and on each measure, the number of errors was low. As the authors noted, gains were maintained, and the intensive treatment group maintained its advantage relative to the comparison group. Parents reported that children in the intensive group

"blossomed", becoming more confident and more verbal.

Van Demark and Hardin (1986) also evaluated 6 weeks of intensive articulation therapy (4 hours daily for 26 days) delivered to children with cleft palate in a residential setting. The children were reevaluated 9 months after the intensive therapy; during that interval, some received therapy at their schools. The subjects were considered to present velopharyngeal competence or marginal competence. The therapy was evaluated in terms of the children's performance on articulation ratings, articulation tests, and other measures. A multiple sound therapy developed by McCabe and Bradley (1975) was used. Multiple sounds were used in therapy each day; therapy involving a given sound could involve the sound in isolation, syllables, words, sentences, or conversation. These units were selected in an attempt to maintain a rate of 80% correct responses. Up to 1000 responses per session were obtained. Half the sessions were individual, and half were delivered to children in pairs. Most of the children were treated by highly experienced clinicians, but some were treated by graduate students working under supervision. Whether the therapy was delivered by the clinician working directly with patients or through students did not appear to influence the results.

Articulation ratings improved to a statistically significant extent over the combined periods of intensive and less intensive or no therapy. However, changes in ratings over either the 6 weeks or 9 months subperiods were not significant. Pretherapy, post-therapy, and 9-month follow-up measures were compared. One measure involved number of sound elements misarticulated. The scores obtained after 9 months of follow-up therapy did not differ significantly from the scores obtained after the 6 weeks of intensive therapy. The authors wrote that only 3 of 13 subjects improved during the follow-up period. They also noted that articulation scores may be insensitive to gains in the direction of less severe misarticulation.

Van Demark and Hardin also studied change in counts of occurrence of different error types and success in production of sounds in different manner of articulation categories. The children moved away from omissions and substitutions, but increased usage of oral distortions. This was justifiably interpreted as speech improvement.

Gains were made in all manner of production categories except nasals, which were close to asymptote performance at the beginning of the study. Fewer gains were observed on a sentence articulation test than on a single-word articulation test. The authors suggested this might reflect the sound samples involved. The authors were disappointed in the amount of improvement achieved; most but not all subjects maintained gains made during the 6 weeks of intensive therapy. They discussed variables that might have limited response to therapy. Some may have presented velopharyngeal insufficiency (one subsequently received a pharyngeal flap), and age may have been a factor. The subjects ranged in age from 6 years, 8 months through 12 years, 0 months. The oldest subject made substantial gains during the 6 weeks of intensive therapy overcoming glottal-stop substitutions and pharyngeal fricatives, but he did not maintain those gains.

The difference in treatment findings reported by Albery and Enderby on the one hand and Van Demark and Hardin on the other could reflect differences in the subjects, in the treatments, in the choice of measures, or other variables.

Kawano et al. (1984) described the response to speech therapy of an individual with cleft palate who substituted a laryngeal fricative for /s/ and /ʃ/ (see Chapter 15). In the course of 4 sessions delivered over a 2-month period, this 20- year-old learned correct placement of both sounds with velopharyngeal closure. The therapy involved manipulation of place of articulation. The patient moved from an oral fricative in small steps to the target fricatives. The authors wrote, "For a correct production of [ʃi], the patient was trained to produced a prolonged whisper [çi] and was also given auditory stimuli of prolonged whisper [ʃi] such as [ʃʃʃ ...] in order to lead to normal Japanese consonant [ʃi]. For [s] sound, he was asked first to relax and protrude the tongue in a flat shape across the lips and to produce whispered [Φu] such as [ΦΦΦ ...] with the tongue pressing lightly against the teeth and to draw back the tongue gradually, thus leading to [θu]. After learning to produce [θu], he was instructed to produce normal Japanese consonant [su] while drawing back his tongue." As indicated in Chapter 15, it is difficult to know how an individual acquires a response such as the laryngeal fricative in the first place. Traditional therapy asks the patient to strive in different ways to produce target sounds; when a sound is produced to the satisfaction of the clinician, the patient is asked to establish it through repetition. Perhaps earlier in life the patient described what happened to produce such a response and someone encouraged that response through feedback and reinforcement. Such a response could be acquired initially through problem solving on the part of a patient who had not yet acquired velopharyngeal competence and who was trying to deliver a response wanted by a clinician. Sequences such as this may result in sounds that are perceptually similar to target sounds. However, such compensations are unwanted when they are noticeably distorted relative to the target sound and when a different combination of services might have resulted in better responses. The patient described was fortunate to meet the skilled clinicians who identified the nature of his laryngeal fricative and then helped him to correct the error.

An instrumental biofeedback therapy for the correction of articulation was described by Michi et al. (1986). These authors employed dynamic palatography in the successful correction of Japanese palatalized articulation and Japanese lateral misarticulation in a 6-year-old girl with a repaired left unilateral cleft and an anterior oronasal fistula of 2 mm diameter. The child was free from audible nasal emission and hypernasality. The palatographic device is commercially available but requires use of a palatal plate custom fitted to the patient. The authors described a therapy plan that included teaching the child: (1) to identify palatographic patterns and to associate them with awareness of tongue position, (2) to understand information on the palatographic display, and (3) to learn correct articulatory movements. The therapy was intended to terminate unwanted articulatory contacts and then to replace them with correct place of articulation. A progression from isolation and syllables through words and sentences to paragraphs and conversation was followed. The authors offer evidence that in the course of 49 hourly sessions over a period of 1 year the child made and maintained substantial articulatory improvement, including the elimination of tongue backing and air stream lateralization. Neither of those misarticulations was likely to self-correct. Progress was more rapid than that made by other children who had therapy that did not involve dynamic palatography.

The studies cited indicate that gains are made with articulation therapy directed to persons who present borderline velopharyngeal insufficiency.

More information is needed about cleft palate patients' changes in articulation with therapy. Studies should be well designed, and the subjects and treatment should be described in detail. Even longitudinal descriptive information would have value if details of subjects and treatment were provided. It is unlikely that any one research study will provide a final answer. The clinician should look to a combination of data and theory for guidance in clinical work. Nonetheless, the short supply of experimental work relative to articulation treatment for cleft palate patients is unfortunate. It is clear that individuals with velopharyngeal insufficiency that is more than marginal in nature do require surgical or prosthodontic treatment of that deficiency.

PRINCIPLES AND THEORY RELATIVE TO ARTICULATION THERAPY

Two of the foundations of speech therapy, clinical experience and experimental data, have been considered thus far. It is appropriate next to consider some general principles and theories that also underlie speech therapy including that directed to the improvement of the disordered articulation presented by patients with cleft palate or related conditions.

The learning theories of psychology have influenced the articulation therapies formulated by speech pathologists. Behavioral psychology has had a particularly strong influence (Mowrer, 1982) and, recently, cognitive psychology has had considerable impact (Muma, 1978). We review the influence of each on articulatory and phonological therapy. An information-processing system of therapy that has both behavioral and cognitive components is described, and suggestions are made relative to the use of phonetic and phonological information in directing articulation therapy.

Behavioral Principles

Many articles and textbooks have described and discussed behavioral learning principles and their application in speech therapy. The topic is discussed here primarily to emphasize its importance to speech work with cleft palate patients. The authors assume familiarity with this information on the part of speech pathologists. However, it may be less well known to persons in some of the other professions serving cleft palate patients. Key learning variables in articulation therapy are: employment of stimuli, choice of response units (speech sounds, syllables, words, features, processes) for use in practice and other therapy activities, reinforcement, and generalization.

The teaching of articulation skills, whether to persons with cleft palate or to persons with developmental misarticulation, involves manipulation of the stimuli that precede a response. Stimuli may be used to teach the patient auditory discrimination, to elicit responses for practice, or for other purposes. Regardless of the response called for in therapy, effective use of antecedent stimuli will enhance that response. Winitz (1969) described stimulus generalization as a phenomenon that can be used in articulation training. Instruction is organized so that responses are conditioned to new stimuli. That is, through learning, the patient produces desired responses in the presence of stimuli that were previously ineffective. In one stimulus-oriented therapy, words in which correct responses occur are paired with words in which a sound of interest is misarticulated. The pairing is done with pictures. Through practice and reinforcement, the correct response generalizes from a correctly articulated key word to training words (Weston and Irwin, 1971). Another clinical technique, the stimulus shift procedure (McLean, 1970; Long et al., 1976) utilizes auditory and visual stimuli to elicit correct articulation of a sound of interest in several words. Then correct articulation is elicited in the same words by use of stimuli that initially would not have been effective.

Choice of response units is important in articulation therapy. By using a series of response units graded for difficulty, the speech pathologist can assist the patient to progress to the desired speech performance without experiencing very much failure. Units for production can also be chosen so that old, unwanted responses are avoided. For example, Gerber (1973) and Winitz (1975) utilized nonsense words in order to avoid triggering the unwanted articulation pattern. Use of a newly created word to refer to an unfamiliar picture or object or assignment of a new meaning to an old word serves to avoid the patient's bias toward use of the well-established articulation error associated with words already in his or her vocabulary (Mowrer and Scoville, 1978).

The clinician may also manipulate events that follow responses. Reinforcers and punishers may be administered; usually, positive reinforcements is employed. The patient is given something he or she values contingent upon a specified response. Negative reinforcement, the removal of a noxious stimulus, and punishment, the removal of something of value to the patient or presentation of an aversive stimulus, may sometimes be useful. Like positive reinforcement, negative reinforcement and punishment, if used, would be made contingent upon a specified response.

Use of behavioral learning principles has been directed to helping patients learn to articulate speech sounds in various contexts, to generalize from articulation of practice material to unpracticed speech, and to maintain newly learned speech behaviors. These principles are especially helpful to the clinician faced with the task of teaching a patient a particular skill or pattern (Bernthal and Bankson, 1988). The study and encouragement of generalization in speech therapy has received much attention in recent years (Elbert and Gierut, 1986; McReynolds, 1987; Fey, 1988; McReynolds and Spradlin, 1989). The potential power of behavioral principles in therapy is demonstrated in a study by Koegel et al. (1988) wherein children taught to self monitor /s/ and /z/ outside the clinic quickly and thoroughly resolved a generalization or carryover problem in which they had used the target sounds correctly in the clinic but not elsewhere. Subject and environmental variables may restrict the power of this procedure (Gray, 1989).

The adoption of behavior-modification procedures moved speech pathologists away from the frequent use of game-playing. This is not to say that play and games have no place in articulation therapy. Shriberg and Kwiatkowski (1982) argued that the clinician should have available a *range* of therapy modes, including play.

Cognitive Principles

A cognitive concept of learning has evolved from information theory, psychophysics, physiology, and psycholinguistics. It utilizes knowledge about attention, memory, and comprehension. This concept is introduced here through consideration of Smith's (1978) views about the child's use of comprehension and hypothesis testing in learning to use language and to read. This viewpoint is then discussed relative to phonological disability and its remediation. This approach is relevant to the enhancement of mature phonological patterns in the cleft palate patient after velopharyngeal sufficiency has been achieved and the ability to produce speech sounds in words has been demonstrated.

Children must comprehend what they are learning; they will ignore that which bewilders them (Smith, 1978). Learning is a natural process based on comprehension; people know much more than what is deliberately taught them. The learner elaborates prior knowledge by relating new information to it. Thus, the child constructs a mentalistic theory of the world from which he or she makes predictions. To develop this theory, the learner must be presented with potentially solvable problems and be given the opportunity to formulate and test hypotheses (make predictions) about the problems. Feedback must be provided to complete the hypothesis testing. Much of the learning that goes into the construction of one's theory of the world is unconscious (Smith, 1978):

> ...*most of our theory of the world, including most of our knowledge of language, whether spoken or written, is not the kind of knowledge that can be put into words... Knowledge which no one can put into words is not knowledge that can be communicated by direct instruction.*

The infant brings meaning to speech by gradually mastering the rules necessary to grammatical utterances in the language to which he or she is exposed. These rules are not spelled out by anyone to the infant; rather the infant and adult share the meaning of an experience. The adult provides language that goes with the meaning and elaborates on language the infant uses in an attempt to express meaning. As Snyder-McLean and McLean (1978) put it, as mother and child interact, they direct their attention to the same stimuli and establish use of the same stimulus-response associations. That is, they establish joint reference for the same experiences.

An adult's response to an utterance by the child may provide feedback that allows the child to test the hypothesis that he has formulated about language and speech. Hypothesis testing and theory building are unconscious; they occur instinctively and the learner will turn away from learning if asked to learn something already known or if the risk of failure is too great. Hypothesis testing carries a risk of being wrong; a learning environment that punishes error may be self-defeating.

In summary, the infant or child learns language best in a situation where he or she can hypothesize a relationship between meaning and an utterance. Testing the hypothesis permits the child to evaluate the data and thus to confirm or modify provisional rules about this relationship (Smith, 1978).

A recent conceptualization of language therapy (Connell 1988) seems to relate to and extend the ideas just presented. The method, induction teaching, was designed to be compatible with a generative view of the nature of language in which meaning is related to language by rules that allow generation of sentences. The method also draws on the theory that language development utilizes an innate induction ability. The therapy is to correspond to a three-step conceptualization of language acquisition wherein the first step is to recognize a pattern, the second step is to explain or understand the pattern, and the third is to use what was learned in the first two steps to hypothesize a rule regarding the correspondence between pronunciation and meaning. Therapy is structured to facilitate pattern recognition and understanding. The induction of rules, however, is left to the learner on the assumption that it is within his or her innate capability. The teaching or therapy is intended to provide the learner with the data needed for hypothesis formulation. The method, which is illustrated by Connell, emphasizes the contrasting of pairs of utterances and meanings. It is challenged by language forms that do not lend themselves to such contrasts. Here Connell refers to the need for triggers for syntactic options within the conceptualization of an innate capacity for language acquisition. His discussion ends with the assertion that the teacher of the child with a specific language impairment should strive "to create a learner who solves grammatical problems efficiently and thereby constructs an appropriate grammar, rather than a learner who increases the frequency of his or her responses" (p. 61).

Phonological Therapy

Discussion of principles and procedures of phonological therapy is warranted since it seems likely that children with cleft palate may demonstrate phonological delay just as may those without a cleft. As indicated earlier, additional data are needed about the frequency of occurrence of such delay in children with cleft palates. On the basis of present information, the speech-language pathologist must give strong consideration in dealing with these children to speech production problems related to structural abnormalities such as velopharyngeal incompetence and malocclusion.

To apply cognitive concepts in phonological therapy for the child with cleft palate, the speech pathologist must first determine that the child has the physiological and phonetic capability of producing the sounds that are to be sequenced. He or she would then provide an environment in which the child can test hypotheses about phonological patterns without fear of embarrassment or other forms of punishment.

Many techniques have been described for use in phonological therapy. Winitz (1975) suggested that the child be presented with comprehension problems for solution. Situations would be structured wherein children could sample and scan "the phonological sequences of their language, making it possible to spot recurring segments." In his view, this experience allows the child to induct the rules of his language. Winitz (1975) would have the mother of a misarticulating child deliberately misunderstand some of what the child says. The mother or clinician is not punishing the child but structuring an environment that encourages the child to formulate an hypothesis about his speech and provides opportunity to test that hypothesis. Winitz (1975) and Winitz and Reeds (1975) would present the learner with short units that can be processed within the capacity of short-term memory. Pronunciation is avoided until syntax and semantics are learned, and training materials are selected to avoid interference as a source of error in learning.

Alerting a child to communication failure may present him or her with a problem about speech and provide an opportunity to solve that problem. However, such therapy is based on the assumption that the child can produce the required speech sounds. Otherwise, unwanted substitutions may result. The role of communication failure in articulation therapy is discussed in a later section of this chapter.

Phonological therapy is sometimes conducted to eliminate the use of phonological processes that are thought to retard a child's progress toward use of adult sound patterns. Several publications (Ingram, 1976; Locke, 1979; Elbert et al., 1980, Weiner, 1981; and Crary, 1982) have described the elimination of processes by alerting the child to communication failure resulting from use of homonyms that occur when phonemic contrasts are not employed. The child who uses "bow" for both "bow" and "boat" has failed to make a phonemic contrast necessary to communication. His word, "bow," functions as a homonym with at least two meanings.

Therapy that successfully eliminates the use of an undesirable phonological process will influence the child's use of all speech sounds that were influenced by that process and facilitate generalization. This application of phonological process is similar to the earlier search for distinctive features that underlie two or more segmental articulation errors (McReynolds and Engmann, 1975). Whether the clinician seeks generalization through modification of processes or through features shared by different speech sounds, the therapy is likely to involve the use of speech sounds as they are distributed in words and running speech. The training may use perception and production and it may stress phonemic contrasts or drill, It is likely to involve the use of sounds from more than one phoneme, but sound-sized segments will be involved in its formulation.

Future advances in phonological therapy may evolve from study of phonemic distinctiveness and from development of improved procedures for study of the child's phonemic inventory. This relates to metalinguistic awareness which Tunmer and Herriman (1984) defined as "...the ability to reflect upon and manipulate the structural features of spoken language, treating language itself as an object of thought, as opposed to simply using the language system to comprehend and produce sentences" (p. 12).

Kamhi and Koenig (1985) wrote that metalinguistic tasks are more demanding on the talker's attention than are speaking and listening, and they speculated that metalinguistic skill may be important in language remediation even though it may not be involved in normal development of language. Chabon and Prelock (1987) differentiated between phonemic awareness and speech sound discrimination. The former, which they regarded as a matter of metalinguistic awareness, involves segmentation of words into sounds or letters. Discrimination, on the other hand, involves a differentiation between words or other speech units that may proceed in the absence of ability to segment words into sounds or to synthesize sounds into words. Chabon and Pre-

lock note that authors have attempted to measure phonemic awareness with different stimuli and different response units and that it is not clear that the measures employed correspond to the phonemic awareness construct. Tomes and Shelton (1989) demonstrated that change in task influences results in research directed to such matters as the child's ability to categorize sounds by place and manner of articulation. Explanation based on tasks of unknown validity consumes a remarkable amount of our attention.

Dean and Howell (1986) described a phonological therapy in which metalinguistic awareness is used as a tool to resolve conflict associated with failure in the expression of meaning and to encourage reflection about the sound system. The child is presumed to have a processing problem rather than an articulatory disorder, and the therapy is directed at the central, organizational level of language. The therapy they describe follows phonological assessment and analysis and involves two interacting phases: (1) development of awareness of structural aspects of language and (2) development of awareness of communicative effectiveness and encouragement of use of repair strategies. Therapy may be conducted within a play context structured to provide information. It is directed to processes rather than to individual sounds, and it utilizes place and manner distinctions. Feedback is not provided about sound production but rather about whether the child has made himself or herself understood. The authors state that although experimental testing of their therapy has not been completed, it is compatible with a body of empirical literature showing that children less then 5 years of age commonly play with, practice, repair, and comment upon the sound structure of the language.

Although many recommendations regarding phonological therapy have appeared in the literature, few of the techniques advocated have been submitted to experimental test.

Two descriptive studies are pertinent here. Gierut (1989) used a subject with cleft palate in a study of a therapy technique involving maximal phonological contrasts. Previous contrast therapy focused on contrasts wherein the learner dealt with syllable or word pairs that differed minimally—perhaps only in one distinctive feature. The maximal opposition therapy technique of contrast treatment "...involves maximal rather than minimal oppositions. In this approach, phonemic distinctions vary along extremes of the broad and multiple dimensions of voice, place, and manner" (p. 9). The author cited evidence that children concentrate on wide sound contrasts before turning to fine-grained distinctions. She also indicated that use of broad contrasts early in therapy is compatible with the viewpoint that children are active and creative in their acquisition of phonology.

The presence of the repaired cleft of the soft and hard palate was not considered important in the child's sound system because he was free from hypernasality and audible nasal emission. Rather, the deletion of initial consonants was considered to reflect a gap in the child's phonological knowledge. He deleted all initial consonants except for /m/, /b/, /w/, and /j/. Those sounds are all voiced and three are bilabial. One is a stop and two are glides; the distinction between oral and nasal sounds is present. The first step of therapy used /s/ because it introduced voicelessness, frication, and a place of articulation posterior to those in use. As success was achieved, a new maximal contrast was introduced. Following work with that contrast, the child was using many initial consonants. The third contrast was selected for fine tuning and involved minimal distinctions.

This paper is of interest here because it describes a therapy technique of a cognitive sort and because the subject is an individual with cleft palate who may present a sound pattern disorder that is more phonological than it is representative of a structural or physiologic disorder. Gierut interpreted unwanted generalization as evidence indicative of phonological knowledge or its absence. "Overgeneralizations suggested that J treated all omitted sounds as equivalent. When J learned that consonants belong in the initial position, it seemingly did not matter which consonant served as the marker" (p. 16).

Tyler et al. (1987) reported change in the sound patterns of four children, two of whom received perception-production minimal pair therapy and two a modified cycles therapy. The therapies combined procedures with long histories of clinical use, including ear training, imitation, and practice. Progress was measured by sampling both phonological processes and speech sounds. The authors present their report as descriptive rather than experimental because no experimental control was employed. Nonetheless, because the subjects made substantial improvement in short periods of time, it is likely that the treatment was effective.

While it is difficult to generalize from the data reported by Gierut and Tyler et al., it appears that articulation-phonological therapy is becoming more efficient in that strong gains are observed with relatively short periods of therapy. Replication and extension research are needed.

Behavioral and cognitive concepts conflict as explanations of normal speech and language acquisition—and other things as well. In a paper that explicates this conflict, Skinner (1989, p. 66) asked, "Is there any field of psychology today in which something does not seem to be gained by adding that charming adjective [cognitive] to the occasional noun?" The word is overused. Nonetheless, concepts and information from these two parts of psychology supplement each other in contributing to the therapy practiced by the speech-language pathologist. We would not choose between them but rather would utilize whatever seemed most appropriate to a particular goal. Next we consider a therapy model that is cognitive in nature but can be employed in a manner compatible with behavioral learning principles.

Perceptual-Motor Information Processing

Information-processing models take the form of boxes and connecting lines. They are useful in so far as they contribute insight and testable hypotheses (Cutting and Pisoni, 1978; Snyder-McLean and McLean, 1978). The model to be discussed here (Fig. 22.1) is an extension of a model presented by Shelton and McReynolds (1979). They in turn drew on a model developed by Marteniuk (1976). They summarized their discussion of Marteniuk's book by writing that his conceptualization of information processing in perceptual-motor performance and learning

...is composed of three basic components: perception, decision, and production. The function of each component is dependent upon short-term memory which not only recodes information for storage and contributes to retrieval of information from long term storage but also participates in the operation of the peripheral sensory system. Perception involves both organization of sensory experience and information selection and prediction. The decision mechanism must select a plan of action suitable to the task faced by the performer, and the production mechanism is concerned with the organization of information

about movement. The production mechanism stores plans of action in a hierarchical order and imposes sequential order on the components of a plan when it is selected for use. Information processing in motor performance requires the performer's attention, and direction of an individual's attention to one operation interferes with attention to other operations. One function of practice is to establish automatic performance thereby decreasing attention demands. Sensory-motor performance and learning involve efficient use of sensory information and decision making as well as execution of the performance.

The model in Figure 22.1 extended in the text that follows may be employed to teach a child to produce speech sounds in context and to establish their automatic use in spontaneous conversation. Following the model, therapy requires the learner to make perceptual responses to stimuli, to plan motor speech responses, and to perform those responses. Not modeled is the important step where the learner evaluates the responses. Auditory and kinesthetic information would feed back to the perceptual mechanism and influence future response planning and execution. Unconscious proprioception would also contribute to performance skill (Shelton, 1989). Perceptual and decision-making activities are incorporated with production and evaluation throughout the course of the therapy. The learner is required to understand the task to be learned and the difference between his or her performance and the desired performance. Thus, cognitive participation on the part of the learner is required. However, the therapy may also make use of behavioral constructs of antecedent events, response units, practice, and reinforcement.

Consider the correction of gross substitutions that continue to be used after successful velopharyngeal surgery. To help a child replace glottal stops and pharyngeal fricatives with more anterior sounds, the clinician could provide perceptual information about the desired articulation and the articulation to be replaced. Both visual and auditory models might be employed to describe the desired articulation and to contrast it with the old pattern. The patient might be asked to plan each production of a target sound in a practice exercise. That is, he or she might be asked to think about where to position the articulators. After each practice response, the patient might

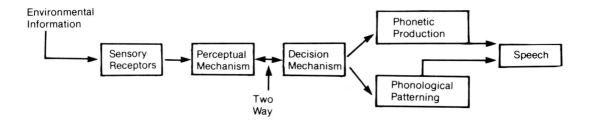

Figure 22.1 Revised perceptual-motor information processing model. (From Shelton RL, McReynolds JV. Functional articulation disorders—preliminaries to therapy. In: Lass NJ, ed. Speech and language: advances in basic research and practice. Vol 2. New York: Academic Press, 1979.)

evaluate that response and contrast it with information produced by the clinician. Feedback from the clinician would help the patient test the hypotheses he or she had drawn. The clinical techniques employed are sequenced as required by the model; however, they can be administered in a manner compatible with behavioral learning.

The decision-making in the therapy just described probably involves information coming down from the higher portions of the central nervous system as well as information coming up from the sensory-perceptual apparatus. Lemme and Daves (1982) (see also Luce and Pisoni, 1987) wrote that top-down processing involves "...the expectations formulated by an individual in response to on-going analysis of the situational context and from the individual's prior knowledge." A top-down component could directly influence the decision, production, and patterning components of the model in Figure 22.1 thus supplementing and interacting with bottom-up components. The cognitive therapy considerations cited earlier are probably top-down in nature.

We would have the perceptual-motor information-processing model account for articulation development with training and for the unusual speech motor skills that are sometimes developed in the absence of instruction or conscious intention. An example is provided by a woman who used the velar tags of her unrepaired cleft of the soft palate to raise and lower the hinged pharyngeal section of her speech appliance (Shelton and McCauley, 1986). She doesn't know how she acquired this skill, and we wouldn't know how to teach it to another person. Her dentist may have fitted the appliance to take advantage of spontaneous movement of the velar tags. However, we think she unconsciously modified those movements in solving the problem of learning to use the appliance skillfully in speech. For another view of motor learning as it pertains to articulation therapy, see Kent and Lybolt (1982).

An appreciation of these principles that underlie articulation therapy may lead a speech pathologist away from applying systems of therapy without regard to the uniqueness of each individual with the complex articulation disorders associated with cleft palate and toward individualized plans of therapy that may be more likely to develop whatever potential for change is present.

THE PRACTICE OF ARTICULATORY-PHONO-LOGICAL THERAPY

Our focus here is on articulation training for patients with velopharyngeal competence or with questionable or marginal incompetence. Plans for articulatory-phonological therapy draw on the clinical views, information, and theory cited above and require consideration of phonetic skills, phonological patterning, and related variables such as velopharyngeal competence. Goals in these three areas may be pursued in parallel (Winitz and Bellerose, 1978). Work on phonetic and phonological goals within a session may interact in a catalytic fashion. If the child is stimulable, phonetic work may be directed early in therapy to sounds that are least likely to be developed spontaneously. Elbert (1984) wrote that the first exemplar (first production of a sound of interest) may reflect the establishment of an "articulatory concept" that may be prerequisite to new acquisitions. Simultaneous work on phonetic and phonological goals encourages generalization or carryover while working on acquisition of phonetic skills. This practice was suggested by Diedrich (1971), and Johnson et al. (1979) reported that children working on /r/ sounds who received acquisition and automatization activities simultaneously made more rapid progress than did children who were given /r/ acquisition training only. This difference was not observed for children working on /s/ sounds.

Planning articulatory-phonological therapy requires consideration of the learner's age. We begin here with consideration of the preschool patient and then consider therapy for the child in the early school years. Therapy for older patients is also considered. Some children require the sort of indirect speech and language instruction described by Brookshire et al. (1981), Hahn (1989), Philips (1979), and Wells (1971). The information presented here, however, involves direct work on the sound system. The therapy described has been used successfully with children as young as 3 years of age at treatment onset. Work by other authors with younger children was cited earlier. Therapy is guided by the patient's speech and response to therapy; this requires continuous assessment of articulation and phonological patterns and periodic reassessment of velopharyngeal function.

The Preschool Child

Many children 3 and 4 years of age can be worked with directly once the clinician establishes a satisfactory relationship with them. Key goals of articulatory-phonological therapy for these children are: (1) development of the ability to produce consonants from different place-manner categories in words and (2) incorporation of those phonetic skills into the child's phonological patterns. Development of sound-production skills through early articulation training may allow the child with a cleft palate to take greater advantage of naturally occurring phonological maturation. Both phonetic and phonological goals may be pursued within a single therapy session. For example, work may be done to establish the phonetic ability to produce sounds from one or more phonemes. The same session may include activities to encourage spontaneous use of other sounds in the phonological pattern. We acknowledge that many children with clefts acquire normal articulatory skills and phonological patterns without benefit of therapy.

In this early training, emphasis is placed on development of the ability to produce both stops and fricatives. This clinical practice is based on the assumption that establishing stopping and frication in a few sounds will contribute to the generalization of those features to other sounds. Bilabial stops may be taught before linguadental stops since their place of articulation is more visible. If velopharyngeal function is questionable, the clinician may choose to avoid working on /k/ and /g/ to avoid encouraging any tendency toward posteriorly placed compensatory articulations. Fricatives, affricates, or both are introduced as gains are made with stops or as stimulability testing indicates the child is ready for one or both of these sound classes. As with stops, we explore first the more visible sounds, the labiodentals. Next one may advance to the linguapalatal sounds. For many children, they are more easily learned than the lingualveolars even though the latter are further forward and hence perhaps more visible. The highly visible linguadental sounds are not taught until it is clear that dentalization of the lingualveolars is not a problem. The exact order of presentation of sounds in these and other sound classes (affricates, glides, and liquids) depends upon the individual's speech pattern, oral structures, and response to stimuli

presented. We sample the child's production of sounds of interest by asking him or her to imitate the sounds in a variety of contexts. If a few correct responses are elicited, we use different contextual variables in a search for contexts in which correct responses can be elicited. Variables to consider include syllable stress, position of the sound in a syllable or word, adjacent sounds, and frequency of occurrence of clusters and words (Kent, 1982). Winitz's (1969) idea of avoiding units that trigger the unwanted misarticulations is also useful.

In general, we recommend use of long-standing speech pathology techniques for teaching children to produce sounds in syllables and words and then to establish automatic use of those sounds in conversation. The therapy will include use of auditory and visual models for imitation, practice and reinforcement of responses in speech material appropriate to the patient's capability, and organization of therapy to encourage generalization from that which is taught in therapy to speech units not used in therapy and to situations outside the clinic. Units employed in therapy may be chosen on the basis of the patient's use of distinctive features or phonological processes. Perceptual as well as motor variables are important in this work. Perceptual training may involve having the child repeatedly listen to syllables or words containing the sounds that are to be learned. Discrimination between the child's better and poorer productions of sounds of interest may be taught. Some perceptual tasks require that the child understand the segmentation of speech into small units. Tasks of this sort may be too difficult conceptually for very young children (Cutting and Pisoni, 1978). Activities such as planning and evaluating responses should be employed only as the child is ready for them.

Sounds may be taught in isolation if the child cannot produce them in syllables or words. This is a controversial issue (Winitz, 1975; Bankson, 1982). Some speech pathologists believe that the individual who always misarticulates a given speech sound will incorporate the correct sound into speech more quickly and easily if it is first taught in isolation. Others believe that the sound should be taught within larger units wherein coarticulation occurs. The definition of what is meant by "isolation" has not been well stated in this controversy. If instruction directed to use of a sound within larger units (i.e., syllables, words) involves stressing the sound of interest by prolongation or increased intensity, then the sound is being isolated from its usual context. As a rule of thumb, for use until more complete empirical information is available, one may teach isolated sound production to the person who always misarticulates a sound of interest—even in imitation of syllables. However, as responses are established in isolation, we shift to larger units—syllables and words—as quickly as possible (Shelton and McReynolds, 1979). We note that the child who cannot produce a sound either in isolation or in context at one time in therapy may be able to do so later. Perhaps therapy directed to other tasks contributes to development of phonetic skills that are not directly taught. Alternatively, maturation of sound production skill may co-occur with but not result from training directed to other tasks. Procedures for teaching production of sounds and incorporating them into contexts are described in drill books, texts, and articles. Work by Buck and Harrington (1949) and Wells (1971) pertains directly to teaching sound production skills to children with cleft palate.

Some children with repaired clefts appear to benefit from activities intended to teach them oral direction of the breath stream. A patient may be asked to feel the breath stream as the clinician produces /p/ sounds, and then to produce /p/ sounds. The productions may be directed to a tissue, thus allowing the child to observe the displacement of the tissue by the breath stream. Excessive pressure should not be encouraged. Hixon et al. (1982) described the use of a straw and a glass of water to measure intraoral air pressure and to provide feedback about the pressure produced. Simultaneous blowing and phonation has been recommended as a therapy to encourage velopharyngeal closure in patients who close during blowing but not speech (Shprintzen et al., 1975). Perhaps this activity also encourages oral direction of the breath stream during speech. Some articulation practice trials may be performed with the nares pinched closed as a means of teaching the child to direct the sound out of the mouth. This technique should not be used so much that the patient learns to depend on nares closure to impound intraoral air pressure.

Various techniques are used to encourage the child's phonological use of newly learned phonetic skills. As was discussed earlier, some involve the child's awareness of his or her communicative effectiveness; others are more behavioral in nature. The "speaker's desire to be understood" is an important contributor to articulation development (Mazza et al., 1979). Elbert et al., (1980) wrote that effective communication is dependent upon the child's ability to perceive and produce phonemic contrasts. They advocated training in the use of contrasts because these are essential to the conveyance of meaning. There is a growing literature on the topic of contrasts and communicative failure.

As mentioned earlier, Winitz (1975) recommended that parents sometimes "misunderstand" the misarticulated speech by responding to the child's speech in a way different from what the child expects. The deliberate misunderstanding of misarticulated speech as a therapy technique requires research and development. Although a number of authors have described articulation change in a positive direction upon questioning or misunderstanding (Gallagher, 1977; Gallagher and Darnton, 1978; Weiner and Ostrowski, 1979) or have noted a relationship between the contribution of a sound to conveyance of meaning and the correctness of its articulation (Leonard, 1971), others have reported more negative results (Prater et al., 1980). Preschool children studied by Shelton et al. (1984) did not alter articulation of target sounds when questioned contingent upon misarticulation. The misarticulated sounds were sounds the children sometimes produced correctly. Investigation is yet to be done to identify the conditions under which "misunderstanding" can serve as a clinical tool. Questions might work best if they direct the child's attention to that which concerns the clinician.

Homonyms that result from the child's misarticulation allow the clinician to help the child to become aware that certain words do contrast with each other and that they must be produced correctly for meaningful communication (Ingram, 1976; Locke, 1979; Weiner, 1981). For example, a cleft palate child said "eye" for "eye," "hi," "pie," and "bye" even though he could easily produce the consonants. He incorporated the consonants into his phonological pattern after experiencing an activity similar to one described by Locke (1979). Pictures of each word were placed on a table. The child indicated to one person which picture he intended to name. He then asked a second person to pick up the picture selected. As the child substituted "eye" for other words pictured, he presumably discovered that he was not getting his message across and he improved his articulation. The same technique was used the with "you" - "shoe" distinction. The same child produced each word as "you," but, in this case, he was not able to produce a correct /ʃ/. He responded to contrast training involving this word pair by using a distorted /ʃ/ in "shoe." This established a phonemic distinction but did not provide the desired response.

It is possible to deal with distortions as well as substitutions through contrast exercises. Distorted sounds may be used in a contrastive way in newly coined words that can be contrasted with English words. The new words may be used to refer to popular items in the child's world such as space ships and aliens. To use this procedure, the clinician must be able to imitate the patient's distortions. Recommendations regarding therapy differ substantially among authors; however, a common feature is that training goals be selected on the basis of a phonological analysis and that sounds employed in therapy be sequenced in such a way that incorrect phonological processes such as the stopping of fricatives and cluster reduction are eliminated.

A behavioral technique to encourage a child's use of newly learned phonetic skills in his or her phonological pattern is to teach parents to monitor their children's speech and to reward correct use of target sounds (Shelton et al., 1972; 1975). Parents may be advised to ask their children to repeat correctly the words in which a target sound was misarticulated. The targets would be sounds the patient could imitate in a variety of contexts and which were sometimes used correctly spontaneously. The parents may require discrimination training to help them identify correct responses. This procedure must be used cautiously because some overzealous parents may hinder learning.

Some 3- and 4-year-old children with cleft palate have severe misarticulation and are likely to require 3 or more years to develop normal articulation, even with therapy. It is important that the therapy be interesting to the child; frustration and boredom may decrease the child's receptivity to therapy later. Therapy should be compatible with the child's ability to accomplish tasks, and within his attention span. The clinician should play a supportive, reinforcing role with the child. The discussion by Shriberg and Kwiatkowski (1982) relative to drill and play is relevant here.

We reiterate that many 3- and 4-year-old children will work actively in response to therapy that combines behavioral and cognitive princi-ples. We sometimes employ token reinforcement wherein a child earns the opportunity to play a game or perhaps to do something with a parent. Some therapy activities are presented in game or other formats that permit lots of practice while helping to maintain the child's participation. No one activity is used so long within a session that the child tires of it. This is less likely to happen if the clinician works on multiple goals—each with a clear beginning and ending—within each session and moves from one part of the room to another. An analogy may be drawn between the therapy room and therapy session, on the one hand, and a stage and a play of three acts on the other. Interest does sometimes sag; attention can often be regained through use of preparatory and imperative commands. The preparatory command tells the child to prepare to execute a performance and the imperative command tells him to do so. The preparatory command could be verbal: get ready to do so and so. A snap of the fingers might then be the imperative command to do it. Preparatory and imperative commands are used to elicit cortical-evoked responses that have been found to be associated with attention (Skinner and Glattke, 1977).

It is important to follow children with palatal clefts closely during the preschool years and to provide each one with the combination of speech therapy, surgery, and dental treatment that is needed to develop essentially normal speech by the time he or she enters school. Some preschool children present unintelligible speech but can build intraoral air pressure for obstruents with little or no nasal emission. These children need articulation therapy. It should not be put off until the child reaches school.

The School-Age Child

Articulatory-phonological therapy guidelines for school-age children are similar to those presented in the previous section for preschool children. Again, we are considering cleft palate children who have velopharyngeal competence or marginal incompetence. Articulatory-phonological therapy is directed at acquisition of speech sounds and their automatic use or incorporation into the phonological pattern. Older children will be able to participate in activities that younger children would not understand. Children of early school age will be more active participants in the formulation and conduct of therapy. At the same time, these children maintain qualities that constitute a readiness for speech acquisition. The sensitive, if not critical, period has not ended.

Most second-grade children are ready to segment the speech stream into sound-sized segments. By this age, children can be given phonetic information and be asked to plan and evaluate articulatory gestures in keeping with the perceptual-motor information-processing model presented earlier (Ruscello and Shelton, 1979). Verbal instructions and information about performance will now be more meaningful.

Instruction in oral direction of the airstream may be effective with children who direct air nasally after secondary velopharyngeal surgery or obturation has provided a mechanism capable of closure.

Whereas the parents of preschool children may be asked to monitor their child's productions of target sounds, the early school child is at least approaching the time when he or she can self monitor, perhaps with some assistance.

As with younger children, care is taken to avoid teaching posterior articulatory placements. That is, the clinician does not want to teach use of the gross substitutions that are so troublesome. Also to be avoided are forceful production of target sounds and facial grimace. If these behaviors are already established and if the velopharyngeal mechanism functions competently, the clinician may undertake their remediation. We assume that the compensatory articulations continue to be used because they have become highly automatic speech behaviors. We would prefer to prevent the establishment of these responses than to have to correct them. Little has been written about the correction of these misarticulations, so their treatment will be a principle-guided, trial-and-error effort. Use of infrequently occurring words or nonsense items as practice material may serve to reduce the likelihood of eliciting the well-established compensatory articulations. One little girl with velopharyngeal competence made excellent progress in the elimination of a pharyngeal fricative until she reached the point of incorporating the anterior place of articulation into commonly used words. Then, she used /s/ plus the pharyngeal production. The solution to this problem was to introduce words that were new to her and that did not signal the old response. One day she was introduced to a slang word she did not know. She was delighted with it and used it correctly at every possible opportunity. Shortly thereafter, the correctly produced /s/ began to appear in conversation.

Dental factors must be considered in planning therapy. Children in the early grades frequently have mixed dentition including missing or partially erupted teeth or dental malocclusions. Children born with clefts of the secondary palate may present maxillary arch collapse that precludes positioning of the tongue within the maxillary arch and resulting lateralization of some fricatives and affricates. Therapy may be deferred if the dental status is expected to improve relatively soon. If not, compensatory therapy goals may be considered; however, the prognosis for improvement with training is often poor.

Throughout therapy, the speech pathologist seeks information regarding the influence of the speech mechanism on response to training. Articulation therapy responses or other speech observations that involve low intraoral air pressure, nasal emission, nares constriction, gross substitutions, or failure to improve speech can be indicators of a physiological fault that warrants surgery or a prosthesis. Certainly, some of these variables can persist after surgery or obturation has provided a velopharyngeal mechanism capable of closure. Nonetheless, it will sometimes be appropriate to discontinue therapy until secondary surgery has been performed and evidence collected that post-surgery articulation training is needed. An obturator may be enlarged if nasal emission continues to be a problem during the course of articulation therapy. If a pharyngeal flap has already been performed, then consideration may be given to widening it. The patient should be given time to learn to use a flap before widening is considered. Few empirical data are available to guide the decision to alter a flap. Revision carries the risk of obstructing the velopharyngeal airway. Obturators have been constructed for patients with pharyngeal flaps. Again, the speech mechanism must be reevaluated from time to time during the course of therapy. Observations made during therapy contribute to understanding the adequacy of the velopharyngeal mechanism. Evidence that the patient is acquiring articulatory responses that were not previously present is supportive of continued training.

The child with a palatal cleft may develop speech that is well articulated and highly intelligible but accompanied by measurable, and perhaps audible, nasal emission and mild-to-moderate hypernasality. This speech behavior is compatible with the existence of marginal velopharyngeal incompetence and occurs in some patients who have had pharyngeal flaps. Some patients present velopharyngeal function that is sufficiently competent to support conscious production of acceptable speech but not automatic use of normal speech. Decisions about whether these patients require further surgery or obturation are sometimes difficult, and the patient or family must decide whether they want either of those treatments. However, many patients with these characteristics do benefit from surgery or prostheses.

The Older Patient

The speech pathologist who specializes in cleft palate and craniofacial disorders probably has fewer cleft palate patients in adolescence and adulthood than was once the case. The services that patients receive earlier in life are effective, and many patients now speak normally by the time they reach adolescence. Nonetheless, there are still patients in this age category who do not speak well, and they merit special consideration. These patients present a great challenge to the speech pathologist. The initial cleft may have been severe, incompetence may persist, and the patient may present especially severe facial disfigurement and occlusal disorder. These patients are likely to respond poorly to speech therapy.

Some adolescent and adult patients have made remarkable adjustments to existing physiological deficits and have better articulation patterns than could be predicted from assessment of the mechanism. Perhaps in attempts to compensate for velopharyngeal deficits, dental malocclusion, midface deficiency, or a combination, they have learned compensatory articulation gestures that produce intelligible but different speech. Furthermore, these abnormal speech patterns are so well learned and automatic that their modification is difficult.

For patients who do not achieve velopharyngeal competence or borderline competence until adolescence or adulthood, the task of acquiring and automating satisfactory articulatory placements is arduous, time-consuming, and expensive. Failure is sometimes experienced, and the patient continues in the use of abnormal speech patterns. There are times when it is best to accept

speech as it is. These patients remind us of the importance of early diagnosis and treatment by members of the cleft palate team. An important goal for all cleft palate specialists is the prevention of such severe speech disorders. In the next section, we briefly consider articulation therapy for persons with velopharyngeal incompetence.

Articulation Therapy for Persons with Velopharyngeal Insufficiency

We are reluctant to initiate articulation therapy for patients with velopharyngeal incompetence that is more than marginal in severity. However, patients are seen who refuse physical management that is needed or for whom management is not available. The health of some patients precludes surgery that could enhance speech. Some patients show so little movement of velum and pharyngeal walls that they are poor candidates for surgery or obturation. Any articulation therapy provided to these individuals is not expected to establish normal speech; rather the goal is to help the patient to do as well as possible.

One goal is to establish correct articulatory placements. This is difficult to achieve for patients who cannot produce the intraoral air pressure required for obstruents. The speech pathologist should avoid asking these patients to produce sounds with good oral air pressure. The attempt encourages the gross substitutions that therapy is intended to correct. For persons who replace several standard sounds with sounds produced further back in the vocal tract, establishment of correct frontal placement of one sound may generalize to other sounds. The backing appears to function as a process that influences sounds from several phonemes. The patient and his or her family should be oriented to the nature of gross substitutions and instructed to avoid them. It is possible that glottal stops and pharyngeal fricatives sometimes become established and reinforced through rewards administered by speech pathologists, parents, teachers, and friends.

Therapy will be guided by stimulability probing and by the patient's response to the training provided. If the individual misarticulates sonorant sounds, such as /r/ and /l/, that do not require high intraoral air pressure, attempts to correct the misarticulation are justified.

Two additional goals of articulation therapy are use of greater mouth opening during speech and use of light articulatory contacts (Shelton et al., 1968). One means of attaining an increased mouth opening during vowels, glides, and liquids is simply to call the patient's attention to that goal and to practice it. A mirror or television monitor may be useful for this purpose. Another technique is to teach exaggerated articulatory movements which lead to greater range of mouth opening and vice versa. A clinical hypothesis in support of teaching intraoral mouth opening was presented by McDonald and Koepp-Baker (1951). Clinical observations indicate that, in the presence of small velopharyngeal openings, increase in mouth opening results in speech that is perceived as more oral. As we have indicated elsewhere, the amount of air that escapes through a velopharyngeal opening is influenced by mouth opening. In some individuals, movement of the mandible and tongue downward may pull the velum down also thus opening the velopharyngeal port.

Use of light articulatory contacts may be taught in a manner similar to that used to establish greater mouth opening. Attention to touch-pressure contacts may be helpful. Training of this sort probably involves reduced expiratory effort. Direct efforts may be made to slow the speech rate. Attention to rate may also encourage greater care in word production, and a slower rate gives the listener more time in which to understand what is being said. Little research has been done to evaluate these techniques. If the speech rate is too slow, the velopharyngeal port will open between words. Training of the sorts described is probably more suitable to older children and adults than to preschool and early elementary school children.

Consideration may be given to teaching compensatory articulation (nonstandard place of articulation) in attempts to achieve intelligibility even though the compensatory placement will be noticeable to conversational partners. The speech pathologist should explore these possibilities and discuss them with patients who might benefit from such assistance.

There are two important warnings to be considered. One is that the patient, the family, and other specialists involved in patient care be well informed about the restricted goals for the therapy. It may be necessary to repeat this information. Otherwise these persons may infer that the speech pathologist continues to be optimistic and that therapy is expected to result in normal speech. There is a danger that its continued use

will serve the delay consideration of additional physical management.

The second warning relates to the first. There is a danger that ineffective therapy will be continued for prolonged periods. Bzoch (1979) referred to patients who had had up to 8 years of speech therapy with little improvement. Continuation of therapy in the absence of improvement is irresponsible. The treatments described in this section should not require very much time. Establishment of these skills on an automatic level may be difficult to achieve. However, these skills do provide the patient with ways to speak better when his or her best oral communication is required.

Again, the speech pathologist must be careful to resist providing therapy beyond the time when no further improvement is to be expected. There are limits to our capabilities, and once we have done our best, within the limits presented by the patient and our resources, we must withdraw from the case with careful explanations to all concerned. The continuation of any therapy is contingent upon evidence of its effectiveness.

Assessment of Response to Therapy

Adaptation of speech therapy to the needs of individual patients is dependent upon the patient's response to the treatment delivered. This response may be assessed by charting the number or percentage of correct responses obtained from repeated articulation samples (Elbert et al., 1967; Wright et al., 1969; Diedrich, 1971; Costello, 1977; Johnson et al., 1979). Charting, which evolved from behavioral research, should maintain a permanent place in the speech pathologist's work with disordered articulation. However, it should be used in a flexible manner. Items used for charting should be selected to sample the behaviors or patterns the clinician is working to develop or to which generalization is expected. Drill books are a good source of materials. For example, Griffith and Miner (1979) organized word lists by speech sound, syllable position, syllable stress, phonetic context, and place-manner-voicing characteristics. Conversational speech samples may be analyzed to obtain longitudinal records of different speech variables, including use of different sounds selected because they share features or are influenced by the same process or processes.

Change in articulation is not effectively assessed by use of speech samples that contain few incorrectly articulated responses or that do not sample misarticulated sounds or other targets as they occur in an adequate number of words. If assessment is intended to measure changes associated with therapy, then data should be gathered rather frequently. Often, charting is used to study sounds that are the direct target of therapy plus phonetically similar sounds that might benefit from the therapy through generalization. For example, if a clinician were teaching a child to produce a target sound in a set of words, the clinician might chart for that child the percentage of correct responses on the training words, or untrained words with the same sound, and on correctness of the sound in reading or conversation. A phonetically similar sound could also be charted as could sounds involved in a particular pattern such as final consonant deletions. Each sample used for charting need not be repeated during each probe session. The clinician should conduct the probing often enough to follow the child's progress. The clinician can select items for response probing that are sufficient in number to allow detection of change without requiring too much time. As the child achieves high percentages of correct responses on training words and demonstrates generalizations of correct production of the target sound in untrained words, the focus of the therapy might be shifted to conversational use of the target sound or sounds. Parsonson and Baer's (1978) discussion of issues in the display of single-subject research data is pertinent here.

Articulation gain may be expressed in terms of the number of items correctly articulated. However, the meaning of a gain may differ, depending on the patient's performance at the beginning of therapy. McCabe and Bradley (1975) evaluate articulation improvement in terms of the percentage of possible change. As they put it relative to a 100-item task:

...a patient with a pre-therapy score of fifty could make a fifty percent change with an actual point change of twenty-five. Another patient with a pre-therapy score of ninety could make a fifty percent change with an actual point change of only five.

This technique is sensitive to the possibility that gain becomes more difficult to achieve as the individual approaches a given goal. However, it is also possible that the initial correct responses are especially difficult to achieve. If so, a weighting to credit early gain, especially from zero correct responses, is also needed.

Van Demark (1971) reported information about several articulation measures for use in assessing the responses of children with palatal clefts to speech remediation. A descriptive scale was devised that contained 27 entries ranging from "consistently correct in conversational speech" through "correct in controlled phrases (less then 50%)" and "correct in isolation (over 50%)" to "unable to discriminate... ." Each child's performance was classified during each therapy period. Where different clinicians provided therapy on the same day, two independent ratings for the day were entered. Charts across days appeared to be sensitive to improvement, and agreement among observers was evident from the similarity of their plots. Van Demark also demonstrated that pre- and post-treatment charts of the percentage of correct responses for all or most consonant sounds provides a visual display of articulation status and change.

Week-to-week response charting should produce an orderly pattern. Where data points are contributed by independent observers to a pattern that follows an orderly curve, confidence in the reliability of the information charted is increased. Evidence that articulation improved more on speech material included in training than on material not included, and evidence that articulation improved more during the period of therapy than during comparable periods when therapy was not provided indicates that the therapy did indeed contribute to the change observed (McReynolds and Kearns, 1982). Van Demark (1971) noted that right-wrong scoring of articulation responses will not capture modification of articulation toward a correct response. The clinician should attempt to describe the child's change in production of target sounds in order to determine the next step in therapy.

The important point about evaluating the effectiveness of articulation therapy is that the information should be utilized in making further treatment decisions. To continue to follow a therapy plan formulated at the time of initial evaluation without informed consideration of the patient's response to the treatment is an error. Information charted must be qualitatively evaluated in terms of what it means relative to resolution of the individual's articulation disorder.

SUMMARY

The child born with a cleft palate requires surgical and dental treatments to establish a mechanism that will support good speech. For many patients, these treatments will suffice and normal speech will develop without therapy; other patients will have disordered speech. The characteristics of disordered speech associated with cleft palate include gross articulatory substitutions and less marked sound substitutions that are perceived as distortions of target sounds. A key function of the speech pathologist working with cleft palate patients with velopharyngeal competence or marginal incompetence is to teach correct articulatory placements and to help in the incorporation of those skills into the child's phonological pattern.

Therapy for the individual patient will be influenced by his or her speech pattern and speech mechanism and will be directed to achievable goals. In general, the principles for articulation therapy for patients with clefts are the same as for other populations of speakers with disordered articulation-phonology. This therapy is based on the clinical experience accumulated by speech pathologists over the years and on the experimental data available. No ultimate therapy has been developed, and the quality of future advances will depend on the quality of the research from which they evolve.

It is important to provide articulation therapy for the patient with cleft palate at the earliest age possible so as to take advantage of the period of natural speech development and to provide the child with a cleft with the best possible speech during the early school years. Articulation-phonology therapy will be part of a multidisciplinary treatment program that involves persons with diverse professional training. Services provided by these specialists must be scheduled in a manner that results in a catalytic or positive interactive effect. Parents will influence the child's response to the treatment provided, and the impact of parental influence will be affected by communication between parents and the professional workers serving their child.

Articulation-phonology therapy will help many cleft palate patients achieve normal speech. However, any therapy with the potential to be helpful also has the potential to be hurtful. Unskilled therapy may teach some of the gross substitutions we strive to prevent or correct. Sometimes the prognosis for improvement is poor, and therapy must be terminated before good speech has been achieved. The speech pathologist must have the courage as well as the knowledge to make this decision.

REFERENCES

Albery L, Enderby P. Intensive speech therapy for cleft palate children. Br J Disord Commun 1984; 19:115.

Bankson NW. Generalization associated with teaching sounds in isolation as compared to syllables. Annual Convention, ASHA, Toronto, 1982.

Bernthal JE, Bankson NW. Articulation and phonological disorders. 2nd ed. Englewood Cliffs: Prentice Hall, 1988.

Berry MF. Correction of cleft palate speech by phonetic instruction. Quart J Speech 1928; 14:523.

Brookshire BL, Lynch JI, Fox DR. A parent-child cleft palate curriculum: developing speech and language. Tigard: CC Publications, 1981.

Buck M. Harrington R. Organized speech therapy for cleft palate rehabilitation. J Speech Hear Dis 1949; 14:43.

Bzoch KR, ed. Communicative disorders related to cleft lip and palate. 2nd ed. Boston; Little, Brown, 1979.

Bzoch KR. Measurement and assessment of categorical aspects of cleft palate language, voice, and speech disorders. In: Bzoch KR, ed. Communicative disorders related to cleft lip and palate. 3rd ed. Little, Brown, 1989:137.

Chabon SS, Prelock PA. Approaches used to assess phonemic awareness: there is more to an elephant than meets the eye. J Child Commun Dis 1987; 10:125.

Chisum L, Shelton RL, Arndt WB, Elbert M. The relationship between remedial speech instruction activities and articulation change. Cleft Palate J 1969; 6:57.

Connell PJ. Induction, generalization, and deduction: models for defining language generalization. Lang Speech Hear Serv Schools 1988; 19:282.

Costello JM. Programmed instruction. J Speech Hear Dis 1977; 42:3.

Crary MA. Phonological Intervention: concepts and procedures. San Diego: College-Hill, 1982.

Cutting JE, Pisoni DB. An information-processing approach to speech perception. In: Kavanagh JF, Strange W, eds. Speech and language in the laboratory, school, and clinic. Cambridge: MIT Press, 1978.

Dean E, Howell J. Developing linguistic awareness: a theoretically based approach to phonological disorders. Br J Disord Commun 1986; 21:223.

Diedrich WM. Procedures for counting and charting a target phoneme. Lang Speech Hear Serv Schools 1971; 5:18.

Elbert M. The relationship between normal phonological acquisition and clinical intervention. Speech Lang Adv Basic Res Pract 1984; 10:111.

Elbert M, Gierut JA. Handbook of clinical phonology: approaches to assessment and treatment. San Diego:College-Hill, 1986.

Elbert M, Rockman B, Saltzman D. Contrasts: the use of minimal pairs in articulation training. Austin: Exceptional Resources, 1980.

Elbert M, Shelton RL, Arndt WB. A task for evaluation of articulation change: development of methodology. J Speech Hear Res 1967; 10:281.

Fey ME. Generalization issues facing language interventionists: an introduction. Lang Speech Hear Serv Schools 1988; 19:272.

Gallagher TM. Revision behaviors in the speech of normal children developing language. J Speech Hear Res 1977; 20:303.

Gallagher TM, Darnton BA. Conversational aspects of the speech of language-disordered children: revision behaviors. J Speech Hear Res 1978; 21:118.

Gerber A. Goal: Carryover; an articulation manual and program. Philadelphia: Temple University Press, 1973.

Gierut JA. Maximal opposition approach to phonological treatment. J Speech Hear Dis 1989; 54:9.

Gray S. Self-monitoring effects on articulation carry-over in school age children. Unpublished Masters thesis. University of Arizona, 1989.

Griffith J, Miner LE. Phonetic context drillbook. Englewood Cliffs: Prentice-Hall, 1979.

Hahn E. Speech therapy for the pre-school cleft palate child. J Speech Hear Dis 1958; 23:605.

Hahn E. Communication in the therapy session: a point of view. J Speech Hear Dis 1960; 25:18.

Hahn E. Directed home language stimulation program for infants with cleft lip and palate. In: Bzoch KR, ed. Communicative disorders related to cleft lip and palate. 3rd ed. Little, Brown, 1989:137.

Hanson ML. Articulation. Philadelphia: WB Saunders, 1983.

Harrison RJ. A demonstrated project of speech training for the preschool cleft palate child: final report. Project No. 6-1167, Grant No. OEG-2-6-061101-1553. US Office of Education, Bureau of the handicapped, HEW, 1969.

Henningsson GE, Isberg AM. Velopharyngeal movement patterns in patients alternating between oral and glottal articulation: a clinical and cineradiographical study. Cleft Palate J 1986; 23:1.

Hixon TJ, Hawley JL, Wilson KJ. An around-the-house device for the clinical determination of respiratory driving pressure: a note on making simple even simpler. J Speech Hear Dis 1982; 47:413.

Hodson BW, Chin L, Redmond B, Simpson R. Phonological evaluation and remediation of speech deviations of a child with a repaired cleft palate: a case study. J Speech Hear Dis 1983; 48:93.

Hubbell RD. Children's language disorders: an integrated approach. Englewood Cliffs: Prentice-Hall, 1981.

Huber MW. A clinical approach to cleft palate speech therapy. West Speech 1957; 21:30.

Ingram D. Phonological disability in children. New York: Elsevier, 1976.

Johnson AF, Shelton RL, Ruscello DM, Arndt WB. A comparison of two articulation treatments: acquisition and acquisition-automatization. Human Commun Can 1979; 4:337.

Kamhi AG, Koenig LA. Metalinguistic awareness in normal and language-disordered children. Lang Speech Hear Serv Schools 1985; 16:199.

Kawano M, Isshiki N, Harita Y, Tanokuchi F. Laryngeal fricative in cleft palate speech. Acta Otolaryngol (Stockh) 1984; 419 (Suppl):180.

Kent RD. Contextual facilitation of correct sound production. Lang Speech Hear Serv Schools 1982; 13:66.

Kent RD, Lybolt JT. Techniques of therapy based on motor learning theory. In: Perkins WH, ed. Current therapy of communication disorders. New York: Thieme-Stratton, 1982.

Koegel RL, Koegel LK, Van Voy K, Ingham JC. Within-clinic versus outside-of-clinic self-monitoring of articulation to promote generalization. J Speech Hear Dis 1988; 53:392.

Lemme ML, Daves NH. Models of auditory linguistic processing. In: Lass NJ, McReynolds LV, Northern JL, Yoder DE, eds. Language, speech, and hearing: normal processes. Vol 1. Philadelphia: WB Saunders, 1982.

Leonard LB. A preliminary view of information theory and articulation omissions. J Speech Hear Dis 1971; 36:511.

Locke JL. Homonymy and sound change in the acquisition of phonology. In: Lass NJ, ed. Speech and language: advances in basic research and practice. Vol 2. New York: Academic Press, 1979.

Logemann JA. Treatment of articulation disorders in cleft palate children. In: Perkins WH, ed. Phonological-articulatory disorders. New York: Thieme-Stratton, 1983.

Long LD, Raymore SL, McLean JE, Brown KH. Procedures manual stimulus shift articulation program. Bellevue: Edmark Assoc, 1976.

Luce PA, Pisoni DB. Speech perception: new directions in research, theory, and applications. In: Winitz H, ed. Human communication and its disorders, a review 1987. Norwood: Ablex Publishers, 1987:1.

Marteniuk RG. Information processing in Motor Skills. New York: Holt, Rinehart, Winston, 1976.

Mazza PL, Schuckers GH, Daniloff RG. Contextual coarticulatory, inconsistency of /s/ misarticulation. J Phonet 1979; 7:57.

McCabe RB, Bradley DP. Systemic multiple phonemic approach to articulation therapy. Acta Symbol 1975; 6:1.

McDonald ET, Koepp-Baker H. Cleft palate speech: an integration of research and clinical observation. J Speech Hear Dis 1951; 16:9.

McLean JE. Extending stimulus control of phoneme articulation by operant techniques. In: Girardeau FL, Spradlin JE, eds. A functional analysis approach to speech and language. ASHA Monographs 14, 1970:24.

McReynolds LV. A perspective on articulation generalization. Sem Speech Lang 1987; 8:217.

McReynolds LV, Engmann DL. Distinctive feature analysis of misarticulations. Baltimore: University Park Press, 1975.

McReynolds LV, Kearns KP. Single-subject experimental designs in communicative disorders. Baltimore: University Park Press, 1982.

McReynolds LV, Spradlin JE, eds. Generalization strategies in the treatment of communication disorders. Toronto: BC Decker, 1989.

McWilliams BJ. Some observation of environmental factors in special development of children with cleft palate. Cleft Palate Bull 1956; 6:4.

McWilliams BJ. Speech and language problems in children with cleft palate. J Am Med Women's Assoc 1966; 21:1005.

McWilliams BJ. Communication problems associated with cleft palate. In: Van Hattum RJ, ed. Communication disorders; an introduction. New York: Macmillan, 1980:379.

McWilliams BJ, Bradley DP. A rating scale for evaluation of video tape recorded x-ray studies. Cleft Palate J 1964; 1:88.

Michi K, Suzuki N, Yamashita Y, Imai S. Visual training and correction of articulation disorders by use of dynamic palatography: serial observation in a case of cleft palate. J Speech Hear Dis 1986; 51:226.

Morley ME. Cleft palate and speech. 7th ed. Baltimore: Williams & Wilkins, 1970.

Morris HL. Evaluation of abnormal articulation patterns. In: Bzoch KR, ed. Communicative disorders related to cleft lip and palate. 3rd ed. Little, Brown, 1989:185.

Mowrer DE. Methods of modifying speech behavior: learning theory in speech pathology. 2nd ed. Prospect Heights, IL: Waveland Press, 1982.

Mowrer D, Scoville A. Response bias in children's phonological systems. J Speech Hear Dis 1978; 43:473.

Muma JR. Language handbook: concepts, assessment, intervention. Englewood Cliffs: Prentice-Hall, 1978.

Parsonson BS, Baer DM. The analysis and presentation of graphic data. In: Kratochwill TR, ed. Single subject research: strategies for evaluating change. New York: Academic Press, 1978.

Philips BJ. Stimulating syntatic and phonological development in infants with cleft palate. In: Bzoch KR, ed. Communication disorders related to cleft lip and palate. 2nd ed. Boston: Little, Brown, 1979:304.

Philips BJ, Harrison RJ. Articulation patterns of preschool cleft palate children. Cleft Palate J 1969; 6:245.

Prater RJ, Strong JC, Kreiling IL. The effects of communication failure on articulatory revision behaviors. Presented at the Annual Convention, ASHA, Detroit, 1980.

Prins D, Bloomer HH. A word intelligibility approach to the study of speech change in oral cleft patients. Cleft Palate J 1965; 2:357.

Ruscello DM, Shelton RL. Planning and self-assessment in articulatory training. J Speech Hear Dis 1979; 44:504.

Schendel LL, Bzoch KR. Advantages of intensive summer training programs. In: Bzoch KR, ed. Communicative disorders related to cleft lip and palate. Boston: Little, Brown, 1970.

Shelton RL. Oral sensory function in speech production and remediation. In: Bzoch KR, ed. Communicative disorders related to cleft lip and palate. 3rd ed. Little, Brown, 1989: 290.

Shelton RL, Hahn E, Morris HL. Diagnosis and therapy. In: Spriesterbach DC, Sherman D, eds. Cleft palate and communication. New York: Academic Press, 1968:225.

Shelton RL, Johnson AF. Parent-clinician interaction in the remediation of disordered articulation. In: Muller DJ, ed. Remediating children's language: behavioural and naturalistic approaches. San Diego: College-Hill Press, 1984.

Shelton RL, Johnson AF, Arndt WB. Monitoring and reinforcement by parents as a means of automating articulatory respones. Percept Mot Skills 1972; 35:759.

Shelton RL, Johnson AF, Willis V, Arndt WB. Monitoring and reinforcement by parents as a means of automating articulatory respones: II. Study of preschool children. Percept Mot Skills 1975; 40:599.

Shelton RS, Lewis M, Spier C. Misunderstanding of children's speech: its relationship to articulation change. Human Communication Canada 1984; 8.

Shelton RL, McCauley RJ. Use of a hinge-type speech prosthesis. Cleft Palate J 1986; 23:312.

Shelton RL, McReynolds JV. Functional articulation disorders—preliminaries to therapy. In: Lass NJ, ed. Speech and language advances in basic research and practice. Vol 2. New York: Academic Press, 1979.

Shelton RL, Ruscello DM. Palatal and articulation training in patients with velopharyngeal closure problems. Annual Meeting of the American Cleft Palate Association, San Diego, 1979.

Shprintzen RJ, McCall RN, Skolnick ML. A new therapeutic technique for the treatment of velopharyngeal incompetence. J Speech Hear Dis 1975; 40:69.

Shriberg LD, Kwiatkowski J. Phonological disorders II: a conceptual framework for management. J Speech Hear Dis 1982; 47:242.

Skinner BF. Recent issues in the analysis of behavior. Columbus: Merrill, 1989.

Skinner P, Glattke TJ. Electrophysiologic response audiometry: state of the art. J Speech Hear Dis 1977; 42:179.

Smith F. Understanding reading. 2nd ed. New York: Holt, Rinehart, Winston, 1978.

Smith JK. Contraindications for speech therapy for cleft palate speakers. Cleft Palate J 1969; 6:202.

Snyder-McLean LK, McLean JE. Verbal information gathering strategies: the child's use of language to acquire language. J Speech Hear Dis 1978; 43:306.

Tomes L, Shelton RL. Children's categorization of consonants by manner and place characteristics. J Speech Hear Res 1989; 32:432.

Trost JE. Articulatory additions to the classical description of the speech of persons with cleft palate. Cleft Palate J 1981; 18:193.

Tunmer WE, Herriman ML. The development of metalinguistic awareness: a conceptual review. In: Tunmer WE, Pratt C, Herriman ML, eds. Metalinguistic awareness in children: theory, research and implication. New York: Springer-Verlag, 1984.

Tyler AA, Edwards ML, Saxman JH. Clinical application of two phonologically based treatment procedures. J Speech Hear Dis 1987; 52:393.

Van Demark DR. Clinical research methodology in evaluating the therapeutic process. Cleft Palate J 1971; 8:26.

Van Demark DR. Some results of speech therapy for children with cleft palate. Cleft Palate J 1974; 11:41.

Van Demark DR, Hardin MA. Effectiveness of intensive articulation therapy for children with cleft palate. Cleft Palate J 1986; 23:215.

Vaughn GR, Clark RM. Speech facilitation: extraoral and intraoral stimulation technique for improvement of articulation skills. Springfield: CC Thomas, 1979.

Weiner F. Treatment of phonological disability using the method of meaningful minimal contrast: two case studies. J Speech Hear Dis 1981; 46:97.

Weiner FF, Ostrowski AA. Effects of listener uncertainty on articulatory inconsistency. J Speech Hear Dis 1979; 44:487.

Wells CF. Cleft palate and its associated speech disorders. New York: McGraw-Hill, 1971.

Westlake H, Rutherford C. Cleft palate. Englewood Cliffs: Prentice Hall, 1966.

Weston AJ, Irwin JV. Use of paired stimuli in modification or articulation. Percep Mot Skills 1971; 32:947.

Winitz H. Articulatory acquisition and behavior. New York: Appleton-Century-Crofts, 1969.

Winitz H. From syllable to conversation. Baltimore: University Park Press, 1975.

Winitz H, Bellerose B. Interference and the persistence of articulatory responses. J Speech Hear Res. 1978; 21:715.

Winitz H, Reeds J. Comprehension and problem solving as strategies for language training. Paris: Mouton, 1975.

Wright V, Shelton RL, Arndt WB. A task for evaluation of articulation change; III: Imitative task scores compared with scores for more spontaneous tasks. J Speech Hear Res 1969; 4:875.

23 | TREATMENT OF VELOPHARYNGEAL INCOMPETENCE

We have discussed surgery and prostheses for treatment of the velopharyngeal mechanism and speech therapy for phonation, resonance, and articulation disorders. Speech therapy for patients with cleft palate has included also techniques intended to improve velopharyngeal function by strengthening muscles or increasing their range of motion or the skill with which they are used (Berry, 1928; Young, 1928; Eckelmann and Baldridge, 1945; Wells, 1945; and Buck and Harrington, 1949).

Interest in therapy for the velopharyngeal mechanism is understandable when it is remembered that normal speech following veloplasty was uncommon as late as 1950 and that some patients continue to present velopharyngeal incompetence, even in 1990. In the early years, when little was known about the anatomical and physiological nature of velopharyngeal valving, the speech pathologist accepted the impossible task of teaching good speech to the patient who lacked the mechanism for it. The assumption was that the patient could increase the bulk and strength of muscles and their range of motion, thus overcoming structural insufficiency. This idea has persisted in the literature and continues to the present day.

Procedures to improve velopharyngeal closure have a long and checkered history. Early descriptions of therapy included components to reeducate and strengthen the palate and components to teach speech skills, particularly articulation. In early clinical work, much use was made of blowing to activate and strengthen the palate.

Speech pathologists have used other activities for muscle training. These include humming, yawning, stimulating the soft palate and the posterior pharyngeal wall with a tongue blade or knitting needle, cheek puffing, practising moving the soft palate in front of a mirror, suctioning liquids through a straw, and many others (Morley, 1970). However, the effectiveness of muscle exercises was unproved. Speech pathologists using these exercises were often frustrated when patients failed to make progress, but no alternatives were available. Thus, they became concerned with learning why treatment was not effective and did pioneer investigations to learn about the velopharyngeal mechanism.

In recent years, investigators have made use of sophisticated technologies to test hypotheses about therapies directed to velopharyngeal function. Nonetheless, there is still little evidence to indicate that muscle exercises or other therapies influence velopharyngeal function.

This continues to be a subject for further research. We need to know whether training procedures do help some persons achieve velopharyngeal function adequate for speech. Perhaps some people are at least helped to develop greater velopharyngeal range of motion. If either of these gains is achieved, what are the treatments and what are the characteristics of the patients who benefit from them? If velopharyngeal movements are developed through therapy, is the use transferred to and maintained in spontaneous speech? Certainly patients are observed to demonstrate remarkable range of motion during speech, even of insufficient velopharyngeal structures. Theoretically an individual should be able to learn precise voluntary control of the velopharyngeal mechanism.

Review discussions have been provided by Cole (1979) and Ruscello (1982, 1989). In this chapter we consider four forms of therapy that have been employed to influence velopharyngeal function: muscle training, articulation training, obturator reduction, and biofeedback.

MUSCLE TRAINING

Clinical Viewpoints

Much of the early therapy for speech problems associated with cleft palate emphasized blowing for the purpose of strengthening muscles, increasing their range of motion, and establishing voluntary control (Kantner, 1947, 1948). Another purpose was to teach oral direction of the air stream. Some patients could learn this skill without apparently altering the velopharyngeal mechanism. Kantner noted that blowing for air stream direction should not be forceful. He offered several cautions relative to blowing exercises. He pointed out that blowing will not exercise the palate unless the palate moves during the exercise; that, even if increased range of motion is achieved, it cannot overcome a large velopharyngeal opening; and that generalization from blowing to speech may not occur. Kantner noted that blowing and palate exercises should be only a small part of speech therapy for cleft palate patients, and he suggested that these exercises be used only in conjunction with speech training.

A paper by McDonald and Koepp-Baker (1951) contributed to the demise of blowing exercises as a therapy method. They pointed out that speech therapy is just as effective without blowing exercises as with them, that it is unlikely that blowing exercises influence palate muscles, and that there are more effective ways to teach oral direction of the breath stream. They also suggested that hypernasality and nasal emission are influenced by the relationship between the size of the openings at the velopharyngeal port and into the oral cavity.

Another criticism of blowing as an exercise for the velopharyngeal mechanism is that the retracted tongue posture associated with blowing may generalize to speech. Children with palatal clefts appear to be prone to use tongue elevation and retraction as a compensation for poor closure anyway (Westlake and Rutherford, 1966). McWilliams and Bradley (1965) reported that blowing exercises could well be harmful for those who produce less velopharyngeal motion during blowing than during speech because of unwanted generalization.

Morley (1970), who had once advocated the use of velopharyngeal exercises in speech therapy for the cleft palate patient, was later critical of them. She noted that such exercises are now seldom required, a reference to the increased effectiveness of surgery undergone by cleft palate patients. She described two patients who achieved velopharyngeal closure through exercise only to relapse within a few months of the termination of the exercises. She noted that therapy directed to improved velopharyngeal function, even when successful, did not by itself alter articulatory movement patterns. Articulation training was also required.

Cole (1979) presented a clinical viewpoint and a literature review about the use of direct muscle training for improving velopharyngeal activity. He recommended muscle training to develop velopharyngeal activity that can be maintained and used in speech and swallowing without undue effort or attention. He said that muscle training is similar to physical therapy in that it involves elicitation and use of reflexes, modification or inhibition of existing motor functions, stimulation of sensory mechanisms, and development of the patient's awareness of sensory cues including those signaling position and movement of structures.

Cole did not say that muscle training should result in velopharyngeal closure during speech regardless of the patient's velopharyngeal structures or function, but he did suggest that any movement achieved may be beneficial to the patient even if surgery or prosthesis proves necessary. He noted that the individual's velopharyngeal structures and function will influence the success of muscle training. The person whose palate is very short is a poor candidate. However, the patient who demonstrates motion in some activities, including gagging or blowing, but not during speech, may benefit. The person who sometimes produces closure during speech is more likely to establish normal closure patterns than are individuals who do not achieve closure. He noted that any gains that are achieved will usually occur early. Increased velopharyngeal motion should be seen within a month, and if no gain has been made in 3 months, additional work will likely be ineffective.

Powers (1986) indicates that physical training methods to improve level of velopharyngeal function for patients with velopharyngeal incompetence, such as palatal stimulation and blowing, are ineffective and can be frustrating for the patient.

Research Evidence

Let us now turn to consideration of research directed to development or assessment of procedures intended to influence velopharyngeal motion. Some articles reporting clinical impressions are reviewed here for their conceptual value, even though they fail to establish that any change in velopharyngeal function occurred or, if it occurred, that it can be attributed to the treatment. Studies that have attempted to employ control groups or features or that have compared different treatments are more useful, and those that have measured the dependent variable, velopharyngeal function, in adequate ways are of special value.

One goal of therapeutic exercise has been to elicit movement or greater range of movement through the triggering of reflexes, to bring that increased range of motion under conscious control, and then to establish it in automatic, skilled speech performance (Yates, 1980). A sequence of this sort was studied by Yules et al. (1968) and Yules and Chase (1969). They sought to establish voluntary function of circumpharyngeal muscles, to cause hypertrophy of those muscles, and to establish use of the muscles in spontaneous speech. The procedure involved extinguishing the gag reflex through repeated tactile stimulation, identifying the patient's threshold for electrical stimuli delivered to the hand at five pulses per second, and using an electrical stimulus of half that threshold value for intraoral stimulation. Stimulation was initially delivered to the tonsillar pillars, and then pharyngeal locations associated with reflexive responses to the stimuli were identified through trial and error.

Training was provided daily for 10-minute periods. Each patient was taught to identify the reflexive response and instructed to elicit it at home using applicator sticks as stimulators. After

cinefluorography showed that the subject had established anterior movement of the posterior pharyngeal wall of 2 mm, an attempt was made to transfer the motion to speech. For this purpose, a device called a Speech-Ometer was constructed. It consisted of microphones placed in proximity to the nares and lips. The signal from each was fed through a stereophonic amplifier to a full-wave bridge rectifier and then to a meter. Deflection of the meter needle indicated whether energy was greater at the nose or at the mouth. The subject was to practice voluntary contractions while using the Speech-Ometer. Volume controls were used to control the sensitivity of the two microphones and thus to control the difficulty the subject faced in maintaining needle deflection toward the oral zone of the meter. Yules et al. (1968) indicated that subjects were able to reduce nasal emission on short tests but that establishment of performance in automatic speech remained to be demonstrated.

Later, Weber et al. (1970) reported follow-up observations of patients who had had the muscle training just described. Of 34 patients, one was described as having significantly reduced nasality. They reported that most patients had no difficulty learning to make voluntary muscle movements after experience with electrical stimulation and could, at will, reduce the amount of nasal air leakage. However, most failed to generalize these actions into their speech.

Tash et al. (1971) studied the ability of four normal children and two with inadequate velopharyngeal closure but no clefts to learn to produce voluntary pharyngeal wall movements during /a/. The six subjects were between 4 and 7 years of age. The two with inadequate velopharyngeal closure showed velopharyngeal gaps during some oral consonants studied by lateral cinefluorography, and they had audible nasal emission. The training program consisted of the following steps: (1) teaching position of the tongue, control of the gag reflex, and elevation of the soft palate, (2) eliciting mesial movement of the lateral pharyngeal walls with touch stimulation and without phonation, (3) developing voluntary mesial movement of the lateral pharyngeal walls without phonation, (4) developing mesial movements of the lateral pharyngeal walls with phonation, (5) developing anterior movement of the posterior pharyngeal wall with phonation, and (6) developing voluntary mesial movement of the lateral pharyngeal walls and anterior movement of the posterior pharyngeal wall with phonation.

Stimulation with a cotton swab was used initially to elicit reflexive movement of the pharyngeal walls. Training was then directed toward having the subject voluntarily produce the movements first while observing him or herself in a mirror and then without the mirror.

Dependent variables included sagittal cinefluorographic assessment of the velopharyngeal mechanism, oral and nasal sound levels, nasal air pressure, and nasality ratings. The subjects learned to move the pharyngeal walls voluntarily, but the treatment did not influence the dependent variables. Thus, as in the studies cited above, skills were learned that were not incorporated into speech. In this study, one subject elevated the larynx and occluded the pharynx as he attempted to produce pharyngeal wall movements. Muscle training can overdrive the larynx and constitute a hazard to the vocal mechanism and to the voice.

Peterson (1973; 1974) conducted another study related to the Yules and Chase research. She used cinefluorography to investigate the responses of three groups of subjects to electrical stimulation of the soft palate. Her subjects included 11 normal subjects, five subjects with palatal pathology who, nonetheless, demonstrated velopharyngeal closure for speech, and five with palatal pathology and velopharyngeal incompetence. A pressure transducer was used with the intraoral stimulating electrode so that the force with which the electrode was applied to tissue could be controlled and different forces could be studied. In addition, tactile stimulation of known force was compared with electrical stimulation. A low voltage generator delivered "faradic wave forms usually associated with motor nerve impulses...." A wave form with rapid rise time was surged in a series of pulses so that intensity built to a maximum and then decreased at the same rate. The velar eminence was stimulated as were locations to its left and right approximately half the distance between the eminence and the anterior faucial pillars. The subjects' sensitivity and discomfort thresholds were determined, and electrical stimulation was applied above and below the discomfort threshold. Tactile stimuli were presented at different forces between 50 and 270 grams. Two subjects with velopharyngeal incompetence showed no response to either tactile or electrical stimulation. Eleven of the subjects, regardless of the group they were from responded only sporadically to the tactile or electrical stimuli. Peterson was skeptical about the clinical application of the current and waveforms she studied at the locations where they were applied. Peterson (1973) concluded that the speech pathologist should not use a particular motor performance such as blowing as an exercise on the assumption that it will elicit a particular motion. Indeed, it may elicit unwanted movement.

Other techniques for enhancing velopharyngeal function have also been studied. Massengill et al. (1968) used blowing exercises with five subjects, sucking exercises with four, and swallowing exercises with four. The subjects, who ranged in age from 8 to 18 years, received articulation training during the study period. Subjects who performed the swallowing exercise reduced velopharyngeal gaps as determined by cephalometric films made before and after treatment. The subjects were asked to monitor the swallowing by placing a finger on the larynx and prolonging the swallow.

Powers and Starr (1974) used exercises with four children who were between 8 and 11 years of age and who had surgically repaired cleft palates. The exercises involved blowing, sucking, swallowing, and gagging. Each task was performed to specified criteria a designated number of times over a 6-week period. Nasality ratings and cephalometric measurements of the velopharyngeal gap observed during the production of a prolonged /i/ were made before and after the therapy program and again 6 weeks later. No gains were made in velopharyngeal function or voice. The authors noted that their procedures were comparable to those which Massengill et al. (1968) found to be successful.

Lubit and Larsen (1969) described an appliance intended to serve as a palatal exerciser. It consisted of a maxillary-retention segment and an attached inflatable bag. Inflation of the bag displaced the velum superiorly and posteriorly and exerted pressure against the posterior wall of the larynx. The authors claimed that 28 patients benefited from use of the exerciser. However, the only data reported were selected radiographs, speech ratings, oral manometer readings, and spectrograms from one individual. In a second report (Lubit and Larsen, 1971), two of four subjects treated continued to show velopharyngeal openings during test sounds even after treatment. The authors offered several conjectures about the physiological mechanisms whereby their exerciser might bring about improved velopharyngeal function. However, the data reported are not adequate to support their conclusion that benefit actually occurred. Also, as Peterson (1974) pointed out, the device would offer resistance to muscles that would serve to depress the velum but not to the levators that elevate the velum.

We must conclude that the bulk of the evidence regarding the effectiveness of muscle training is negative. The better the controls and measurements in these studies, the more negative the results. At least some clinical claims of success in enhancing velopharyngeal function with muscle training probably reflect the relatively easy task of establishing conscious voluntary motion in the velum or lateral pharyngeal walls. The value of such motions remains to be shown. No one to date has demonstrated in sizable samples the development through muscle training of velopharyngeal movements as remarkable in range of motion and skill of execution as those required for normal speech. Perhaps improved technology and methodology will give a more favorable result in the future.

We consider therapeutic exercise for velopharyngeal function to be experimental and do not recommend it.

ARTICULATION THERAPY

On occasion, the opinion is expressed that articulation training may influence velopharyngeal function. Westlake and Rutherford (1966) noted that both clinician and client prefer to work directly on speech with improved velopharyngeal function as a dividend. Few experimental data are available that pertain to the influence of articulation training or other speech instruction on velopharyngeal function. Nylen (1961) reported that speech therapy was associated with alteration of velopharyngeal function as assessed through frame-by-frame measurement of cinefluorographic films. However, this section of his monograph was essentially anecdotal, and the therapy wasn't described. Prins and Bloomer (1965) reported that palatopharyngeal function as measured with a manometer during oral blowing did not improve during the course of an 8-week intensive, residential speech program that included procedures intended to strengthen velopharyngeal function, to direct the air stream orally, and to improve place of articulation. Word

intelligibility did improve, but not to the point where any subject eliminated all errors on the intelligibility measure used.

Shelton et al. (1969) used sagittal cinefluorography to determine whether articulation improvement with therapy was accompanied by changes in velopharyngeal function. They studied size of the velopharyngeal gap, forward movement of the pharyngeal wall, distance between the tongue and the atlas of the first cervical vertebra, and the distance between the tongue and the posterior wall of the pharynx. No evidence was found that articulation training influenced any of the measurements made.

Morley (1970) noted that velopharyngeal function may improve spontaneously for as long as 8 months following surgery; if articulation training is delivered during that period, it should not necessarily be credited with any improvement in velopharyngeal function.

Articulation therapy delivered to persons with velopharyngeal insufficiency may result in unwanted effects. Speech clinicians offering articulation instruction to young children with velopharyngeal dysfunction should take care not to teach tongue support of the velum nor pharyngeal substitutions. These unwanted compensations might be taught inadvertently since the lingual postures employed are not easily observed.

Trost-Cardamone (1986) suggests that forms of phoneme-specific failure of velopharyngeal closure are responsive to articulation training. Riski (1984) regards such misarticulations as "functional velopharyngeal incompetence," and advises that this condition can be identified by screening techniques for the observation of nasal emission and be confirmed by aerodynamic assessment. He also recommended specific therapy techniques. However, these discussions are not directly relevant here, since we do not consider patients of this type to demonstrate physiologic velopharyngeal incompetence. Because some glottal stops have been observed to be produced with an open velopharyngeal port, Hoch et al (1986) would deliver therapy to teach use of oral stops. They would do this before any secondary surgery was provided. They would first identify non-movement of the velopharyngeal mechanism during glottal stops by use of videonasopharyngoscopy. Their sequence of therapy techniques begins with use of whispering and aspiration to establish voiceless stops in syllables. They assert that velopharyngeal movement patterns associated with stops can be observed reliably over repeated examinations; their subject identification and treatment procedures deserve attention in well controlled applied research.

In conclusion, research evidence relative to the influence of articulation therapy changing velopharyngeal function is weak and neither supports nor rules out a relationship. Research is needed that tests the influence of particular articulation training techniques on velopharyngeal function as they are delivered by themselves and in concert with other therapeutic methods. On the basis of clinical experience, it seems likely that identification of a treatment effect would require relatively long-term therapy and that 4 to 6-year-old children may be the most promising subjects. Until this work is done, articulation therapy should be employed where needed to change articulation. However, its use as a procedure for influencing velopharyngeal function is not warranted.

MODIFICATION OF PROSTHETIC SPEECH APPLIANCES

Prosthetic speech appliances may be constructed to fit between the repaired cleft palate and the pharyngeal walls. Effective use of the appliance requires that the patient move the pharyngeal walls to contact the pharyngeal segment of the appliance. The prosthodontist leaves space between the pharyngeal walls and the pharyngeal segment for nasal respiration; that space must be closed during speech, presumably by pharyngeal wall movement.

A number of authors have reported clinical impressions that prosthetic speech appliances sometimes stimulate increased movement of the velopharyngeal muscles (Harkins and Koepp-Baker, 1948; Cooper et al., 1960, McGrath and Anderson, in press). Rosen and Bzoch (1958) attributed movement gains of this sort to the resistance the speech appliance offers to the muscles; strength is increased by working muscles against resistance. Whether or not increase in strength actually occurs with obturation is a matter of conjecture. Rosen and Bzoch also noted that tissues may swell around a speech bulb because of allergy or infection or that it may be necessary to reduce the size of a speech bulb simply because initially it was made too large. In a series of papers, Blakeley (1960, 1964, 1969),

Blakeley and Porter (1971) and Weiss (1971, 1972) reported that gradual reduction of the pharyngeal section of an obturator can result in increased velopharyngeal movement and that sometimes the movement has sufficient range that the speech appliance can be discarded without adverse influence on speech. In 1960, Blakeley reported his experience with a child who developed good speech with training over a 3-year period during which she wore a prosthetic appliance. At the end of the time, the appliance was removed, and she maintained good articulation. Her voice was described as slightly hypernasal. Blakeley noted that once good speech is obtained, it does not easily deteriorate.

In 1964, Blakeley described three patients who underwent obturation and speech therapy. Speech bulb reduction was performed every 30 to 90 days as the patients improved in voice and articulation. A listening tube was used to guide removal of acrylic. In Blakeley's procedure, small amounts of acrylic were removed until a change in nasal resonance or nasal emission was noted. These three patients underwent pharyngeal flap surgery following the appliance reduction, with the expectation that increased pharyngeal wall motion as a result of obturator reduction could result in better speech with the pharyngeal flap. The question of how they would have responded had the pharyngeal flap been done to begin with remains unanswered.

Blakeley described the obturator-reduction procedure further in 1969. The obturator is fitted when the child is 3 to 4 years of age so that the child is able to impound oral air pressure during part of the period of articulation development. The appliance program is supplemented by speech therapy, especially as the child begins to develop fricatives and affricatives. For the hypernasal child, the appliance is constructed so that it is large enough to produce hyponasality. Otherwise, the child may relax the velopharyngeal valving mechanism and maintain hypernasality. Obturator reduction is initiated when the child shifts to oral speech.

Blakeley noted that pharyngeal compensation to a reduction should occur in 4 to 6 months. His goal in reducing the size of the obturator is to challenge the pharynx just enough so that it compensates for the increased space. He avoids reducing the bulb so much that the patient ceases to compensate and turns the mechanism off. Blakeley indicated that appliances should be reduced in their lateral dimensions more than from front to back.

Obturator reduction appears to be effective in developing velopharyngeal motions in some patients. Weiss (1971), a colleague of Blakeley's, reported success in removing obturators from 23 of 125 patients without apparent detrimental effects on speech. Blakeley (1969) reported that 30 percent of the remaining patients underwent pharyngoplasty after their appliances were reduced to the limits of their ability to compensate. One child had a poor speech result when the pharyngeal flap replaced the obturator. The other operations were successful. Weiss (1972) wrote that mild hypernasality and nasal emission were present in some of the patients who were considered to have achieved satisfactory velopharyngeal function through obturator reduction. Blakeley and Porter (1971) reported success in improving velopharyngeal function through obturator reduction in a 9-year-old boy with palatal paralysis and pharyngeal weakness.

A key question relative to obturator reduction is how to predict which individuals will develop good velopharyngeal function with obturation and maintain it when the obturator has been reduced and perhaps removed. Wong and Weiss (1972) addressed this question by comparing the records of one group of patients who maintained normal speech after discarding their obturators with those of another group who could not discard their obturators without deterioration in speech and voice quality. In the first group, obturator-reduction therapy had been initiated at an average age of 88 months compared with 126 months in the second group. Types of cleft palate and noncleft velopharyngeal insufficiency were similarly distributed in the two groups, and they were similar in articulation and nasality. The study did not determine any means for predicting the response of a particular patient to obturator reduction.

Recently McGrath and Anderson (in press) have described their clinical program of prosthetic treatment of velopharyngeal incompetence using both palatal lift and pharyngeal bulb appliances. They consider the method to have particular merit as a presurgical step to estimate the eventual benefit from velopharyngeal surgery. They also regard the method to have potential value for increasing velopharyngeal motion, "sometimes to the extent of acquiring a competent system." They report a success rate of 95% in 200 patients but provide no supporting data.

In work motivated by Blakeley's research, Shelton et al. (1968, 1971a) studied obturator reduction in 19 subjects. They eliminated as subjects six other persons who produced measurable nasal air pressure during speech even when their obturators were temporarily enlarged with pharyngeal paste. Before the investigators initiated reduction, they checked each subject's obturator for fit. Cephalometric radiographs were used to guide the removal of acrylic that appeared to be unnecessary. The obturators were to allow no more than 2 cm H_2O of nasal air pressure during stops and fricatives. When pharyngeal paste was placed on the pharyngeal section of the appliance, that paste was contacted but not wiped clean by the velopharyngeal structures as the patients spoke and changed head posture.

The subjects in this study ranged in age from 6 years, 7 months, to 18 years, 6 months. Most of the subjects underwent from one to three reductions, and 4 to 15 weeks passed between reductions. No reduction in articulation scores was noted even for sibilants and plosives. Nasal air pressure was slightly increased at the end of the study. Subjects were studied by sagittal cinefluorography before and after the obturator reduction. Two of the 19 subjects were observed to produce greater pharyngeal wall movement in the postreduction films. Sometimes subjects appeared to achieve closure around the pharyngeal section of the appliance by changing craniocervical posture or by displacing the speech bulb. Perhaps more positive results would have been obtained had multiview radiographs or endoscopy been employed, had the subjects been younger, had they been studied longer, and had they been unable to displace the appliance. No pharyngeal reflex of the upper portion of the posterior pharyngeal wall was observed.

In a third study, Shelton et al. (1971b) assessed two cleft palate children and one child with velopharyngeal insufficiency as they wore "exchangeable speech appliance sections." These pharyngeal sections were constructed around acrylic cores that housed set screws. Consequently, each pharyngeal section could be removed from and returned to the carrier wire that attached to the maxillary (retainer) portion of the prosthetic appliance. Each child was provided with three or four exchangeable pharyngeal sections. The first was fitted by the same muscle trimming, speech testing, and x-ray procedures that were used in the previous study. The other sections were 2 or 4 mm narrower or shorter than the first. Each subject was studied for a period of 6 to 14 months, during which time he or she was seen approximately once a month. At the beginning of the study, each subject's articulation, nasal sound level, and nasal air pressure were measured with each obturator section in place and with the appliance removed. Oral sound pressure level was also measured. However, the subject was asked to monitor that value and to hold it as constant as possible. These measures were repeated under each obturator condition at each monthly visit, and the subject was shifted to a smaller pharyngeal section for home use if he appeared to have adapted as indicated by speech and water manometer information. Sagittal cinefluorographic films were made of each subject at the beginning and end of the study and were used to count pharyngeal wall movements. A subject possessed only one pharyngeal section at any one time.

Measurements made at the beginning of the study showed a relationship between section size and dependent variables. Best performance accompanied the largest section. Throughout the study the performance of each subject with the appliance removed was inferior to performance with any of the pharyngeal sections in place. No subject improved on all of the four dependent variables under any one of the section conditions. From study of the cinefluorographic films, the authors inferred that one subject developed posterior pharyngeal wall movement under one or two section conditions. The authors did not consider any observed gains in velopharyngeal function made by these patients to have been of much clinical value. Shelton et al. noted that a subject's performance may vary as a result of adaptation to the study, fatigue, and allergy.

Although the three reports in this series do not support obturator reduction as a technique for improving speech and velopharyngeal closure, neither do they prove that the technique does not influence velopharyngeal motion to some extent. They do indicate that, because any changes that occur are probably small, they can be difficult to detect. The time available to the subjects for adaptation was less than that used in Blakeley's studies. The greater the duration of treatment, the greater is the opportunity for uncontrolled variables to confound a study. In spite of these findings, Shelton and his colleagues had the clinical experience of reducing the appliance in one young man to the point where he was judged to need it no longer. At the time obturation was started, his speech reflected insufficient velopharyngeal closure. It seems possible that the technique may be applicable to some patients, but we do not yet know which ones.

Support was given to the use of obturator reduction by information published by Warren (1965) and Mazaheri and Mazaheri (1976). Warren described the application of his oral-nasal differential air pressure and nasal air flow instrumentation in fitting obturators. He presented information about a postsurgical cleft palate patient who had very low oral-nasal differential air pressure (indicating that pressure was as great in the nose as in the mouth) and high nasal air flow prior to obturation. Warren described the patient's palate as short and immobile. The initial appliance fitting was intended to establish light contact between the pharyngeal muscles and the appliance during swallowing. The appliance was enlarged after the patient had worn it for about 2 months. However, a velopharyngeal orifice of approximately 60 mm^2 remained during the production of non-nasal consonants. Four months later, an oral-nasal pressure difference had been established and nasal flow during oral consonants had dropped to essentially zero. Pressure-flow data indicated that, at that time, the patient had a velopharyngeal orifice of 1.7 mm^2 during production of /b/. It appeared that the patient had learned to close the velopharyngeal muscles around the appliance in a pattern appropriate to the phonetic context of the speech being produced. No speech training was mentioned.

Mazaheri and Mazaheri (1976) described palatal lift appliances and combined lift and pharyngeal-section appliances constructed for three patients with velopharyngeal structural insufficiency and one with acquired neurogenic deficiency of the velopharyngeal mechanism. The treatment period was less than 1 year for each patient. Three of the four patients received speech therapy during the period of appliance therapy. In each case, velar movement was absent prior to treatment and marked afterwards. This observation was based on sagittal cephalometric radiographs, which might have produced incomplete data. Two of the four patients showed closure on the post-treatment radiographs. The authors stated that some patients were able to abandon their appliances. For others, the treatment was to supplement secondary velopharyngeal surgery.

Studies reporting increase in velopharyngeal motion as the result of reduction programs have extended over a long period of time. Sometimes no direct evidence of closure or of increased range of motion has been reported. Descriptions of speech change tend to be impressionistic and possibly biased. Use of obturation to enhance accomplishment of closure seems to involve skilled motion rather than muscle hypertrophy or strength. The patient described by Warren learned to close the pharyngeal structures around an obturator even though he did not completely close off the passage into the nasopharynx. Apparently it was not necessary that the appliance offer resistance to muscles in order to influence velopharyngeal function. It is not clear that clinical success achieved through the manipulation of obturators supports the use of muscle training without obturators as a clinical procedure. Nor would we be justified in inferring that all patients respond to obturator manipulation in the same way. Perhaps some individuals benefit through muscle strength and hypertrophy, others through skilled motion, others through a combination, and others not at all.

We consider use of obturator reduction for the improvement of velopharyngeal function to be experimental. Nonetheless, the ability of some persons to achieve closure and to speak well after obturator reduction where audible nasal emission and hypernasality were serious problems prior to obturation is not to be ignored. The fact that clinicians and investigators in several centers have reported that obturators could be removed after a period of use and good speech maintained without the appliance suggests that a phenomenon of improved velopharyngeal function does occur with obturation in some patients. Appliance reduction appears to be a more promising technique of developing velopharyngeal motion and incorporating it into speech than are the other procedures reported in this chapter.

INFORMATION FEEDBACK

Biofeedback was defined by Davis and Drichta (1980) as "an intervention technique that uses electronics to monitor and amplify body functions that may be too subtle for normal awareness." Instruments provide the learner with information about subliminal body functions in a direct and rapid manner. According to Davis and Drichta, biofeedback differs from other techniques in that information is provided directly to the patient during performance, and the information is available to the patient to use as he or she chooses.

The term *biofeedback* is used here to refer to the use of information derived from performance about performance to improve performance. However, departing from the Davis and Drichta definition, we accept descriptive information provided by a clinician as a form of biofeedback therapy. The emphasis is on providing the patient with information about performance rather than on reinforcement. Usually the learner watches or listens to information obtained through endoscopy, aeromechanical measures, auditory recordings, electromyography, or other instruments.

Procedures intended to improve velopharyngeal function by supplying information to the patient about that function are found in the early attempts at speech habilitation for the cleft palate patient. Moser (1942) discussed use of cold mirrors, water manometers, and stethoscopes for this purpose. Kantner (1937) noted that, in therapy, these devices work best with individuals who sometimes achieve velopharyngeal closure even though they do not do so in automatic speech. In a landmark study, Masland (1946) coupled pneumoscopes to the nose and mouth of patients and used the devices in conjunction with a kymograph to record and display oral and nasal air pressure. Masland's patients wore prosthetic speech appliances, and it was hoped that they would learn to close the velopharyngeal sphincter against the pharyngeal segments of the appliances. The patients were to accomplish this by monitoring their pressure traces during the production of /pV/ syllables. Four case studies were presented. The subjects were variable in their success at reducing nasal emission; two eliminated the nasal air leakage on oral consonants and two reduced the frequency of occurrence of the leakage.

Monitoring of velopharyngeal movements and postures by kinesthesis has also been recommended in the clinical literature. Westlake and Rutherford (1966) advocated that the patient voluntarily move the velopharyngeal muscles while attending to sensory cues. One of the authors noted that he could feel tightness in the velopharyngeal mechanism upon contracting it, but could not feel contact between the velum and the pharyngeal walls. Heightened awareness of one's body functions without benefit of instrumentation may be a form of biofeedback, but it is outside the definition offered by Davis and Drichta (1980) referred to earlier.

TEACHING VELOPHARYNGEAL MOTIONS

Teaching Normal Subjects

It is well established that people can learn to make voluntary motions of the velum and pharyngeal walls. Whether or not the motions learned can be helpful in speech is less clear. In a series of studies, Shelton and associates found that normal persons quickly learn voluntary elevation of the velum (Shelton et al., 1970a, 1970b).

In the first study, four normal school children aged 8 to 12 and five normal young adults were asked to observe and feel palate elevations as they phonated. They used a mirror to practice relaxation of the velum and positioning of the tongue so that the palate could be seen. To train voluntary palatal movement, the experimenter asked the subject to open the mouth and to elevate the velum. The experimenter described to the subject movements of the palate and of adjacent structures. After the first five trials, each subject was given 5 minutes in which to practice palatal elevation before a mirror. Then the subjects executed five more trials. Both children and adults made voluntary palatal movements on some trials prior to the initiation of training. After the first 10 training trials plus 5 minutes of practice, the mean number of correct responses on a 10-block trial was 8.5 for children and 9.6 for adults.

In the second study, two normal subjects were instructed to elevate the soft palate to different heights on command. Tape-recorded numbers from 1 to 7 were played to the subjects who were to elevate the palate slightly upon hearing the number 1, to produce an extensive elevation in response to the number 7, and to respond proportionately to the intervening numbers Electromyography, incorporating suction surface electrodes, measured action potentials in the velum. Velar motions produced by the subjects were rated by two observers on a 7-point scale. Information analysis of the ratings and of measures of the peak amplitudes and duration of the action potentials indicated that the subjects were able to elevate their palates to about two different heights, not seven. Either the subjects were incapable of discrete degrees of velar elevation, or the measurements made were not sensitive to them. Nonetheless, the subjects could elevate their palates on command.

Shelton et al. (1975) used an oral panendoscope attached to a videorecorder to provide feedback in teaching velopharyngeal movements. Three normal subjects learned to position themselves on an endoscope and to observe their velopharyngeal ports displayed on a television screen. Each subject attempted closure on 10 nonspeech trials initiated by fixation of the larynx and then on 10 additional trials wherein reflexive movements elicited by touch pressure cues were to be imitated. The subjects readily learned to utilize the feedback system to perform the task under investigation. The neck of each subject was videotaped in profile during the study by use of a second television system. Each male subject elevated his larynx during all trials under each condition. The laryngeal motions of the female subject could not be evaluated from the tape. However, she produced muscle contractions in the neck area and elevated her shoulders suggesting hypertension in the laryngeal area.

Siegel-Sadewitz and Shprintzen (1982) described successful use of a nasopharyngoscope to teach a normal individual to change her pattern of velopharyngeal closure from circular to coronal thus increasing medial motion of the lateral pharyngeal walls.

Teaching Patients with Velopharyngeal Valving Disorders

Moller et al. (1973) used a strain gauge transducer to monitor and train velar movement during /u/ in a 12-year-old boy with speech and radiographic evidence of a short velum and velopharyngeal insufficiency. The transducer was cemented to a maxillary molar so that a sensor tip touched the middle third of the velum in the midline and followed its movement. Other instrumentation enabled the researchers to record the subject's responses, to display them to the subject, to compare them with a criterion level set by the investigators, and to reward correct responses. Training was provided three times a week for a total of 15 sessions. Responses during training were compared with baseline information. Sagittal cephalometric radiographs indicated that the boy increased movement of his velum during phonation of /u/ but that the size of the velopharyngeal gap was not reduced. The configuration of the boy's posterior pharyngeal wall changed during treatment apparently because adenoid atrophy was occurring at the same time. The authors noted that information about motion of the lateral pharyngeal walls might have been useful.

Tudor and Selley (1974) attached a U-shaped orthodontic wire to an acrylic base plate. It was positioned to touch and lift the resting soft palate. The authors inferred that the wire provided patients with information about the location of the palate and contributed to their development of voluntary velar movement. They also made an electrical visual aid in which two electrodes connected to a control box, replaced the wire loop used in the earlier appliance. When the soft palate elevated, breaking contact with the electrodes, a light went out. The authors had the patient wear the palatal training appliance all day. The purpose of the electrical visual aid was to replace speech therapy and practice. The patient was asked to feel the appliance and to lift the velum away from it. The authors recommended this procedure for patients of all ages if they fail to achieve velopharyngeal closure because of weakness or poor coordination. Five of 11 patients who had had dysarthria for 2 years ceased to drool and established intelligible speech within 3 weeks of using this procedure. The authors presented this information as a preliminary report and included neither pre- nor post-treatment data.

Later Selly et al. (1987) stated that use of the U-shaped palatal training appliance results in resensitization of the velum-to-tongue contact and consequently reduced tongue humping. That in turn results in a more open oral tract and increased opportunity for the air and sound streams to exit orally. Stuffins (1989) described use of the palatal training appliance with 26 patients and reported substantial success.

Shprintzen et al. (1975) described and evaluated a therapy intended to develop velopharyngeal closure during speech from velopharyngeal closure present during blowing and whistling. The authors presumed that subjects who close the velopharyngeal port during blowing and whistling but not during speech probably learned to leave the velopharyngeal muscles turned off as they developed speech prior to surgical provision of a structurally sufficient closure mechanism.

Four subjects were studied; they were 4, 8, 10 and 19 years of age. Two had place of articulation within normal limits. A third omitted /s, z, ∫, f, and t∫/, and another produced hypernasality, facial grimace, glottal stops, and distortions of /s/ and /z/. For each subject the authors reported the frequency of occurrence of nasal emission during passages studied and the percentage of speaking times during which nasal emission was evident. Nasal emission was studied with a scape-scope. The treatment involved a series of steps roughly as follows:

1. Determine that the patient achieves closure during blowing or whistling.
2. Teach the patient to blow or whistle and phonate simultaneously. Identify nasal air leakage with a scape-scope or other device and reward trials free from nasal emission on a continuous basis.
3. Continue phonation but fade blowing-whistling. Use /i/ because of its similarity to blowing in tongue configuration and location. Reward correct responses but punish nasal air emission.
4. Combine nonnasal vowel with two nonnasal consonants in CVC syllables.

Initially all satisfactory responses were reinforced. However, as a child progressed, the schedule of reinforcement and punishment was altered. During the training, each subject was asked to sense his or her performance kinesthetically or auditorily. In time, the use of the scape-scope was discontinued in favor of auditory monitoring by the clinician. Perceptually satisfactory responses were rewarded, and a home program was instituted.

All four subjects improved their velopharyngeal function as indicated by their velopharyngeal pattern observed from the videofluorographic tape and evidence of reduced nasal air leakage. One subject, an individual with hearing loss, retained mild hypernasality and nasal snorting. The other three subjects developed essentially normal function. Treatment duration ranged from 22 sessions administered over 13 weeks to 36 sessions administered over 15 weeks.

In 1989, Shprintzen wrote that today he would include observation of sustained /f/ and /s/ in a project of this sort because some individuals who do not otherwise close the velopharyngeal port during speech do close during those productions.

Investigators in Japan have reported success in developing velopharyngeal closure in patients with palatal clefts through use of biofeedback provided by a nasofiberscope. Miyazaki et al. (1974) described change in subjects' velopharyngeal function from pre- to post-training observations. Initially, the subjects were classified as having one of four closure patterns: complete closure only during swallowing, complete closure on swallowing and blowing, complete closure during swallowing, blowing, and non-nasal consonants, and complete closure during swallowing and blowing and on plosives, fricatives, and some vowels. Patients were treated once or twice monthly for more than 6 successive months. The subjects differed in their pretreatment closure patterns, but none had the most adequate pattern of closure. At the end of the study, 16 of 37 patients had closure that was considered to be the best or most adequate, and the others had improved their patterns. The authors concluded that patients who achieve closure during blowing can also achieve closure easily during phonation. No experimental control features were reported for this study.

Nishio et al. (1976) described a study related to that of Miyasaki et al. Most of their subjects initially achieved closure during swallowing but had to learn to close during blowing and phonation. Once closure was present in blowing, the authors found that it took less than 1 month to develop closure for plosives and fricatives. The duration of treatment averaged 3.4 and 5.6 months for two different subject groups.

Another study from Japan used similar procedures and again reported positive results (Yamaoka et al., 1983). Again the procedure involved a progression from activities including swallowing and blowing in which closure occurred initially to speech activities in which closure did not occur. An element of self-training is involved. The authors referred to the value of the patient having a feeling of closure during either blowing or obstruent production.

These are unexpected findings. Since velopharyngeal closure in swallow involves a different mechanism than that employed in speech, generalization of closure from swallow to speech is not anticipated.

In another biofeedback study Shelton et al. (1978) taught two adolescent subjects to position themselves on an oral endoscope coupled to a video camera and playback system. One subject had a surgically repaired cleft lip and palate and a pharyngeal flap, and the other had velopharyngeal insufficiency in the absence of cleft palate. The subjects were taught to monitor their own velopharyngeal closure on the television screen, and they were instructed to attempt to increase the range of velopharyngeal motion during the production of syllables. An experimenter observed each subject's performance and offered interpretations and suggestions. The subjects approximated closure frequently as the study progressed. However, performance gains were not established on an automatic level, and the subjects' clinical speech problems were not resolved.

Shelton and Ruscello (1979) summarized descriptive information regarding treatment of several patients with hypernasality, audible nasal emission, or both. With one exception, these patients all had cleft palate or velopharyngeal insufficiency. One adolescent had a 50 dB bilateral, congenital, neural hearing loss. Attempts were made to improve velopharyngeal function by having the subjects monitor their performance either by oral videoendoscopy or by the pen trace of an oscillograph displaying nasal air flow. Where misarticulation was also a problem, subjects were given articulation training. One subject with cleft palate who had normal hearing was taught to monitor his nasal air flow through a hearing aid with the microphone placed under his nose.

Shelton and Ruscello reported that these patients did not benefit from biofeedback. The boy with the hearing loss reduced nasal airflow during training sessions but at the cost of unwanted change in other speech behaviors. Other subjects were reported to have reduced the production of nasal noises during /sk/, /st/, and other clusters as they participated in articulation training. The nasal snort or fricative seems more amenable to elimination than does audible nasal emission. This is perhaps because the snort involves an articulatory maneuver.

Hoch et al. (1986) referred to their nasopharyngoscopic feedback therapy with nine patients. They reported success with all patients except one with a neurological disorder. Witzel et al. (1989) reported improved velopharyngeal function for speech in three patients who had recently undergone secondary velopharyngeal surgery and who received videonasopharyngoscopic biofeedback therapy and articulation therapy. The authors described the biofeedback therapy as a useful adjunct to speech therapy techniques. They cited the need for investigation of precise treatment protocols under circumstances where confounding variables are controlled. In these case studies, subjects were asked to observe their velopharyngeal ports through the nasopharyngoscope and to close the velopharyngeal ports by means of whatever worked—blowing, whistling, swallow-ing, squeezing throat muscles—and to attend to sensations associated with the movement. Ther-apy progressed through nonspeech movement of the lateral walls to movement during articulation. Sounds were identified that were associated with the greatest range of lateral pharyngeal wall motion, and therapy was addressed to increase motion during those sounds and then during other sounds. Two patients completed therapy, and one dropped out. The two patients who completed the therapy were described as making substantial improvement in velopharyngeal func-tion and in speech. One was reexamined a year post treatment and was observed to close ports on each side of a pharyngeal flap completely and "appropriately" during connected speech. The authors emphasized the need for further experi-mental testing of biofeedback treatment.

Dalston and Keefe (1987) described use of a microcomputer in conjunction with the photode-tector for monitoring and modifying velopharyn-geal movements. They cited unpublished prelimi-nary evidence from a small number of normal and cleft palate speakers to the effect"…that the computer-based biofeedback treatment approach described in this paper enables subjects to modify velopharyngeal behaviors and, where appropr-iate, reduce or eliminate hypernasality and nasal emission of air…" (p. 167).

Tonar has also been used in biofeedback research with individuals with clefts. An indicated elsewhere, reduction in nasalance may involve improved velopharyngeal function or other ad-justments of the speech mechanism. Fletcher (1978) outlined incremental steps from low vowels and sonorants to obstruents for biofeedback with Tonar for the reduction of nasalance in 19 subjects with clefts, in four subject subgroups. Members of one group achieved and maintained a normal nasalance level. One member of the fourth group failed to respond to the treatment. Members of the intermediate groups achieved but either failed to maintain normal nasalance or improved but not enough to reach the targeted nasalance level.

The research reviewed here is encouraging if only because many independent observers have reported positive findings. Additional research should be addressed to the establishment and maintenance of velopharyngeal function compe-tent for speech performance that is indistinguisha-ble from that of persons free from clefts or other disability. Treatments should be refined to the

point where techniques can be selected that are appropriate to the individual patient and where treatment outcome can be predicted. This re-search should probably be structured within a model of speech motor control or perceptual-motor performance and learning.

TRENDS SHOWING IMPROVED VELOPHARYNGEAL FUNCTION

Speech pathologists are familiar with trends toward improved articulation as children mature and toward loss of adenoid tissue about the time of puberty. Children may learn to make better use of the velopharyngeal mechanism, and in very young children structural relationships change greatly with maturation. If velopharyngeal func-tion is subject to improvement through learning, we might expect a trend toward improved velo-pharyngeal function in reports of longitudinal observations of patients with clefts. There may be such a trend, but it is weak. Indeed, investigators have been more alert to loss of velopharyngeal competence with age and with loss of adenoid tissue.

Shelton and Ruscello (1979) reported that two children whom they did not treat, but fol-lowed longitudinally, eliminated, nasal airflow over a period of 1 or 2 years. These children, one of whom presented cleft palate and the other velopharyngeal insufficiency of unknown origin, had received speech training at school during the period in which the observations were made.

Van Demark and Morris (1983) reported longitudinal articulation scores and ratings of velopharyngeal competence, articulation, and na-sality in three clinical groups of subjects: compe-tent, borderline competent, and incompetent. Various patterns were identified. The borderline group was characterized as variable in compe-tence ratings. Of special importance here, howev-er, was the observation that some subjects in this group "…showed marginal competency until about age seven and then achieved competency and maintained it…" Relative to loss of velopha-ryngeal closure with adenoid atrophy, the authors stated, "…some subjects may develop additional movements which facilitate closure and thus alle-viates [sic] the need of additional surgery, while other patients may not."

Karnell and Van Demark (1986) studied three groups of subjects. Group A scored below

20% correct on the Iowa Pressure Articulation Test (IPAT) at age 4 years and received secondary operative management by 8 years of age. Group B scored below 20% on the IPAT at age 4 and did not receive secondary management by age 8. Members of group C scored above 20% at age 4 and did not receive secondary operative management. Velopharyngeal competence was rated with a three-category descriptive scale: competence, marginal competence, and incompetence. The number of patients from each group in the velopharyngeal competence category increased through about 10 years of age. This trend continued but at a slower pace for Group A members, whereas it leveled off for C and reversed somewhat for B. These data indicate that some individuals do improve velopharyngeal function or competence over time.

Van Demark et al. (1988) identified trends from the annual evaluation of children with palatal clefts whereby articulation and resonance improved over time even in children who eventually required secondary velopharyngeal operations. Velopharyngeal competence ratings and lateral radiograph ratings showed that children who received secondary surgery after 10 years of age had improved velopharyngeal competence between 4 and 4.5 years, which remained constant through the eighth or ninth year, and then deteriorated slightly. Data from these three Iowa studies probably reflect variability in both subject performance and in measurement. However, they suggest a group trend, though weak, toward improved velopharyngeal competence.

Observations of nasal resonance reported by Fox et al. (1988) indicated that children tended to move to more acceptable resonance after about 5 years of age. This observation could reflect improved use of the velopharyngeal mechanism.

A study of Siegel-Sadewitz and Shprintzen (1986) described change—but not necessarily improvement—in velopharyngeal function with structural maturation. They observed and described subjects' velopharyngeal closure patterns before and after puberty and adenoid involution. Their subjects were 20 children with normal velopharyngeal mechanisms, five with repaired cleft palate, and five with unrepaired submucous clefts. The latter 10 children had normal speech and were free from velopharyngeal insufficiency. The subjects were studied by means of multiview videofluoroscopy and nasopharyngoscopy. Subjects were classified in terms of velopharyngeal

closure pattern—e.g., sagittal, coronal, circular. Many subjects changed pattern from prepubertal to postpubertal observations. Some subjects showed contact of the lateral pharyngeal walls in midline below the velum prior to puberty. After puberty and maturation of the velopharyngeal mechanism, lateral wall displacement toward midline was less extensive but resulted in contact with the velum. These authors concluded here and in other papers that learning does influence velopharyngeal function.

Shelton and McCauley (1986) described velopharyngeal movements of a woman who wore a hinged speech prosthesis for the treatment of an unoperated cleft of the secondary palate. The authors noted that the appliance may have been constructed to take advantage of existing movements, but they thought that learning probably influenced the woman's skillful use of the appliance. She would bump the hinged section of the appliance with her tongue and catch it with the velar halves and maintain it in an elevated position. That elevation was sometimes maintained through nasal consonants. The patient's speech was indistinguishable from normal.

The uvula is sometimes removed to relieve snoring, sleep apnea, or both (Kuehn, 1986; Kuehn and Dalston, 1988). Finkelstein et al. (1988) describe change in velopharyngeal function in 27 patients who underwent uvulopalatopharyngoplasty. Their patients were endoscoped daily in the first postoperative week and then monthly until examiners and patient were satisfied with the outcome. Each patient was classified into one of four closure patterns (coronal, circular, circular and Passavant's ridge, or sagittal). Over time, lateral wall movement increased in five patients from the coronal group. No one developed a Passavant's ridge. Thus, a subset of the patients did alter their velopharyngeal movement patterns. Study of patients undergoing this operation offers opportunity for new observations of velopharyngeal function. The operation removes tissue considered to be unnecessary to velopharyngeal function and dangerous to the patient. Comparison of the results with those of primary and secondary velopharyngeal operations should be supplementary.

In this section, once again, we see reason to expect change in velopharyngeal function over time and the suggestion that learning does influence velopharyngeal function. But this evidence is weak.

DISCUSSION

Skeletal muscle is subject to conscious control, and it should be possible to teach skilled motion of the velopharyngeal structure within any limitations imposed by tissue deficiency, impaired innervation, or both. It is evident that some cleft palate patients do learn remarkable velopharyngeal motions and that a few apparently can reduce, though not eliminate, both nasal emission and hypernasality. Normal persons and some patients with cleft palates readily learn to make movements of the velum and perhaps of the pharyngeal walls. However, demonstrations of some increase in velopharyngeal motion often is not associated with resolution of the patient's clinical problem. No standard criteria have been established for identifying potential candidates for biofeedback training or for performing such training. The speech pathologist would be hard pressed to predict with any precision the response of individual patients to biofeedback treatments.

If biofeedback is to be useful, it must be used with techniques capable of establishing skilled patterns of opening and closing the velopharyngeal port during running speech. Unless normal velopharyngeal function in automatic speech is achieved, the patient will continue to have disordered speech. Even if the size of the velopharyngeal opening is reduced, an opening large enough to impair speech may remain.

As indicated earlier, another objective may be to increase range of motion and a more nearly normal sequence of velopharyngeal movements to enhance the patient's response to some other treatment such as a pharyngeal flap (Cole, 1979, McGrath and Anderson, in press). However, there are no reported data to support that contention.

We interpret present findings to indicate that a number of variables must be considered in further development and evaluation of these methods. For example, the way in which biofeedback information is presented to the patient may influence treatment effectiveness. Yates (1980) wrote that feedback may be presented continuously or noncontinuously, during a trial or at the end of a trial. The information may be binary, or it may reflect gradations of performance. These variables have not been studied relative to velopharyngeal function training.

Choices about feedback mode must be made. The literature reviewed earlier does not offer clear guidance regarding choice of feedback display for teaching velopharyngeal function. Some authors appear to assume that direct observation of the velopharyngeal mechanism as through a nasopharyngoscope is necessarily the form of feedback most likely to be effective. However, Hixon (personal communication) has suggested that a display reflecting a parameter controlled by the velopharyngeal mechanism, such as resistance or air flow, might be more effective than display of the muscles themselves or their electrical activity. We postulate that different modes of information feedback are not mutually substitutable for use in rehabilitation of the cleft palate patient.

It seems likely that some of the information feedback in velopharyngeal therapy is of poor quality. Scope devices sold for this purpose are so sensitive to nasal air flow that small amounts of leakage, perhaps clinically insignificant flow, will produce large displacement of the indicator piston. Auditory observation by the clinician and description to the patient of the patient's performance is a weak form of biofeedback therapy. Feedback of the information about oral air pressure may differ in effectiveness from feedback of information about nasal air flow or other forms of feedback. Warren (1986) has suggested that the velopharyngeal mechanism serves a pressure-regulating function. If that is the case, oral air pressure feedback might be especially deserving of investigation. For example, research might be conducted to determine whether an individual can learn to increase intraoral air pressure during obstruent production. If the performance was successful, nasal air flow should not be increased and preferably should not exist. Many questions remain about how best to use biofeedback as therapy for velopharyngeal function.

Clearly, there are important choices to be made in patient selection. Patients who demonstrate normal velopharyngeal function, but inconsistently, are likely to be excellent choices. On the other hand, the inconsistency may stem from a physiologic deficiency. Still less certain, based on present knowledge, is whether patients with consistent velopharyngeal incompetence, even though marginal in extent, can be expected to benefit.

As indicated earlier, duration of therapy may also be an important treatment variable. Shprintzen et al. (1975) and Miyazaki and associates (1974) reported success in treatment periods ranging from roughly 3 to 6 months. Reports of increased velopharyngeal motion with obturator reduction have involved longer periods of time. As a rough rule of thumb, we might expect biofeedback to be effective within a 6-month period, if at all. However, investigators might consider use of longer study periods. Some individuals alter velopharyngeal function very quickly. A boy who emitted /s/ and /z/ nasally but who otherwise spoke orally was scheduled for velopharyngeal surgery. With a few minutes of training, he learned to modify the sounds to oral /s/ and /z/ and then to produce /s/ and /z/ in words and syllables.

The choice of a response unit for use in therapy is an important issue. Should feedback monitoring utilize nonspeech activities, words, sentences, or something else? If possible, response units should be chosen that do not trigger old, unwanted responses. Much that has been written about ways to avoid competition between old and new activities in articulation therapy may be relevant here (Winitz, 1969; 1975).

Finally, some clinicians and speech scientists suggest that velopharyngeal therapy is well-established and a matter of course. Perhaps this is a reflection of the emphasis on aggressive marketing that currently characterizes the practice of many professions in the United States. Regardless, much of the research concerning velopharyngeal therapy was directed to goals short of resolution of a clinical problem, and some was descriptive in nature and characterized by lack of experimental control and questionable measurement practices. Evidence in support of therapy for velopharyngeal function is weak but sufficiently promising to warrant further research. As stated by Ruscello (1989), in future research, subject variables that may relate to response to treatment should be identified, and the treatment itself should be specified in detail and followed carefully. Variables that might confound the research should be controlled. Ruscello also stated that this research should be well-founded conceptually and that investigators should strive to understand the mechanisms involved in subject response to such therapy. Indeed, to the current authors it appears that publications in this area have moved away from consideration of motor performance-learning theory or other theory that might guide a cumulative research effort. We appear to be slipping back to the practice of an earlier era in speech-language pathology of accepting the opinions of authorities as truth.

SUMMARY

We have considered articulation therapy, muscle training, obturator reduction, and biofeedback as possible treatments for the development of adequate velopharyngeal function or improvement of that function. Clinical research and clinical reports support obturator reduction and biofeedback enough to warrant their continued study. However, no single procedure can be recommended for routine clinical application.

In the future study of procedures for increasing velopharyngeal function, investigators should continue to be especially careful to differentiate between subjects who fail to achieve closure because of an inadequate mechanism and those who fail to achieve closure for other reasons. Care should also be taken to avoid pushing the patient to learn something that for him or her is impossible.

The clinician cannot be certain that an individual patient is making the best possible use of the speech mechanism, and we know of no precise way to distinguish between those who might acquire adequate use of the velopharyngeal mechanism through training and those who cannot. Individuals who sometimes close the velopharyngeal port during speech or during blowing or whistling would appear to be the most likely candidates for velopharyngeal valving therapy. However, even they may differ from each other in the extent to which they achieve closure and would surely differ in their prognoses for response to training.

A theoretical framework is needed for future experimental work regarding the development of velopharyngeal closure through behavioral means. It is possible that closure may be achieved in some individuals through trial-by-trial learning directed by the speech pathologist who provides stimuli, feedback, and reinforcement. Others may discover means of achieving closure unconsciously as they struggle and problem-solve to speak intelligibly. Each of these two learning forms, the first termed bottom-up and the second top-down, can be conceptualized within a perceptual-motor, information-processing model of motor performance and learning. This model is discussed in Chapter 22. It seems applicable to research in velopharyngeal function as well as in articulation. Until that research is carried out, we remain skeptical about the benefits of therapy directed at improving velopharyngeal valving for speech.

REFERENCES

Berry MF. Correction of cleft-palate speech by phonetic instruction. Quart J Speech 1928; 14:523.

Blakeley RW. Temporary speech prosthesis as an aid in speech training. Cleft Pal Bull 1960; 10:63.

Blakeley RW. The complementary use of speech prostheses and pharyngeal flaps in palatal insufficiency. Cleft Palate J 1964; 1:194.

Blakeley RW. The rationale for a temporary speech prosthesis in palatal insufficiency. Br J Disord Commun 1969; 4:134.

Blakeley RW, Porter DR. Unexpected reduction and removal of an obturator in a patient with palate paralysis. Br J Disord Commun 1971; 6:33.

Buck M, Harrington R. Organized speech therapy for cleft palate rehabilitation. J Speech Hear Dis 1949; 14:43.

Cole RM. Direct muscle training for the improvement of velopharyngeal activity. In: Bzoch KR, ed. Communicative disorders related to cleft lip and palate. 2nd ed. Boston: Little, Brown, 1979:328.

Cooper HK, Cooper JA, Mazaheri M, Millard RT. Psychological, orthodontic, and prosthetic approaches in rehabilitation of the cleft palate patient. In: Dental Clinics of North America Philadelphia: WB Saunders, 1960.

Dalston RM, Keefe MJ. The use of a microcomputer in monitoring and modifying velopharyngeal movements. J Comp Users Speech Hear 1987; 3:159.

Davis SM, Drichta CE. Biofeedback: theory and application to speech pathology. In: Lass NJ, ed. Speech and language: advances in basic research and practice. Vol 3. New York: Academic Press, 1980:283.

Eckelmann D, Baldridge P. Speech training for the child with a cleft palate. J Speech Dis 1945; 10:137.

Finkelstein Y, Talmi YP, Zohar Y. Readaptation of the velopharyngeal valve following the uvulopalatopharyngoplasty operation. Plast Reconstr Surg 1988; 82:20.

Fletcher SG. Diagnosing speech disorders from cleft palate. New York: Grune and Stratton, 1978.

Fox DR, Lynch JI, Cronin TD. Change in nasal resonance over time: a clinical study. Cleft Palate J 1988; 25:245.

Harkins CS, Koepp-Baker H. Twenty-five years of cleft palate prosthesis. J Speech Hear Dis 1948; 13:23.

Hixon TJ. Personal communication.

Hoch L, Golding-Kushner K, Siegel-Sadewitz VL, Shprintzen RJ. Speech therapy. Sem Speech Lang 1986; 7:313.

Kantner CE. Four devices in the treatment of rhinolalia aperta. J Speech Hear Dis 1937; 2:73.

Kantner CE. The rationale of blowing exercises for patients with repaired cleft palates. J Speech Dis 1947; 12:281.

Kantner CE. Diagnosis and prognosis in cleft palate speech. J Speech Hear Dis 1948; 13:211.

Karnell MP, Van Demark DR. Longitudinal speech performance in patients with cleft palate: comparisons based on secondary management. Cleft Palate J 1986; 23:278.

Kuehn DP. Causes of velopharyngeal incompetence. J Child Commun Dis 1986; 10:17.

Kuehn DP, Dalston RM. Cleft palate and studies related to velopharyngeal function. In: Winitz H, ed. Human communication and its disorders: 1988 annual review. Vol 2. Norwood: Ablex, 1988.

Lubit EC, Larsen RE. The Lubit palatal exerciser: a preliminary report. Cleft Palate J 1969; 6:120.

Lubit EC, Larsen RE. A speech aid for velopharyngeal incompetency. J Speech Hear Dis 1971; 36:61.

Masland MW. Testing and correcting cleft palate speech. J Speech Hear Dis 1946; 11:309.

Massengill R Jr, Quinn GW, Pickerell KL, Levinson C. Therapeutic exercise and velopharyngeal gap. Cleft Palate J 1968; 5:44.

Mazaheri M, Mazaheri EH. Prosthodontic aspects of palatal elevation and palatopharyngeal stimulation. J Prosth Dent 1976; 35:319.

McDonald ET, Koepp-Baker H. Cleft palate speech: an integration of research and clinical observation. J Speech Hear Dis 1951; 16:9.

McGrath CO, Anderson NW. Prosthetic treatment of velopharyngeal incompetence. In: Bardach J, Morris HL, eds. Multidisciplinary management of cleft lip and palate. Philadelphia: WB Saunders, in press.

McWilliams BJ, Bradley DP. Ratings of velopharyngeal closure during blowing and speech. Cleft Palate J 1965; 2:46.

Miyazaki T, Matsuya T, Yamaoka M, Nishio J. A nasopharyngeal fiberscope (film). Boston: American Cleft Pal Assoc. 1974.

Moller KT, Path M, Werth LJ, Christiansen RL. The modification of velar movement. J Speech Hear Dis 1973; 38:323.

Morley ME. Cleft palate and speech. 7th ed. Baltimore: Williams & Wilkins, 1970.

Moser HM. Diagnostic and clinical procedures in rhinolalia. J Speech Hear Dis 1942; 7:1.

Nishio J, Yamaoka M, Matsuya T, Miyazaki T. How to exercise the velopharyngeal movement by the velopharyngeal fiberscope. Jap J Oral Surg 1974; 20:450. Abstracted. Cleft Palate J 1976; 13:310.

Nylen BO. Cleft palate and speech: a surgical study including observation on velopharyngeal closure during connected speech, using synchronized cineradiography and sound spectrography. Acta Radiol 1961; Suppl 203.

Peterson SJ. Velopharyngeal function: some important differences. J Speech Hear Dis 1973; 38:89.

Peterson SJ. Electrical stimulation of the soft palate. Cleft Palate J 1974; 11:72.

Powers GR. Cleft Palate. Austin: Pro-Ed, 1986.

Powers GL, Starr CD. The effects of muscle exercises on velopharyngeal gap and nasality. Cleft Palate J 1974; 11:28.

Prins D, Bloomer HH. A word intelligibility approach to the study of speech change in oral cleft patients. Cleft Palate J 1965; 2:357.

Riski JE. Functional velopharyngeal incompetence: diagnosis and management. In: Winitz H, ed. Treating articulation disorders: for clinicians by clinicians. Baltimore: University Park Press, 1984:223.

Rosen MS, Bzoch KR. The prosthetic speech appliance in rehabilitation of patients with cleft palate. J Am Dent Assoc 1958; 57:203.

Ruscello DM. A selected review of palatal training procedures. Cleft Palate J 1982; 19:181.

Ruscello DM. Modifying velopharyngeal closure through training procedures. In: Bzoch KR, ed. Communicative disorders related to cleft lip and palate. 3rd ed. Boston: Little, Brown, 1989:338.

Selley WG, Zananiri M-C, Ellis RE, Flack FC. The effect of tongue position on division of airflow in the presence of velopharyngeal defects. Br J Plast Surg 1987; 40:377.

Shelton RL, Beaumont K, Trier WC, Furr ML. Videoendoscopic feedback in training velopharyngeal closure. Cleft Palate J 1978; 15:6.

Shelton RL, Chisum L, Youngstrom KA, Arndt WB, Elbert M. Effect of articulation therapy on palatopharyngeal closure, movement of the pharyngeal wall, and tongue posture. Cleft Palate J 1969; 6:440.

Shelton RL, Harris KS, Sholes GN, Dooley PM. Study of nonspeech voluntary palate movements by scaling and electromyographic techniques. In: Bosma JF, ed. Second Symposium on Oral Sensation and Perception. Springfield: CC Thomas, 1970a:432.

Shelton RL, Knox AW, Elbert M, Johnson TS. Palate awareness and nonspeech voluntary palate movement. In: Second Symposium on Oral Sensation and Perception. Springfield: CC Thomas, 1970b:416.

Shelton RL, Lindquist AF, Arndt WB, Elbert M, Youngstrom KA. Effect of speech bulb reduction on movement of the posterior wall of the pharynx and posture of the tongue. Cleft Palate J 1971a; 8:10.

Shelton RL, Lindquist AF, Chisum L, Arndt WB, Youngstrom KA, Stick SL. Effect of prosthetic speech bulb reduction on articulation. Cleft Palate J 1968; 5:195.

Shelton RL, Lindquist AF, Knox AW, Wright VL, Arndt WB, Elbert M, Youngstrom KA. The relationship between pharyngeal wall movements and exchangeable speech appliance sections. Cleft Palate J 1971b; 8:145.

Shelton RL, McCauley RJ. Use of a hinge-type speech prosthesis. Cleft Palate J 1986; 23:312.

Shelton RL, Paesani A, McClelland KD, Bradfield SS. Panendoscopic feedback in the study of voluntary velopharyngeal movements. J Speech Hear Dis 1975; 40:232.

Shelton RL, Ruscello DM. Palatal and articulation training in patients with velopharyngeal closure problems. Annual Meeting of the American Cleft Palate Association, San Diego, 1979.

Shprintzen RJ. Research revisited. Cleft Palate J 1989; 26:148.

Shprintzen R, McCall GM, Skolnick L. A new therapeutic technique for the treatment of velopharyngeal incompetence. J Speech Hear Dis 1975; 40:69.

Siegel-Sadewitz VL, Shprintzen RJ. Nasopharyngoscopy of the normal velopharyngeal sphincter: an experiment of biofeedback. Cleft Palate J 1982; 19:194.

Siegel-Sadewitz VL, Shprintzen RJ. Changes in velopharyngeal valving with age. Internat J Pediatr Otorhinolaryngol 1986; 11:171.

Stuffins GM. The use of appliances in the treatment of speech problems in cleft palate. In: Stengelhofen J, ed. Cleft palate the nature and remediation of communication problems. Edinburgh: Churchill, Livingstone, 1989.

Tash EL, Shelton RL, Knox AW, Michel JF. Training voluntary pharyngeal wall movements in children with normal and inadequate velopharyngeal closure. Cleft Palate J 1971; 8:277.

Trost-Cardamone JE. Effects of velopharyngeal incompetence on speech. J Child Commun Dis 1986; 10:31.

Tudor C, Selley WG. A palatal training appliance and a visual aid for use in the treatment of hypernasal speech. Br J Disord Commun 1974; 9:117.

Van Demark DR, Hardin MA, Morris HL. Assessment of velopharyngeal competency: a long-term process. Cleft Palate J 1988; 25:362.

Van Demark DR, Morris HL. Stability of velopharyngeal competency. Cleft Palate J 1983; 20:18.

Warren DW. A physiologic approach to cleft palate prosthesis. J Prosth Dent 1965; 15:770.

Warren DW. Compensatory speech behaviors in individuals with cleft palate: a regulation/control phenomenon? Cleft Palate J 1986; 23:251.

Weber J Jr, Jobe RP, Chase RA. Evaluation of muscle stimulation in the rehabilitation of patients with hypernasal speech. Plast Reconstr Surg 1970; 46:173.

Weiss CE. Success of an obturator reduction program. Cleft Palate J 1971; 8:291.

Weiss CE. The significance of Passavant's pad in postobturator patients. Folia Phoniatr 1972; 24:51.

Wells CG. Improving the speech of the cleft palate child. J Speech Hear Dis 1945; 10:162.

Westlake H, Rutherford C. Cleft Palate. Englewood Cliffs: Prentice Hall, 1966.

Winitz H. Articulatory acquisition and behavior. New York: Appleton-Century-Crofts, 1969.

Winitz H. From syllable to conversation. Baltimore: University Park Press, 1975.

Witzel MA, Tobe J, Salyer KE. The use of videonasopharyngoscopy for biofeedback therapy in adults after pharyngeal flap surgery. Cleft Palate J 1989; 26:129.

Wong LP, Weiss CE. A clinical assessment of obturator-wearing cleft palate patients. J Prosth Dent 1972; 27:632.

Yamaoka M, Mastuya T, Miyazaki T, Nishio J, Ibuki K. Visual training for velopharyngeal closure in cleft palate patients; a fiberscopic procedure (preliminary report). J Maxillofac Surg 1983; 11:191.

Yates AI. Biofeedback and the modification of behavior. New York: Plenum Press, 1980.

Young EH. Overcoming cleft palate speech; help for parents and trainers. Minneapolis: Hill-Young School, 1928.

Yules RB, Chase RA. A training method for reduction of hypernasality in speech. Plast Reconstr Surg 1969; 43:180.

Yules RB, Welch J, Urbani J, Elliott R. Untraining nasality. Annual Meeting of the American Cleft Palate Association, Miami Beach, 1968.

INDEX

Note: Page numbers followed by *f* refer to figures; page numbers followed by *t* refer to tables.